AF750790

Atlas of Customized TMJ-Cranio-Jaw Prosthesis

Chi Yang
Editor

Harry Schwartz • Zixian Jiao • Pan Lisa
Associate Editors

Atlas of Customized TMJ-Cranio-Jaw Prosthesis

Managing Temporomandibular Joint Disorders

Springer

PMPH
PEOPLE'S MEDICAL PUBLISHING HOUSE

Editor
Chi Yang
Department of Oral Surgery
Shanghai Ninth People's Hospital, Shanghai
Jiao Tong University School of Medicine
Shanghai, China

Associate Editors
Harry Schwartz
UCLA Health Sciences Center, LA, USA

Zixian Jiao
Shanghai Ninth People's Hospital
Shanghai Jiao Tong University, School of
Medicine, Shanghai, China

Pan Lisa
International Medical College Asia
Taipei, China

ISBN 978-981-95-0610-1 ISBN 978-981-95-0611-8 (eBook)
https://doi.org/10.1007/978-981-95-0611-8

© People's Medical Publishing House, PR of China 2025

This work is subject to copyright. All rights are solely and exclusively licensed by the Publisher, whether the whole or part of the material is concerned, specifically the rights of reprinting, reuse of illustrations, recitation, broadcasting, reproduction on microfilms or in any other physical way, and transmission or information storage and retrieval, electronic adaptation, computer software, or by similar or dissimilar methodology now known or hereafter developed.
The use of general descriptive names, registered names, trademarks, service marks, etc. in this publication does not imply, even in the absence of a specific statement, that such names are exempt from the relevant protective laws and regulations and therefore free for general use.
The publishers, the authors, and the editors are safe to assume that the advice and information in this book are believed to be true and accurate at the date of publication. Neither the publishers nor the authors or the editors give a warranty, express or implied, with respect to the material contained herein or for any errors or omissions that may have been made. The publishers remain neutral with regard to jurisdictional claims in published maps and institutional affiliations.

This Springer imprint is published by the registered company Springer Nature Singapore Pte Ltd.
The registered company address is: 152 Beach Road, #21-01/04 Gateway East, Singapore 189721, Singapore

If disposing of this product, please recycle the paper.

This book is dedicated to Shanghai Jiao Tong University School of Stomatology on its 90th anniversary.
I would also like to dedicate this book to the following people, who have influenced my work:

Academician Wei-Liu Qiu, the pioneer, on his 90th birthday
Academician Ke-Rong Dai, developer of the osteoarticular prosthesis
Academician Zhi-Yuan Zhang, leader of the discipline
Harry and Mei-Ling Schwartz

Foreword

I first visited the Shanghai Ninth People's Hospital in 1978 and met Prof. Weiliu Qiu, who was head of the Department of Oral and Maxillofacial Surgery. He was an experienced head and neck surgeon and a pioneer in the field of microvascular reconstructive surgery of the oral cavity. Over the years, we maintained a good relationship. When Prof. Qiu told me in 1999 that he would like to recommend a promising young man to come to Los Angeles for an exchange visit, I agreed without hesitation. That young man was the editor-in-chief of this book, Prof. Chi Yang.

Prof. Yang was appointed as an international scholar at UCLA and a visiting scholar in maxillofacial surgery at Kaiser Permanente Medical Group. During the year of his visit, he became both a colleague and a friend. We were doing about five orthognathic surgeries per week at that time, but only one to two TMJ surgeries per month. Joint surgery happened to be his main area of interest. I taught him a lot about orthognathic surgery, but almost nothing about TMJ surgery. In fact, he taught me a great deal about joints. I introduced him to several American specialists in the field of TMJ surgery and arranged for him to observe endoscopic surgeries in the orthopedic department of our hospital. The orthopedic department's knee and shoulder treatment techniques and equipment laid a good foundation for his future development of endoscopic TMJ disk repositioning techniques and customized instruments. This is a treatment innovation for which he is now internationally renowned.

During Prof. Yang's stay in the United States, I introduced him to a US manufacturer of custom-fitted TMJ prostheses. Due to a number of factors, the use of their devices in China did not work out. Since then, Prof. Yang has collaborated with experts in the fields of bioengineering and manufacturing to develop a series of clinically stable and reliable customized prostheses. These devices are based on anatomical and kinetic analyses of the joint, combined with material selection and testing. Prof. Yang illustrates the development of these prostheses with detailed case reports. The reader is taken through the history, examination, planning, design, surgery, outcome, and follow-up for each case.

For me, the most interesting part of this work is the "Combined Prosthesis." Most of the TMJ replacements I have done in the United States include a metal condyle and neck, and a high-molecular-weight polyethylene fossa. In Prof. Yang's practice, there are tumors and other lesions involving the TMJ, the adjacent mandible, the base of the skull, or all three structures. The design and application of the "Combined Prosthesis" has made the reconstruction of these extensive lesions more precise, efficient, and reliable.

Prof. Yang also lays out his vision for the future. This includes surface modification of prosthesis for muscle attachment and osseointegration, and the use of artificial intelligence in prosthesis design to facilitate fit and function. I look forward to his follow-up work in these areas and hope to see the publication of related achievements.

Harry C. Schwartz
Professor, Emeritus Chief of Oral & Maxillofacial Surgery
Kaiser Permanente Medical Group
UCLA Health Sciences Center
Los Angeles, CA, USA

Preface

I spent the last year of the Millennium as an International Scholar at UCLA in Los Angeles. When I returned to China in 2001, I began writing several times, but without success. Many things in life do not go as expected. Twenty years have gone by, and I have nearly reached the age of 60. According to the Chinese saying, "Accumulating soil into a mountain, accumulating water into an abyss." I have gained a great deal of experience. I have found my voice. I am finally ready to write.

This book is the author's first monograph. It presents our experience with customized prostheses for temporomandibular joint (TMJ) defects. It features both skull base defects and mandibular defects. It brings together experimental studies since 2009, and our clinical experience at the Ninth People's Hospital affiliated to Shanghai Jiao Tong University School of Medicine in the past 6 years, demonstrating the development and manufacture of various types of prostheses and their clinical applications. The book covers six aspects of our work: customization, concept, design, materials, process, and installation. It reviews the way in which we approached the difficult areas of virtual design, special processing technology, digital precision, positioning, installation, and more.

I. *The significance of custom-made or adapted prostheses*
   (a) The customized TMJ prosthesis is a part of the modern trend in adapting complex bone and joint reconstruction to the needs of the individual patient. It is an important embodiment of precision medicine.
   (b) The TMJ has a complex structure, with undulating bone surface morphology and large individual differences among patients. This can lead to difficulties in the placement of a standard stock prosthesis, including the following:
      - Bone grafting may be required to seat a stock prosthesis. This is done empirically and can still result in improper seating. Even with digital guides, errors are possible.
        - Bone removal may be required to seat a stock prosthesis. This is usually done by grinding, a process that can be difficult and time-consuming. It can be prone to complications, such as nerve damage.
        - Two incisions are required to complete the approach. Especially the incision posterior or inferior to the mandible can injure the facial nerve or can leave an unsightly scar.
        - Intermaxillary fixation is required prior to attachment of the condylar component. This is time-consuming. It increases the risk of post-operative infection because of the need to alternate between the sterile surgical field and the mouth.
        - When placing screws to attach the condylar component, there is a risk of causing numbness of the lower lip because of damage to the inferior alveolar nerve.
        - If the defect is too large, no stock prosthesis is available.
        - In order to overcome these disadvantages, a custom-made prosthesis is necessary.

II. *The TMJ Union Concept and Combined Prosthesis*

The origin of the term TMJ union concept is as follows: The TMJ is the articulation between the skull base and the mandible. The articular fossa is part of the skull base, at the inferior portion of the temporal bone. The distance to the brain can be as little as 1 mm at its thinnest point. Also, the condyle is the proximal portion of the mandible.

Guided by this concept, custom-made prostheses designed by the author can be categorized as follows:

(a) Total joint prostheses.
(b) Combined TMJ—cranial base prostheses.
(c) Combined TMJ—mandibular prostheses.
(d) Other craniomandibular prostheses related to TMJ surgery. These include the articular eminence blocking prosthesis for chronic dislocation and custom plates for mandibular reconstruction or orthognathic surgery that is done in conjunction with total joint reconstruction.
(e) Future developments in prosthetic design that are still in the experimental stage.

III. *Prosthesis Design and Optimization*

The development of TMJ prostheses started with a hemi-articular design, then evolved to the total joint prosthesis. The original devices were entirely metal, then evolved to a metal-to-plastic pairing. The US Food and Drug Administration currently approves two TMJ prostheses, the Biomet stock prosthesis and the TMJ Concepts custom prosthesis. These devices have outstanding performance, with long-term efficacy of more than 94%. However, further development can and will take place in the coming years in order to address several issues:

1. Intelligent design of individualized motor function surfaces.
2. Retention and restoration of muscle function.
3. Precise intraoperative positioning of the prosthesis.

In the coming decade, the prosthesis will gradually change from one with standardized and modular design to one with individualized, digital, and intelligent design. Expansion into new fields, with new concepts, new technologies, and new materials will permit reconstruction of the skull base and/or adjacent mandible to be combined readily with total joint reconstruction.

IV. *Material Progress*

In addition to the evolution in design, advancements in the development of biomaterials are an important factor in the development of the joint prosthesis. Early workers reported the use of precious metals, nickel-chromium, polymethyl methacrylate, tetrafluoroethylene, and other materials. The toxicity of some metal ions and excessive wear and tear often led to failure. Having studied the development of successful large joint prostheses in orthopedics, current TMJ prostheses pair a highly cross-linked ultra-high molecular weight polyethylene (UHMWPE) joint socket with a cobalt-chromium-molybdenum alloy joint head. The two approved prostheses in the United States use this material pairing. In addition, teams are studying the use of polyether ether ketone (PEEK), pure titanium, and tantalum alloys in joint prostheses. These are areas for future development.

V. *Prosthesis Manufacturing*

The process for manufacturing TMJ prostheses has evolved gradually. Initially casting or forging were used for the metallic components. Currently, CAD/CAM technology and finishing are used throughout the world for custom-made prostheses. Our team utilizes a combination of finishing and 3D printing. We focus on 3D printing technology for materials such as cobalt-chromium-molybdenum alloy, UHMWPE, PEEK, tantalum alloy, and other materials. We believe that 3D printing will be the primary method of processing and production in the near future.

VI. *Precise Installation of the Prosthesis*
The prerequisite for accurate installation of a custom-made prosthesis is accuracy in performing osteotomies and bone contouring at the recipient site. We utilize virtual design to manufacture custom cutting and installation guides, which provide this accuracy. They enable precise installation of the custom-made prosthesis. The benefits of this process include the following:
(a) Precise planning of a resection and creation of a surgical defect helps avoid recurrence of pathologic lesions.
(b) The process permits accurate installation of the prosthesis, which is necessary for ideal occlusion of the teeth, a requirement for normal jaw function. It avoids the need for revision surgery due to poor alignment.
(c) The process simplifies what can be a complex surgery, turning it into a series of steps, like building blocks.
(d) The process reduces surgical trauma and bleeding by decreasing unnecessary dissection of soft tissues and bone removal.
(e) The process diminishes the risks of surgery and helps avoid major complications caused by the proximity to important nerves and blood vessels, the middle cranial fossa, the ear canals, and other structures.
(f) The process shortens operative time, due to all of the above advantages.

Since our team began research in 2009, Zhang Shanyong and others have used five-axis finishing technology to manufacture devices for animal experimentation. We have confirmed the accuracy and safety of devices manufactured in this way. In 2015, the author led the team to integrate 3D printing technology for the design and manufacture of the first generation of devices for clinical use in patients. The first were implanted in 2016. As of the current time, 102 devices of various designs have been placed. After a maximum of 6 years follow-up, the results are encouraging, and have led to the development of the first domestic group standard of the "Patient Fitted Artificial Temporomandibular Joint" (T/CAMDI 027–2019). In addition to our unit, devices have been placed at units in Zhejiang, Hebei, Guangzhou, Shanxi, and Moscow. Ten additional devices will be implanted in the near future.

Numerous disciplines are involved in the development of prosthetic devices. These include materials science, engineering, computer science, and numerous biologic sciences. We are in constant pursuit of optimized design, adapted materials, and advanced manufacturing processes. Clinical application of these devices primarily involves the specialties of oral and maxillofacial surgery, otolaryngology, neurosurgery, and plastic surgery. The sub-specialties of oral and maxillofacial surgery involved include TMJ surgery, oncologic surgery, reconstructive surgery, and orthognathic surgery. A preoperative multidisciplinary conference is often required in order to develop a reasonable treatment plan prior to the implantation of a complex joint prosthesis.

Although some of the devices described have not yet received government approval, the author decided to write this volume based on the outcomes in the initial follow-up period. The intention is to promote the development of TMJ-cranial-mandibular reconstruction by reporting the encouraging results of various customized prostheses from development and manufacturing to clinical application.

The book explains our newer design concepts and clinical applications. We hope that understanding our work will stimulate upstream cooperation from our peers in the pursuit of newer concepts, biomaterials, and processes. Deeper cooperation in product development will be a great advantage for our patients, some of whom suffer from what once was considered irreparable defects of the TMJ and skull base.

We hope to stimulate midstream cooperation from manufacturers involved in this field, who may consider investment in developing and marketing this series of products.

Finally, we hope to stimulate upstream cooperation from hospitals and surgeons, who may have patients who could benefit from one of these devices. The patient is the ultimate beneficiary of these products. Clinical application of all devices described in this book has been in compliance with medical ethics, regulations, and procedures prescribed in the following legal codes: SH9H-[2015] No. 18, SH9H-2018-T52-1, SH9H-2019-T267-1, SH9H-2019-T315-1, SH9H-2020-T15-1, SH9H-2020-T111-1. We look forward to working with domestic and international colleagues and conducting multi-center clinical studies for further validation and development of these devices.

Special Acknowledgments

1. Special thanks to our leaders, Academician Wei-Liu Qiu and Academician Zhi-Yuan Zhang. Without their tireless support and dedication over the past 30 years, especially their active advocacy in pioneering innovations, exploring the unknown, and troubleshooting challenging problems, my team and I would not exist.
2. Thanks to the orthopedic 3D printing center, headed by Academician Ke-Rong Dai, and especially the pivotal role played by Director Wen-Bo Jiang. Their successful experience in producing custom-made orthopedic joint prostheses and hip joint-pelvis prostheses has been a great reference for us. All prostheses in this book were manufactured in this center.
3. Thanks to the 30 years of success of the two TMJ prostheses that are approved in the United States! In 2002, accompanied by Prof. Harry Schwartz, Xudong Wang and I visited TMJ Concepts in Ventura, California. We were received by Prof. Louis G. Mercuri, one of the founders of the company, and Dave Samson, the manager. We not only visited the production line for customized prostheses, but we discussed the feasibility of developing the Chinese market. In 2003, the company agreed to provide three joints at no cost. Samson came to Shanghai Ninth People's Hospital, where the author operated the first customized TMJ replacement in China. In 2005, after negotiation, Zimmer Biomet agreed to provide five stock TMJ prostheses for a clinical trial. The inventor, Prof. Peter Quinn came to Shanghai to perform the first Biomet stock TMJ replacement with the author and Xiao-Hu Zhang. This is how the history of TMJ replacement in our country began. After long-term follow-up, the efficacy of these prostheses is over 94%. The excellent results encouraged us to develop our own product. We would also like to thank Dr. Larry Wolford, who pioneered simultaneous TMJ replacement and orthognathic surgery. He has been invited to our country twice to give lectures. He invited Shan-Yong Zhang and others to visit him in Texas. He has provided us with very useful help in doing this work.
4. Special thanks to Harry and Mei-Ling Schwartz! Dr. Schwartz is the Chief of Maxillofacial Surgery at Kaiser Permanente Medical Group and an Adjunct Professor at UCLA. He was my teacher and close friend during my stay in the United States, and my orthognathic surgical skills originated with him. In his department, I also operated on TMJ tumors, performed arthroscopic disc repositioning, repaired condylar fractures, performed costochondral grafts, did surgery to prevent chronic condylar dislocation, and more. He gave me several monographs, including my favorite "Bone Tumors." When I returned to China, he gave me many surgical instruments, including a cheek-piercing bone hook, which my team and I still use. Their kindness and contributions will never be forgotten!
5. Thanks to the many related disciplines in our hospital! In addition to Orthopedics, there are Prof. Hao Wu, Prof. Zhaoyan Wang, and their teams in the Department of Otolaryngology-Head and Neck Surgery. There is Prof. Zhilin Guo in the Department of Neurosurgery. There is Prof. Yue He in the Department of Oral and Maxillofacial Head and Neck Oncology. We thank them for their selfless help in TMJ-skull base tumor surgery and TMJ-mandibular reconstruction. This also highlights the advantages of working in a general hospital.

6. Thanks to our research and development collaborators! They are:
   (a) For materials and processing, Prof. Ai-Dang Shan and Prof. Ke Chen's team from Shanghai Jiao Tong University School of Material Science and Engineering
   (b) For product testing, Prof. Hai-Ming Zhang's team, Engineer Xiao-Lin Tian and Engineer Hai-Yi Qin
   (c) For processing and post-processing, General Manager Ya-Jun Shen's team from Shanghai ShengShi Medical Device Company
   (d) For digital structure design, Prof. Xiao-Wen Zhao's team from Shenzhen Excellent Company
   (e) For intelligent design, Prof. Sheng-Hui Liao's team from Central South University
7. Thanks to our research and development collaborators who are in the experimental stage! Prof. Li-Jing Yang's team from Ningbo Institute of Materials Research, Chinese Academy of Sciences, Academician Mei-Fang Zhu's team from Dong Hua University, and Academician Wen-Jiang Ding's team from the School of Materials Science and Engineering, Shanghai Jiao Tong University.
8. Thank you to my team! There is no substitute for the role of the key members. Dr. Ji-Si Zheng, as the most important member, who participated in the development, manufacturing, postoperative follow-up, and efficacy evaluation of all the prostheses. This is a great credit. Prof. Min-Jie Chen for his outstanding contribution in the combined TMJ-skull base reconstructive surgery and combined TMJ-mandibular reconstructive surgery. Prof. Shan-Yong Zhang for his hard work in the initial experimentation, and his promising achievements in developing metal and non-metallic biomaterials. Dr. Xiao-Han Liu's talent in drawing and her hard work and dedication. Dr. Qian-Yang Xie's excellent work in TMJ-orthognathic surgery virtual planning. Prof. Duo-Hong Zou's guidance in seeking research and development partners and his hands-on experimental work, which makes us look forward to future products. Thank you to Dr. Da-He Zhang, Jia-Yi Li, and Xu-Zhuo Chen for your great graphic processing work. Thank you to Nurse Yi Luo for taking surgical photos and archiving the cases.
9. Thanks to my family for their constant support.

Lastly, I sincerely welcome suggestions and criticism from all sides. This fosters continual improvement in my work.

Shanghai, China Chi Yang

Contents

The History of Temporomandibular Joint Diseases and Their Treatment

1

Chi Yang, Jisi Zheng, Dahe Zhang, Xiaohan Liu, and Minjie Chen

The temporomandibular joint (TMJ) is composed of matching hinges on both sides of the jaw, right and left, which, most importantly, provide rotational and sliding movements to masticate food and to articulate speech. It is one of the most complex joints in the human body in terms of its anatomy and movements. TMJ diseases are among the most common clinical diseases in dentistry, aside from caries, periodontal disease, and malocclusion. Diseases such as anterior joint disc displacement, condylar dislocation, condylar fracture, condylar resorption, osteoarthritis, ankylosis, tumors or tumorlike lesions, congenital malformations, developmental malformations, and acquired deformities fall within the scope of surgical treatment. For patients who do not respond to non-surgical treatments, whose joints cannot be preserved, or who exhibit significant clinical symptoms or secondary moderate-to-severe dentofacial deformities, TMJ prosthetic joint replacement may be one of the most effective solutions to restore joint function and improve aesthetics.

The origin and development of understanding of TMJ and its diseases, from terminology to diagnostic and therapeutic approaches, is largely informed by the valuable experience of bone and joint surgery in orthopedics, most importantly hip and knee surgery. The history of the development of TMJ surgery at the Ninth People's Hospital affiliated to Shanghai Jiao Tong University School of Medicine is no exception.

International research on TMJ prostheses has had a history of more than 60 years, and it has evolved from semi-joint prostheses to total joint prostheses with metal and polymer materials. Research in China on TMJ prostheses has had a history of 30 years, but at the beginning, it was mostly an experimental study. However, since 2009, the author's team has conducted basic research on TMJ prostheses and their clinical applications, and we have developed a series of individually customized TMJ and craniomandibular prostheses, such as the total TMJ prosthesis, TMJ-skull base combined prosthesis, TMJ-mandibular combined prosthesis, customized fixation plates in orthognathic surgery, and condylar dislocation prosthesis.

However, before describing the benefits of our TMJ and maxillary prostheses, it is necessary to, firstly, clarify the definition and classification of TMJ diseases. Following, we wish to review the history of the development of TMJ surgery abroad and in China, as well as to describe the experience of our team in utilizing innovative concepts of TMJ surgery, advancing the development of TMJ prostheses, and applying the related innovative technologies. Therefore, this chapter will first provide an overview of the basic concepts and the history of TMJ surgery, presenting a full picture to support the subsequent chapters.

1.1 Fundamentals of TMJ Diseases

Chi Yang and Jisi Zheng

The structure and basic functions of the temporomandibular joint (TMJ) are well established. However, there is still no unified view of the role of the articular disc, which will be discussed further shortly. The high prevalence and variety of TMJ diseases have led to different domestic and international classifications, but none of them has been focused on diseases of the TMJ itself and the concomitant or secondary diseases (e.g., dental and mandibular malformations, joint-craniofacial diseases, joint-mandibular diseases). For this reason, Sect. 1.1 of this chapter reviews the definitions and national and international classifications of TMJ diseases, and then explains the new classification developed by our team, one which is guided by the concept of placing the joint specifically at the center of the classification. This new

Chi Y. (✉) · Jisi Z. · Dahe Z. · Xiaohan L. · Minjie C.
Shanghai Ninth People's Hospital, Shanghai Jiao Tong University School of Medicine, Shanghai, China

© People's Medical Publishing House, PR of China 2025
Chi Y. (ed.), *Atlas of Customized TMJ-Cranio-Jaw Prosthesis*, https://doi.org/10.1007/978-981-95-0611-8_1

"Yang's" classification is the basis for the subsequent divisions of chapters throughout the book.

1.1.1 Definition of the TMJ

The temporomandibular joint (often referred to as "TMJ" or "joint" for short in this book) is also known as the craniomandibular joint. It is the only movable articulated connection of the mandible to the skull base and the only joint in the whole body that has both left and right hinges, and these move in conjunction with each other. On each end of the mandible—both left and right—there is a condyle, a fossa, and an articular disc situated between the condyle head and the fossa. This disc is enclosed within a flexible capsule composed of membranes and muscles. The articular disc moves forward with the condyle when the mouth is opened. This mechanical structure not only allows bending and rotational movement (like the main movement of other joints in the body, such as the knee or elbow). Rather, the TMJ also has a large anterior-posterior gliding movement, which is of great significance in maintaining normal oromaxillofacial function, and without which, there would be no wide mouth opening, no forward jaw extension, and no sideways movement, as is used in vigorous chewing. This joint not only dominates mandibular movement but also is essential to crucial life functions such as speech, mastication, facial expression, and respiration.

The articular disc plays an important role in all this movement, and it is believed to have at least the following functions:

- Regulating the volume and morphological gap between the condyle and fossa so that they fit together while in action
- Cushioning and spreading the load of the joint
- Enhancing the stability of the joint during mastication
- Providing lubrication and nutrition to the articulating surfaces
- Preventing the degeneration of the condyles and fossae
- Promoting the normal growth of the mandible in children and adolescents

Among these elements of the TMJ, the articular disc, condyle, and lateral pterygoid muscle constitute a closely related complex (referred to as the disc-condyle-muscle complex), which is of great significance in maintaining the physiological function of this joint.

1.1.2 Definition and Classification of TMJ Diseases

For the classification of joint diseases, there are different views at home and abroad, and there is still no unified conclusion. But for a general overview, the author has categorized them into narrow and broad definitions based on the extent of the lesion. TMJ diseases in the narrow sense are lesions that occur within the joint or intracapsular pathologies. In a broader sense, TMJ diseases refer to lesions occurring in the joints and surrounding musculoskeletal and neuromuscular tissues; in addition to intra-articular lesions, they also include related musculoskeletal lesions and diseases. TMJ surgery focuses on the treatment of intracapsular and associated skeletal lesions.

1.1.2.1 Classification by the American Society of TMJ Surgeons (ASTMJS)

There are many international classifications of temporomandibular diseases, and these vary from author to author. The most influential classifications are Research Diagnostic Criteria for Temporomandibular Disorders (RDC/TMD, 1992) and its later version Diagnostic Criteria for Temporomandibular Disorders (DC/TMD, 2014).

There has been no uniform classification of TMJ diseases in China, but according to the material of the Peking University School of Stomatology, such diseases can be basically divided into nine categories:

1. TMJ disorders
2. Joint cysts and tumors of various kinds
3. Ankylosis of joints
4. Trauma and fracture
5. Infections
6. Developmental anomalies
7. Dislocations
8. Systemic diseases affecting the joints
9. Other diseases

The last refers to those diseases that are commonly seen in the outpatient clinic with the complaint of difficulty in opening the mouth, i.e., some related diseases such as hypertrophy or osteochondroma of the coronoid process.

This listing is closely related to the classification of the American Society of TMJ Surgeons, broadly including intra-articular and extra-articular pathology.

1.1.2.2 Yang's Proposal for a New Classification of TMJ Diseases

Taking the joint as the focus of the classification, our surgery team at the Ninth People's Hospital of Shanghai Jiao Tong University School of Medicine has proposed, firstly, a binary differentiation, a classification concept contrasting the "joint extension complex" (Fig. 1.1) to the "joint surrounding complex" (Fig. 1.2).

The "joint extension complex" is also known as the "joint-jaw-occlusion-airway" complex. These four items are joined because the TMJ is the proximal end of the mandible, and through the mandible, it connects to the far end of the complex, the occlusion, i.e., the association of the upper and lower teeth. So, the combination "joint-jaw-occlusion" is the trinity of the structure of points involved in the mechanical function. But because mandibular retraction often accompanies TMJ diseases and can lead to narrowing of the upper airway, "airway" is included in the name of the complex since the crucial function of respiration must always be kept in mind in the design of the treatment. It is proposed that the complex be treated in combination because primary diseases of the joint can lead to imbalance of the other three components of the complex, and so resolution of the disorder involves combined diagnosis and treatment of the complex (Fig. 1.1).

The "joint surrounding complex," also known as the "joint-skull base-ear-infratemporal fossa (ITF)" complex, refers to the area of the joint impinging on the skull base, bordering the ear canal at the back, and adjoining the infratemporal fossa (Fig. 1.2).

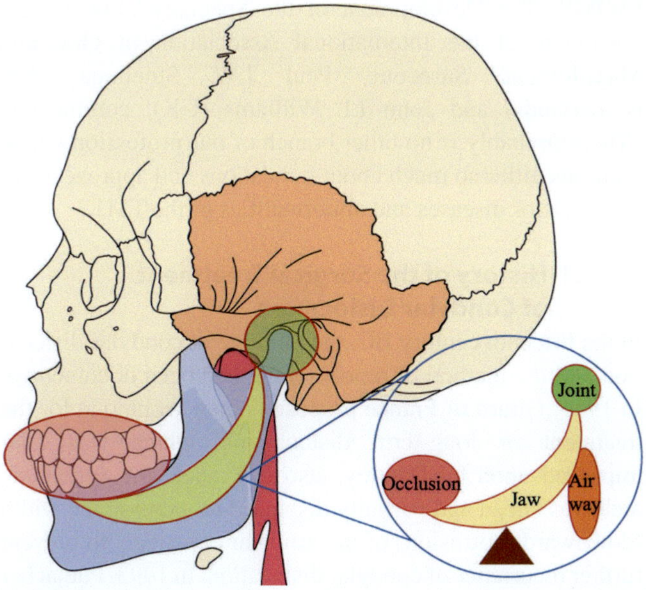

Fig. 1.1 The "joint-jaw-occlusion-airway" complex concept. In this schematic diagram, the TMJ is accented in green, the mandible in yellow, the occlusion in pink, and the airway in red. The complex is the region extending down from the condyle

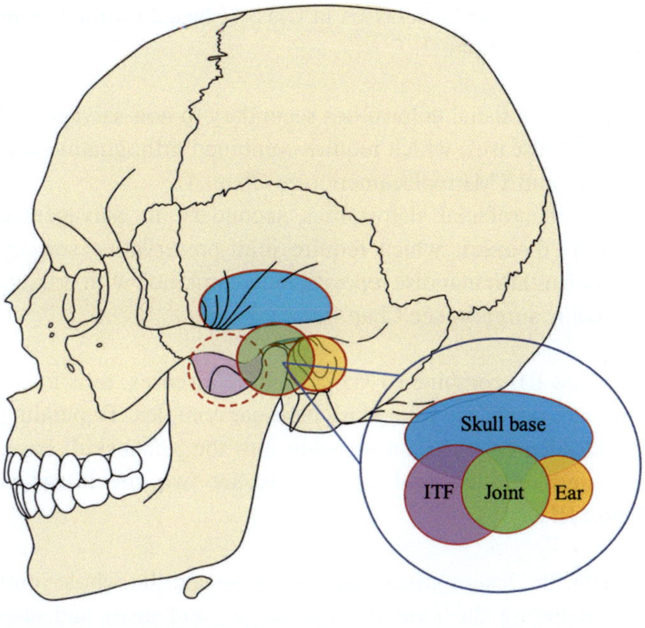

Fig. 1.2 The "joint-skull base-ear-infratemporal fossa" complex. In this schematic diagram, the TMJ area is circled in green, the cranial base in blue, the ear in yellow, and the infratemporal fossa in purple. The infratemporal fossa is partly hidden behind the condyle and beneath the skull base. The complex is the surrounding region around the condyle

Taking the new conceptualization, differentiating the joint extension complex and the joint surrounding complex as the guiding idea, the author proposes a new classification of TMJ and related skeletal diseases, which may be concluded as "Yang's Classification," which is composed of four major categories, as follows.

Class I, TMJ diseases, refers to intra-capsular lesions. This category includes joint disc displacement, osteoarthritis, condylar resorption, ankylosis, condylar dislocation, condylar fracture, and joint tumors. See Chap. 3 for total joint prosthesis treatment and Chap. 10 for condylar dislocation treatment.

Class II, dentofacial deformities secondary to TMJ diseases, also known as TMJ-originated dentofacial deformities, refers to deformities caused by primary joint diseases. All types of intracapsular joint diseases may lead to such conditions, such as condylar resorption, TMJ ankylosis, condylar fracture, condylar dislocation, condylar hypertrophy, and condylar tumors. Severe mandibular retrognathia, or micrognathia, can also lead to narrowing of the upper airway. Thus, the problems to be addressed in this group of diseases are joint structure and function, bone and soft tissue deformities of the maxillofacial region, occlusal disorders, and even respiratory disorders. Class II falls under the category of the joint-jaw-occlusion complex and requires multidisciplinary integration, such as TMJ surgery, orthognathic surgery, and orthodontics.

There are two subclasses in Class II based on the health status of the joints:

- IIa, dentofacial deformities secondary to non-salvageable TMJ diseases, which require combined orthognathic surgery and TMJ replacement (see Chap. 4)
- IIb, dentofacial deformities secondary to salvageable TMJ diseases, which require joint-preservative surgery such as articular disc repositioning combined with orthognathic surgery (see Chap. 5)

Class III, combined TMJ-skull base diseases, falls under the category of the joint-skull base-ear complex. Depending on the degree of lesion invasion into the joint, skull base, ear, and infratemporal fossa, there are two subclasses in Class III:

- IIIa, the lesion affects the skull base and the whole joint (including the joint fossa, condyle, and disc) and also involves the ear canal and infratemporal fossa, and the purpose of surgical treatment is to remove the lesion completely and to rebuild the structure and function of the total joint and skull base (see Chap. 6).
- IIIb, the lesion affects the skull base and the joint fossa, and the disc-condyle-lateral pterygoid muscle complex is normal. The aims of surgical treatment are to remove the lesion, preserve the disc-condyle-muscle region, and rebuild the structure and function of the skull base and joint fossa. Combined joint-skull base pathology often requires a combination of joint surgery, otolaryngology, and neurosurgery (see Chap. 7).

Class IV, combined TMJ-mandible diseases, belongs to the joint-jaw-occlusion complex. In terms of onset and progression, while primary disease may originate in the joint and spread to other mandibular regions, it is more common for lesions elsewhere in the mandible to encroach upon or extend near the joint:

- IVa, combined TMJ-mandibular lesions where the joint is non-salvageable, with surgical treatment aimed at removing the lesion and reconstructing the TMJ-mandibular structure and function (see Chap. 8).
- IVb, subcondylar mandibular lesions near the joint, but the joint can be preserved, with surgical treatment aimed at removing the lesion, preserving the disc-condylar-muscle complex, and reconstructing the mandibular structure and function (see Chap. 9). Such a joint lesion requires a combination of joint surgery, mandibular reconstructive surgery, and oral implantology.

It can be seen in the above classification that Class I is purely TMJ diseases and Classes II–IV are TMJ diseases combined with other pathologies, with the distinction of whether they fall under the joint-jaw-occlusion complex or the joint-skull base-ear complex, and these four categories form the basis for the subsequent classification and clinical application of TMJs and craniomandibular prostheses in this book.

1.2 History of TMJ Surgery

Chi Yang, Dahe Zhang, and Xiaohan Liu

The history of TMJ surgery has been a long and progressive process, and its development has been accompanied by continuous innovation in diagnostic and treatment concepts, examination methods, material sciences, and surgical approaches. It encompasses the efforts and contributions of scholars from many countries.

1.2.1 History of TMJ Surgery Worldwide

The development of TMJ treatment can be traced globally back to more than 3600 years ago. Starting with the discovery and treatment of condylar dislocation, treatment later focused on TMJ ankylosis, joint tumors, disc displacement, osteoarthritis, congenital deformities, and condylar fractures. Although great strides have been made in all areas, controversy persists. In 2012, in a review of "50 years of IAOMS: The Development of the Specialty," two former presidents of the International Association of Oral and Maxillofacial Surgeons, Paul J.W. Stoelinga (The Netherlands) and John Ll. Williams (UK), commented, "There probably is no other branch of our profession where opinions differ so much about indications and approaches as there are for diseases and abnormalities of the TMJ."

1.2.1.1 History of the Surgical Treatment of Condylar Dislocation

In the fifteenth century BC, the etiology of condylar dislocation and the method of repositioning had been documented. In 1943, Girard of France proposed a new technique for the treatment of long-term dislocations, which was later improved upon by Dautrey, also in France: the zygomatic arch was sliced and partially displaced to increase the width (downward protrusion) of the articular eminence, to prevent further recurrence of condylar dislocation. In 1993, Puelacher (Austria) and Waldhardt (Austria) reported inserting a small titanium plate to augment the articular eminence and treat recurrent dislocations.

1.2.1.2 History of Surgical Treatment of Ankylosis

In 1816, Howship (UK) reported a case of "ankylosis of the TMJ secondary to lymphatic tuberculosis." Since 1827, some scholars have proposed methods such as gap surgery or interstitial implantation, but high recurrence rates and facial deformity have not been resolved. 1920 saw the first reconstruction of the TMJ by Gillies (UK) using free rib cartilage. In 1998, Nitzan (Israel) suggested that for ankylosis of the joints with preserved condylar processes on the medial side of the joints, a lateral arthroplasty could be performed.

In the same period, the introduction of artificial total joint prostheses was a revolutionary innovation with encouraging results seen in long-term follow-up. The now more established view of surgical treatment is to use rib cartilage grafts in the growth spurt period of children and adolescents, but total joint prostheses in adults.

1.2.1.3 History of the Surgical Treatment of Tumors

In 1873, Adams (UK) mentioned that the condyle and the mandibular body on the same side could become hyperplastic or hypertrophic, leading to facial deformity. In 1883, Heath (UK) reported that the occlusal relationship and facial shape could be restored by removing the condyle and part of the mandibular ramus. In 1899, Eckert (Germany) reported a case of condylar osteoma leading to obvious deviation of the mandible, and the mandible was restored to its normal position after removal of the osteoma. After that, surgical repair was reported for tumors originating from the TMJ region, including osteochondroma, synovial chondroma, giant cell tumor of bone, and giant cell tumor of tendon sheath. Through to the middle of the twentieth century, some scholars reported the surgical resection of joint tumors, but surgeons lacked the techniques of reconstruction.

Later, with the development of digital medicine and material science, autologous bone or prosthesis was used for reconstruction. For defects limited to joints, the tumor was resected and the joint reconstructed with rib cartilage or total joint prosthesis; when the defects were large, TMJ-skull base prostheses, TMJ-mandibular prostheses, and such were needed to be designed and fabricated for reconstruction.

1.2.1.4 History of the Surgical Treatment of Articular Disc Displacement

250 years ago, William Hey (UK) first introduced the term "internal derangement" of the knee, defined as a localized mechanical trauma of the meniscus that interferes with smooth (normal) joint function. Meanwhile, in 1983, Bell (USA) introduced the term "temporomandibular disorders" at the American Dental Association meeting, and this term encompasses the problem of dislocation of the articular discs and the associated musculoskeletal structures and has been used ever since.

In 1887, Annandale (UK) first reported the procedure of articular disc repositioning, and in 1909 and 1929, Lanz (NL) and Wakeley (UK) reported the procedure of articular disc resection.

In 1957, Henny (USA) and Baldridge (USA) introduced high condylectomy. In 1961, Ward (UK) proposed subcondylar osteotomy (condylar resection). In the 1970s, some scholars began to refocus on articular disc reposition surgery, but the lack of instruments capable of fixating the disc resulted in a low surgical success rate.

In 2001, Mehra (USA) and Wolford (USA) reported on the use of Mitek anchor for articular disc repositioning, and in 2002, Wolford (USA) reported on the use of articular disc repositioning combined with orthognathic surgery to treat anterior disc displacement associated with dentofacial deformity.

The introduction of arthroscopy was a major technological leap. Diagnostic arthroscopy was first reported by Ohnishi (Japan, 1975). Subsequently, in 1991, Ohnishi (Japan) and McCain (USA) described arthroscopic disc repositioning techniques.

The International Consensus Conference on TMJ Surgery of 1992, sponsored by the American Association of Oral and Maxillofacial Surgeons, stated that "TMJ arthroscopy is a proven approach to the treatment of temporomandibular disorders, and that for those patients who have been treated with arthroscopic or open surgery, it can be used in a variety of ways, such as in the treatment of TMD. For intracapsular lesions that can be resolved with either arthroscopic or open surgery, arthroscopic surgery is superior because of the minimal damage to normal structures."

1.2.1.5 History of the Surgical Treatment of Degenerative Arthritis

In 1856, Humphrey (UK) reported a case of condylectomy for TMJ arthritis. In 1873, Adams (UK) described rheumatoid arthritis of the TMJ. It is only in recent decades that such diseases have achieved consensus in nomenclature with the term degenerative arthritis, also known as osteoarthritis. There has been a proliferation of non-surgical and surgical methods of treatment; non-surgical treatments include the use of splints, physical therapy, and medicines; surgical treatments include articular disc repositioning and total joint replacement.

1.2.1.6 History of the Surgical Treatment of Congenital Anomalies

From the second half of the nineteenth century to modern times, scholars found that TMJ deformities and deficiencies were associated with congenital malformations such as the first and second branchial arch syndrome and Treacher Collins syndrome. In 1969, Pruzansky (USA) put forward the typology of mandibular hypoplasia; in 1988 and 1991, Kaban (USA) and Vento (USA), respectively, supplemented it and used it widely in clinical practice. Surgical techniques have been developed for the correction of jaw deformities and TMJ reconstruction, including orthognathic surgery, rib cartilage grafting, distraction osteogenesis, and total joint replacement.

1.2.1.7 History of the Surgical Treatment of Condylar Fractures

Condylar fracture includes intracapsular fracture, condylar neck fracture, and subcondylar fracture, which can cause ankylosis of the affected side of the joint and shortening of the height of the mandibular ramus and may also lead to occlusal disorders and joint dysfunction. In 1952, MacLennan (USA) proposed that the goal of condylar fracture is to ensure the range of mandibular activity and to restore the normal occlusion as soon as possible. In 1974, Sanders (USA) described the conservative and surgical treatment options for condylar fractures. Nowadays, the more mature view of surgical treatment is that fractures with insignificant displacement of the fracture fragment and no significant occlusal disturbances can be treated conservatively; surgical intervention should be considered for severely displaced and dislocated fractures with significant occlusal disturbances, and the most challenging fractures are intracapsular fractures, as well as those in children, since their normal growth may be compromised by the fracture.

1.2.2 Contemporary International Organizations of TMJ Surgeons

The establishment of national and international organizations for TMJ surgery has been a great impetus to the development of the discipline. They are:

- American Society of TMJ Surgeons (ASTMJS): founded in the summer of 1986 by Clyde Wilkes and 11 colleagues in Key West, Florida, the professional organization was established in 1988, when Dr. Qiu Weiliu became an international member, the first from China. In 2003, Yang Chi also became an international member.
- European Society of TMJ Surgeons (ESTMJS): founded in 2009 at the initiative of Piero Cascone (Italy) and Gerhard Undt (Austria), in close collaboration with the ASTMJS in Rome, Italy. Yang Chi has been its only international member from China.
- Japanese Society of TMJ Surgeons (JSTMJS): established on May 25, 2013.
- Latin American Society of TMJ Surgeons (LASTMJS): established on May 22, 2019, during the 24th International Conference on Oral and Maxillofacial Surgery (ICOMS). The society was inaugurated at the Windsor Barra Hotel in Rio de Janeiro when its new auditorium was opened.
- Indian Society of TMJ Surgeons (ISTMJS): inaugurated in Kochi in 2019.
- The TMJS Collaborative Group of the Specialized Committee of Oral and Maxillofacial Surgery, the Chinese Stomatological Association, was established in 2012, with Yang Chi as the head of the group. Later, following the written request of higher-level authorities, the Chinese Stomatological Association no longer set up secondary branches, so the group has been inactive.

1.2.3 History of TMJ Surgery in China

1.2.3.1 History of Surgical Treatment of Condylar Dislocation in China

The development of TMJ surgery is documented as early as the Tang Dynasty. Specifically, in 652 AD, Sun Simiao described the manifestations of acute dislocations and the operation of manipulative repositioning in a medical text of 30 volumes entitled *Qian Jin Yao Fang (Essential Prescriptions Worth a Thousand Gold).*

In modern times, Zhou Shuxia (1965) introduced a method for the surgical treatment of old dislocations, and Zhong Yongchi (1983) proposed the "intermaxillary repositioning method." For recurrent dislocations, Hua Shaochen (1982) used zygomaticotemporal notch bone grafting; Qiu Weiliu, Hu Qingang, and Ha Qi (1990) used endoscopic synovial sclerotherapy, which was introduced in international monographs; Xu Yandi (1992) used injection of a sclerosing agent into the extracapsular articular eminence; and Yang Chi, Qiu Weiliu, and Ha Qi (1999) used arthroscopic sclerotherapy in conjunction with suture traction.

1.2.3.2 History of Surgical Treatment of TMJ Ankylosis

Zhang Disheng (1954) reported surgical treatment for TMJ ankylosis; in addition, numerous early medical researchers carried out pioneering exploration, e.g., Zhou Shuxia (1959), Song Ruyao (1964), Qiu Weiliu (1980), Dong Yaojun (1983), and Hong Min (1986), who all reported their experiences. The focal issues were surgical methods, recurrence rates, and age at surgery. Regarding the treatment of ankylosing maxillofacial deformities and respiratory disorders, Qiu Weiliu et al. (1985) reported a horizontal osteotomy of the mandibular ramus anteriorly and an "L"-shaped rib graft. In the past 30 years, a large number of younger generation, such as Yang Chi (1999), Long Xing (2002), Zhang Yi (2006), He Dongmei (2006), Li Zubing (2009), Li Jihua (2013), and Zhu Songsong

(2016), have moved forward on this work, and their efforts have been directed at preventing recurrence, correcting dentofacial deformities, and resolving respiratory stenosis. In 2008, Yang Chi proposed a classification and treatment strategy for TMJ ankylosis itself and secondary dentofacial deformities, emphasizing the importance of preserving condyle and articular disc structures, as well as a combined diagnostic and treatment plan for joint-mandibular-occlusal-respiratory disorders.

1.2.3.3 History of the Surgical Treatment of Tumors

For neoplastic diseases in the TMJ region, there are more case reports by scholars in China, for example, Yao Hengrui et al. (1985), Mao Tianqiu et al. (1989), Liang Yufu et al. (1990), Qiu Weiliu and Yang Chi et al. (1997), Hu Min et al. (1998), and Qiu Yating and Yang Chi et al. (2010), who presented the early case reports of various types of tumors occurring in the TMJ region. For the treatment of joint tumors, the early-stage research was mostly addressed to open surgery with simple removal, but some scholars began to consider the issues of concurrent reconstruction, simultaneous orthognathic surgery to align the maxilla and mandible, minimally invasive treatment, and digital applications for improved precision in surgery. For example, Mao Tianqiu (1989) and Hong Min (1989) proposed immediate joint reconstruction after removal of osteochondroma of the condylar process; Wang Xing (1999) proposed the surgical treatment of osteochondroma of the condylar process in combination with correction of malformation of the maxillofacial region. Several key points are that Sun Jian (2006) in a national meeting proposed early ideas of resection and repair methods for treating giant cell lesions of bone in the skull base-TMJ region, Yang Chi (2011) proposed minimally invasive treatment of arthroscopically assisted synovial chondromatosis in the TMJ area, and further to that, Yang Chi (2011) in a national meeting proposed computer-assisted treatment of condylar osteochondroma combined with correction of maxillofacial deformity. In conclusion, research on systematic classification and surgical treatment in the field of joint tumors has proceeded, but still more in-depth clinical and basic research is needed. Among these efforts, since 2004 Yang Chi has put together a more systematic classification and elaboration of surgical strategies for TMJ tumors and tumorlike lesions.

1.2.3.4 History of the Surgical Treatment of Articular Disc Displacement

As early as 1965, Que Bingyan reported articular cartilage disc and post-disc lax tissue resection; Hongmin et al. (1985) reported lateral pterygoid muscle stripping; Ha Qi, Qiu Weiliu, and Zhang Xize (1986) reported high condylectomy and/or articular disc removal; Zhang Zhenkang et al. (1987) reported articular disc reposition and repair, disc removal, and silicone implantation; Hong Min et al. (1991) reported position adjustment and decompression surgery outside the joint; in 1995, Zeng Rongsheng and Long Xing, respectively, reported endoscopic lavage for loosening of adhesions; Gu Zhiyuan (1996) reported arthrocentric irrigation and closure therapy; Wang Dazhang (1996) reported on his observations and evaluation of endoscopic surgical treatment of intra-joint TMJ disorders at the founding conference of the Chinese Stomatological Association and the Sixth National Academic Conference of Stomatology; and Yang Chi et al. (1998) reported endoscopic sclerotherapy in combination with suture traction.

At the beginning of the present century, Zhang Shanyong (2010), Yang Chi (2012), Cai Xieyi (2012), Chen Minjie (2012), He Dongmei (2015), and Liu Xiaohan (2019) reported arthroscopic disc reposition and suture surgery and open anchorage of the disc. In 2012, when the author's team reported a modified arthroscopic disc reposition and suture technique (first applied in 2001 and continuously improved since then), arthroscopic disc reposition and suture returned to the public eye. This technique has led to a quantum leap in the treatment of disc displacement by eliminating the need for an anchorage screw; instead, the disc is repositioned and sutured to the soft tissues behind the joint with a special suture. This procedure has been widely reported to have high success rates and stability. Meanwhile, the author's team has focused on articular disc displacement and condylar resorption, and resulting dentofacial deformity in the case of adolescents, specifically what may be the relevant factors of causation for adolescents and how it should be treated. They have advocated a combined treatment plan of articular disc repositioning and orthodontics applying functional devices. Shen Pei and Xie Qianyang, respectively, published the results of the randomized controlled trials and natural outcome correlation analysis. In the case of adults with disc displacement and condylar resorption that has caused dentofacial deformity, joint instability, and maxillofacial deformity can be addressed with joint surgery and orthognathic surgery.

1.2.3.5 History of the Surgical Treatment of Osteoarthritis

In the early and middle stages of osteoarthritis, if the articular disc meets the conditions for preservability, it can be effectively repositioned. But in the case of patients in the advanced stages of the disease, the principle of surgical treatment is similar to that of orthopedics: joint replacement is used when non-surgical treatments such as medications are ineffective and there are persistent clinical symptoms, or when the affliction is accompanied by severe mandibular retraction. Qiu Yating (2010) reported endoscopically assisted replacement of the joint with costochondral graft (CCG), Zhang Shanyong (2015) and He Dongmei et al.

(2019) reported replacement with a standard prosthesis, and Zheng Jisi (2019) reported endoscopically assisted replacement with an individually customized prosthesis. Zhang Shanyong and Chen Xuzhuo et al. (2020) reported the clinical efficacy and imaging evaluation of personalized TMJ fossa prostheses connected with heterogeneous materials.

1.2.3.6 History of the Development of Surgical Treatment of Congenital Anomalies

In 1957, Song Ruyao and Zhang Guangpu reported facial deformity and developmental asymmetry due to condylar hyperplasia (hypertrophy) and overgrowth of one side of the face. With the rise of orthognathic surgery in the 1980s, surgical treatment has advanced by leaps and bounds. Domestic scholars have also reported on the diagnosis and treatment of congenital malformations such as shortness of one side of the face caused by the first and second branchial arch syndrome in fetal development; the treatment has especially been aided by the gradual development of computer-assisted surgical techniques, which has improved the accuracy of orthognathic surgery and distraction osteogenesis.

1.2.3.7 History of the Surgical Treatment of Condylar Fractures

In 1988, Zou Zhaoju et al. suggested, through 100 cases with long-term follow-up, that treatment of children should be conservative, but for adults, surgery should be considered. Hong Min et al. (1990) and Wu Xianggen et al. (1991) reported the management of condylar longitudinal fractures and advocated surgical treatment; otherwise, osteoarthritis could be secondarily applied. In 2001, Zhang Yi proposed that for the condylar neck and subcondylar type of fracture with displacement and dislocation, treatment through anatomical repositioning plus small splints should be sufficient, taking into account also the internal fixation and stability.

In 2008 and 2010, after years of exploration and accumulation, Yang Chi's team proposed a new classification of intracapsular fractures of the condyle based on coronary CT, summarizing the absolute and relative indications for conservative and surgical treatment of intracapsular fractures of the condyle. The key point of surgery is to preserve the integrity of the "disc-condyle-muscle complex," emphasizing that free replantation can easily lead to complications such as osteoarthritis and ankylosis.

1.3 History of TMJ Prostheses

Chi Yang, Dahe Zhang, and Xiaohan Liu

The advent of the TMJ prosthesis is an important milestone in the development of TMJ surgery. The application of TMJ prostheses internationally and in China has followed a similar course, maturing from the development of inter-joint space implants to hemiarticular prostheses to total joint prostheses, showing a change in design concepts. Advances in materials science and manufacturing technology and the related experience of developing orthopedic joint prostheses have been instrumental in this process.

1.3.1 The International History of TMJ Prosthesis Development

The use of prostheses in TMJ treatment can be traced back to more than 180 years ago and can be broadly categorized into three phases: exploration, establishment, and maturity.

1.3.1.1 Exploratory Phase

As early as 1840, Carnochan (USA) implanted small blocks of wood into the post-resection space of ankylosed joints to prevent the recurrence of ankylosis. In 1933, Ridson (Canada) utilized gold foil; Eggers (USA) in 1946 and Goodsell (USA) in 1947 used tantalum foil; and in 1957, Smith and Robinson (USA) used stainless steel plates, which were implanted into the ankylosed joint space to prevent re-ankylosis.

It was not until 1960 that Robinson (USA) first introduced the concept of hemiarticular prosthesis design with his anatomically designed stainless steel socket prosthesis. After that, following this precedent, Christensen (USA) designed an articular fossa prosthesis of cobalt-chromium-molybdenum cast plate, Kriens (Germany) chose silicone to manufacture the articular fossa prosthesis, Hahn (USA) utilized acrylic and cobalt-chromium-molybdenum mesh to make a condylar prosthesis, Kent (USA) used cobalt-chromium alloy to make a mandibular prosthesis, and so on. However, due to the greater risk of bone resorption in hemiarticular prostheses and following the experience of problems with large orthopedic articulating prostheses, the design and application of total articulating prostheses have gradually predominated.

1.3.1.2 Establishment Phase

In 1965, Christensen (USA) added a mandibular prosthesis to the cobalt-chromium-molybdenum alloy articulating fossa prosthesis, which led to the development of the total joint prosthesis design concept. However, due to the limitations of material development, most subsequent total joint prostheses opted for metal-to-metal materials, such as the pure metal total joint prostheses developed by Momma (Germany, 1977), Kummoona (Iraq, 1978), and Kent (USA, 1972, 1983, 1986). Among them, the most famous one is the Vitek-Kent total joint prosthesis, which was later withdrawn from use by the US Food and Drug Administration, with a letter citing severe particle detachment, foreign body reaction, tissue destruction, and intractable orofacial pain produced by the implantation of the prosthesis. This incident became known as a major disaster in the history of the development of TMJ prostheses.

1.3.1.3 Maturity Phase

The development of cobalt-chromium-molybdenum alloys, titanium alloys, and polymer materials has led to the development of two products that have matured in terms of design, materials, and manufacturing concepts, namely, individually customized total joint prosthesis and standard total joint prosthesis. Among them, the development of the customized total joint prosthesis can be traced back to 1989. It consisted of a joint fossa component manufactured of titanium alloy and ultrahigh-molecular-weight polyethylene, and a mandible component composed of titanium alloy and cobalt-chromium-molybdenum alloy. This prosthesis was approved by the US Food and Drug Administration in 1999. The standard total joint prosthesis, which consisted of an ultrahigh-molecular-weight polyethylene joint fossa component and a mandibular component of cobalt-chromium-molybdenum alloy, with the addition of a titanium slurry coating that promotes osteointegration, obtained approval by the US Food and Drug Administration in 1995. These two types of total joint prostheses are now widely used.

1.3.2 History of the Development of TMJ Prostheses in China

The research and development of domestic TMJ prosthesis is slightly later than that of foreign countries, and it is roughly divided into three stages: exploration, application, and independent research and development.

1.3.2.1 Exploratory Stage

As early as the 1990s, Zhang Yi et al. (1993) from the School of Stomatology, Peking University, carried out experimental studies on the design and related properties of condylar prostheses with 3D adjustable structures and verified their material properties and biocompatibility in animal experiments. Since then, other scholars have explored the design and utilization of the articular fossa prosthesis, surface coating of prostheses, bioceramic materials, polymer materials (such as polyether ether ketone), biomechanical analysis, and 3D anatomical measurements, but most of them are hemiarthroplasties and are in the experimental stage.

1.3.2.2 Application Stage

In 2004, Tang Youchao and Tian Weidong of West China College of Stomatology, Sichuan University, applied Medicon or Betlach condylar prostheses for condylar restoration after resection of benign mandibular tumors. Later, some scholars applied other types of hemiarthroplasties in clinical trials.

In 2003, Yang Chi and Zhang Xiaohu of the Ninth People's Hospital of Shanghai Jiao Tong University School of Medicine recognized the need for personalized total joint prostheses for the treatment of severe osteoarthritis, as had been developed abroad, but these could not be applied in China due to the restriction of laws and regulations. In 2005, Yang Chi et al. introduced the standard total joint prosthesis into China and applied it; after that, the standard total joint prosthesis was approved by the China Food and Drug Administration (CFDA), which opened the way to promote the use of it in China. Given this availability, Sichuan University West China College of Stomatology, Peking University College of Stomatology, and Beijing Friendship Hospital of Capital Medical University also utilized imported standard total joint prostheses.

1.3.2.3 Independent Research and Development Stage

Since 2009, the TMJ team of the Ninth People's Hospital of Shanghai Jiao Tong University School of Medicine has been committed to research on and independent development of the total joint prosthesis. In 2009, Zhang Shanyong et al. developed a sheep total joint prosthesis and carried out animal experiments to validate the stability and effectiveness of its in vivo implantation.

In 2015, a study was done of the measurements of the anatomical structure of the normal Chinese adult craniomaxillofacial bones ($N = 400$) and the trajectory of the mandibular movement ($N = 90$); the data was collected with infrared motion capture technology in fine detail and mined. The team designed a total joint prosthesis that conforms to the joint anatomy and movement. The manufacture of the prosthesis uses an individually customized design of composite materials, with ultrahigh-molecular-weight polyethylene for the joint fossa component, cobalt-chromium-molybdenum alloy for the condyle head, and titanium alloy for the mandible component. The team incorporated 3D printing technology into the design and manufacture of the total joint prosthesis; in 2016, they utilized this self-developed 3D-printed total joint prosthesis in several clinical cases. This technology has been applied to patients who were regularly followed up on, for the longest time of 8 years, and the results of implantation have been found to be stable. In 2016, a metal/non-metal joining process was developed which utilizes stir friction welding technology to enable a secure joining of titanium alloys and ultrahigh-molecular-weight polyethylene, to manufacture durable and stable joint sockets with improved osteointegration.

Guided by the conceptualization of the joint extension complex and the joint peripheral complex, the team has also developed many kinds of 3D-printed protheses: the TMJ-skull base combined prosthesis, the skull base-fossa prosthesis, the TMJ-mandibular combined prosthesis, the customized fixation plates in orthognathic surgery, the mandibular reconstruction plate, and the condylar dislocation prosthesis, in order to meet the need for repair and reconstruction in all kinds of difficult and complex cases. Up to this point, the author's team has successfully constructed a series of Chinese TMJ and craniomandibular prosthesis products, and they have been clinically proven to be safe and effective.

We have also put into place a standardized workflow with communications among the several institutions, to ensure the efficient design, processing, testing, and application of the prostheses, and their performance has equaled or even exceeded the performance of international products of the same kind. The author's team has gone through 8 years of R&D and iteration of multiple generations of prostheses, obtained 26 domestic and international patents, and established four group standards. Their products have been utilized in 10 provinces and cities, such as Beijing, Xi'an, Zhejiang, Guangdong, Shanxi, Hebei, and Shandong, as well as 12 hospitals in Moscow, Indonesia, and other cities and countries.

1.3.2.4 Evaluation of the Efficacy of the TMJ Prosthesis

The American Academy of Oral and Maxillofacial Surgeons in its 95th edition of the Oral and Maxillofacial Surgery Guide has the following stipulations concerning the efficacy evaluation and follow-up time of total TMJ prosthesis implants:

- The follow-up period should be at least 2 years.
- The patient should be self-consciously pain-free or feel only slight pain.
- The patient's mandibular motor function should improve, including minimum postoperative mouth opening of 25 mm, or an increase of more than 10 mm compared with the preoperative condition.
- The patient should have improvement in masticatory function, with a normal or almost normal diet.
- The patient should have a functionally normal and stable occlusion of the upper and lower teeth.

The minimum follow-up period for all types of prostheses in the whole book was set at more than 2 years, and the postoperative efficacy evaluation indexes were recorded according to these criteria.

1.4 Innovations in TMJ Surgery at Shanghai Jiao Tong University School of Medicine

Chi Yang and Minjie Chen

TMJ surgery is one of the most effective ways to treat joint diseases, and it represents a high level of diagnosis and treatment of these diseases. In the 1990s, Qiu Weiliu explicitly urged the development of TMJ surgery in China, suggesting that the relevant medical practitioners concentrate their efforts on all diseases and secondary dental and maxillofacial deformities occurring in this joint. These include defects such as disc displacement, condylar resorption, condylar fracture, articular ankylosis, condylar dislocation, and articular tumors, tumorlike lesions, and cysts. For this purpose, Qiu Weiliu set up a specialized ward in 1993 at the Ninth People's Hospital affiliated to the Shanghai Jiao Tong University School of Medicine. To date, the accumulated total number of joint surgeries done amounts to 15,250 patient cases with 21,172 sides of the face treated, and in the last year, 2023, the annual volume of joint surgeries was 2168 cases and 3103 sides of the joints (Fig. 1.3). Only the work of the Department of Oral Surgery of the Ninth People's Hospital is shown on the chart below.

1.4.1 Innovations in TMJ Surgery at the Department of Oral Surgery of Shanghai Ninth People's Hospital

For TMJ diseases in Class I of Yang's new classification, i.e., intracapsular lesions, the improved and innovative surgical methods include: arthroscopic surgery, open disc reposition surgery, TMJ ankylosis surgery, condylar fracture surgery, condylar dislocation, joint tumor surgery, and total joint prosthesis replacement surgery.

1.4.1.1 Innovations in Minimally Invasive Arthroscopic Surgery

1. Arthroscopic disc reposition and suture: we have researched and developed suture devices, radiofrequency coblator, created arthroscopic horizontal mattress suture method, and taken the lead in introducing coblation technology to release the anterior attachment of the disc. The success rate of disc repositioning at more than 2 years' magnetic resonance imaging (MRI) follow-up is 95.3%.
2. Arthroscopic synovial chondromatosis removal: systematically proposed the indications for the operation, the surgical methods for tiny and huge loose bodies.

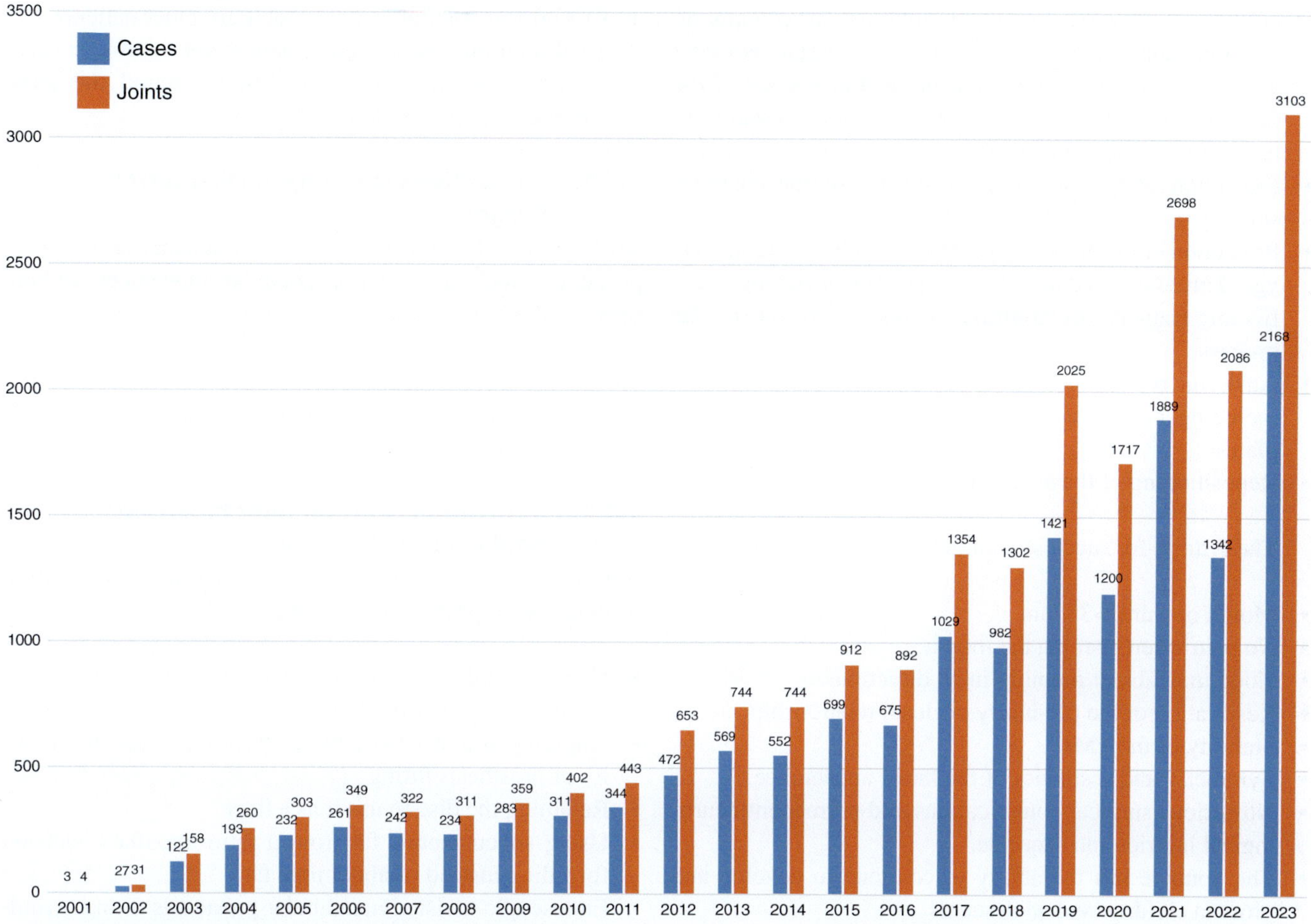

Fig. 1.3 Statistics on TMJ surgery at the Department of Oral Surgery of Shanghai Ninth People's Hospital affiliated to the Shanghai Jiao Tong University School of Medicine from 2001 to 2023. The blue bars are the number of patients, and the orange bars are the number of joints

3. Endoscopic-assisted arthroplasty: combined with CCG reconstruction, utilizing endoscopy and transbuccal techniques. The CCG fixation was accomplished using only a preauricular incision, avoiding a posterior mandibular incision. Similarly, applying this method to total joint prosthesis fixation not only avoids submandibular incision but also eliminates the need for intermaxillary ligation.

1.4.1.2 Innovations in Open Disc Repositioning Surgery

Technical improvements to the articular disc anchorage procedure are proposed, including adequate anterior attachment release of the disc, overcorrection of the disc position, and free fat grafting within the anterior attachment release area to prevent recurrence, resulting in long-term stabilization of the position of the disc after the procedure. The technique of disc suturing technique under small incision is reported, which adopts similar suturing techniques and instruments as arthroscopic disc repositioning suture, and has the advantages of easy operation, wide indications, and easily popularized.

1.4.1.3 Innovations in Ankylosis Surgery

The classification of joint ankylosis and corresponding treatment plan are proposed, especially emphasizing preserving the remaining condyle and disc structure on the medial side of the fusion bone as much as possible and using temporal fascia fat flap or abdominal fat to fill the lateral gap after removing the fusion bone by lateral arthroplasty, which significantly reduces the recurrence of joint ankylosis comparing with the non-filling and occlusal muscle flap filling.

1.4.1.4 Innovations in Condylar Fracture Surgery

The improved classification of intracapsular fracture and the corresponding treatments are proposed, and the five key points for successful surgery are:

- Adequate exposure (modified anterior auricotemporal incision, anterior approach to the superficial temporal vascular bundle for better exposure and protection of the facial nerve, applicable to both internal and external fractures of the condylar capsule)
- Protection of the cartilaginous surface of the condylar surface
- Protection of the blood supply of the condylar lateral pterygoid muscle, avoiding extensive peeling or freeing of the fracture fragment to minimize the resorption of condylar process
- Anatomic repositioning of the fracture and stable fixation including bicortical long screws and/or small titanium plates
- Repositioning of the articular disc

The criteria for successful surgery are:

- Mouth opening >35 mm.
- No pain when opening the mouth.
- Good mandibular mobility in all directions.
- Restoration of the pre-injury occlusal relationship.
- Stability of the TMJ.
- Symmetry and aesthetics of the facial appearance.
- No serious surgical complications and permanent neurological injuries and sequelae.
- The condyle has the ability to continue to develop and grow in children and adolescents.

1.4.1.5 Innovations in Joint Tumor Surgery

Surgery for preservation of joints:

1. Osteochondroma resection with preservation of condyle
2. Surgical approach of condylar neck or subcondylar osteotomy to expose the tumor of infratemporal fossa, which emphasizes the importance of the integrity of the "disc-condylar-muscle complex" in preserving the structure and function of the joints
3. Surgical approach of preservation of occlusal muscle with attachment of zygomatic arch to expose the tumor of infratemporal fossa

The above improvements are aimed at not only complete resection of the tumor but also preservation of normal joint structure and function, as well as considering maxillofacial appearance.

1.4.1.6 Innovations in Joint Reconstruction Surgery

Create a method of pedicled hemi-sternoclavicular joint to solve the following problems:

1. CCG reconstruction is not suitable for elder patients.
2. Total joint prosthesis replacement is not suitable in cases such as poor nutritional conditions around the joint, chronic infection, and large defect area.

1.4.1.7 Innovations in Condylar Dislocation Surgery

An "L"-shaped small titanium plate implantation was proposed to block the anterior condylar movement without opening the joint capsule. Subsequently, two types of prosthesis for condylar dislocation were independently developed, respectively, for the blocking of anterior condylar motion and the widening of the joint eminence, to prevent condylar dislocation (see Chap. 10).

1.4.1.8 Innovations in Total Joint Prosthesis Replacement Surgery

Improvements in standard total joint prosthesis installation techniques are proposed, including:

- Using digital guides designed to guide prosthesis positioning and bone trimming
- Applying articular fossa bone graft to increase the stability of prosthesis fitting
- Retaining the disc to use it as a liner
- Using subcutaneous fat from a retro-maxillary incision for filling instead of abdominal fat
- Endoscopic-assisted mandibular prosthesis fitting, avoiding post-mandibular incisions
- Preservation of the lateral pterygoid muscle attachment

Among them, the digital guide plate-assisted total joint prosthesis installation was included in the monograph *Atlas of Temporomandibular Joint Surgery* by Peter D. Quinn, 2nd edition (2015). Subsequently, the customized total joint prosthesis was independently developed to achieve precise joint replacement (see Chap. 3).

1.4.2 Innovations in Combined TMJ-Orthognathic Surgery

Surgical treatment for dentofacial deformity secondary to TMJ diseases, i.e., arthrogenic dentofacial deformity, which is classified as Class II in Yang's new classification, mainly includes: anterior displacement of the disc and condylar resorption, ankylosis of the joints, congenital joint deformity or absence, joint tumor, and so on. For salvageable joints, joint preservation surgery is used, and orthognathic surgery is performed in the same period or in stages to correct the jaw deformity. For non-salvageable joints, joint replacement with simultaneous or staged orthognathic surgery is used, and simultaneous combined surgery is mostly used for adults.

1.4.2.1 Staged Orthognathic Surgery for Children or Adolescents with Anterior Disc Displacement

In children or adolescents with anterior disc displacement, the regeneration of the condyle is often seen after disc reposition, and this corrects or improves the jaw deformity. However, for some people who still have a more obvious dentofacial deformity in adulthood, orthognathic surgery is then used to correct it (see Chap. 5).

1.4.2.2 Simultaneous Orthognathic Surgery for Adult Joint Disc Repositioning

For joints that can be preserved, concomitant orthognathic surgery with articular disc reposition is used to relieve the dentofacial deformity while stabilizing the joint morphology and position to prevent recurrence after orthognathic surgery. In orthognathic surgery, in order to achieve precise positioning of the osteotomy bone block and precise control of the condylar position, customized bone fixation plates have been independently developed and used for fixation in orthognathic surgery (see Chap. 5).

1.4.2.3 Simultaneous Orthognathic Surgery with Autogenous Bone Replacement

For joints that cannot be preserved, simultaneous orthognathic surgery with autologous bone reconstruction is used to treat dentofacial deformities secondary to joint diseases, restoring the joint's motor function and solving the problems of dental and maxillofacial deformities and airway narrowing at the same time.

1.4.2.4 Simultaneous Orthognathic Surgery for Total Joint Prosthesis Replacement

For non-salvageable joints, standard total joint prosthesis or personalized total joint prosthesis replacement with simultaneous orthognathic surgery is used (see Chap. 4).

1.4.3 Innovations in TMJ-Skull Base Reconstructive Surgery

For TMJ-skull base combined diseases in Class III of Yang's new classification, the following treatments are designed according to the extent of lesion invasion.

1.4.3.1 Total Joint-Skull Base Combined Reconstruction

For a total joint that cannot be preserved, meaning that the disease encroaches on the skull base, articular fossa, and condylar process, autologous bone repair of TMJ and skull base is proposed as a repair and reconstruction technique. The skull base and articular fossa are repaired by using a temporal bone flap or a free iliac bone flap and the condylar process by using CCG or a hemi-sternoclavicular joint. The temporal fascial fat flap is used as an interposition, and the dead space is filled with free fat. But to avoid taking autogenous bone, as an alternative, a customized TMJ-skull base combined prosthesis has been designed and applied for the repair of such defects (see Chap. 6).

1.4.3.2 Skull Base-Fossa Reconstruction

For the preservation of the articular disc and condyle, meaning that the lesion only invades the skull base and articular fossa, and the condyles and articular disc are normal, a technique of repairing and reconstructing skull base-articular fossa lesions with preservation of the disc-condylar-muscle complex is proposed. The zygomatic arch and/or condylar process are temporarily severed, and the tumor of the skull base-articular fossa is sufficiently exposed and completely resected, and then the skull base and articular fossa are repaired using temporal bone flaps or free iliac flaps, with temporal fascial fat flaps acting as an interlayer, and free fat is used to fill the dead space before fixing the temporarily severed zygomatic arch and/or condyle. But to avoid taking autogenous bone, as an alternative, skull base-fossa prostheses are also designed for the repair of such defects (see Chap. 7).

1.4.4 Innovations in TMJ-Mandible Reconstructive Surgery

For the combined TMJ-mandibular diseases in Class IV of Yang's new classification, the following treatments are performed according to the extent of the lesion encroachment:

1.4.4.1 Innovations in TMJ-Mandibular Combined Reconstruction Surgery

For TMJ and mandibular combined diseases in children and adolescents, it is appropriate to reconstruct the joint-mandible with extra-long double-layered CCG; in adults, a customized TMJ-mandibular combined prosthesis combined with iliac or vascularized fibula flap reconstruction and dental implants at a later stage are used to achieve the form and function of the TMJ-mandibular-facial-occlusal reconstruction (see Chap. 8).

1.4.4.2 Innovations in Mandibular Reconstructive Surgery with Condylar Preservation

For mandibular lesions adjacent to the condyle, mandibular reconstruction with preservation of the "disc-condylar-muscle complex" is proposed, which ensures the blood supply to the condyle and the integrity of the cartilaginous surface of the condyle and the normal position of the articular disc. In children and adolescents, extra-long ribs are preferred; in adults, iliac or vascularized fibula flaps are used in combination with a customized mandibular reconstruction plate (see Chap. 9). Preservation of the "disc-condylar-muscle complex" means preservation of normal joint function.

2 Application Fundamentals of Temporomandibular Joint-Related Cranium and Jaw Prosthesis

Chi Yang, Jisi Zheng, Wenbo Jiang, and Yaxing Bao

The temporomandibular joint (TMJ) and craniomaxillofacial prostheses serve as critical approaches for reconstructing bone and joint defects in the craniomaxillofacial region. The fundamental basis for prosthesis design derives from anatomical characteristics, kinematic patterns, and biomechanical properties of the joint. These parameters guide the prosthesis design, material selection, and manufacturing processes. Subsequently, the prostheses undergo rigorous physicochemical performance testing to evaluate compliance with international standards, followed by sterilization and packaging. This developmental process requires iterative clinician-engineer collaboration and continuous refinement to ultimately develop TMJ and craniomaxillofacial prostheses that meet both anatomical compatibility and physiological functional requirements.

Here in this chapter, we will first review the several kinds of prostheses that can be applied to the TMJ and related lesions. Then we will proceed to discuss several dimensions of our recent research and development. The first is a detailed study of the characteristics of anatomy and movement of the TMJ for a sample of the Chinese population. Related to this is a stress analysis of the structures of bones, which must be understood in carrying out the design of prostheses to reinforce or to substitute for the bones and their functions. In the case of the TMJ, this is a joint that must perform complex sliding movements in opening of the mouth plus side-to-side movements of the jaw, but these movements may also need to be powerful and repeated with great stress. So, the design of the core components of the prostheses must meet these demanding specifications. With this context given as a requirement, we will discuss the manufacturing procedures and the materials and proceed from that to rigorous testing of these products.

Last in this chapter, we will present a flow chart of the complex interactions among patients, doctors, technicians, and institutions in our medical system that are necessary for providing these devices to those who need them.

Chi Y. · Jisi Z. (✉)
Shanghai Ninth People's Hospital, Shanghai Jiao Tong University School of Medicine, Shanghai, China

Wenbo J.
Clinical and Translational Research Center for 3D Printing Technology, Medical 3D Printing Innovation Research Center, Shanghai Ninth People's Hospital, Shanghai Jiao Tong University School of Medicine, Shanghai, China

Yaxing B.
Gaofeng Medical Equipment (Wuxi)Co., Ltd, Wuxi, China

2.1 Definition and Classification of TMJ and Related Craniomandibular Prostheses

Chi Yang and Jisi Zheng

This section introduces the definition of TMJs and related craniomandibular prostheses; it then briefly presents the range of joint and craniomandibular prostheses, explaining this in the form of diagrams, as well as their indications and expected therapeutic outcomes.

2.1.1 Definition of TMJ and Related Craniomandibular Prostheses

"TMJ and related craniomandibular prosthesis" is a general term for a variety of prostheses designed according to the needs of reconstruction following resection of joints, skull base, and/or mandible due to defect or lesion, to restore the joint function and craniomandibular bone and shape. Customized prostheses have become the major trend in this kind of surgery, and these are the focus of this book's exposition.

© People's Medical Publishing House, PR of China 2025
Chi Y. (ed.), *Atlas of Customized TMJ-Cranio-Jaw Prosthesis*, https://doi.org/10.1007/978-981-95-0611-8_2

2.1.2 Classification of Customized TMJ and Craniomandibular Prostheses

The schematic diagram on the title page of this book personifies the most challenging diseases encountered in our clinical experience, along with the corresponding reconstructive prostheses. The design concept draws on the style and metaphor of the two-faced god of ancient Roman mythology, Janus. The left face represents the past (the disease), and the right face foretells the future (the outcome). It was said of Janus that "He is the god of the beginning and the end, symbolizing the beginning and the end of all things." The author hopes that the present medical studies that are the product of the joint efforts of our colleagues can put an end to irrational and ineffective reconstruction methods and open the future of scientific exploration. Hopefully, this book can serve as a catalyst for a new standard of medical reconstruction, aiding those with serious afflictions. We hope to figuratively transform the diseased left face of the past into the reconstructed right face of the future.

In this first section of Chap. 2, this general representation is further refined to show the types of prostheses that are to be introduced in this book. There are seven major categories of prostheses covered in this book:

- The first category, total joint prostheses, is used to repair simple TMJ lesions accompanied by severe jaw deformities that require concurrent orthognathic surgery (Fig. 2.1); see Chaps. 3 and 4.
- The second category, customized fixation plates in orthognathic surgery, for fixation of the mandible or maxilla during TMJ and simultaneous or staged orthognathic surgery, including the "H" or "Y" plate for fixation following a Le Fort I procedure on the maxilla, the genioplasty plate, and the condylar-stabilized mandibular sagittal splitting plate (Fig. 2.2), as described in Chap. 5.
- The third category, TMJ-skull base combined prostheses, is used for the repair of TMJ-skull base diseases (Fig. 2.3); see Chap. 6.
- The fourth category, skull base-fossa prostheses, is used to repair skull base-fossa lesions (Fig. 2.4), as described in Chap. 7.
- The fifth category, TMJ-mandibular combined prostheses, is used to repair TMJ-mandibular combined lesions (Fig. 2.5); see Chap. 8.
- The sixth category, mandibular reconstruction plates, is used to repair proximal TMJ-mandibular lesions and is intended to preserve the condyle and its surrounding attachments (Fig. 2.6); see Chap. 9.
- The seventh category, prostheses for preventing condylar dislocation, includes condylar dislocation blocking plates and eminence lengthening prostheses (Fig. 2.7), as described in Chap. 10.

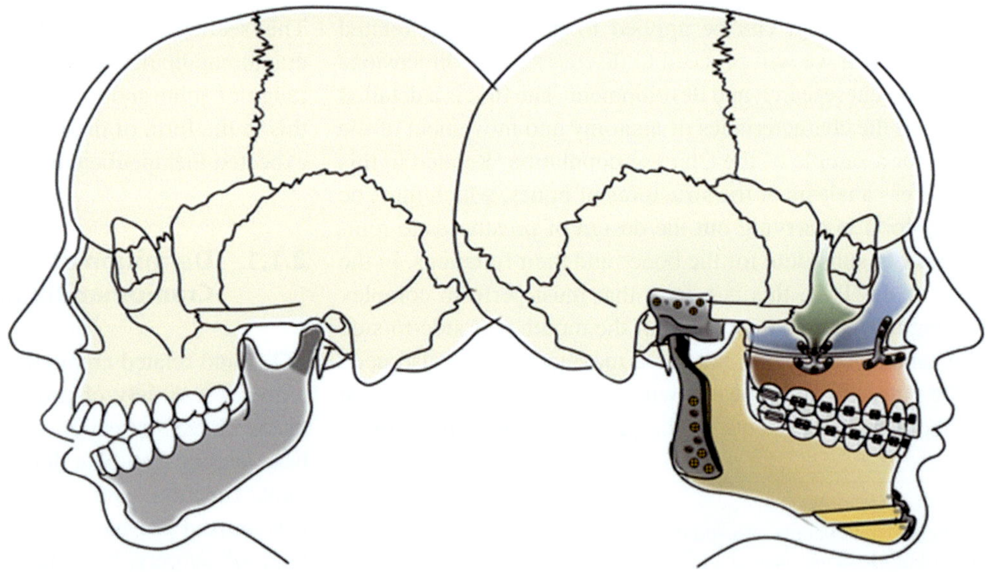

Fig. 2.1 Orthognathic surgery with simultaneous implantation of a total joint prosthesis (see Chaps. 3 and 4). The left image shows the diseased state, arthrosis (dark gray) accompanied by mandibular retrognathic deformity of the jaw (gray). The right image represents orthognathic reconstruction: a total joint prosthesis (dark gray) to replace the TMJ, Le Fort I procedure (orange) with fixation using H and Y plates, and genioplasty (yellow anterior) to advance the chin. The total joint prosthesis also extends the lower jaw forward

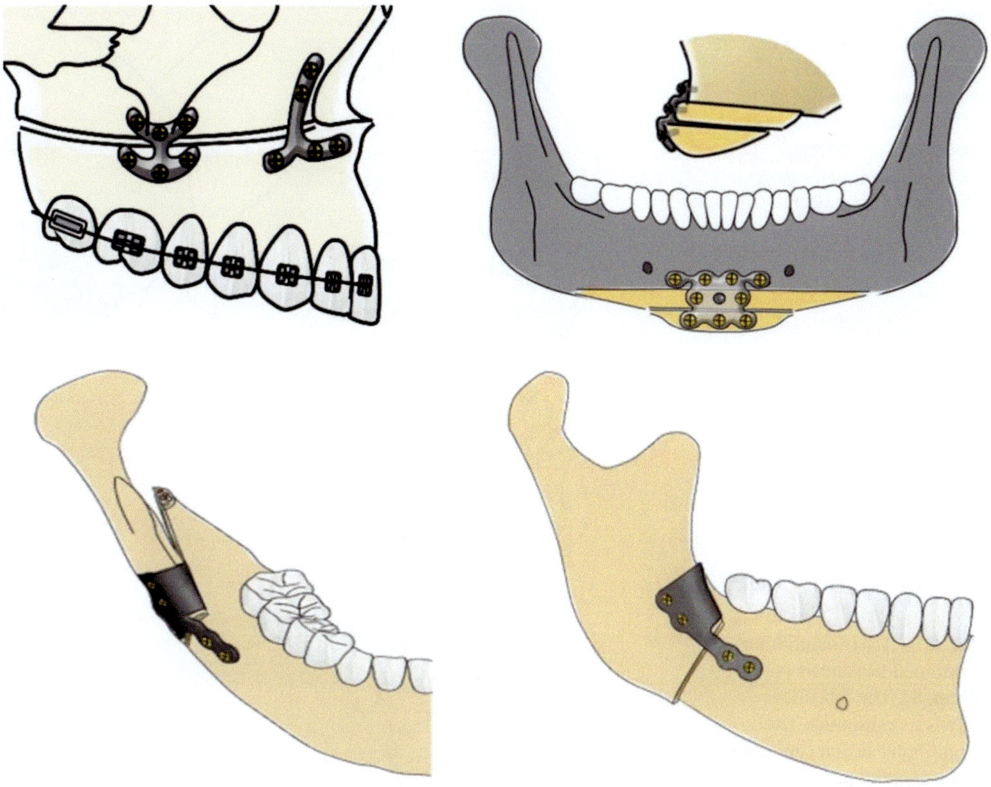

Fig. 2.2 Orthognathic surgical fixation plates (see Chap. 5). (**a**) An H and Y shape plate (gray) designed for fixation after maxillary Le Fort I osteotomy. (**b**) Genioplasty fixation plate (gray) designed for fixation of chin bone. (**c** and **d**) Condylar-stabilized mandibular sagittal split plate (gray) designed for condylar stabilization after mandibular sagittal split

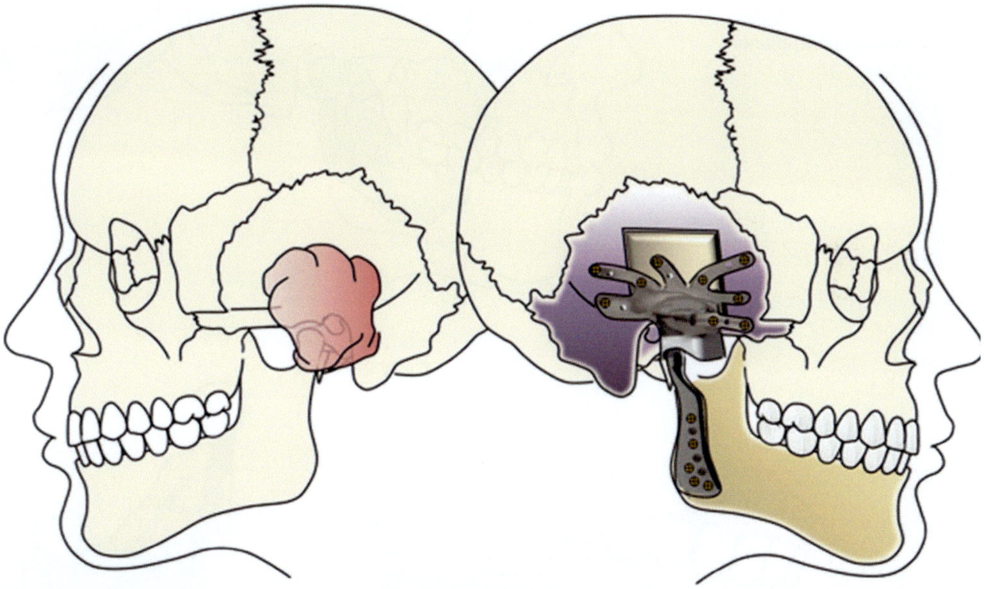

Fig. 2.3 TMJ-skull base combined prosthesis (see Chap. 6). The left image shows a continuous TMJ-skull base lesion (pink); the right image represents reconstruction with a TMJ-skull base combined prosthesis (dark gray)

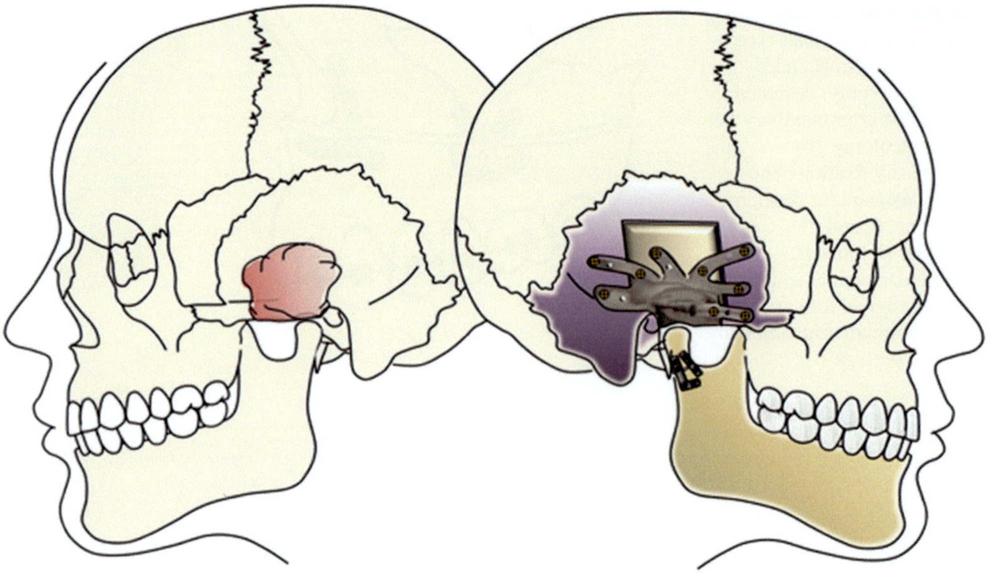

Fig. 2.4 Skull base-fossa prosthesis (Chap. 7). The left image shows a skull base-fossa lesion (pink); the right image represents a skull base-fossa prosthesis reconstruction (dark gray). The condyle has been preserved

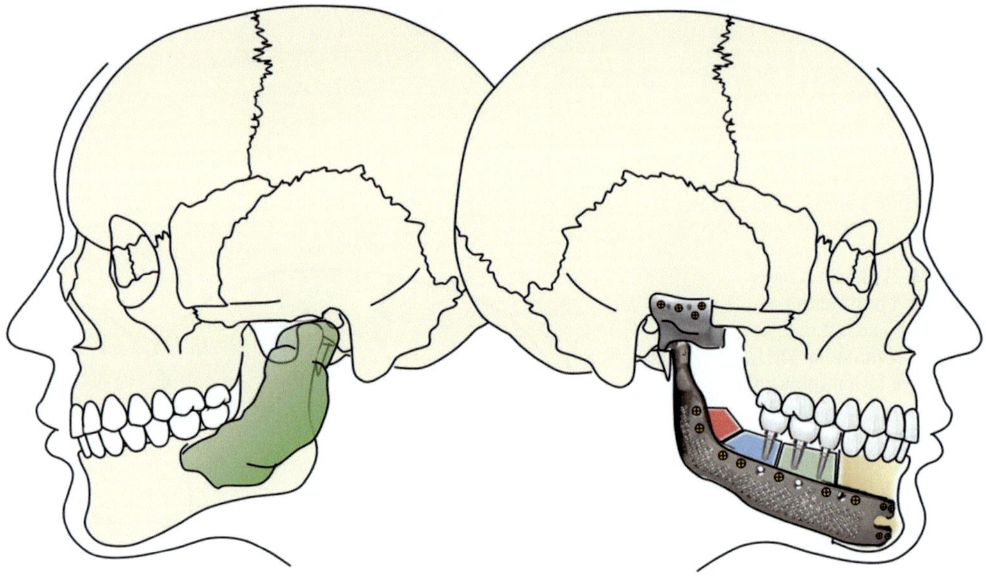

Fig. 2.5 TMJ-mandibular combined prosthesis (see Chap. 8). The left image shows a continuous TMJ-mandibular lesion (green); the right image represents a prosthetic reconstruction of the TMJ-mandibular combined prosthesis (dark gray), an autogenous bone graft (pink, blue, and light green), and dental implants (light gray)

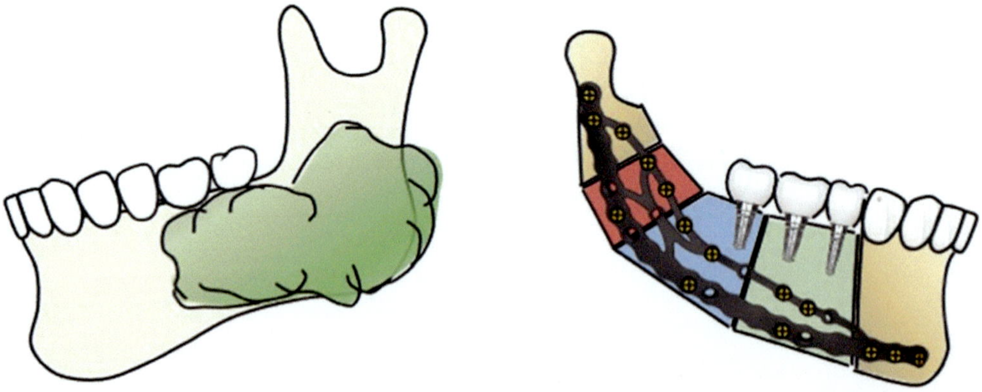

Fig. 2.6 Mandibular reconstruction plate (see Chap. 9). Illustration of a mandible reconstruction with dental implant restoration utilizing a customized mandibular reconstruction plate (dark gray), autogenous bone grafts (pink, blue, and green), and dental implants (light gray) that work together to restore the mandibular bone structure and contour, while preserving the normal fossa and the condyle

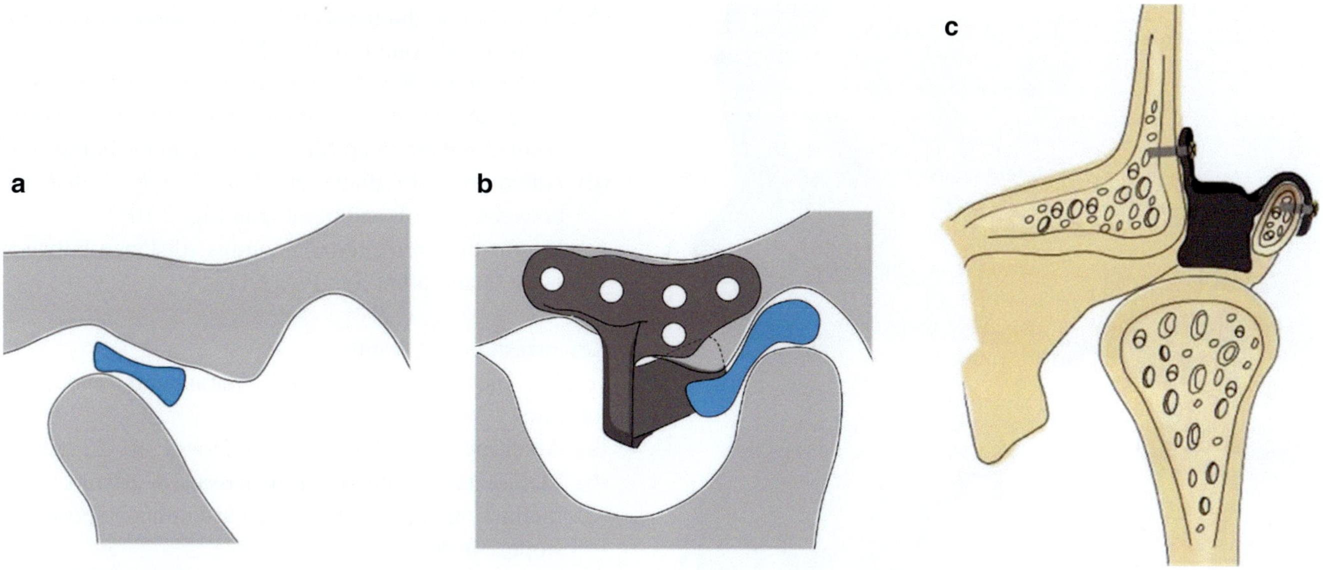

Fig. 2.7 Customized prostheses for preventing condylar dislocation (see Chap. 10). (**a**) The left TMJ is shown. The condyle and disc (blue) moved past the eminence, and the condyle has been dislocated. (**b**) An implanted condylar dislocation blocking plate (dark gray) stops the condyle and disc from excessive anterior movement. (**c**) The right TMJ is shown. Eminence lengthening prosthesis (black, sagittal view). The prosthesis is located in the gap between the zygomatic arch and the temporal bone, extending downward slightly more than the eminence, impeding dislocation. Both types of prostheses avoid surgical disturbance of the disc and capsule

2.2 The Research and Development Process for Customized Prostheses: Surveys of TMJ Anatomy of the Chinese Population

Beginning in 2009, the author of this book has brought together a team for research and development on customized TMJ and craniomandibular prostheses. This team has carried out comprehensive basic research, including prosthesis design, manufacturing, testing, and other preclinical research and development and finally optimized the prosthesis models and surgical techniques through repeated clinical application and feedback following evaluation of the results. The following sections of Chap. 2 describe the results of this research and development on many fronts, from precise study of anatomy for a sample of the Chinese population to scientific design of the core components of the prostheses, to materials innovation and durability testing.

2.2.1 Determining the General Anatomical Specifications for Customized TMJ Prostheses

The research and development of TMJ and craniomandibular prostheses must be based on a foundation of preliminary basic research. The theoretical basis for prosthesis design requires an in-depth analysis of joint anatomy, joint movement, and stress distribution.

Two surveys were carried out, the first covering the basic dimensions of the TMJ structures and the second survey on the movement of the TMJ.

2.2.1.1 Measurement and Analysis of TMJ-Craniomandibular Anatomical Data

The source of the empirical data for the TMJ structures is summarized as follows:

1. A total of 400 patients (aged ≥18 years) with partial edentulism who sought implant restoration at the Department of Oral Surgery, Ninth People's Hospital affiliated to Shanghai Jiao Tong University School of Medicine between 2012 and 2015, were selected. Their craniomaxillofacial computed tomography (CT) data were exported in DICOM format and imported into specialized software to reconstruct 3D models of the craniomaxillofacial structures.
2. Key measurement parameter descriptions:

   For the points of reference, see the following four figures (Figs. 2.8, 2.9, 2.10, and 2.11). The following anatomical parameters were measured:

   (a) Anteroposterior diameter of the fossa (distance between point A and point D in Fig. 2.8)

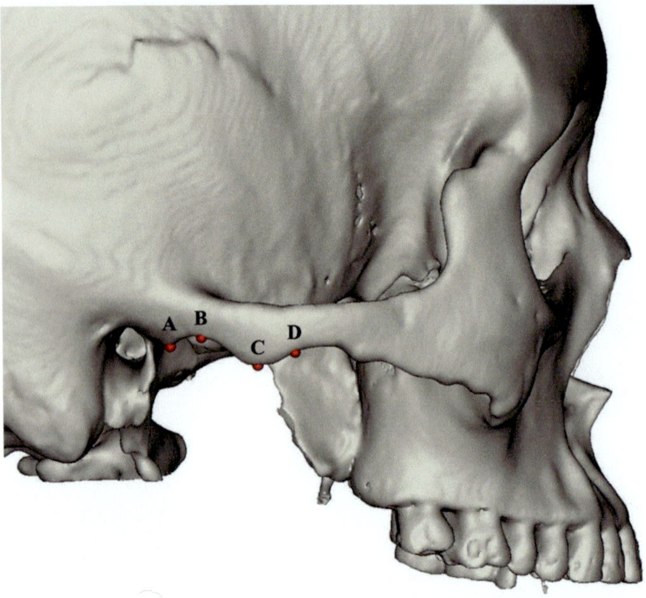

Fig. 2.8 Anatomical landmarks of eminence and fossa. Point A: the posterosuperior apex of the fossa (tangential point where the posterior wall of the glenoid fossa intersects a plane parallel to the Frankfort horizontal plane). Point B: the laterosuperior apex of the fossa (tangential point where the lateral wall of the fossa intersects a plane parallel to the Frankfort horizontal plane). Point C: the lowest point of the eminence (inferiormost point where the eminence intersects a plane parallel to the Frankfort horizontal plane). Point D: the anterior point of the articular eminence (anterior most point where the anterior slope of the articular eminence intersects a plane parallel to the Frankfort horizontal plane)

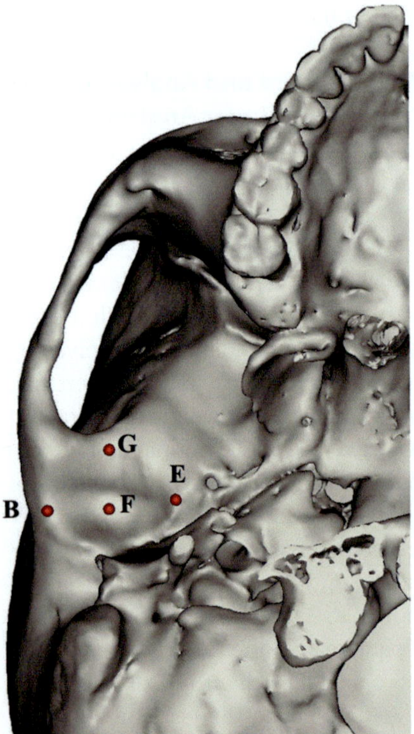

Fig. 2.9 Anatomical landmarks of eminence and fossa. Point B: the laterosuperior point of the fossa. Point E: the medial point of the fossa. Point F: the superior apex of the fossa. Point G: the anterior point of the fossa

(b) Mediolateral diameter of the fossa (distance between point B and point E in Fig. 2.9)
(c) Inclination angle of the articular eminence posterior slope (angle between the line connecting point B and point C and the Frankfort horizontal plane in Fig. 2.9)
(d) Anteroposterior diameter of the condyle (distance between point P and point Q in Fig. 2.10)
(e) Height of the mandibular ramus (distance between point O and point S in Fig. 2.11)

3. Key measurement results:

   The measured anatomical parameters were as follows:

   (a) Anteroposterior diameter of the fossa: 20–22 mm
   (b) Mediolateral diameter of the fossa: 18–20 mm
   (c) Inclination angle of the articular eminence posterior slope: 30–40°
   (d) Anteroposterior diameter of the condyle: 8–12 mm
   (e) Height of the mandibular ramus: 45–65 mm

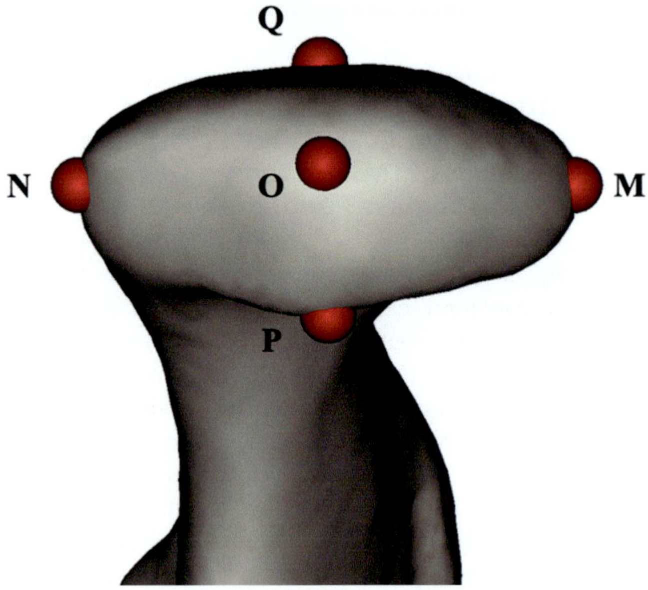

Fig. 2.10 Anatomical landmarks of condyle. Point O: the superior apex of the condyle (tangential point where the condylar head intersects a plane parallel to the Frankfort horizontal plane). Point N: the most lateral point of the condyle. Point M: the most medial point of the condyle. Point P: the anterior point of the condyle (tangential point where the anterior condylar border intersects a vertical plane parallel to line MN and perpendicular to the Frankfort horizontal plane). Point Q: the posterior point of the condyle (tangential point where the posterior condylar border intersects a vertical plane parallel to line MN and perpendicular to the Frankfort horizontal plane)

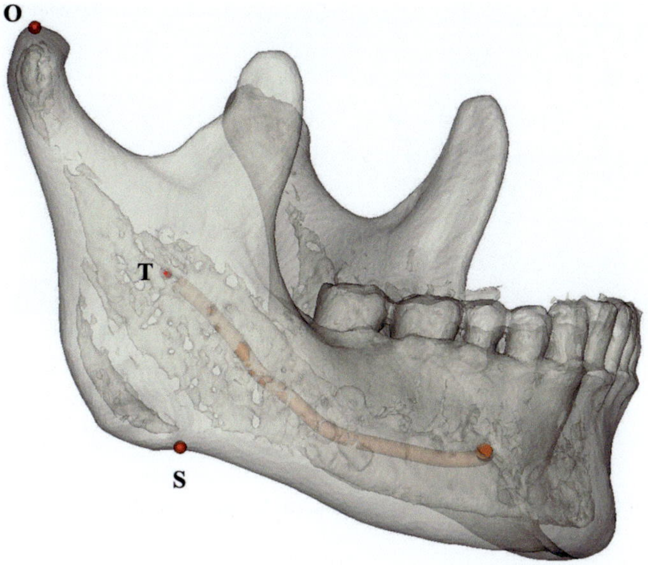

Fig. 2.11 Anatomical landmarks of the mandible. Point O: the superior apex of the condyle. Point T: the mandibular foramen point. Point S: the antegonial notch. Measurement points marked on the mandibular ramus

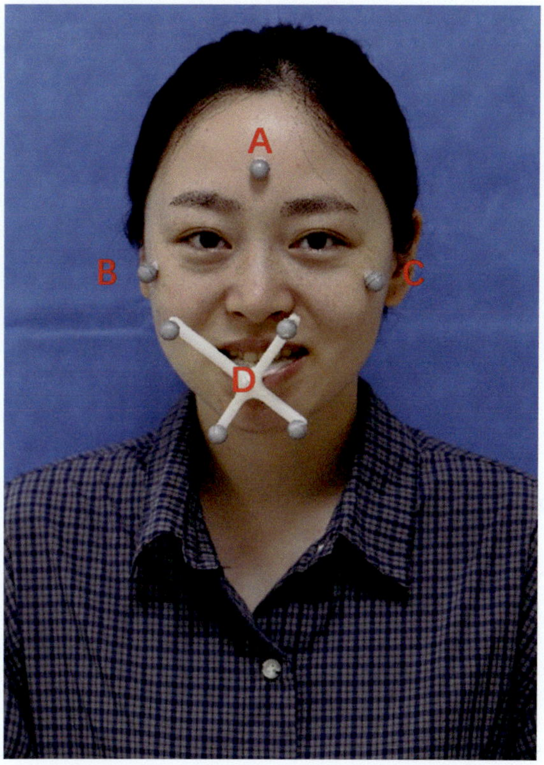

Fig. 2.12 Infrared motion capture technology setup. (**a**) Frontal marking points. (**b**, **c**) Zygomatic marking points. (**d**) Mandibular marking points and brackets

2.2.1.2 Measurement and Analysis of Joint Motion Parameters

1. Sample source: this study enrolled 90 patients (aged ≥18 years) with partial edentulism who sought implant prosthetic treatment at the Department of Oral Surgery, Ninth People's Hospital affiliated to Shanghai Jiao Tong University School of Medicine between 2014 and 2015.
2. Motion parameter acquisition and analysis

   Infrared motion capture technology was employed to record mandibular movements during maximum mouth opening/closing, protrusion, lateral excursions, and unilateral mastication (Figs. 2.12 and 2.13). The kinematic data were subsequently integrated into 3D reconstructed models to calculate condylar movement trajectories.
3. Key measurement results

   Kinematic parameters: anteroposterior movement range, 20–24 mm; mediolateral movement range, 18–22 mm; condylar movement arc (inferoanterior trajectory), 1/6π to 2/9π (equivalent to 30–40°) (Fig. 2.14).

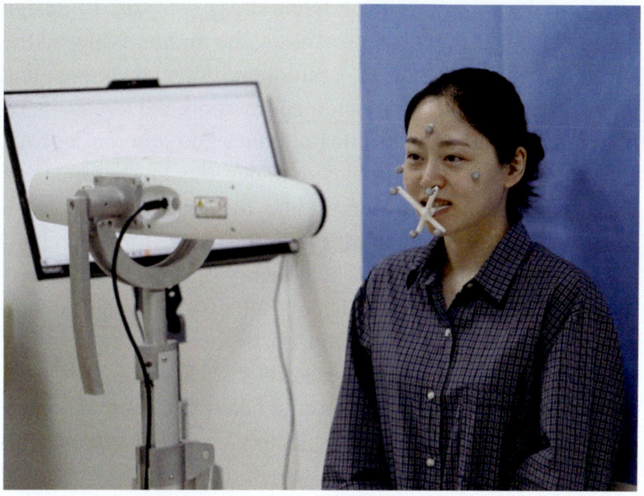

Fig. 2.13 Data capture of various types of mandibular movements. These include maximal mouth opening and closing, anterior extension, lateral movement, and unilateral mastication

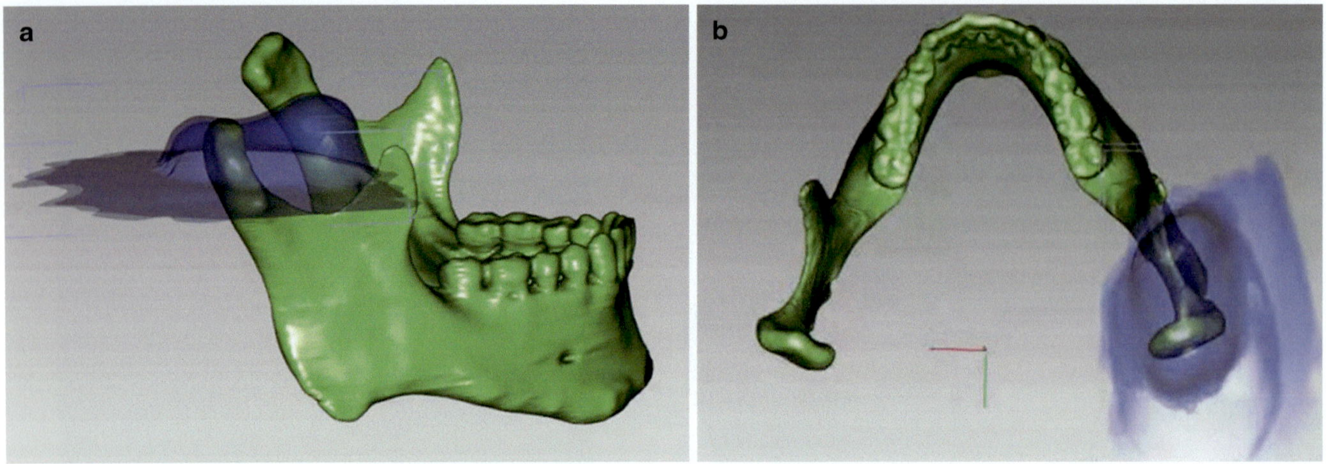

Fig. 2.14 Maximum changes in the 3D position of the condyle during various types of mandibular movement. (**a**) Lateral view. (**b**) Top view

2.3 The R&D Process for Customized Prostheses: Stress Analysis and Sizing of Extension Parts

The size and shape of the extension component relies heavily on the understanding of the joint-craniomaxillary stress distribution, and its fixation plate or wing should be designed on the line of stress distribution to facilitate craniomaxillofacial and articular stress conduction.

Normal joint-craniomandibular stress analysis: to design the extension parts of the prosthesis, the author explored the stress distribution of the craniomaxillofacial bones and joints. Using the 3D finite element method, the stress distribution of the craniomaxillofacial bones and joints of normal Chinese people was simulated under the environment of maximum masticatory force. The mechanical conduction routes are similar to the traditional maxillary "three mechanical buttresses" and the classical theory of mandibular external oblique conduction. The results of this simulation analysis provide a mechanical basis for the design of the extension parts of the prosthesis.

Sample source: CT data from a healthy adult male's craniomaxillofacial region were selected, imported into specialized software, and reconstructed into a 3D model of the required craniomaxillofacial structures.

Finite element analysis: using 3D finite element methodology, stress distribution across normal adult craniomaxillofacial bones and joints was simulated under maximum masticatory load conditions.

Key analysis results: the stress transmission pathways aligned with classical biomechanical theories.

Anterior maxillary route: from upper anterior teeth → piriform aperture → nasal root → frontal bone (analogous to the canine buttress)

Anterior zygomatic route: from upper posterior teeth → zygomaticoalveolar crest → lateral orbit → frontal bone (analogous to the anterior zygomatic buttress)

Posterior zygomatic route: from upper posterior teeth → zygomaticoalveolar crest → zygomatic arch → articular eminence → cranial base (analogous to the posterior zygomatic buttress)

External oblique ridge route: from lower posterior teeth → external oblique ridge → mandibular notch → condyle → cranial base

Mandibular ramus route: from mandibular angle → mandibular ramus → condyle → cranial base (Figs. 2.15 and 2.16)

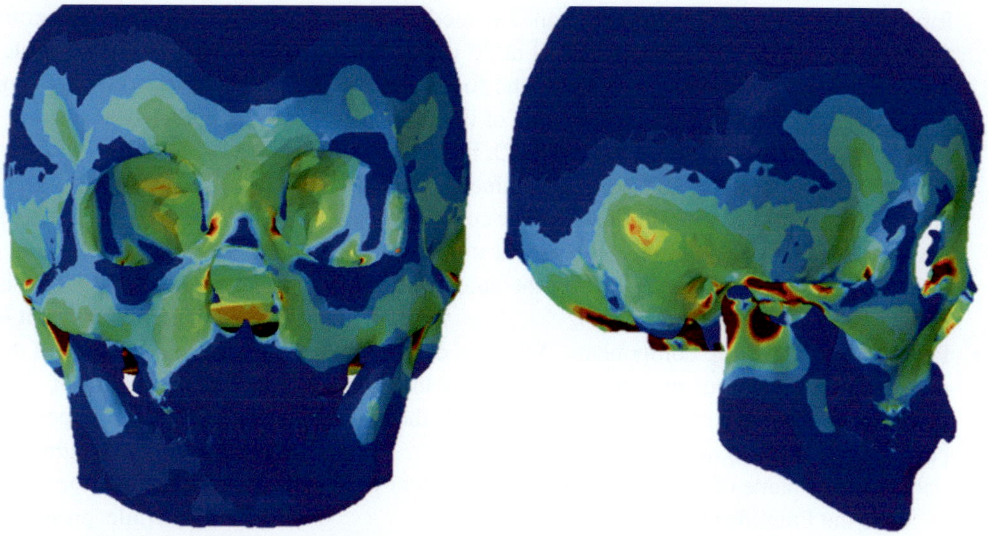

Fig. 2.15 Stress distribution in the craniomaxillofacial bones and TMJ. Red, orange, and yellow are high. Green is medium. Blue is low. (**a**) Frontal view. (**b**) Lateral view

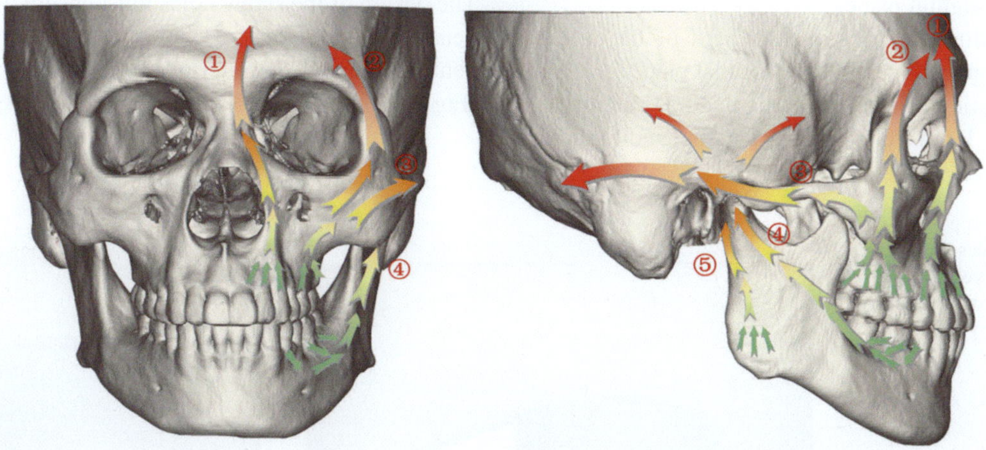

Fig. 2.16 The pathways of mechanical stress in the craniomaxillofacial bones and TMJ. ① Upper anterior teeth → piriform aperture → nasion → frontal bone; ② upper posterior teeth → zygomatic buttress → lateral orbital rim → frontal bone; ③ upper posterior teeth → zygomatic buttress → zygomatic arch → articular tubercle → articular fossa → mastoid process → occipital bone; ④ lower posterior teeth → external oblique ridge of mandible → sigmoid notch → condylar process → skull base; ⑤ mandibular angle → posterior border of mandible → condylar process → skull base. (**a**) Frontal view. (**b**) Lateral view

2.4 The R&D Process: The Design of Core Components for Customized TMJ and Craniofacial Prostheses

The design of personalized TMJ and craniofacial prostheses primarily involves the design of core components and extension components.

The core components refer to the functional surfaces or regions responsible for relative motion between the fossa and the condylar head. These components bear the prosthesis's rotation, sliding, force transmission, and wear, making them the most critical parts of the personalized TMJ and craniofacial prostheses.

The extension components refer to the parts that extend from the core components to surrounding bone structures, including the zygomatic arch, cranial base, temporal bone, mandibular ramus, and mandibular body. These components play a role in repairing defects and securing the prosthesis in place.

The design principles and steps for the prostheses discussed in this book are introduced in detail below.

2.4.1 Design of Core Components

- Shaping of the core components: the dimensions and shape of the core components are determined based on key anatomical and movement parameters of the joint. The anteroposterior diameter of the fossa component is set at 22 mm, based on the anteroposterior distance of the fossa and the condyle's range of motion. The mediolateral diameter of the fossa component is set at 20 mm, determined by the mediolateral distance of the fossa and the condyle's range of motion. The curvature of the joint surface is defined as 1/6π (equivalent to 30°), based on the posterior slope angle of the articular eminence and the condyle's anterior-inferior motion arc. The condylar head component is shaped as a quasi-cylindrical structure with a diameter of 10 mm, determined by the anteroposterior diameter of the condyle (Fig. 2.17).

- Positioning of the core components: After the core component has been sized, its correct position in the joint defect needs to be determined. Positioning of the core component (red) is based on the following:
  - The upper plane of the articular fossa component parallels the Frankfort horizontal plane.
  - The lateral plane of the articular fossa component parallels the sagittal plane.
  - The anterior and posterior surfaces of the articular fossa component parallel the coronal plane.
  - The posterior edge of the articular fossa component should be 3 mm from the bony external auditory canal.
  - The glenoid fossa component should be positioned as superiorly as possible while ensuring the placement of two rows of zygomatic arch fixation screws (Fig. 2.18)

2.4.2 Design of Extension Components

Taking a total joint prosthesis as an example, the shape of the zygomatic arch component is determined by the length from the posterior projection of the fossa to the zygomaticotemporal suture, the width of the zygomatic arch, and the stress distribution. The shape of the mandibular component is determined by the height of the mandibular ramus, the width of the posterior edge of the mandible, and the stress distribution, while preserving the masseteric tuberosity to facilitate the reattachment of the masseter muscle (Fig. 2.19). The design of the screw holes must ensure that each component has at least five screw holes, and the mandibular component must avoid the inferior alveolar neurovascular bundle (Fig. 2.20).

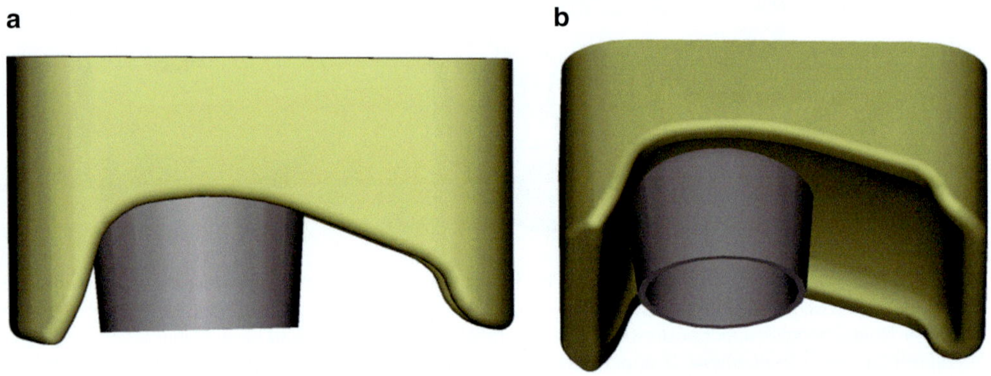

Fig. 2.17 Core component design. This includes the fossa component (yellow) and the condylar head component (gray). (**a**) Frontal view. (**b**) View from below

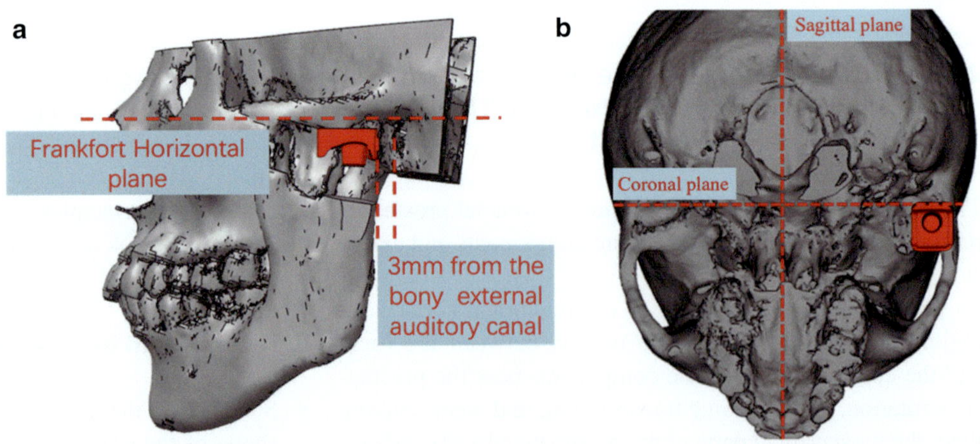

Fig. 2.18 Positioning of core components (red). (**a**) Lateral view. (**b**) Cranial base view

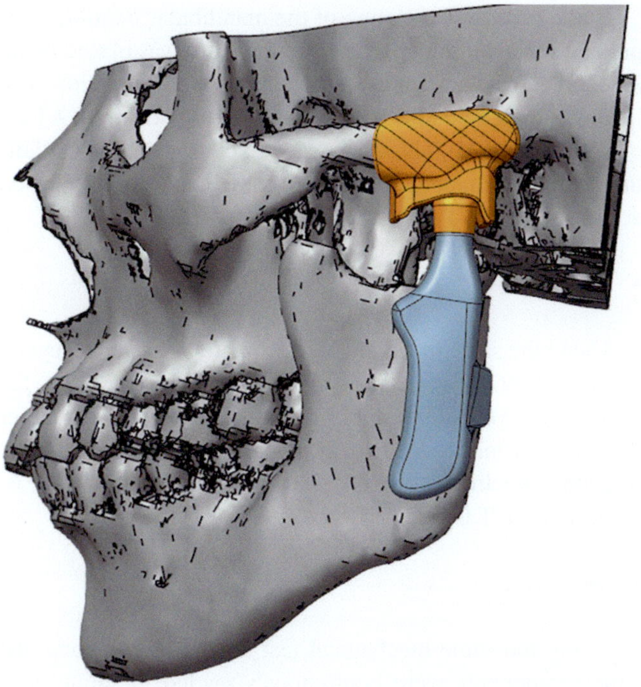

Fig. 2.19 Design of extension components. This includes the zygomatic arch component of the fossa prosthesis (upper part in yellow) and the mandibular component of the mandibular prosthesis (blue), which is designed with reference to the craniomaxillofacial bone and joint stress distribution

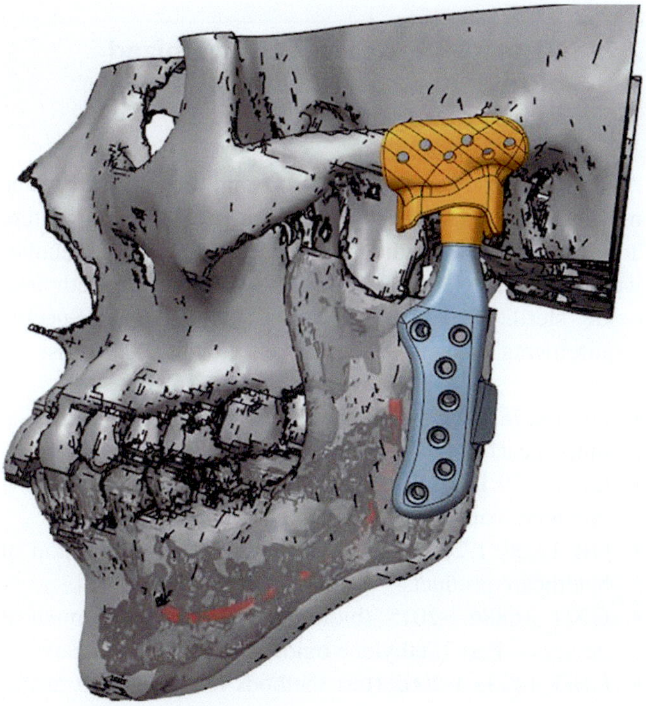

Fig. 2.20 Screw hole design. The location of the screw holes should be determined to facilitate fixation and refer to the craniomaxillofacial bone and joint stress distribution design

2.5 The R&D Process for Customized Prostheses: Manufacturing and Materials

2.5.1 Customized TMJ and Craniomandibular Prosthesis Processing

The fabrication of the prostheses discussed in this book adheres to the relevant international, national, and industry standards for surgical implants. The materials selected include titanium alloy powder, cobalt-chromium-molybdenum alloy, and ultrahigh-molecular-weight polyethylene (Fig. 2.21). The manufacturing process involves a combination of five-axis precision machining and metal 3D printing (Fig. 2.22). The condylar head component and the mandibular component are connected using Morse taper joints and assembled into the mandibular prosthesis. Specific guidelines are followed according to standards such as YY/T 0640-2016 and GB/T 16886.1-2011.

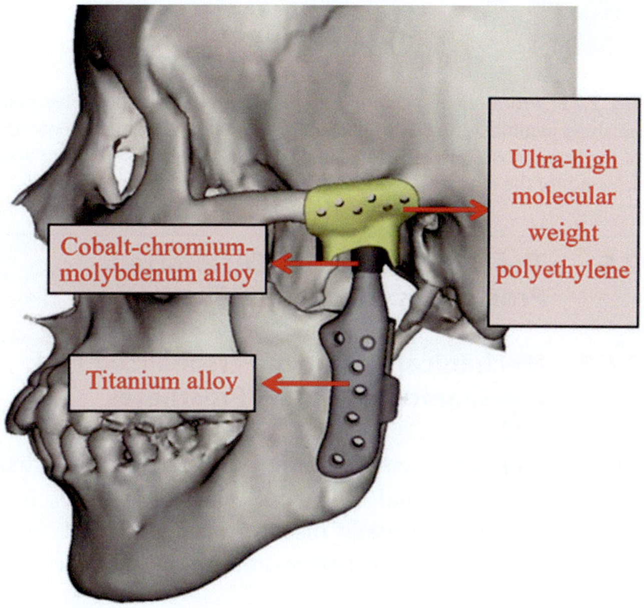

Fig. 2.21 Material selection for each component of the prosthesis. Highly cross-linked ultrahigh-molecular-weight polyethylene was selected for the fossa prosthesis, cobalt-chromium-molybdenum alloy for the condylar head component, and titanium alloy for the mandibular component

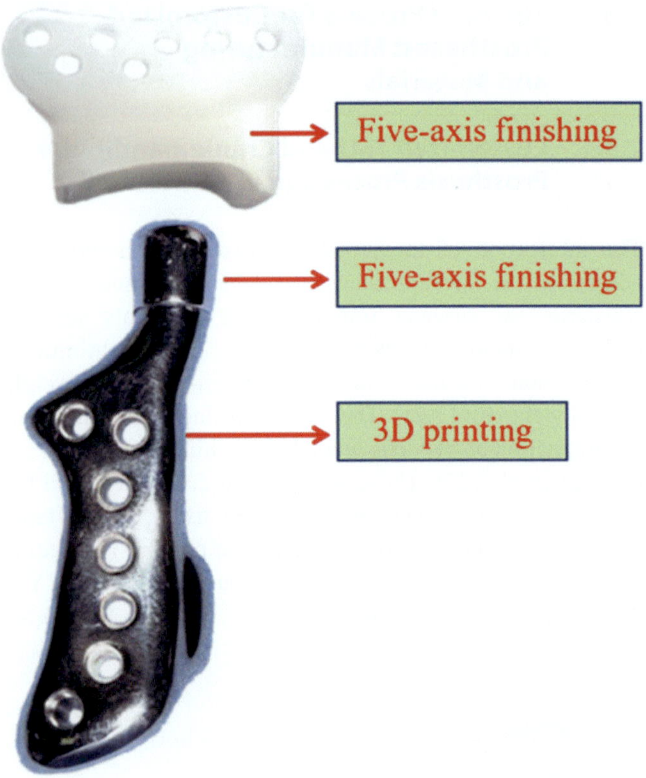

Fig. 2.22 Prosthetic processing and manufacturing methods. Five-axis finishing manufacturing was selected for the condylar head components of the fossa prosthesis and mandibular prosthesis, and 3D printing was selected for the mandibular components of the mandibular prosthesis

2.6 The R&D Process for Customized Prostheses: Mechanical Testing

2.6.1 Mechanical Testing of Personalized TMJ and Craniomandibular Prostheses

The mechanical performance of the prostheses has been first analyzed and optimized using finite element analysis, followed by testing for static mechanics, fatigue, and wear according to relevant standards to ensure clinical application requirements are met.

- Finite Element Analysis

Finite element analysis: the distribution of stresses in each component of the prosthesis was modeled in a simulated environment of maximum masticatory force. It was determined that the maximum stress is far less than the yield strength of each component.

- Mandibular Prosthesis Static Mechanical Testing

Static mechanical testing of the mandibular fixation component: the mandibular fixation component was placed in the mechanical test apparatus in the anatomical orientation. The load was increased until bending or fracture occurred. A load of no less than 2500 N was needed to cause mechanical failure of the component. Specific guidelines were followed according to YY/T 0809.10-2022.

- Fatigue Test

Using the same mechanical test apparatus as above, cyclic loading of 497 N was carried out at a frequency of 12 Hz, for 10 million cycles. No cracks could be detected with either the electron microscope or the metallographic microscope. Specific guidelines were followed according to YY/T 0809.6-2010 and YY/T 0809.8-2010.

- Wear Test

Using the same mechanical test apparatus as above, the core components were continuously cycled in saline, at a load of 9 kg, for 5 million cycles. It was determined that the surface wear rate does not exceed 0.01 mm/million cycles, and the volume wear rate does not exceed 0.39 mm^3/million cycles. Specific guidelines were followed according to YY/T 0651.2-2008 and YY/T 1426.2-2016.

2.7 The R&D Process for Customized Prostheses: Sterilization and Packaging

After the prosthesis is processed and manufactured, the metal components shall be sterilized by high-temperature and high-pressure methods, while the ultrahigh-molecular-weight polyethylene components shall undergo ethylene oxide sterilization and pass biological testing. Specific requirements shall comply with the following standards:

- GB 18278.1-2015 (sterilization of healthcare products—moist heat)
- GB 18279.1-2015 (sterilization of healthcare products—ethylene oxide)
- GB 18280.1-2015 & GB 18280.2-2015 (sterilization of healthcare products—radiation)
- GB/T 16886.7-2015 (biological evaluation of medical devices—Part 7: ethylene oxide sterilization residuals)
- GB/T 14233.1-2005 (test methods for infusion, transfusion, and injection equipment for medical use—Part 1: chemical analysis methods)

The sterilized products shall be labeled with the word "STERILE" and properly packaged to maintain sterility under specified storage, transportation, and handling conditions. Relevant requirements shall comply with standards such as YY/T 0640-2016 (aseptic processing of medical devices).

2.8 The Flow Chart of General Process of Digital Design and Application of Customized Prostheses

Jisi Zheng, Wenbo Jiang, and Yaxing Bao

The design and manufacturing of joint and craniomaxillofacial prostheses shall adhere to the shared principles of medical-engineering integration, interaction, and collaboration. The applying institution must submit complete patient data. Currently, the prosthesis and related product designs are developed by our institution (the author's unit), and upon approval by the applying institution, the processes of manufacturing, quality control, and post-processing are implemented. The final products, along with the surgical design drawings, are delivered to the applying institution (Fig. 2.23).

- Information Collection and Assessment

The physicians at the requesting hospital shall collect comprehensive patient data, including clinical symptoms, clinical examinations, and imaging examinations such as maxillofacial and occlusal photographs, maxillofacial CT scans, TMJ MRI (magnetic resonance imaging), panoramic radiographs, lateral and frontal cephalograms, and dental models.

Additional examinations such as temporal cone beam CT (CBCT) or iliac/fibular CT scans may be required when necessary. Subsequently, physicians from both the requesting institution and our clinical team will jointly evaluate the surgical indications, feasibility, and necessity of prosthesis application (Fig. 2.23a).

- Prosthesis Design and Development

The author's team utilizes computer-aided design (CAD) and computer-aided manufacturing (CAM) technologies to develop a surgical resection plan, personalized prosthesis, and surgical guides based on the patient's clinical data.

Physicians from the requesting hospital, our clinical team, and engineers conduct regular design reviews and discussions to ensure the prosthesis design aligns with both surgi-

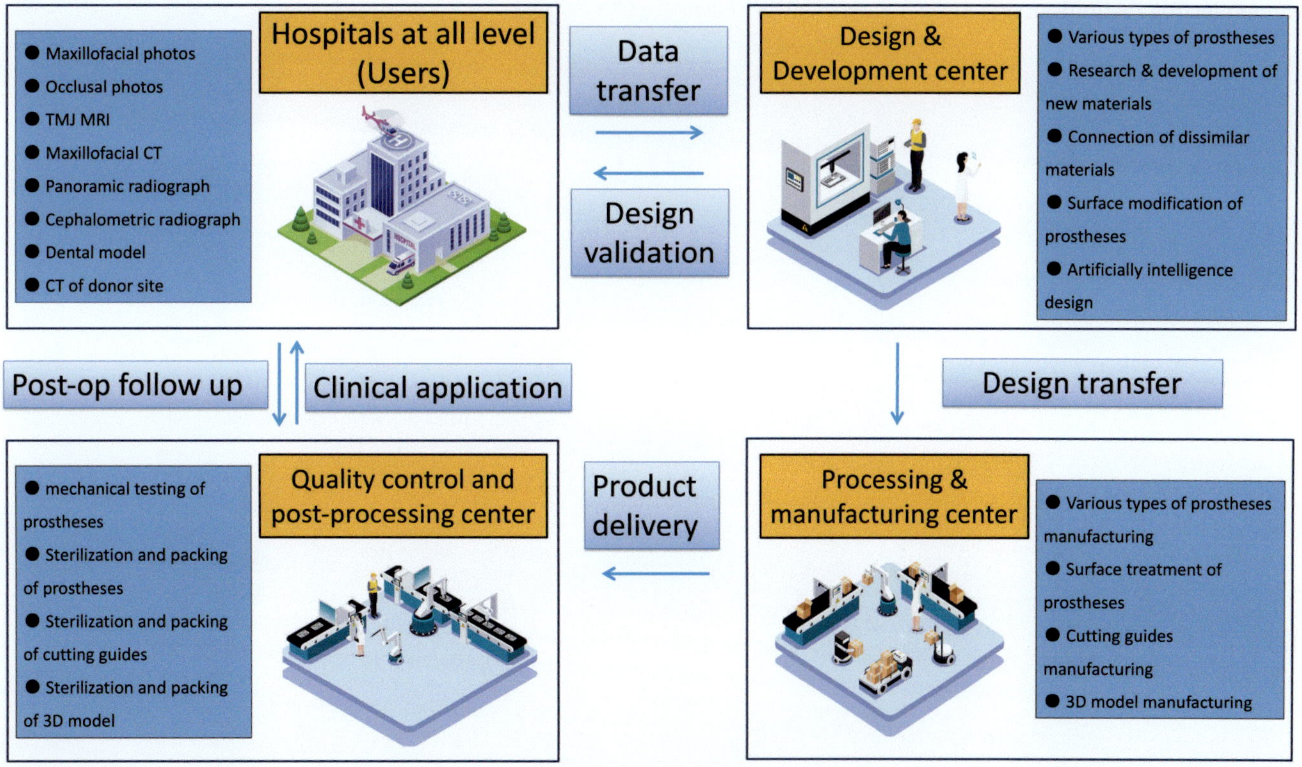

Fig. 2.23 Flow chart process for medical application, manufacturing, and surgical implantation of customized joint and craniomandibular prostheses

cal requirements and patient expectations. Based on these collaborative evaluations, the surgical plan, prosthesis, and cutting guides are further refined or modified to accommodate the patient's individual anatomical characteristics and clinical needs (Fig. 2.23b).

- Prosthetics Fabrication and Manufacturing

Upon approval of the surgical plan, prosthesis, and guides by both physicians and engineers, the manufacturing center initiates production of the customized prosthesis and surgical guides using either 3D printing technology or computerized numerical control (CNC) machining, completing the fabrication process (Fig. 2.23c).

- Quality Control and Post-processing

The manufactured prostheses undergo post-processing procedures including cleaning, polishing, and sandblasting, followed by stringent quality control inspections. These inspections cover appearance, surface defects, surface roughness, internal quality, dimensional accuracy, and mechanical testing of samples. All quality control measures strictly comply with the T/CAMDI 027-2024 standard. Subsequently, the prostheses undergo trial fitting on skull models to verify their positioning and fit accuracy. Only after meeting all requirements are they sterilized, packaged, and delivered to the requesting institution.

Special note: during delivery, the requesting surgeon, our clinical team physicians, and engineers must emphasize detailed communication regarding specific implementation steps of the surgical plan, fundamental principles of surgical guide usage, and basic procedures for prosthesis installation.

- Surgical Performance and Instruction

During the surgical procedure, the surgeon performs the operation according to the predetermined surgical plan. First, the positioning guide is used to assist in the precise resection of pathological tissues, followed by priority fixation using the pre-drilled screw holes left by the positioning guide to ensure accurate prosthesis installation.

It is strongly recommended that our team's surgeons provide on-site guidance or assistance during the initial cases to ensure optimal implementation.

- Postoperative Follow-up and Evaluation

In the initial postoperative phase, under the guidance of our expert team, patients undergo systematic follow-up and clinical evaluation to monitor prosthesis performance and rehabilitation progress. All outcomes are promptly relayed to our surgical team and engineering specialists, enabling data-driven refinements for future optimization.

3 Prosthetic Reconstruction of TMJ Diseases

Chi Yang, Jisi Zheng, and Shanyong Zhang

This chapter addresses Yang's Modified Classification Category I, temporomandibular joint (TMJ) diseases. For severe TMJ diseases, prosthetic reconstruction or replacement is one of the most effective methods of restoring form and function to that joint. Since the 1950s, the TMJ prosthesis has gradually developed from a semi-articular prosthesis to a total TMJ prosthesis (referred to as total joint prosthesis) in the 1990s and has been more widely used in clinical practice. At present, there are two mature total joint prostheses abroad. The author's team independently developed a personalized total joint prosthesis.

In this chapter, based on the definition and classification of TMJ diseases that cannot be preserved, and the introduction of traditional repair and reconstruction methods, we focus on the innovative repair and reconstruction methods and digital design process of personalized total TMJ prostheses, and we verify their safety and effectiveness through clinical applications.

3.1 Overview of Reconstruction of TMJ Diseases

Chi Yang and Jisi Zheng

Joint replacement is indicated for the reconstruction of joint defects or loss due to a variety of joint diseases in which joints cannot be preserved. This section will describe the definition, classification, and traditional methods of prosthetic reconstruction for non-salvageable joint diseases of the temporomandibular joint (TMJ), with an emphasis on the types of designs, indications, contraindications, and digital design process for personalized total joint prostheses.

Chi Y. (✉) · Jisi Z. · Shanyong Z.
Shanghai Ninth People's Hospital, Shanghai Jiao Tong University School of Medicine, Shanghai, China

3.1.1 Definition of Non-salvageable TMJ

The non-salvageable TMJ diseases that cannot be preserved refer to joint conditions that are unresolvable through non-surgical methods or joint-preserving surgeries. Total joint replacement may be considered if these disorders are progressive, present significant clinical symptoms, lead to moderate-to-severe dentofacial deformities, and/or are accompanied by upper airway stenosis, severely impacting the patient's quality of life. Such conditions include mid-to-late-stage osteoarthritis, severe condylar resorption, ankylosis, comminuted fractures, joint tumors, and first and second branchial arch syndromes.

3.1.2 Classification of Non-salvageable TMJ

Joint defect or deficiency refers to the partial or complete loss of joint bone structure due to congenital factors, disease progression, surgical resection, or other causes. Based on the extent of the lesion, joint bone destruction and defect locations can be classified as follows:

3.1.2.1 Condylar Lesions

This includes lesions or defects within the range from the condylar head to above the mandibular foramen. The management of lesions in this range does not involve the inferior alveolar neurovascular bundle, and the design options and fixation methods for repair and reconstruction are essentially the same (Fig. 3.1). Options include autogenous bone grafting and total joint prosthesis replacement.

3.1.2.2 Articular Fossa Lesions

This includes defects of the internal and lateral margins of the articular fossa, the articular eminence, and the posterior portion of the zygomatic arch. When the area of defects in this range is less than 50% of the total size of the articular fossa (Fig. 3.2), the residual articular fossa or articular eminence can be preserved, and most of them do not require

© People's Medical Publishing House, PR of China 2025

Chi Y. (ed.), *Atlas of Customized TMJ-Cranio-Jaw Prosthesis*, https://doi.org/10.1007/978-981-95-0611-8_3

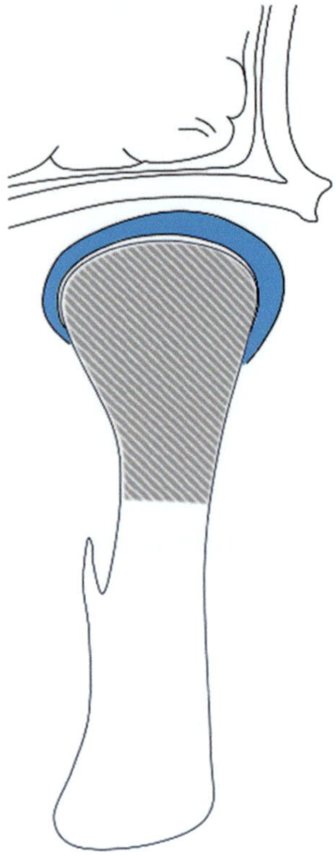

Fig. 3.1 Extent of condylar defect (from the top of the condyle to the mandibular foramen). The articular disc is shown in blue, and the dotted line shows the extent of the defect involved

bone repair and can be filled with soft-tissue flaps (e.g., temporal fascia fat flap, free fat).

3.1.2.3 Total Joint Lesions

The condylar head and disc are simultaneously affected, suitable for total joint prosthesis repair and reconstruction (Fig. 3.3).

3.1.3 Traditional Reconstruction Methods for Non-salvageable TMJ Diseases

Traditional repair and reconstruction methods can be categorized into autologous bone reconstruction or reconstruction with a prosthesis according to the materials utilized and partial or total joint replacement according to the extent of surgery.

Autogenous bone replacement types are:

1. Condyle replacement with costochondral graft (CCG), hemi-sternoclavicular joints, or coronoid process
2. TMJ fossa replacement with ilium or temporal bone

3.1.3.1 Autologous Bone Replacement

Replacement of condyle with autogenous coronoid process, CCG (Fig. 3.4a), and pedicled hemi-sternoclavicular joint (Fig. 3.4b) and replacement of articular fossa with autoge-

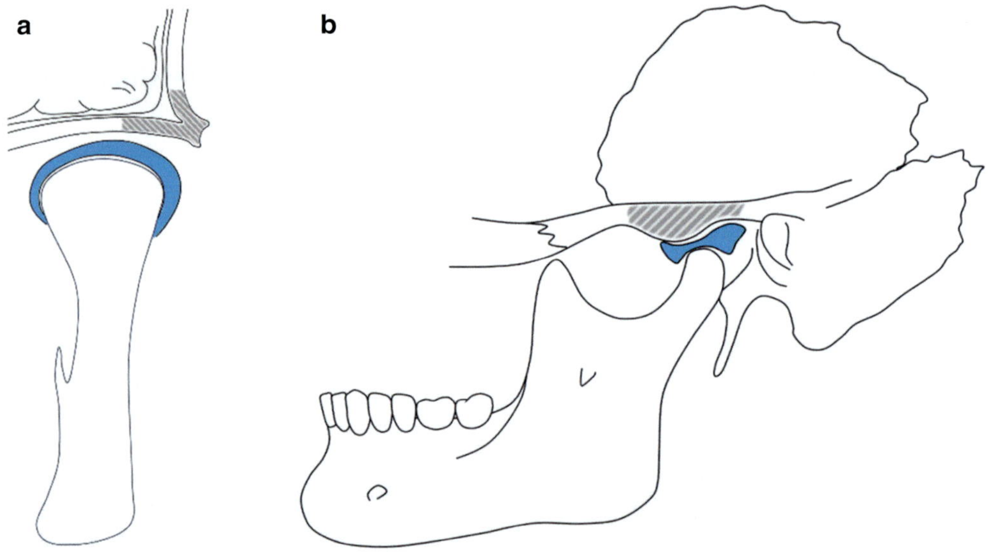

Fig. 3.2 Extent of joint fossa and joint eminence defects, with affected area less than 50% of the joint fossa. The articular disc is shown in blue, and the dashed line shows the extent of the defect involved. (**a**) Extent of the joint fossa defect. (**b**) Extent of the joint eminence defect

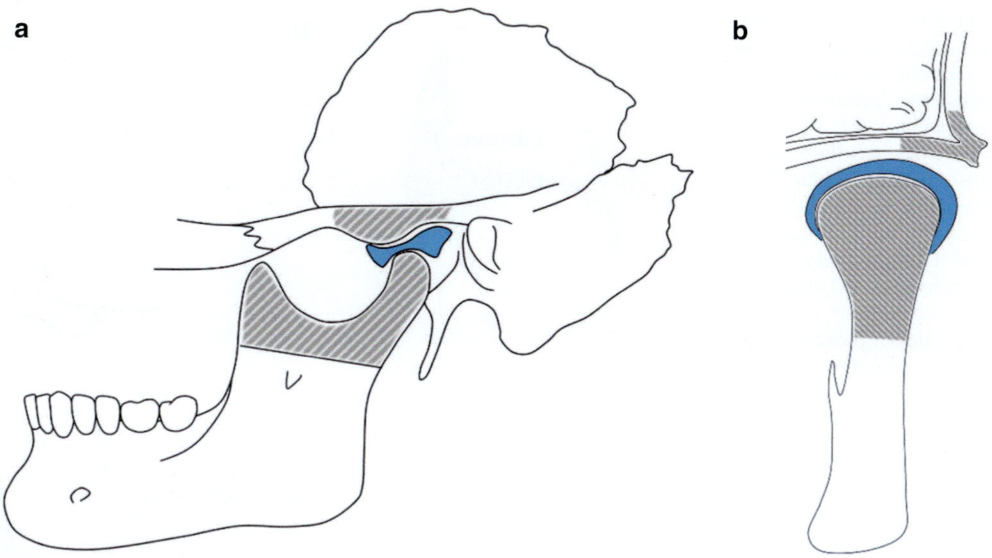

Fig. 3.3 Extent of joint defect. The gray line shading marks the extent of the defect. The articular disc is shown in blue. (**a**) Sagittal view. (**b**) Coronal view

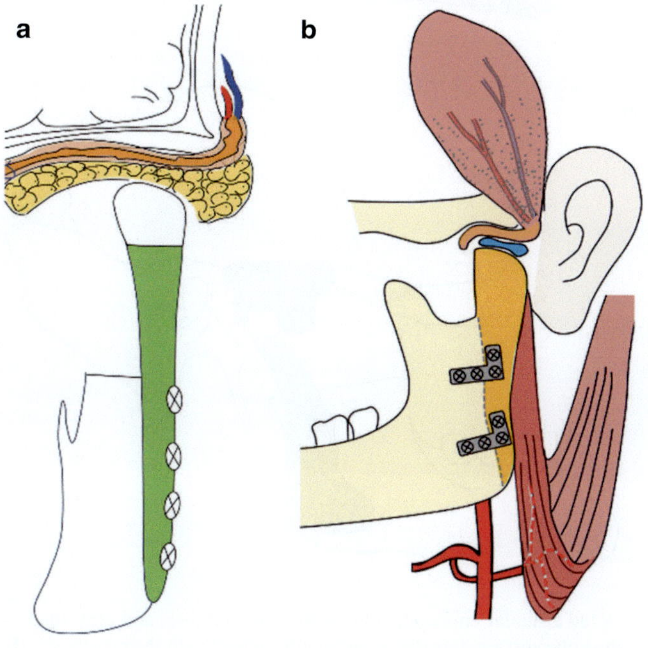

Fig. 3.4 Autologous bone replacement of condyles. (**a**) CCG replacement of condyle, where yellow is the temporalis fascia adipose flap, light green and its upper white color is the CCG, dark blue is the vein, and red is the artery. (**b**) Pedicled hemi-sternoclavicular joint replacement of condyle: yellow is the pedicled hemi-sternoclavicular joint, blue is the articular disk, and gray is the titanium plate

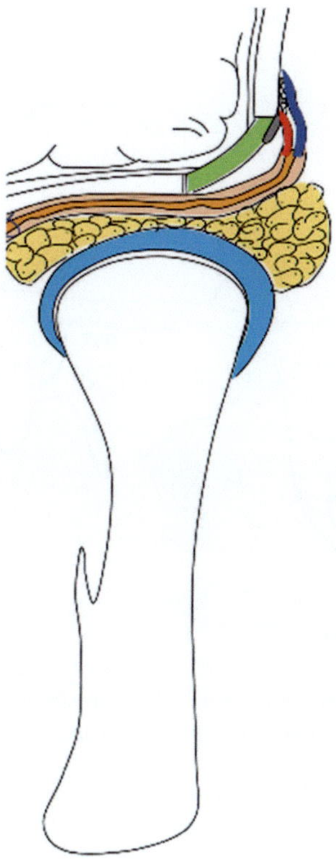

Fig. 3.5 Autologous bone replacement of the articular fossa. Green is the ilium or temporal bone, yellow is the temporal fascia fat flap, gray is the titanium plate, light blue below the fat is the disc, dark blue is the vein, and red is the artery

nous ilium or temporal bone (Fig. 3.5). It requires a bone donor area, more complex surgical operation, and risks of resorption and instability of autogenous bone.

3.1.3.2 Replacement of the Joint with Prosthesis

An articular fossa prosthesis can be used to replace the articular fossa (Fig. 3.6a) and a condylar prosthesis to replace the condyle (Fig. 3.6b). But condylar replacement alone carries the risk of bone resorption in the articular fossa and skull base, or even protrusion of the prosthesis into the skull.

Simultaneous replacement of the articular fossa and the condyle is a total joint prosthesis replacement (Fig. 3.7). There are two types of total joint prostheses available: standard or custom-made total joint prostheses. Standard total

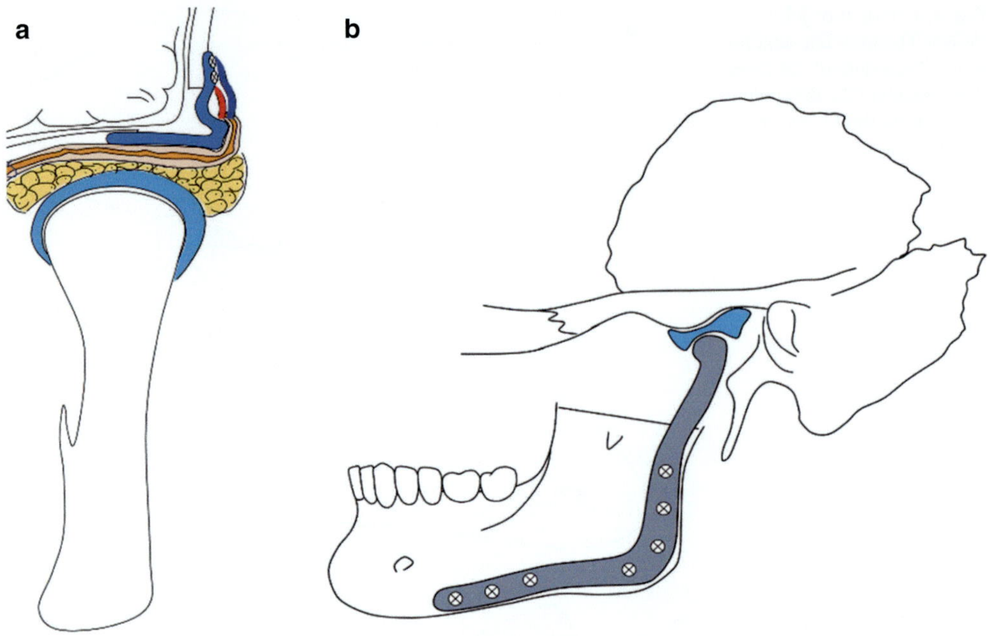

Fig. 3.6 Replacement with a prosthesis. (**a**) Replacement of the articular fossa with a prosthesis. Yellow is the temporalis fascia fat flap, blue above the fat is the articular fossa prosthesis, blue below the fat is the articular disc, dark blue above is the vein, and red is the artery. (**b**) Replacement of the condyle with a prosthesis, with gray as the condylar prosthesis and blue as the articular disc

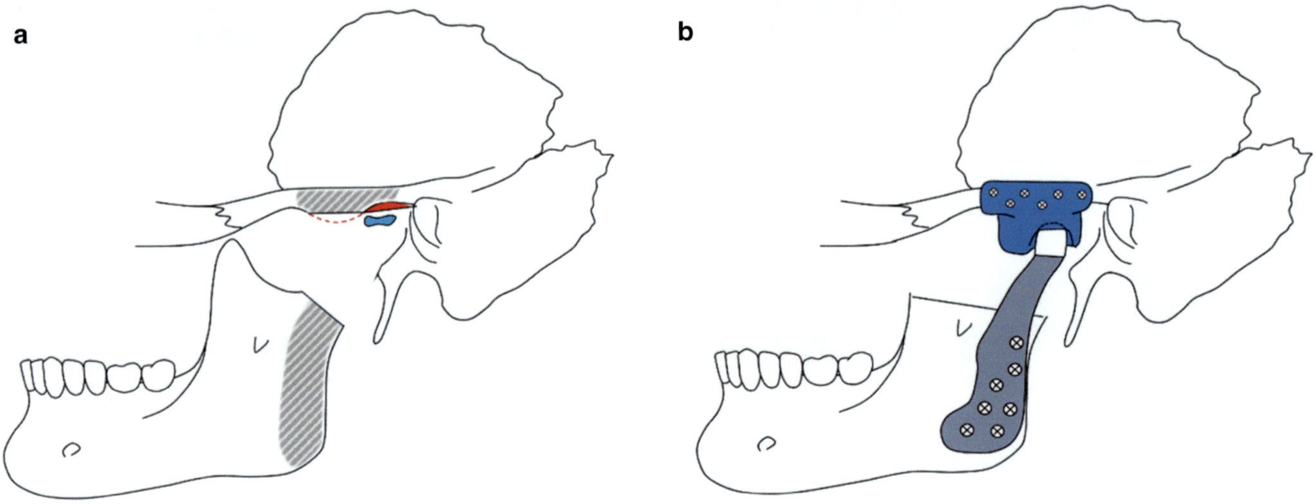

Fig. 3.7 Total joint replacement with a prosthesis (standard type). (**a**) Prosthesis implantation bed preparation: partial resection of the articular eminence to prepare for implantation of the articular fossa prosthesis and at the same time bone surface smoothing of the articular eminence, condylectomy, and smoothing of the mandible. Red is the partial resected articular eminence, blue is the articular disc, and gray shading is the bone surface area that is surgically shaped to fit the prosthesis. (**b**) Standard total joint prosthesis replacement outcome: blue is the articular fossa prosthesis, and gray and white are the mandibular prosthesis

joint prostheses, the finished product, are usually available in large, medium, and small sizes; personalized total joint prostheses are customized to fit the patient's joint and surrounding bone structural characteristics. Both types of prosthesis have been made earlier outside of China. Surgery applying the standard total joint prosthesis needs to grind down the bone surface to make the prosthesis match the bone structure; the procedure is difficult to operate, with low precision and poor stability of the prosthesis resulting. In the past, the foreign customized total joint prosthesis could not be used in China due to restrictive laws and regulations on imports.

3.1.4 Innovative Reconstruction with Customized Total TMJ Prosthesis

Following in-depth investigation of the design of the two American prostheses and rich clinical experience in application of this technology, as well as examination of the structural and kinetic characteristics of Chinese TMJ anatomy, the author has combined digital design and the 3D printing manufacturing process to develop new types of personalized total joint prostheses. The full surgical preparation and process involve digitally designed surgical guides, endoscopic-assisted fixation, and other key technologies, with the aim of realizing a precise, efficient, and stable total joint prosthesis replacement. Calling on the joint defect model, the design of the surgical operation, and prosthesis design principles, this chapter introduces the design of three types of customized total joint prostheses, and potentially more, to meet different clinical needs.

3.1.4.1 Types of Total Joint Prosthesis Design

3.1.4.1.1 Classic Total Joint Prosthesis

The overall shape of this prosthesis is close to that of the total joint prosthesis developed earlier in the United States and elsewhere, and of course, it consists of two parts, a fossa prosthesis and a mandibular prosthesis. The difference is that the fossa prosthesis used here is made of ultrahigh-molecular-weight polyethylene, and the mandibular prosthesis is made of cobalt-chromium-molybdenum alloy for the articular head and titanium alloy mandibular parts, which are produced to individual specifications with 3D printing technology. The classic surgical plan has been used to install the prostheses, i.e., two incisions (anterior auriculotemporal and retromandibular) with intermaxillary ligation (Fig. 3.8).

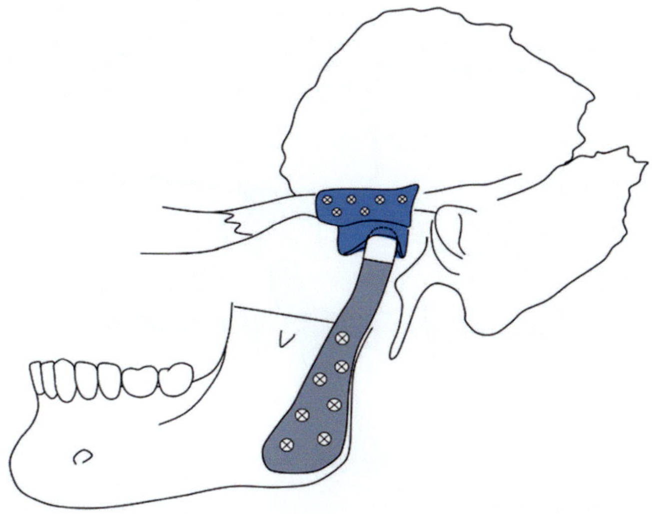

Fig. 3.8 Classic total joint prosthesis. The blue color is the customized articular fossa component of the prosthesis made of ultrahigh-molecular-weight polyethylene, the gray color is the mandibular component made of titanium alloy, and the white color is the cobalt-chromium-molybdenum alloy condylar head component

3.1.4.1.2 Mandibular Prosthesis Component Extension Design for Precise Positioning on the Mandible

The mandibular prosthesis component extension has anterior and posterior positioning wings, an innovative design of curling edges that wrap around and hold on to the bone, thus facilitating precise positioning during surgery. Combined with endoscopic fixation techniques, only an anterior auriculotemporal incision and a small transbuccal incision are required, eliminating the need for intermaxillary ligations and achieving minimally invasive results with minimal risk of infection (Fig. 3.9).

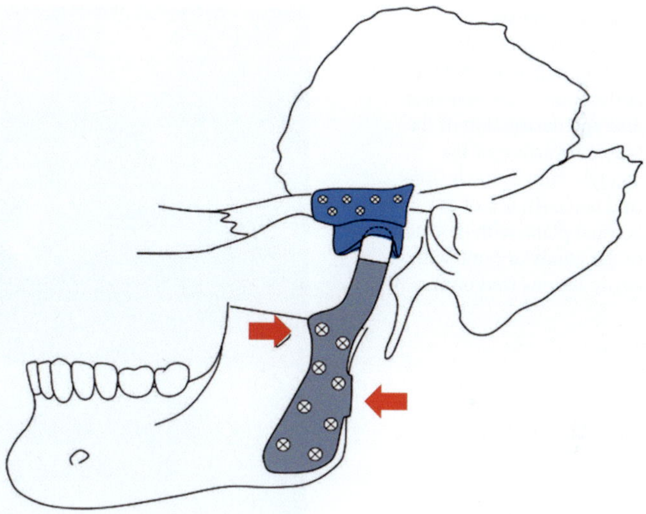

Fig. 3.9 Total joint prosthesis with wings on the mandible component to facilitate positioning. The blue is the fossa prosthesis made of ultrahigh-molecular-weight polyethylene, the gray is the titanium alloy mandibular component, and the white color at the top of the mandible component is the articulating head component made of cobalt-chromium-molybdenum alloy. The mandible component has shallow wings on it located at the front-top and back-middle edges (indicated by the red arrows) to aid in positioning during surgery as well as to provide secure fixation of the mandibular prosthesis

3.1.4.1.3 Metallic/Nonmetallic Fossa Prosthesis to Aid Osseointegration

The joint fossa prosthesis is composed of both metallic and nonmetallic materials, with zygomatic arch component made of titanium alloy to hold the ultrahigh-molecular-weight polyethylene articulating fossa component in place. The friction welding process has been engineered to achieve a solid metallic/nonmetallic connection, suitable for dealing with large joint defects in future development. In this case, the articular fossa prosthesis with special surface characteristics can aid osseointegration with the patient's own bone for long-term stabilization (Fig. 3.10).

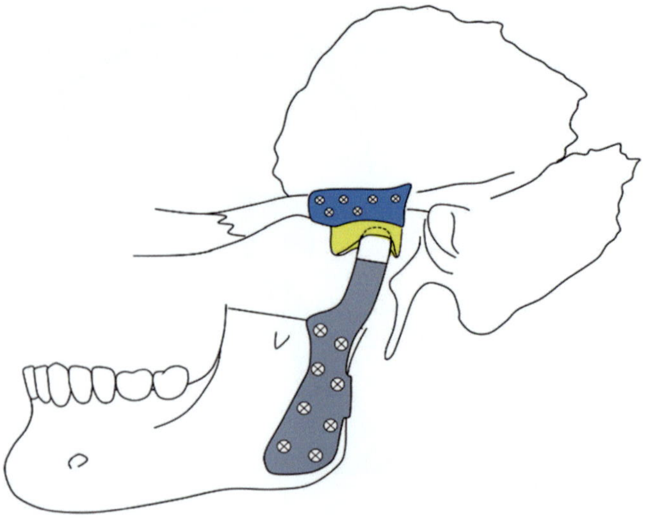

Fig. 3.10 Metallic/nonmetallic total joint prosthesis with titanium alloy zygomatic arch component (blue) and ultrahigh-molecular-weight polyethylene fossa component (yellow), manufactured with joining by friction welding. The gray is the mandibular component (metallic), and the white is the condylar head (also metallic)

3.1.4.2 Indications and Contraindications for the Application of a TMJ Prosthesis

3.1.4.2.1 Indications for Application of the Total Joint Prosthesis

See the US Food and Drug Administration (FDA) certification report, the clinical consensus on total joint prosthesis implantation published by the British Association of Oral and Maxillofacial Surgeons and Japan, and our team's many years of clinical tests. Specifically, condylar, fossa, and eminence lesions caused by the following diseases are indications:

- Severe osteoarthritis that fails to respond to conservative treatment and has significant persistent symptoms (Fig. 3.11)
- Idiopathic condylar resorption that qualifies as a non-salvageable joint, with moderate to severe dentofacial deformities (Fig. 3.12)

Fig. 3.11 Severe osteoarthritis. (**a**) MRI of joint with displacement and perforation of the articular disc and destruction of the articular surface of the condyle with cystic lesions (red box). (**b**) CT of the coronal plane with destruction of the condylar bone with cystic lesions (red box)

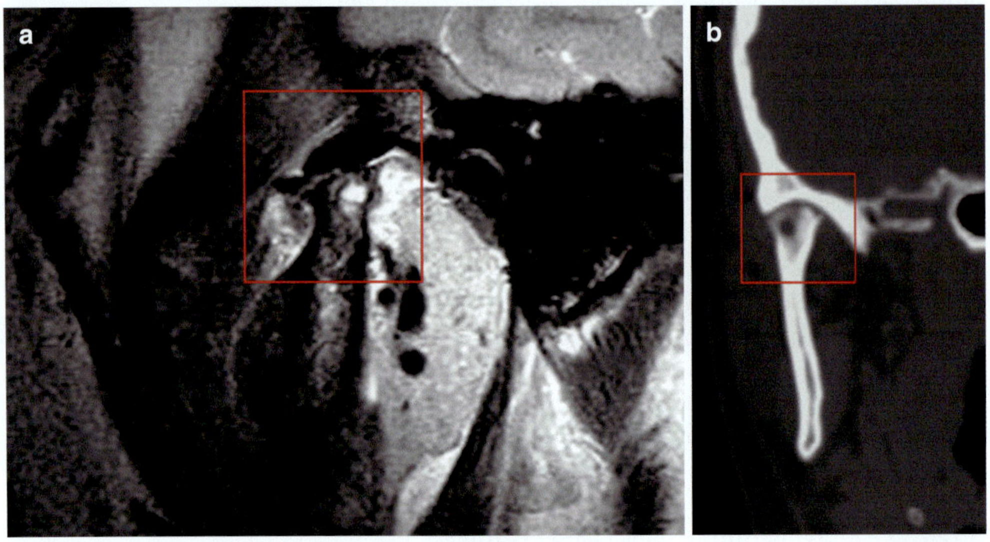

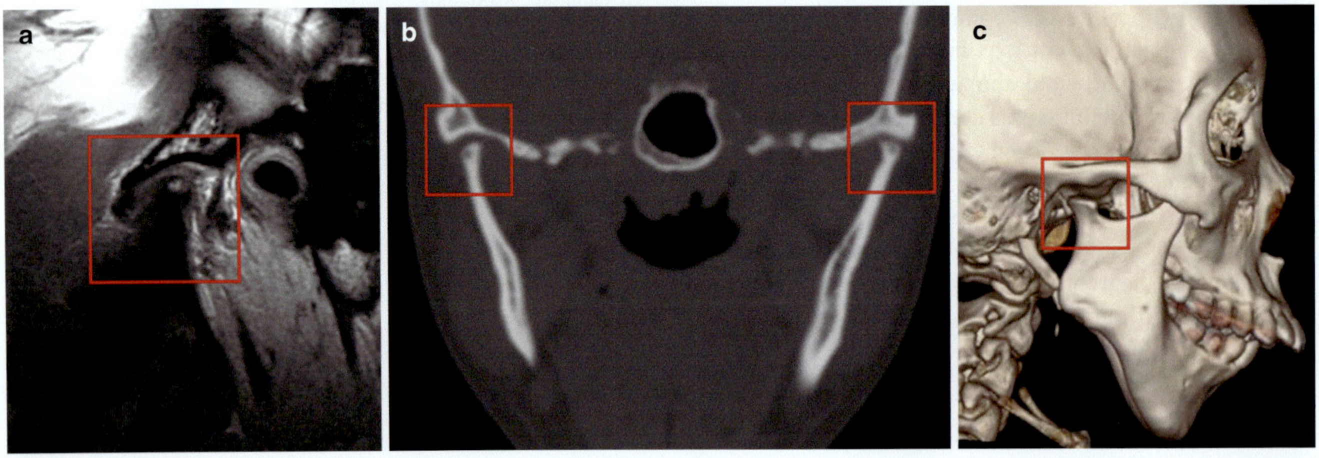

Fig. 3.12 Idiopathic condylar resorption. (**a**) Joint MRI with displaced articular discs and condylar shortening (red box). (**b**) Coronal CT with bilateral condylar shortening and absence of bone marrow (red box). (**c**) CT representation with condylar shortening (red box) and severe clockwise rotation and retrognathia of the mandible

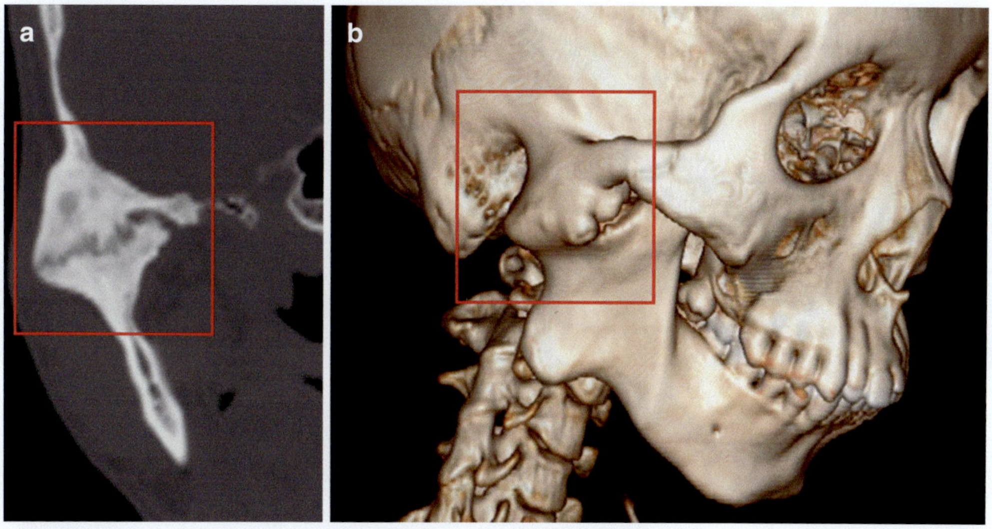

Fig. 3.13 TMJ ankylosis. (**a**) Coronal CT scan, showing bony fusion (red box). (**b**) 3D reconstruction representation of cranium, showing bony fusion (red box) and mandibular retrognathia

- Ankylosis of the joint with no or non-salvageable residual condylar on the medial side (Fig. 3.13)
- Resorption of the bone graft or re-ankylosis after autologous bone grafting (Fig. 3.14)
- A comminuted condylar fracture that cannot be surgically repositioned and is expected to result in ankylosis of the joint and severe shortening of the mandibular ramus, causing even dentofacial deformity (Fig. 3.15)
- Arthritic diseases in the static phase or chronic phase of rheumatoid arthritis (Fig. 3.16)
- Joint tumors and tumorlike lesions that have affected the condyle (Fig. 3.17)

3.1.4.2.2 Contraindications for Application of the Prosthesis

- Absolute contraindications:
  1. Allergy to titanium alloy, cobalt-chromium-molybdenum alloy, or ultrahigh-molecular-weight polyethylene materials used in the prosthesis.
  2. Acute infectious diseases, or chronic diseases in acute phase
  3. Uncontrolled systemic diseases
- Relative contraindications:
  1. Those whose bones are nearing maturity during growth and development
  2. Those with controlled acute or chronic infections
  3. Those with non-severe bruxism
  4. Those with a controlled stage of systemic disease
  5. Use with caution in those with poor nutritional conditions, e.g., osteonecrosis after radiotherapy

3.1.5 The General Process of the Digital Design for Customized Total Joint Prosthesis

The overall process of preparation for the manufacture of the prosthesis and its installation in surgery, exemplified by that for the most common condylar lesion, consists of three stages: virtual surgical planning, designing the prosthesis and cutting guides, and other surgical procedures. (See the following subsections A, B, and C and Fig. 3.18, outlining all steps in sequence; note that the sequence on the schematic figure is not all left to right and repeats some parts of the figure, so follow the arrows.)

3.1.5.1 Virtual Surgical Planning: Plan the Removal of the Lesion and Create the "Defect Model" Where the Prosthesis Will Be Implanted

- Plan the scope of the lesion: first, import the patient's CT data into the design software; create the required three-dimensional model of the patient's maxillofacial region, and mark the extent of the defect (Fig. 3.18a1).
- Plan the osteotomy lines for removal of the lesion:
  - Subcondylar osteotomy line: the osteotomy is usually made below the condyle to safely remove the lesion while considering the space needed for the prosthesis installation.
  - Articular eminence osteotomy line: the osteotomy line should also be devised to facilitate the removal of the lesion while leaving enough bone to hold the fossa

Fig. 3.14 Failure of autogenous bone graft. (**a**) Coronal CT scan, showing bony fusion of CCG to articular fossa (red box). (**b**) 3D reconstruction representation of bony fusion (red box)

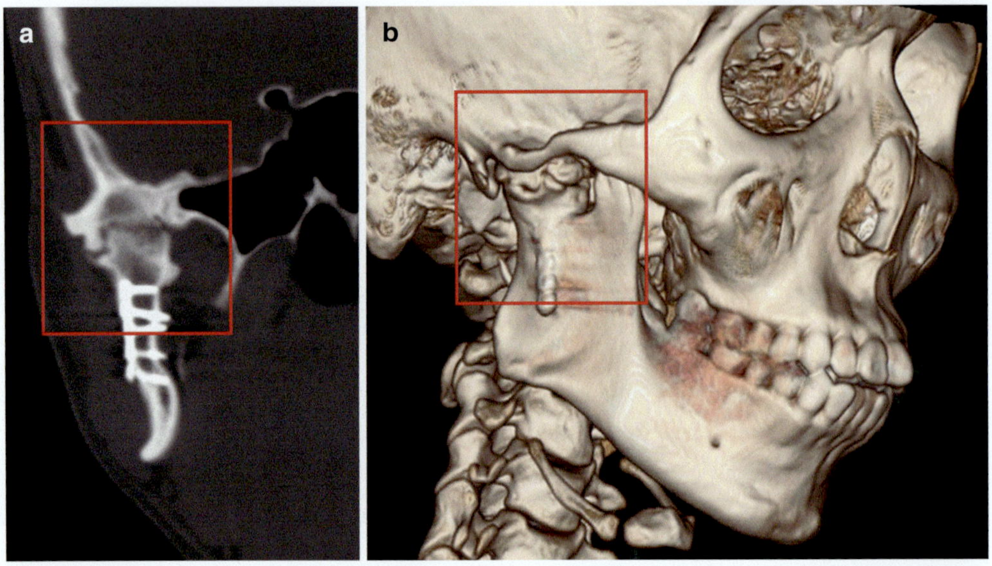

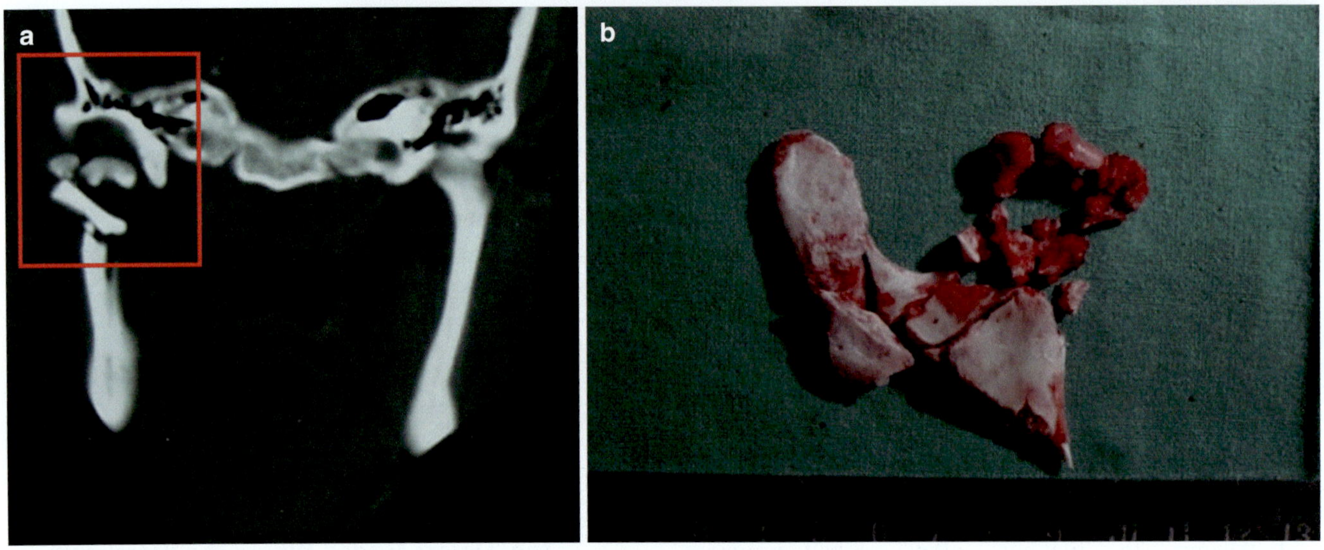

Fig. 3.15 Comminuted condylar fracture. (**a**) Coronal CT scan, comminuted fracture of the right condyle (red box). (**b**) Actual specimen of comminuted bone fragments of the condyle and coronoid process

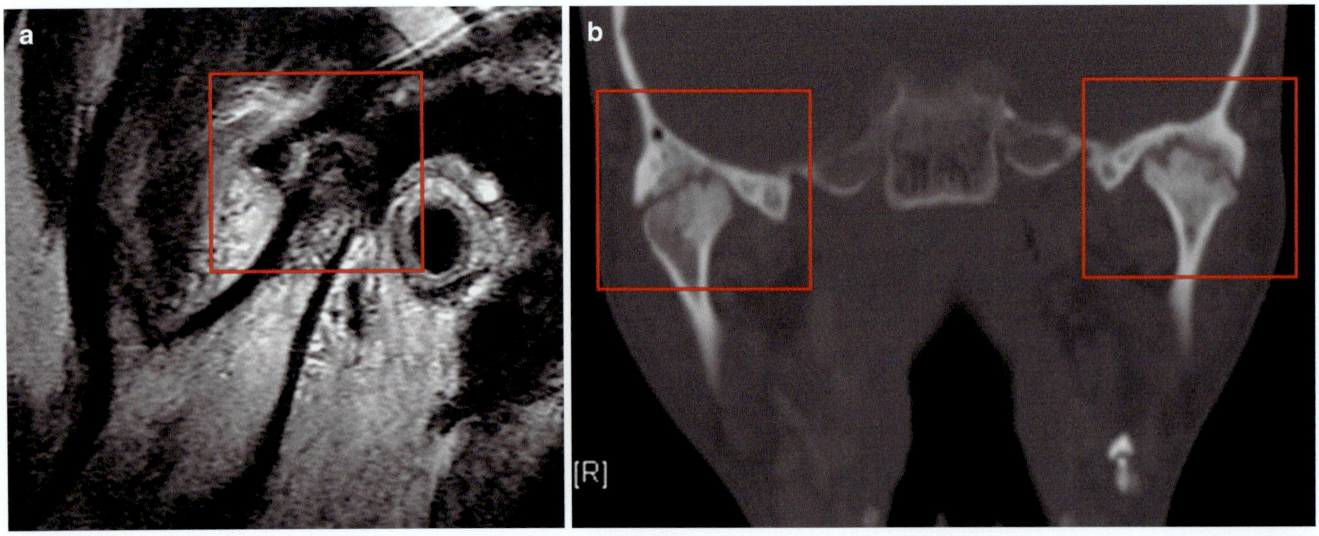

Fig. 3.16 Rheumatoid arthritis. (**a**) MRI of joints with absent articular discs and significant bone destruction (red box). (**b**) Coronal CT scan with bilateral joint ankylosis and bone destruction (red boxes)

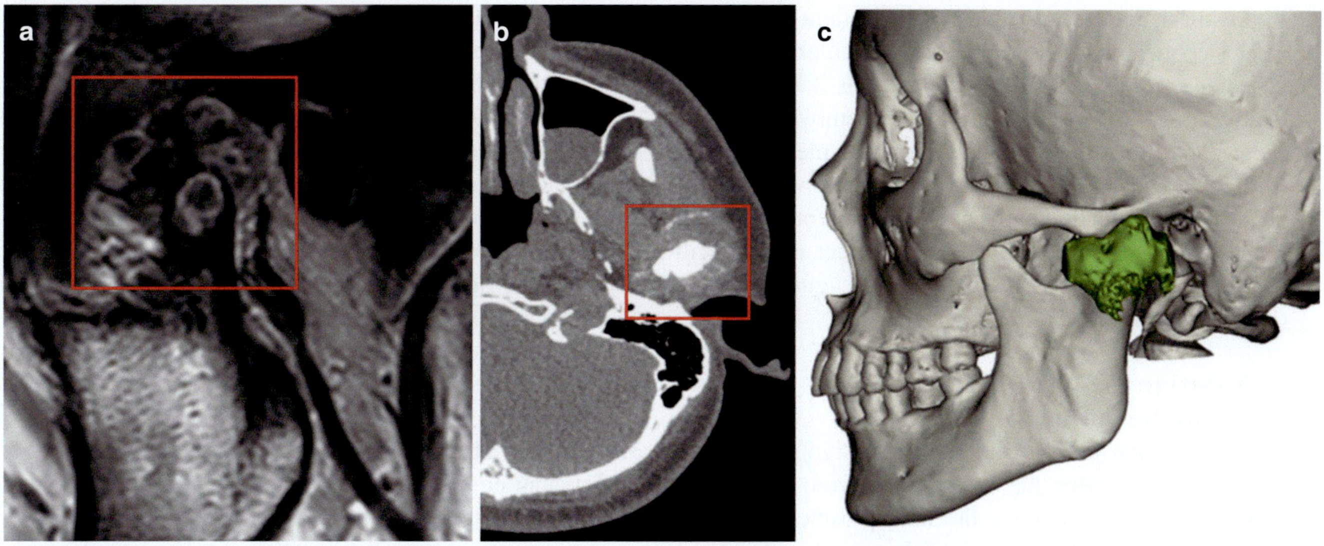

Fig. 3.17 Joint tumors. (**a**) MRI of joint with massive growths in the joint cavity and condylar destruction (red box). (**b**) Axial CT scan slice with peri-condylar calcified lesions and condylar sclerosis (red box). (**c**) 3D reconstruction of the lesions (green)

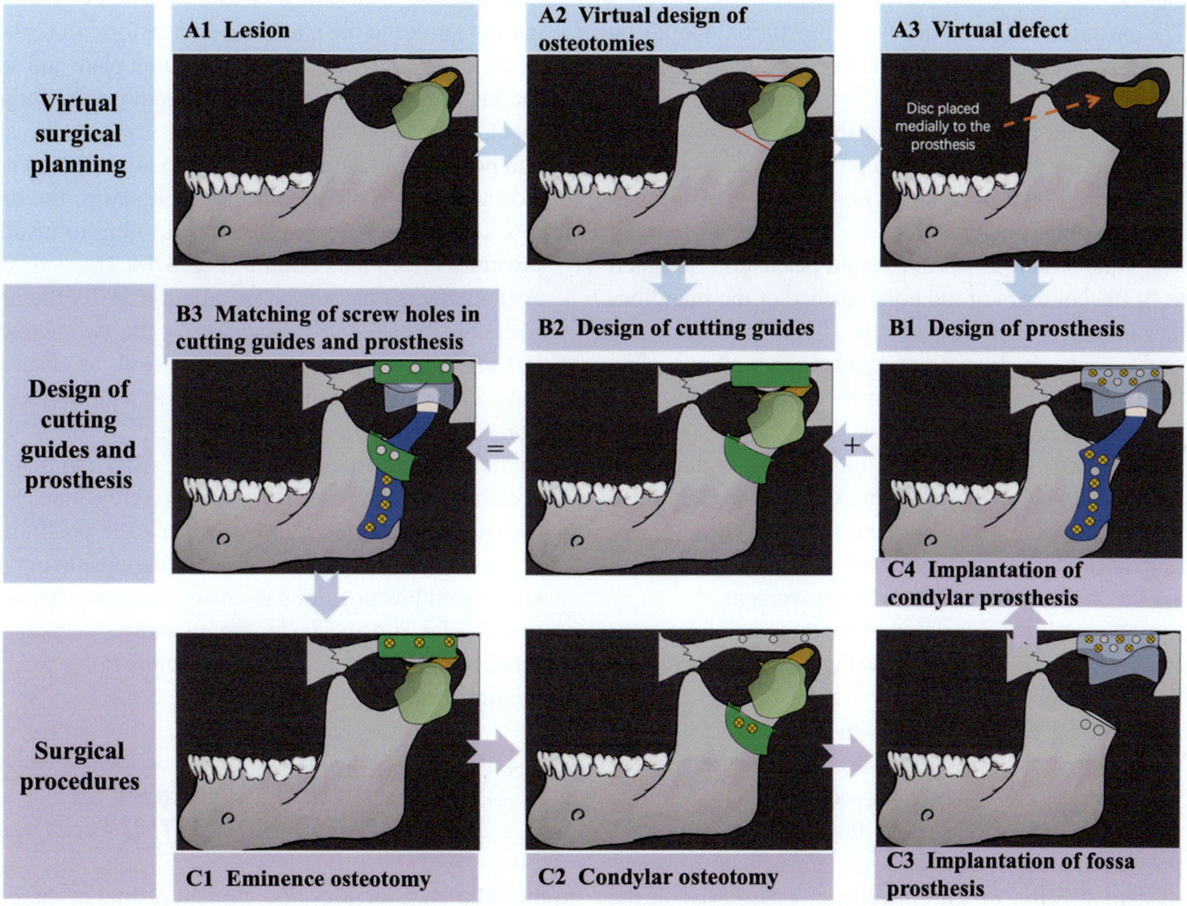

Fig. 3.18 Digital design of total joint prosthesis and its surgical implantation: (**a1**) Define the scope of the defect (green) from CT scan data, making a 3D model of the patient's cranium. (**a2**) Design the osteotomy lines for removal of the defect and preparation for prosthesis implantation. (**a3**) Obtain the "defect model" resulting from osteotomy, i.e., the space for the prosthesis. (**b1**) Design the articular fossa prosthesis (light blue) and mandibular prosthesis (blue) based on the "defect model." (**b2**) Design the two cutting guides based on the osteotomy lines (green), to be used for precise positioning. (**b3**) Transfer the positions of the prosthesis screw holes to the cutting guides. (**c1**) Actual surgery: use a cutting guide to assist articular eminence osteotomy. (**c2**) Use a cutting guide to assist subcondylar osteotomy. (**c3**) Implantation of the articular fossa prosthesis component. (**c4**) Implantation of the mandibular prosthesis component

prosthesis in place, especially if the patient's condition is accompanied by ankylosis, articular eminence lesion, or steep articular eminence (Fig. 3.18a2).

- Establishment of defect model. Plan to remove the lesion according to the osteotomy lines, and take measurements from the model and adjust them according to what should be the best for function of the prosthesis and/or for correction of craniofacial deformity. This "defect model" will be used for prosthesis and cutting guide design (Fig. 3.18a3 to b1).

3.1.5.2 Design the Total Joint Prosthesis and the Cutting Guides

- Design the total joint prosthesis: the design of the total joint prosthesis uses the information from the defect model in order to produce the final prosthesis product shown in Fig. 3.18b1, with the following key points of consideration:
  - The fossa prosthesis should have its horizontal plane set at 0° to 10° relative to the Frankfort horizontal plane.
  - The posterior edge of the fossa prosthesis should be 3 mm to 5 mm away from the bony external auditory canal.
  - The condylar head component should be positioned at the posterior end of the fossa prosthesis when the jaw is closed, as well as centered in the fossa prosthesis to allow smooth movement.
  - The mandibular prosthesis should be custom designed to fit the contours of the bone surface of the mandibular ramus.
  - The articular fossa prosthesis and the mandibular prosthesis require at least five screws each for stable fixation to the bone.
  - After the design of the total joint prosthesis has been completed and tested by fitting on a 3D-printed head model, there should be further review and communication between doctors and engineers and, if needed, another round of revision and improvement.
- Design the cutting guides. Following the plan of the osteotomy lines to remove the defect (Fig. 3.18a2), design the cutting guides during surgery:
  - Subcondylar cutting guides, which have the following three functions: first, position and guide the cutting path during the osteotomy; second, assist accurate installation of the prosthesis; third, the cutting guides provide at least two screw holes that will serve in permanent fixation of the mandibular prosthesis on the jawbone (Fig. 3.18b2).
  - Articular eminence cutting guides, which have the same functions as the subcondylar cutting guides mentioned before: cutting path guidance, accurate installation of the prosthesis, and confirming the fixation position of the articular fossa prosthesis on the zygomatic arch (also Fig. 3.18b2).
  - Design the screw holes of cutting guides to match the screw holes planned for prosthesis: overlay the images that correspond to Fig. 3.18b1 (prosthesis) and B2 (guides) to determine the screw hole positions that are to be shared by the two. The lengths of the screws must also be measured on the cranium or jaw. The goal is that not only is the osteotomy accurate, but also the prosthesis can be installed precisely and quickly without the need for intermaxillary ligation (Fig. 3.18b3).

3.1.5.3 The Steps of the Surgical Procedure

1. Articular eminence osteotomy: Attach the eminence cutting guides to the zygomatic arch and perform the osteotomy to allow space for installation of the articular fossa prosthesis. Then remove the guide and the small bone block (the articular eminence) that was cut off (Fig. 3.18c1).
2. Subcondylar osteotomy: First, attach the subcondylar cutting guides to the mandible and perform the osteotomy of the condyle; then, remove the guide plate and separate the lateral pterygoid muscle, and remove the large bone block containing the lesion. Next, separate the anterior and posterior attachments of the articular disc on its outer side and turn it sideways, and then suture the articular disc to the inner side to serve as a lining to insulate the prosthesis from the cranium (Fig. 3.18c2).
3. Articular fossa prosthesis installation: Affix the articular fossa prosthesis with screws using the two screw holes left after the osteotomy guide removal, to ensure accuracy, and then fix the other three to four screws in the bone (Fig. 3.18c3).
4. Mandibular prosthesis installation: Affix the mandibular prosthesis with screws using the two screw holes left after the osteotomy guide removal. Check the position of the articulating head and the occlusal relationship in the open and closed jaw positions to ensure accuracy. Then fix the mandibular prosthesis to the mandible securely using three to four screws in the other screw holes prepared in the prosthesis (Fig. 3.18c4).

3.2 Reconstruction Techniques with Customized Total TMJ Prosthesis

In the following sections, the clinical results of three different personalized total joint prostheses are illustrated in three clinical cases.

The prosthesis in Case A is of international classic design, consisting of a customized ultrahigh-molecular-weight polyethylene fossa prosthesis and a cobalt chromium molybdenum and titanium alloy mandibular prosthesis. The surgery was performed using a modified anterior auriculotemporal and retromandibular incision with intermaxillary ligation to stabilize the positions of the fossa prosthesis and the mandibular prosthesis.

The prosthesis in Case B demonstrates a shape innovation, one in which the prosthesis can be positioned more accurately during surgery by adding wings to the posterior and upper anterior edges of the mandibular prosthesis component. This innovation is combined with digitally designed cutting guides to set precise screw holes, as well as the use of an endoscope to assist in fixation of the mandibular prosthesis, which avoids the need for retromandibular incisions and intermaxillary ligations.

The prosthesis in Case C shows a technological innovation in materials, using friction welding to prepare a titanium alloy and ultrahigh-molecular-weight polyethylene jointed fossa prosthesis to achieve osseointegration of the fossa prosthesis with the fossa bone and to prevent loosening of the prosthesis, as well as to provide long-term stabilization.

3.2.1 Case A. Design and Application of an International Standard Design Total Joint Prosthesis

- Patient information: male, 76 years old.
- Complaint: right preauricular pain with limited mouth opening for more than 2 years.
- History: the patient had right preauricular pain, weakness of mastication, and restriction of mouth opening for 2 years, and 6 months of non-surgical treatment was ineffective.
- Past history: history of high blood pressure, controlled by long-term medication, most recently 140/74 mmHg. History of old myocardial infarction, no specific treatment, taking one pill daily of Chinese medicine for heart protection. History of removal of intestinal polyps 12 years ago. History of removal of lipomas from the legs 14 years ago. History of drug and food allergy denied.
- Clinical examination: face was basically symmetrical, there was no facial swelling, and mouth opening was limited to 18 mm, with some deviation to the left. Deep overbite of front teeth, but occlusion was stable in the mouth; the periodontal and dental conditions could be summarized as shown in Fig. 3.19. Preauricular pain was scored 8 on the visual analogue scale (VAS) scale of zero to ten (0 means no obstacle to eating, 10 means unable to eat).
- Imaging examination: a panoramic scan showed that the right condyle was shorter than the left one (Fig. 3.20); MRI showed that the right joint had anterior disc displacement without reduction, perforation of the disc and abnormality of the condyle, and effusion in the articular cavity (Fig. 3.21), and CT showed that the right condyle was abnormal and had suffered severe destruction (Fig. 3.22).
- Diagnosis: osteoarthritis of the right TMJ.

3.2.2 Case A. Diagnostic Imaging

3.2.3 Case A. Treatment Plan

- Overall treatment plan: right-side defect resection of condyle and reconstruction with a customized total joint prosthesis of standard international design.
- Virtual surgical planning:
  - Design of the resection scope: (1) the diseased condyle (from the condylar head to the subcondylar process) and (2) the lower part of the articular eminence.

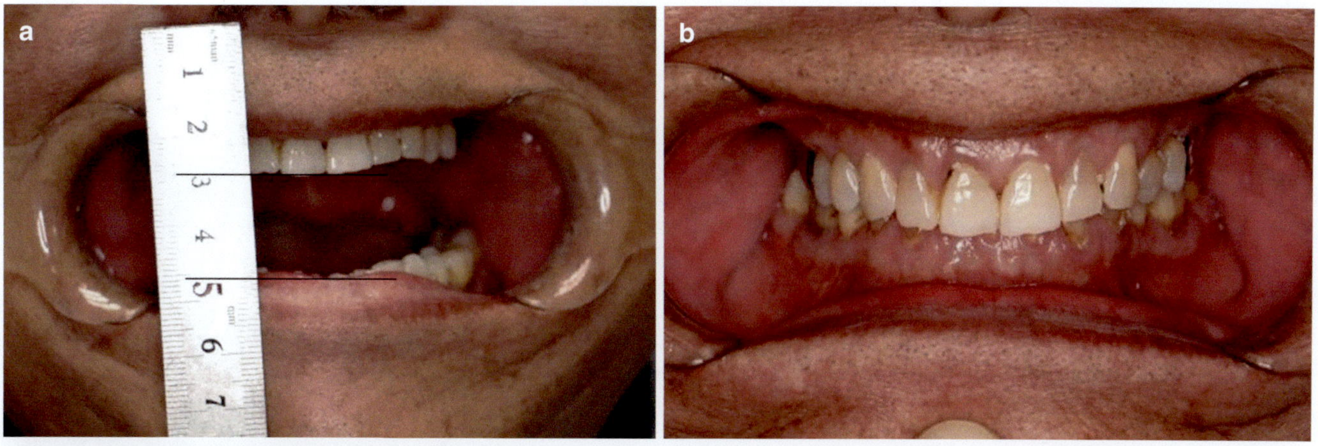

Fig. 3.19 Case A. Clinical examination. (**a**) Maximum interincisal opening was 18 mm, with slight deviation to the right (left). (**b**) There was a deep overbite with stable occlusal contacts

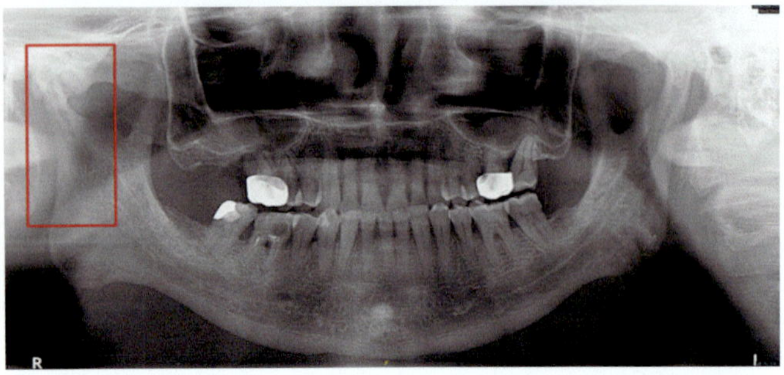

Fig. 3.20 Case A. Panoramic view. The red box highlights the right condyle, the right condyle is short, and the lower dental midline is deviated to the right

– Digital simulation of the surgery: Design a condylar osteotomy line on the sigmoid notch; set an articular eminence osteotomy line on the zygomatic arch to remove the articular eminence. Mark the resectioned area of the cranium to obtain a model of the space that will be left after osteotomy, the "defect model" (Figs. 3.23 and 3.24).

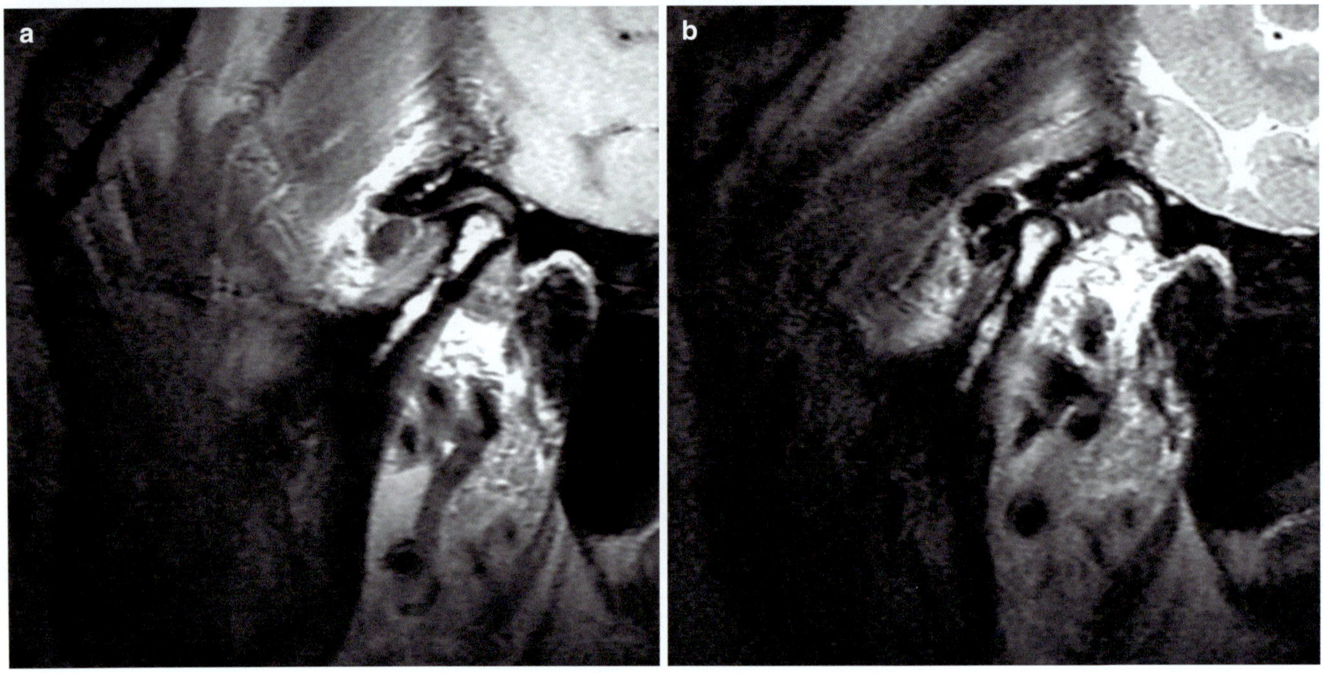

Fig. 3.21 Case A. TMJ MRI. There is severe resorption of the right condyle. The disc is anteriorly displaced and non-reducing. There is deformation, shortening, and perforation of the posterior region of the disc. (**a**) Closed position. (**b**) Open position

Fig. 3.22 Case A. 3D reconstruction of the maxillofacial CT. There is severe resorption of the right condyle

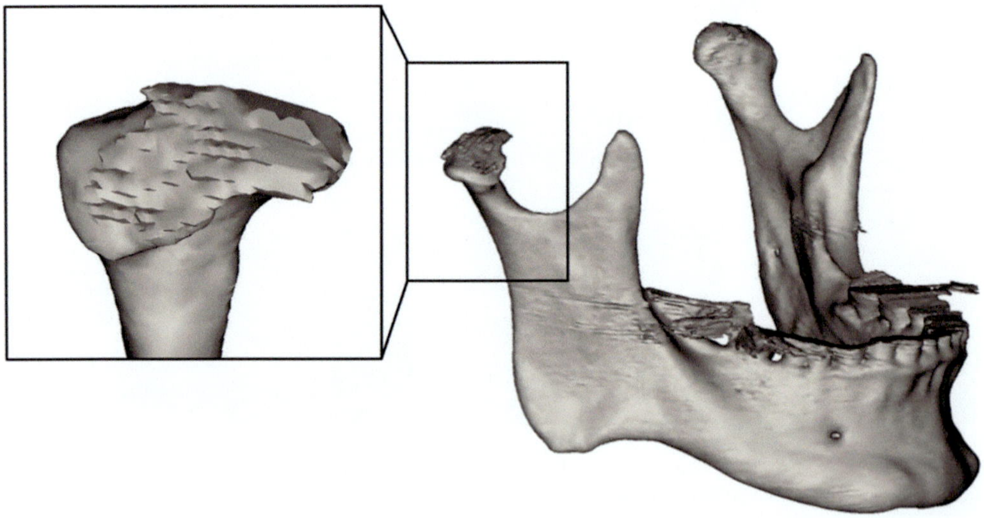

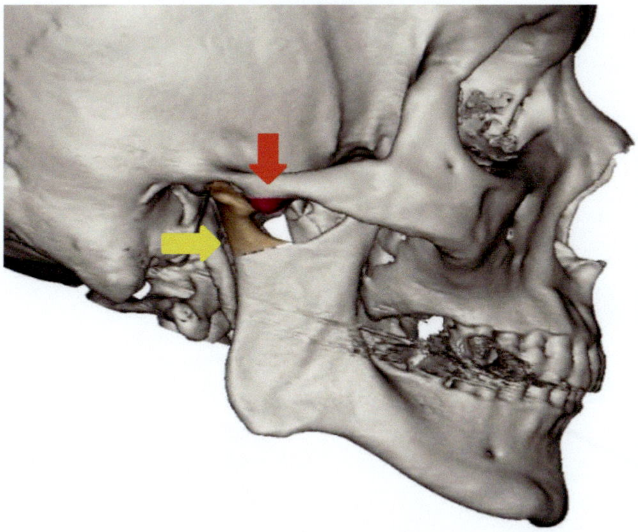

Fig. 3.23 Case A. Articular eminence osteotomy line (red arrow) and subcondylar osteotomy line (yellow arrow) design. The brown and red areas are the scope of resection

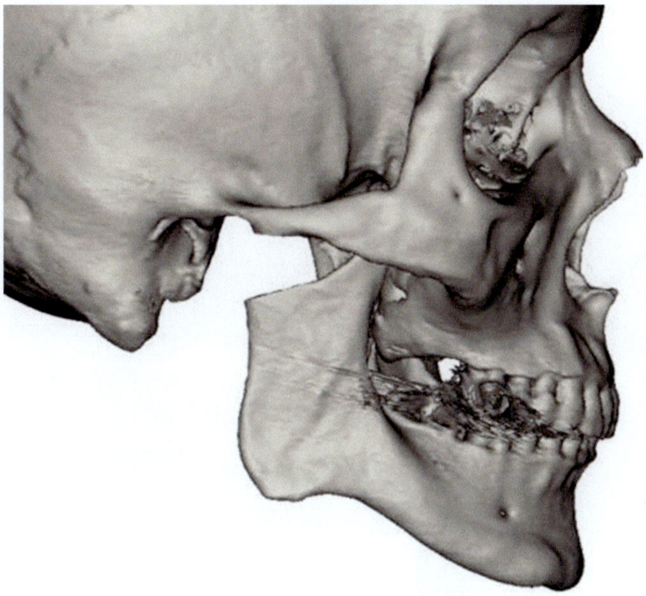

Fig. 3.24 Case A. Post-excision model. The virtual defect after osteotomies

3.2.4 Case A. Design and Processing of the Classic Total Joint Prosthesis Components and the Cutting Guides

- Design of the classic total joint prosthesis
  1. Import and placement of core components: import and place the fossa core component and the condyle head core component, as described in Sect. 2.4.1 in Chap. 2 (Fig. 3.25).

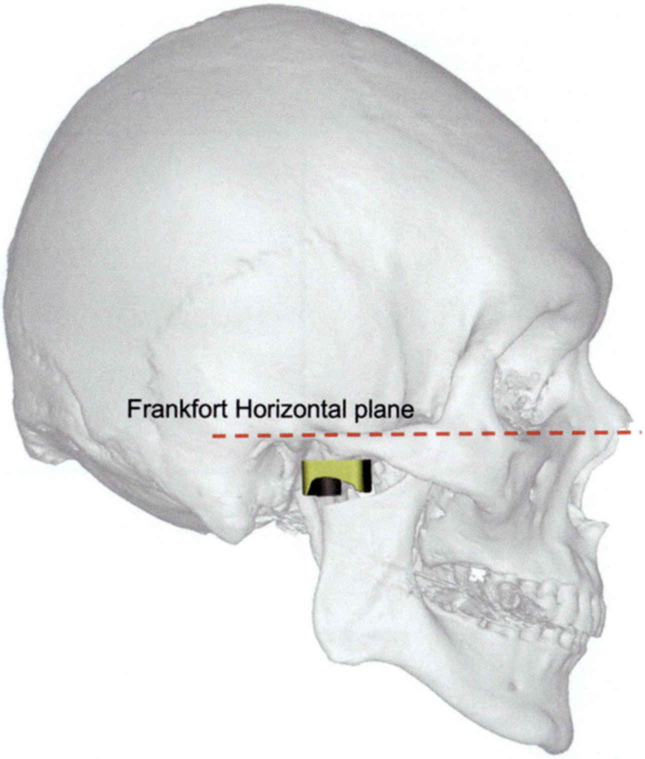

Fig. 3.25 Case A. The correct position of the fossa prosthesis (yellow) and the condyle head (dark gray) of the mandibular prosthesis is determined. The articular head is in the posterior position of the fossa prosthesis

- Design of the articular fossa and mandibular extension prosthesis

The design principles are described in Sect. 2.4.2 in Chap. 2. For the design of the fossa prosthesis, the extension part should fit closely to the fossa and zygomatic arch bone surfaces, with at least six screw holes (Fig. 3.26); for the design of the mandibular prosthesis, the extensions should fit closely to the mandibular ramus surfaces, with at least six screw holes (Fig. 3.27).

3. Screw hole depth measurement: after the prosthesis design is completed, estimate the length of each screw to be used in the fossa prosthesis and mandibular prosthesis (Fig. 3.28).

- Fabrication and test fitting of the prosthesis

The fabrication process is described in Sect. 2.5 in Chap. 2. After fabrication of the prosthesis, a trial fitting is performed on the head model of the patient to observe whether the articular fossa prosthesis and the mandibular prosthesis fit the bony surfaces and are stable. It is also necessary to ensure that the joint head of the mandibular prosthesis is correctly located in the posterior median position of the fossa prosthesis (Fig. 3.29).

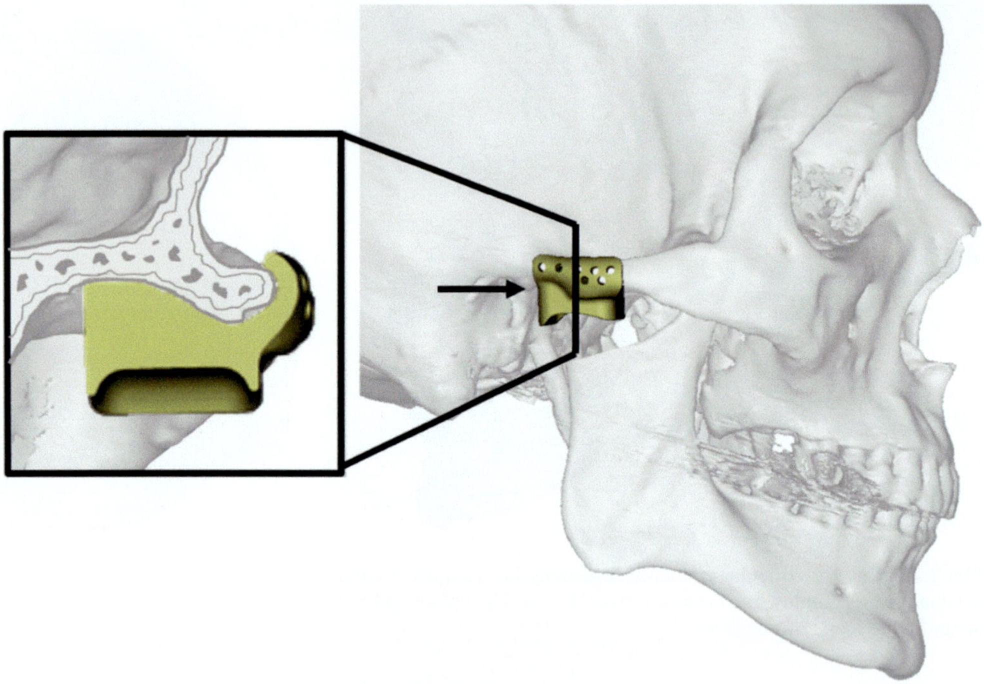

Fig. 3.26 Case A. Design of the zygomatic arch fixation component and the fossa component. The components fit precisely to the surface of the fossa and the zygoma and have at least six screw holes

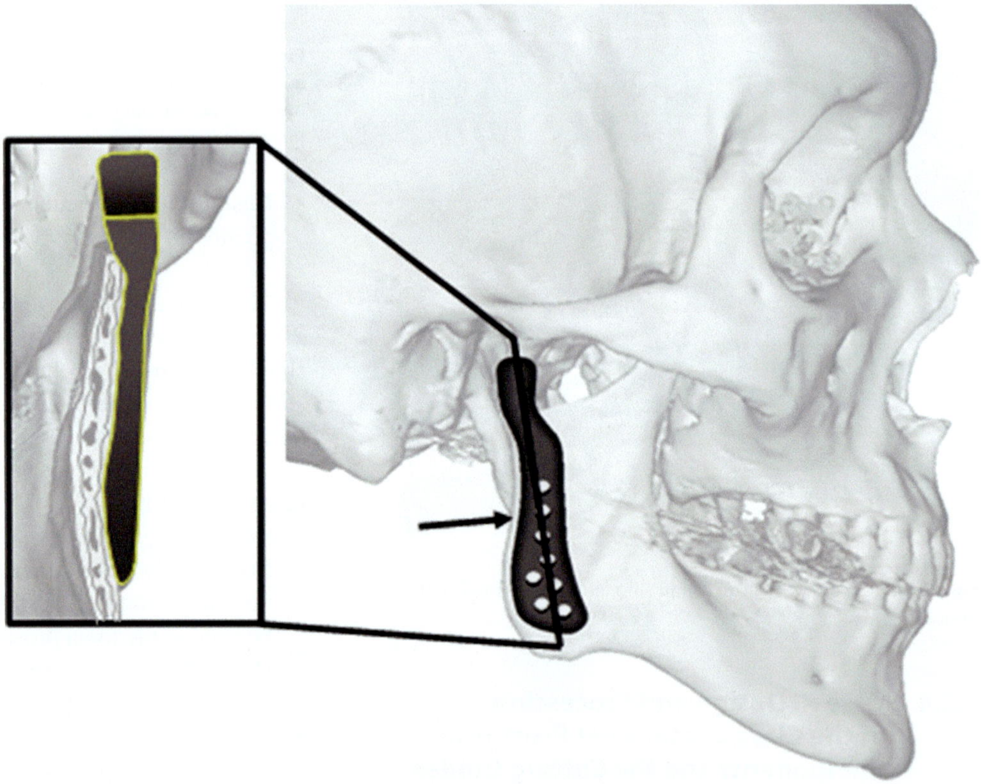

Fig. 3.27 Case A. Design of the mandibular fixation component. The extension component fits precisely to the surface of the ramus and has at least six screw holes

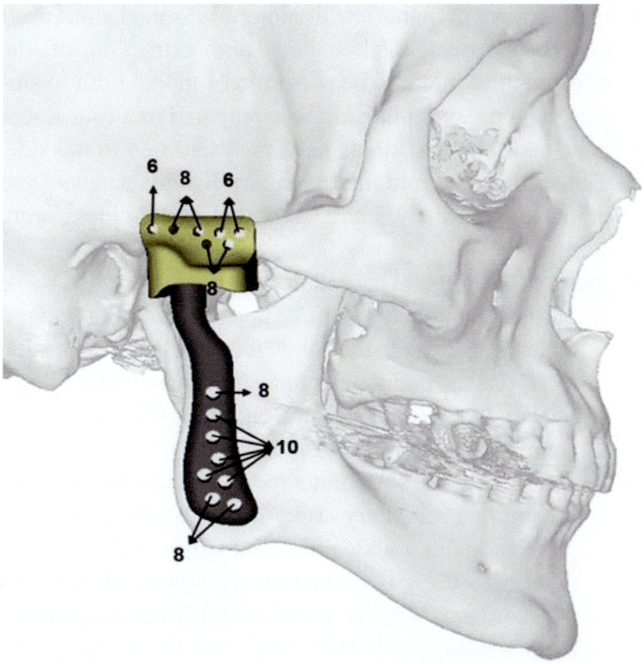

Fig. 3.28 Case A. Measurement of screw lengths. After the prosthesis has been designed, the thickness of the prosthesis plus the thickness of the underlying bone equals the length of the screw to be implanted in each hole

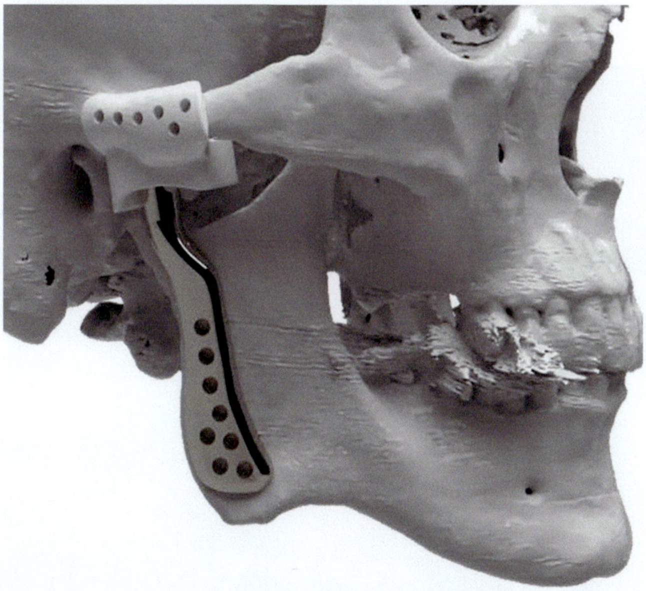

Fig. 3.29 Case A. After the prosthesis has been manufactured, a CT-based skull model is used to check whether the fixation components fit precisely to the bone surfaces. It is important to be certain that the condylar component is in the middle posterior position of the fossa component

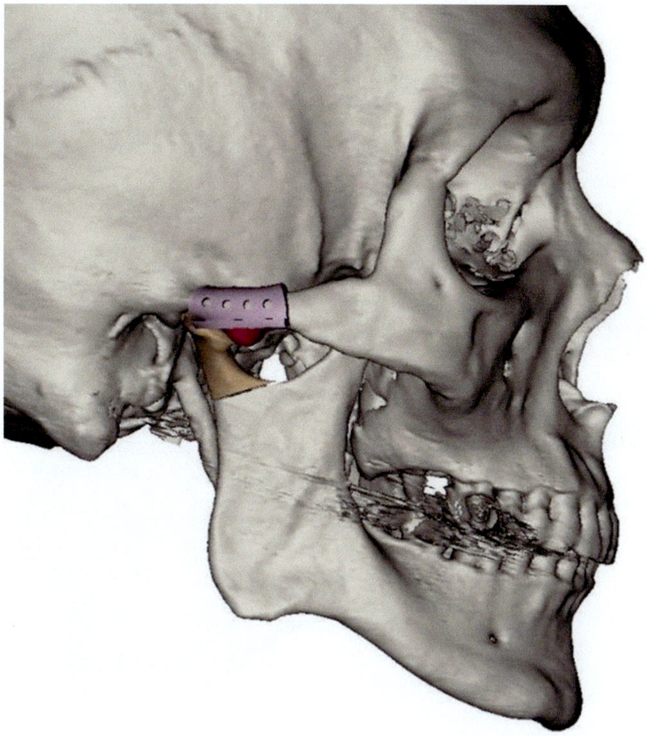

Fig. 3.30 Case A. Cutting guide for eminence osteotomy. The cutting guide is designed according to the anatomy of the eminence and zygoma for precise osteotomy of the articular eminence

- Design of the cutting guides for surgery
  1. Eminence cutting guide design: the guide is designed in accordance with the eminence osteotomy line to achieve precise removal of the bone during surgery and the correct positioning of the screw holes (Fig. 3.30).
  2. Subcondylar cutting guide design: the guide is designed in accordance with the subcondylar osteotomy line to achieve the precise removal of the diseased bone during surgery and the correct positioning of the screw holes (Fig. 3.31).

3.2.5 Case A. Surgical Procedure

- Preoperative laboratory tests: complete blood count (CBC), coagulation profile, urinalysis, stool routine test, fasting plasma glucose (FPG), liver and renal function tests, infectious disease screening (HIV/HBsAg/HCV/TP), electrocardiogram (ECG), chest radiography (CXR), etc.

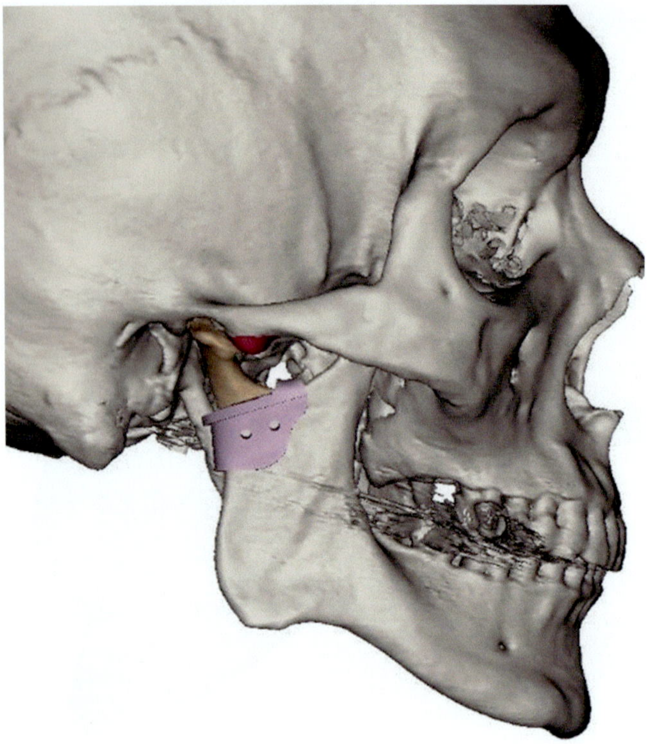

Fig. 3.31 Case A. Cutting guide for subcondylar osteotomy. The cutting guide is designed according to the anatomy of the upper ramus for precise ostectomy of the diseased condyle

- Preoperative preparation: signing of informed consent. If necessary, periodontal scaling and extraction of the affected third molar to be performed 1 month prior to surgery. The preauricular skin was prepared in a four-finger area, and female patients have their hair tied to the side. Titanium screws and intermaxillary ligation screws were prepared routinely, and the cutting guides were sterilized.
- Steps of the surgical procedure
  1. Surgical approach: modified anterior auriculotemporal incision to expose the joint; retromandibular incision to expose the mandibular angle and mandibular ramus.
  2. Subcondylar osteotomy: the cutting guide for the subcondylar osteotomy is installed and fixed in place with two screws; the auriculotemporal vascular bundles and the internal maxillary artery of the condylar neck are protected with a wide periosteal stripper. The subcondylar osteotomy is performed with an oscillating saw in accordance with the position and direction indicated by the cutting guide (Fig. 3.32), and the diseased condyle is resected (Fig. 3.33).

1. Eminence osteotomy: the cutting guide for the eminence osteotomy is affixed, and then an oscillating saw is utilized to perform the osteotomy in the position and direction indicated by the guide (Fig. 3.34).

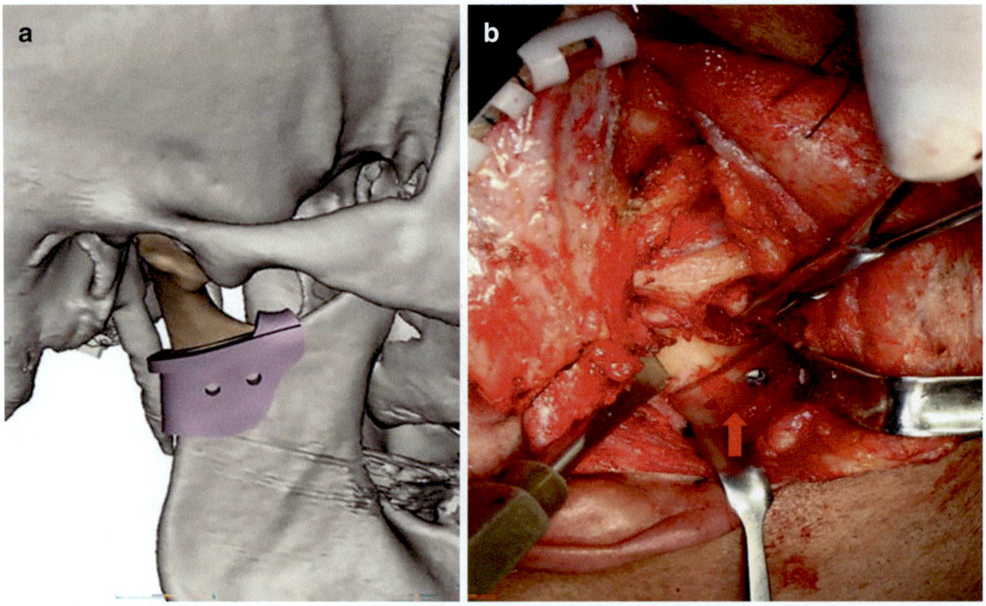

Fig. 3.32 Case A. The cutting guide (pink) assists the subcondylar osteotomy on the mandible (red arrow). (**a**) Design. (**b**) Actual

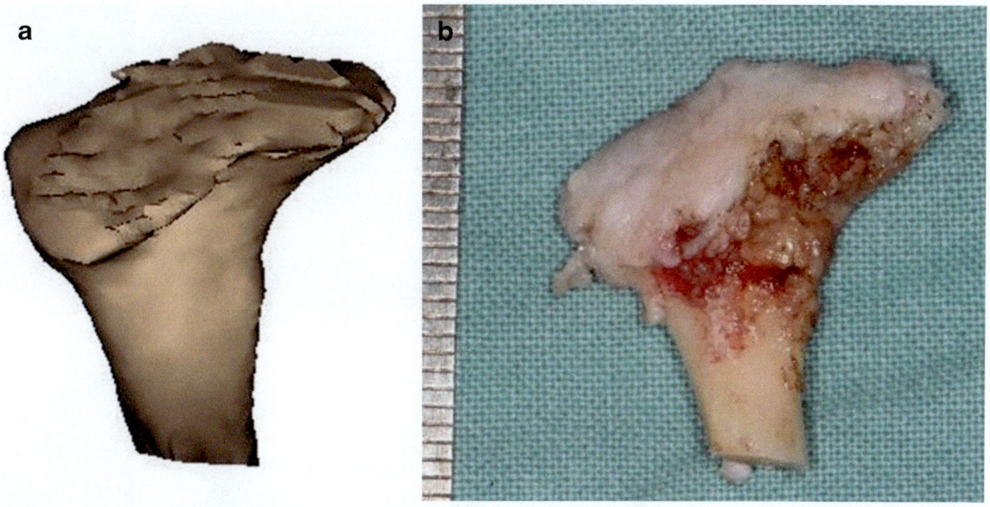

Fig. 3.33 Case A. Precision excision of the condyle. (**a**) Virtual plan. (**b**) Surgical specimen

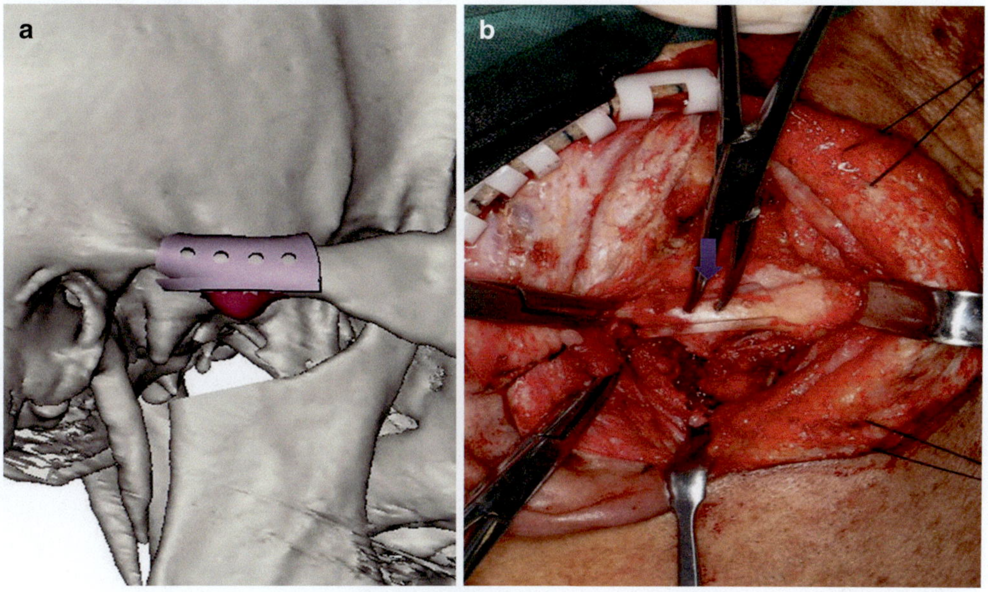

Fig. 3.34 Case A. Use of a cutting guide for eminence osteotomy. The cutting guide (purple arrow) is digitally designed to fit the zygomatic arch. A clamp or screws hold it in position. The osteotomy is performed with a oscillating saw. (**a**) Virtual plan. (**b**) Operative view

2. Prosthesis implantation:
   - Secure the fossa prosthesis on the zygomatic arch, using the two screw holes of the eminence cutting guide for positioning. The fossa prosthesis should be secured in place with at least five screws, matching each to the pre-measured screw hole depth and screw length (Fig. 3.35).
   - After intermaxillary ligation to maintain the correct position of occlusion, the mandibular prosthesis is inserted through the retromandibular incision, and at least five screws are used to secure it to the bone, matching each to the pre-measured screw hole depth and screw length (Fig. 3.36).
   - After fixation of all the screws, the intermaxillary ligation is released, and the head of the joint is checked to ensure that it is positioned posteriorly in the middle of the fossa and that the occlusal relationship is stable.
   - Finally, take 1 cm × 3 cm of free fat from under the skin at the retromandibular incision, encircle the neck of the mandibular prosthesis with it, and suture it to secure it in position.
   - Insert a surgical drainage tube and close the incision layer by layer (Fig. 3.37).
   - Special emphasis should be placed avoiding infection during alternating operations inside and outside the mouth, so there is a need for two sets of equipment, and when the surgeon alternates the site of operation, there must be change of surgical gowns and gloves, as well as re-sterilization of the surgical area, and the operation should proceed in strict accordance with the principle of asepsis, to prevent postoperative infection.

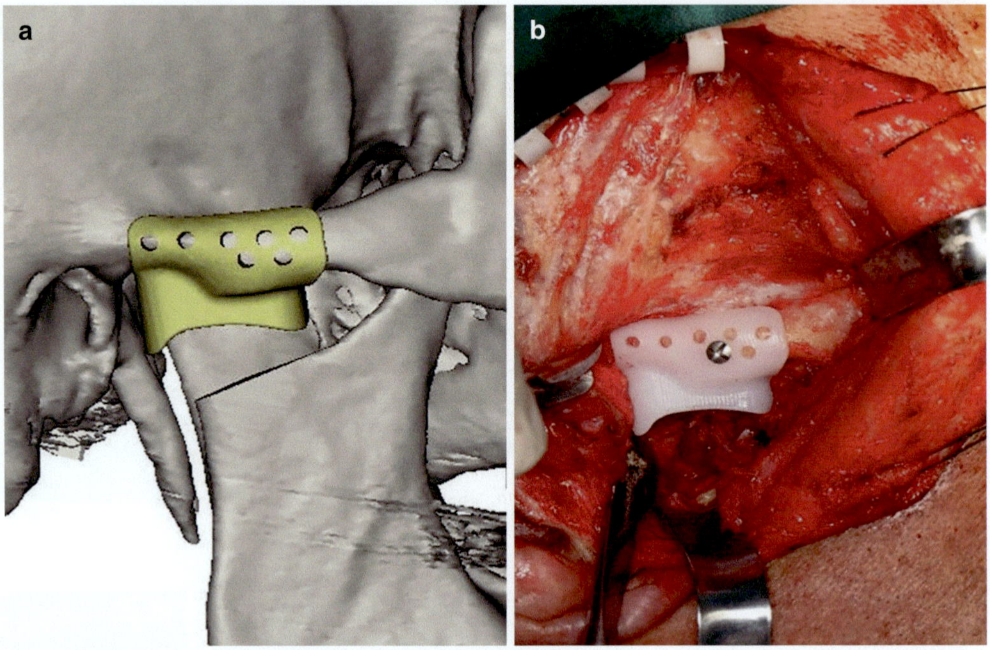

Fig. 3.35 Case A. Implantation of the fossa prosthesis. At least five screws are used to secure the prosthesis. Screw lengths have been pre-measured. (**a**) Virtual plan. (**b**) Operative view

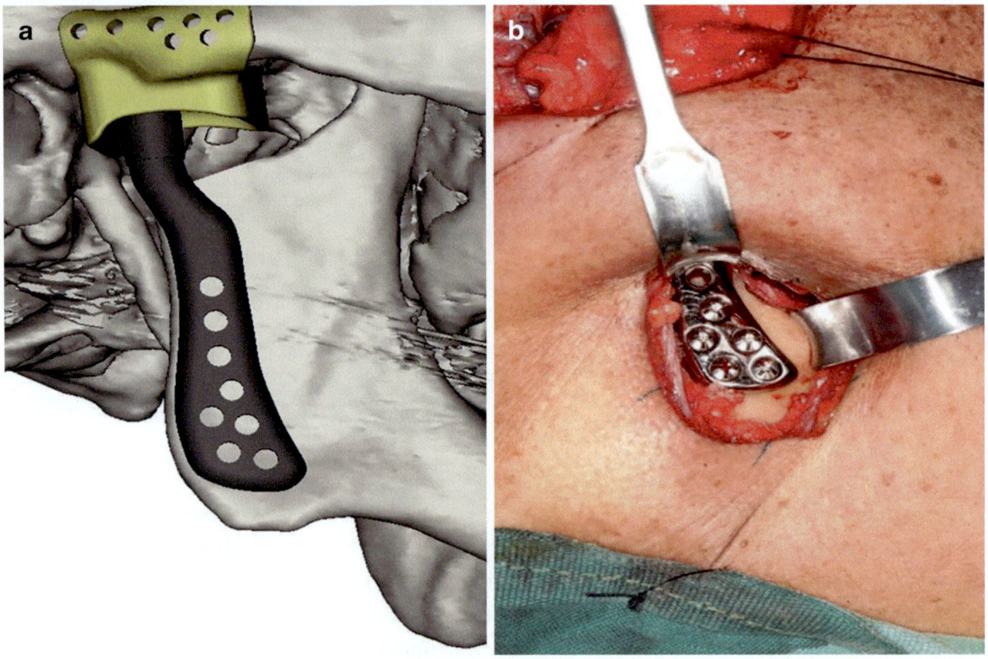

Fig. 3.36 Case A. Implantation of condylar prosthesis. After intermaxillary fixation, at least five screws are used to secure the prosthesis. Screw lengths have been pre-measured virtually. (**a**) Virtual plan. (**b**) Operative view

- Postoperative orders and nursing care
  Routine anti-inflammatory, anti-edema, and nutritional support therapy is administered. The negative-pressure drain is removed 2–3 days postoperatively, and the dressing is changed. Head and facial compression bandaging is maintained for 1 week. Sutures are removed 7–10 days after surgery. Follow-up imaging includes panoramic radiography, lateral and posteroanterior cephalograms, and CT scans. A sour-free diet should be observed for 1 month postoperatively.

- Follow-up: in the postoperative period, the condition of the patient was followed up several times. There was an aesthetic evaluation of facial shape, a functional evaluation of mouth opening, and an evaluation of the prosthesis in terms of safety and accuracy in positioning.

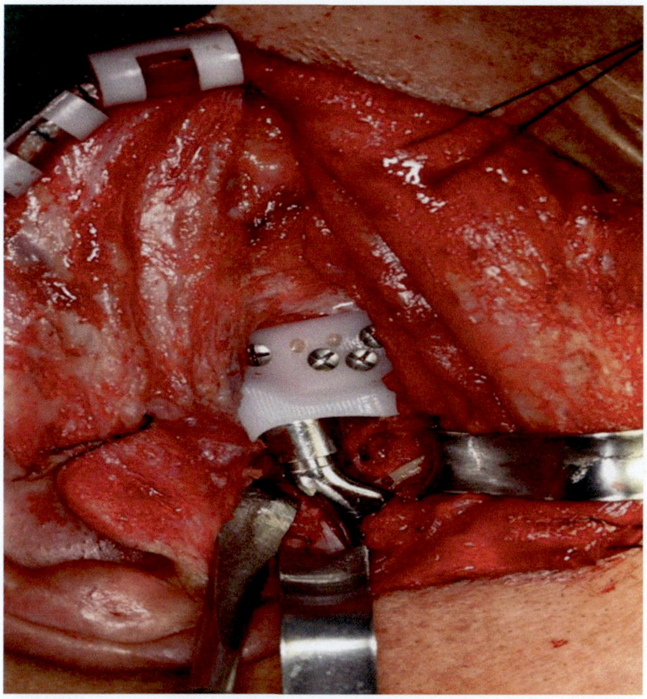

Fig. 3.37 Case A. Confirmation of position of the prosthesis and wound closure. After the prosthesis has been secured, intermaxillary fixation is removed, and the fossa-condyle position is checked. The condyle must be in the mid-posterior portion of the articular fossa prosthesis. The occlusion must remain unchanged

3.2.6 Case A. Postoperative Analysis of the Prosthesis Implantation Precision

The osteotomy guides were accurately positioned during surgery, and the prosthesis was fitted smoothly (Fig. 3.38). The comparison between the preoperative design and the postoperative CT 3D scans showed that the prosthesis position was precise (Fig. 3.39). The analysis of the postoperative prosthesis fitting error showed that the error in the core component was 0.57 mm, and the overall error in the prosthesis was 1.25 mm (Figs. 3.40 and 3.41).

3.2.7 Case A. Long-Term Follow-Up and Prognosis

- 6-year postoperative follow-up
  1. No discomfort reported; facial contour appears normal without abnormalities, and the surgical site shows no signs of redness, swelling, or other adverse reactions.
  2. Preauricular pain improved, with VAS score reduced to 1.
  3. Maximal interincisal opening (MIO): improved to 35 mm, with 6 mm lateral movement to the affected side and 4 mm lateral movement to the healthy side, while the mouth opening was deviated to the affected side by 4 mm.
  4. Chewing function: normal diet.
  5. Occlusal relationship: stable, the same as before surgery (Fig. 3.42).
  6. Prosthesis evaluation: the prosthesis was free of complications such as infection, rejection, loosening, displacement, fracture, osteogenesis outside of normal structures, and allergy (Fig. 3.43).

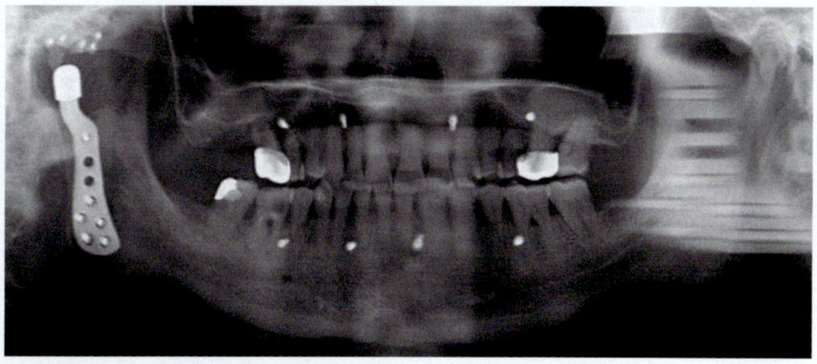

Fig. 3.38 Case A. Immediate postoperative OPG

3.2.8 Case A. Advantages and Disadvantages

- Advantages
  1. Safety and effectiveness of the clinical application of the prosthesis: during 6 years of follow-up, the clinical symptoms improved, the mandibular motor function improved, the masticatory function was normal, the original occlusal relationship was maintained, and there were no adverse reactions or complications.
  2. The processing concept is more advanced, using 3D printing to manufacture the customized total joint prosthesis.
  3. Improvement of symptoms and recovery of important functions, including basic disappearance of pain, significant improvement of mandibular motor function, increase in mouth opening, and maintenance of the original occlusal relationship.
- Disadvantages
  1. The articular fossa prosthesis does not form osseointegration with the bony surface and is only held in place by screws, with a theoretical risk of prosthesis loosening.
  2. Can a posterior mandibular incision be omitted, and a single preauricular incision be used to complete all surgical procedures?
  3. It might be explored whether the prosthesis can be fitted accurately without intermaxillary ligation, which would make the surgery faster and simpler and reduce the risk of postoperative infection.

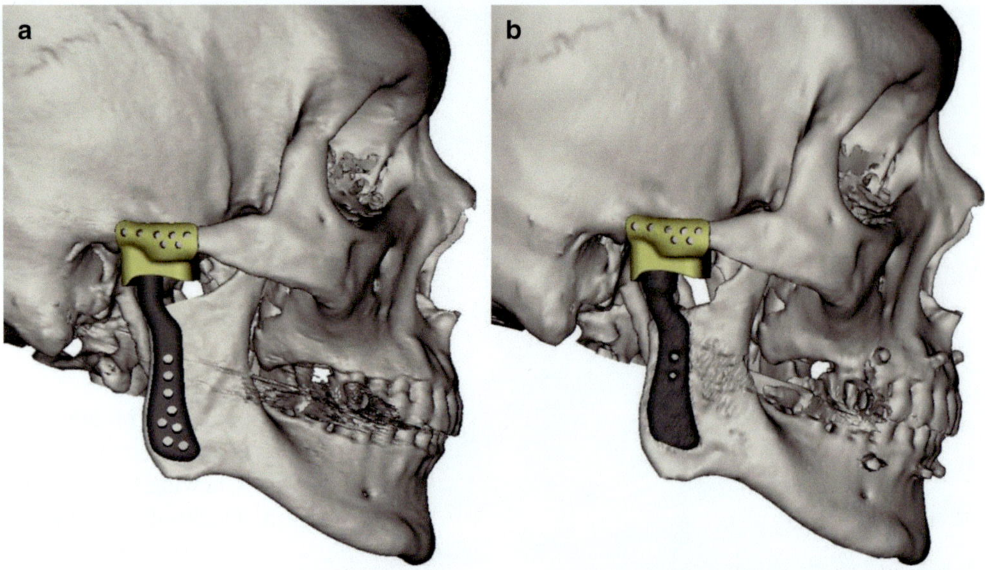

Fig. 3.39 Case A. Comparison of CT 3D scans showing precise prosthesis placement. (**a**) Preoperative design. (**b**) Immediate postoperative result

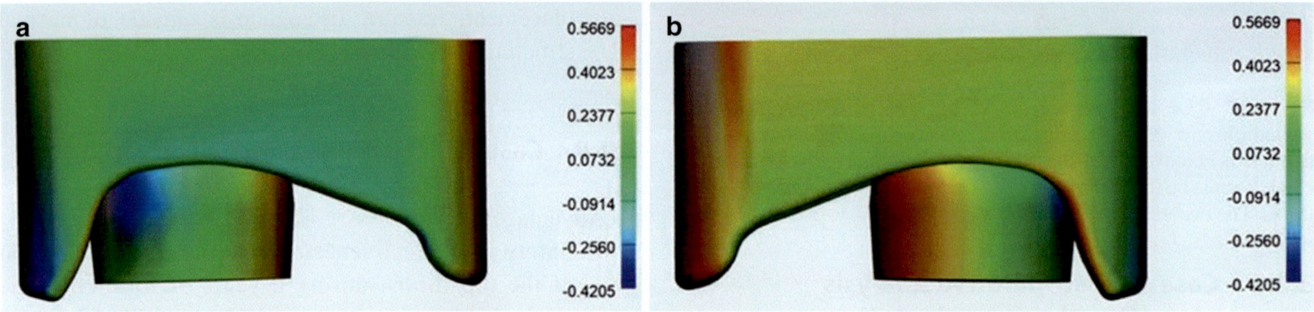

Fig. 3.40 Case A. Prosthetic core error of 0.57 mm. (**a**) Lateral error. (**b**) Medial error

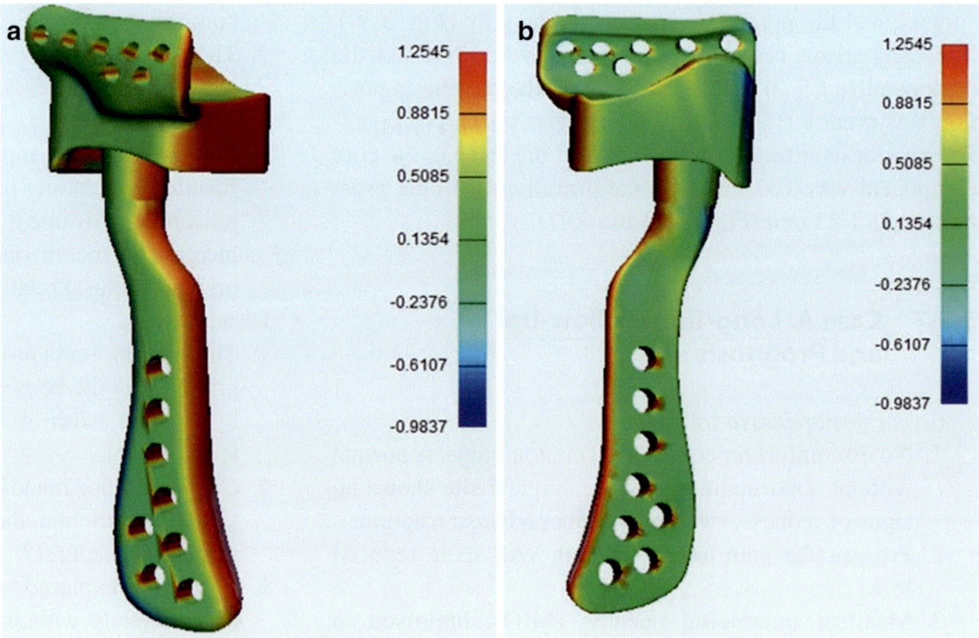

Fig. 3.41 Case A. Overall prosthesis error of 1.25 mm. (**a**) Lateral error. (**b**) Medial error

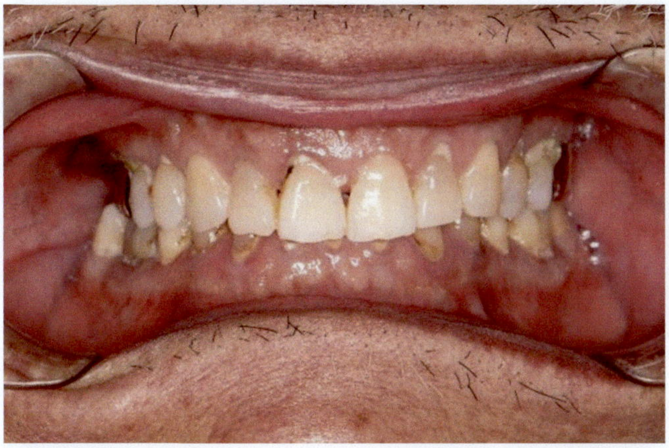

Fig. 3.42 Case A. Stable intraoral occlusal relationship at 6 years postoperatively\

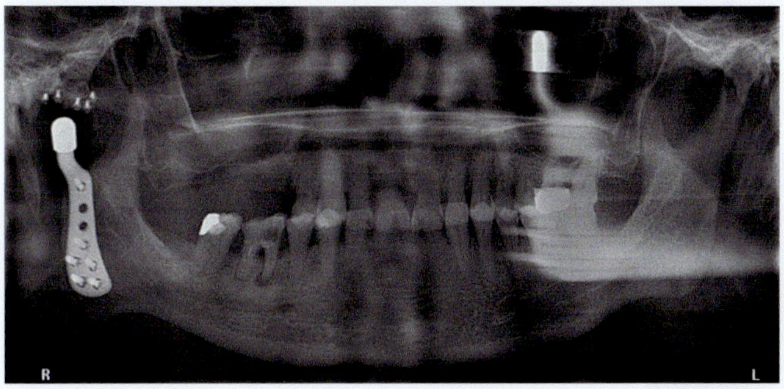

Fig. 3.43 Case A. 6-year postoperative panoramic view

4. The prosthesis error analyzed in this case includes not only the implantation error but also the manufacturing error and fitting error, and the resulting calculation is the sum of the three errors, which is a problem that exists in the calculation of all the prosthesis implantations in this book. To attain greater precision, this is a complication that urgently needs to be solved.

3.3 Design and Surgical Technique Innovation: A Total TMJ Prosthesis with Mandibular Self-Positioning Design

3.3.1 Case B: Implantation of a Total TMJ Prosthesis with Mandibular Self-Positioning Design and One Less Surgical Incision

- Patient information: female, 51 years old.
- Complaint: right preauricular pain with limited mouth opening for more than 2 years.
- History: the patient reported a 2-year history of unexplained right preauricular pain accompanied by limited mouth opening and mandibular deviation to the left.
- Past medical history: sustained fractures of the clavicle, right thigh, and lower leg due to trauma 19 years ago, with good postoperative recovery. No history of systemic diseases. No known drug or food allergies.
- Clinical examination. Facial appearance: leftward deviation without significant swelling. Right preauricular region: tenderness present, with a pain VAS score of 5 (Fig. 3.44). Mouth opening: restricted, with a maximal interincisal opening (MIO) of 20 mm and leftward deviation upon opening. Intraoral examination: stable occlusion; periodontal and dental conditions were satisfactory (Fig. 3.45).
- Imaging examination: MRI showed right condylar hyperplasia, perforation of the disc, and disappearance of the disc body (Fig. 3.46); CT showed abnormal morphology of the right condyle (Fig. 3.47).
- Diagnosis: suspected right condylar hyperplasia.
- Postoperative pathology. Microscopic description: osseous hyperplasia with proliferation of surface bone, cartilage, and fibrous tissue, along with localized surface bone

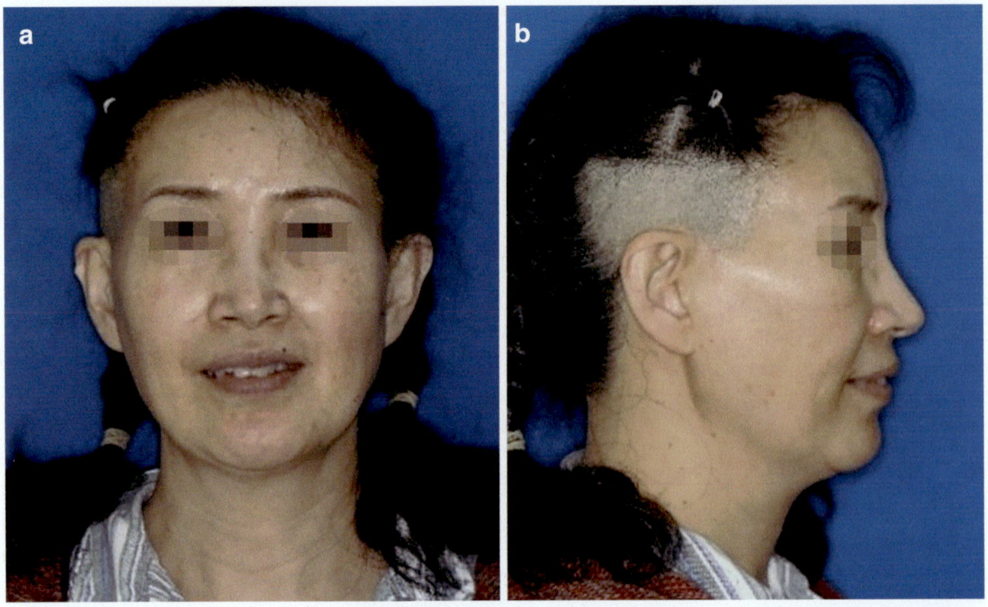

Fig. 3.44 Case B. Facial examination. There is fullness in front of the right ear. (**a**) Frontal view. (**b**) Lateral view

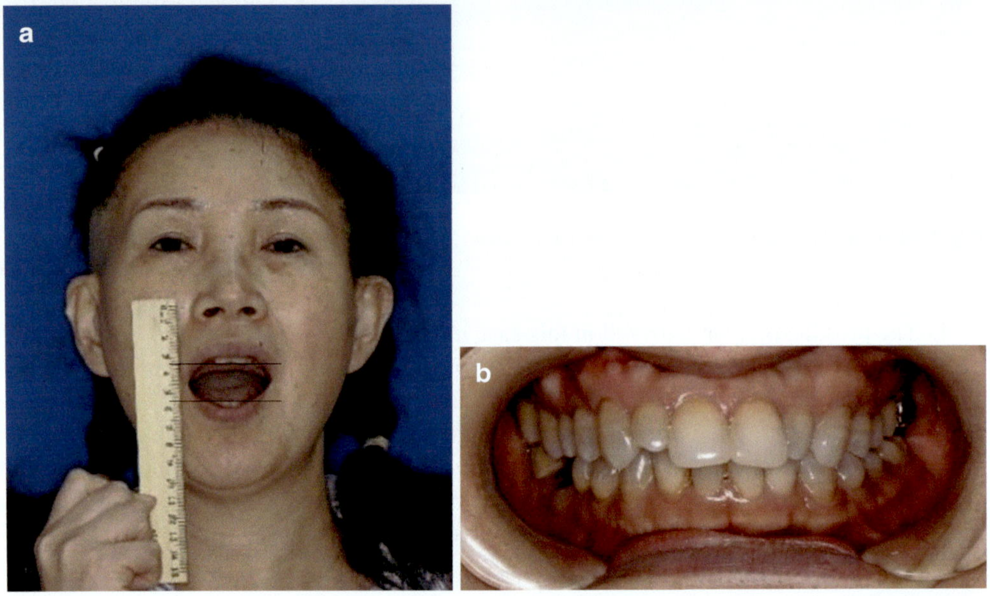

Fig. 3.45 Case B. Intraoral examination. (**a**) Maximum interincisal opening was 20 mm. (**b**) Occlusal relationship was stable

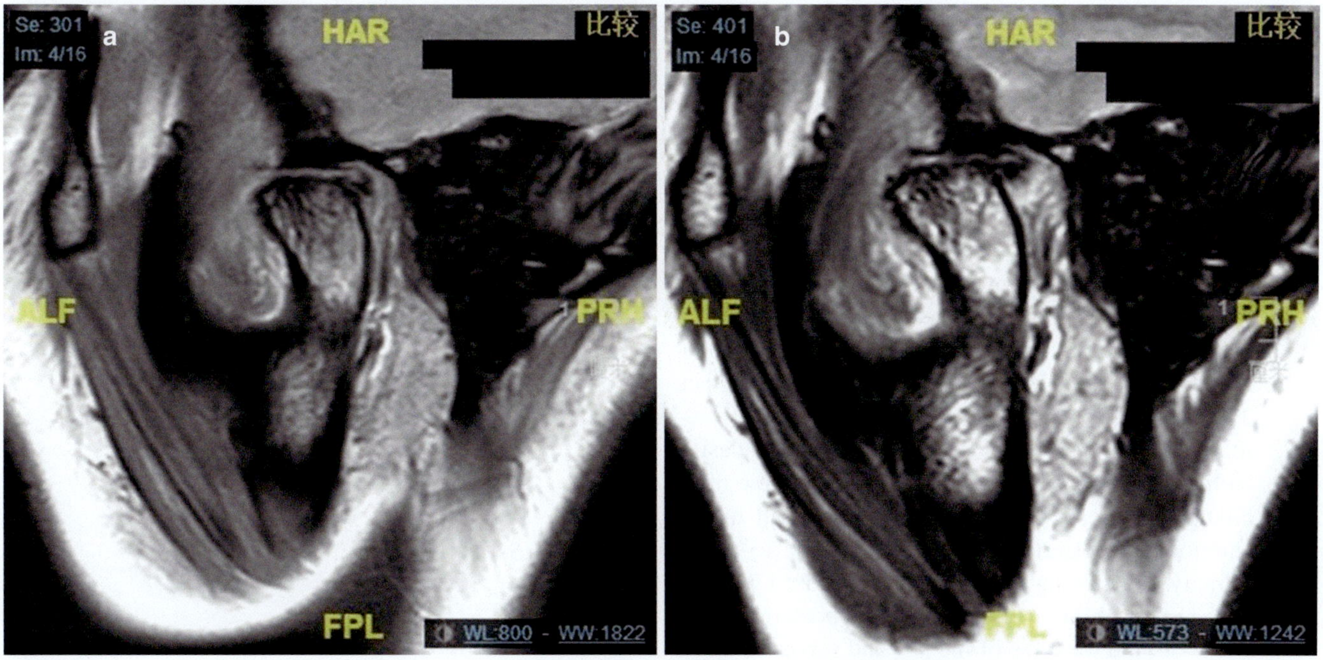

Fig. 3.46 Case B. TMJ MRI. Hypertrophy and flattening of the right condyle, with thinning and perforation of the disc. (**a**) Closed position. (**b**) Open position

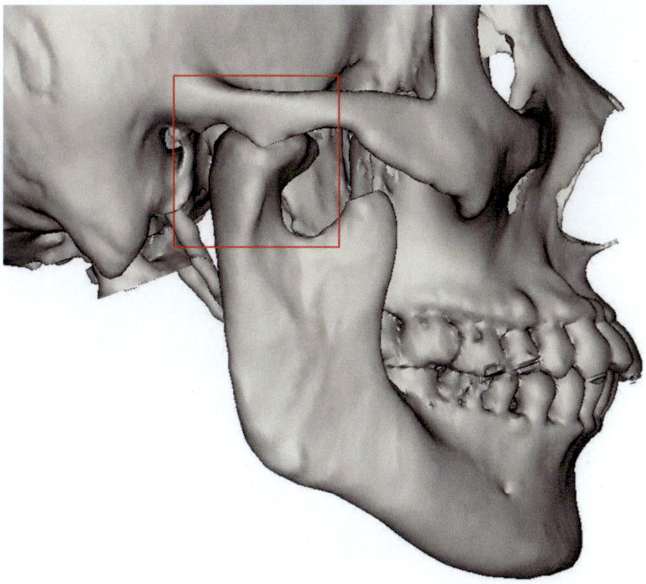

Fig. 3.47 Case B. 3D reconstruction of the maxillofacial CT. Hypertrophy of the right condyle (red box)

resorption and hyperplasia. Pathological diagnosis: "right condyle" hyperplasia.

3.3.2 Case B. Diagnostic Imaging

3.3.3 Case B: Treatment Plan

- Overall treatment plan: excision of the right condyle and reconstruction of the TMJ with a customized total joint prosthesis (new design with self-positioning mandible prosthesis)
- Virtual surgical planning:
  - Design of the resection scope: resection of the diseased condyle from the condylar head to the subcondylar process; removal of the lower half of the articular eminence

– Digital simulation of the surgery: the same as described in Sect. 3.2.3, Digital Simulation of the Surgery

3.3.4 Case B: Design and Processing of the Prosthesis and the Cutting Guides

- Design of the mandibular prosthesis component
  1. Placement of the core components is described in Sect. 2.4.1 in Chap. 2.
  2. Mandibular extension design is described in Sect. 2.4.2 in Chap. 2.

     In addition to the typical total TMJ prosthesis design with fossa and mandible components, this new mandibular prosthesis has been fitted with small upper-anterior and posterior extensions, "wings" to aid in primary positioning during surgery and to provide long-term stability (Fig. 3.48). The posterior wing wraps around the edge of the jaw and serves to fix its precise position; the upper anterior flange closely follows the contours of the bone.
  3. Measurement of screw length: measure the thickness of the prosthesis plus the mandibular bone to determine the length of the screws at each point (Fig. 3.49).

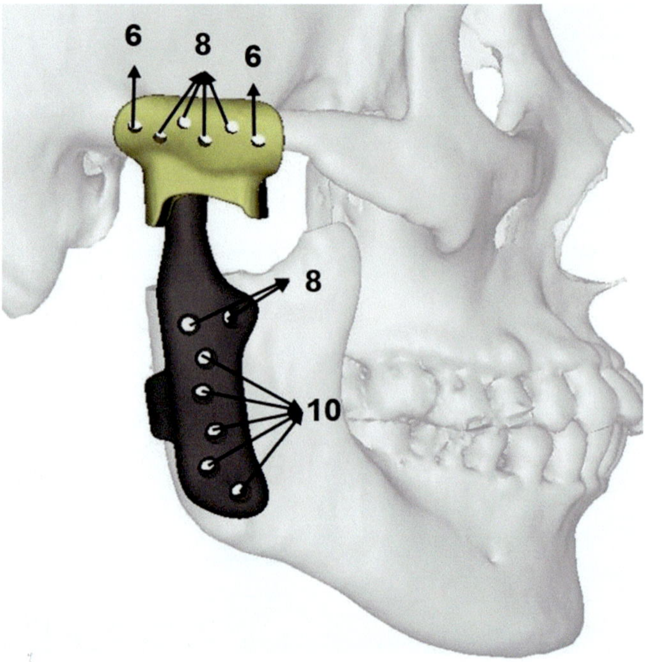

Fig. 3.49 Case B. Screw length measurement (mm)

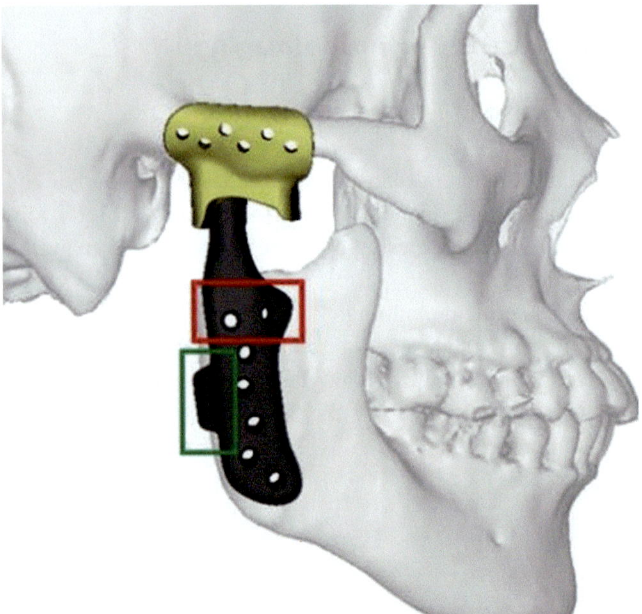

Fig. 3.48 Case B. Self-positioning wing plate. The mandibular fixation component fits precisely to the surface of the ramus. Two holes (red rectangle) in the upper portion of the fixation component are the same holes used to stabilize the cutting guide. The posterior wing plate (green rectangle) surrounds the posterior border of the ramus. These allow for autonomous positioning of the condylar prosthesis, without intermaxillary fixation

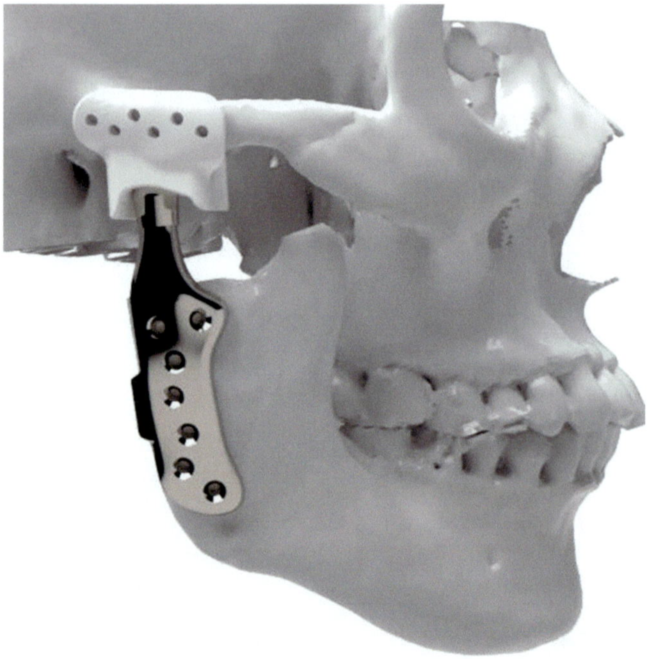

Fig. 3.50 Case B. Prosthesis test fitting on the skull model of the patient

- Fabrication and test fitting of the prosthesis

  See Chap. 2, Sect. 2.5 (Fig. 3.50).

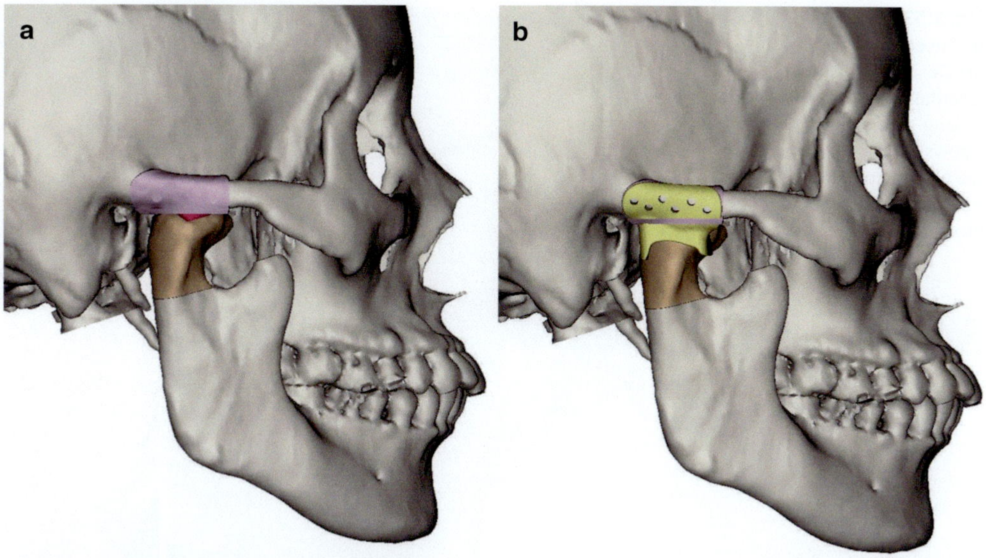

Fig. 3.51 Case B. Eminence cutting guide. (**a**) Cutting guide (pink) design. (**b**) Articular fossa prosthesis (yellow) screw holes and guide plate (pink, pictured underneath) screw holes are in the same position

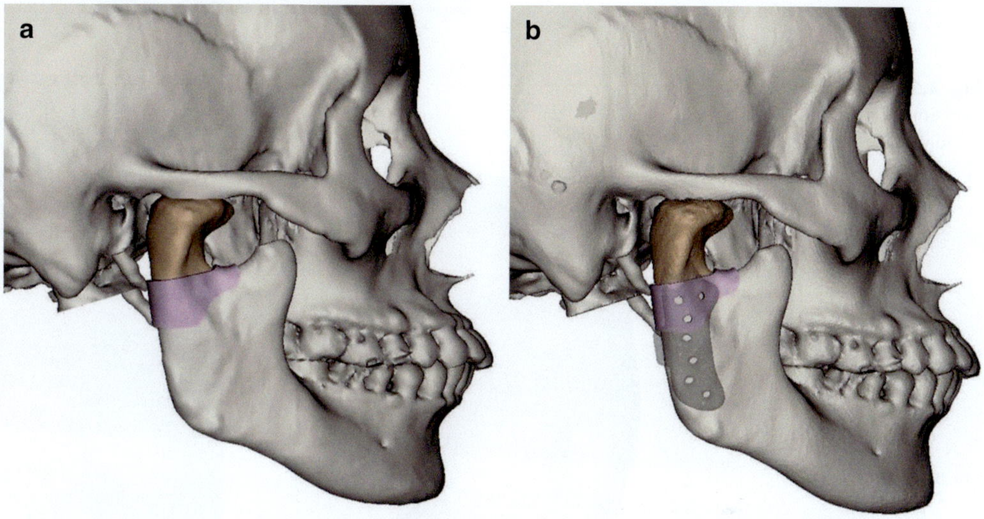

Fig. 3.52 Case B. Subcondylar cutting guide. (**a**) Guide plate (pink) design. (**b**) Guide plate (pink) screw holes and mandibular prosthesis (gray) screw holes are in the same position for at least two screws at the top. Another four screw holes are placed farther down on the mandible prosthesis extension

- Design of the cutting guides
  1. Eminence cutting guide design: the guide is designed to follow the osteotomy line, and the fossa prosthesis screw hole positions are transferred to the guide (Fig. 3.51).
  2. Subcondylar cutting guide design: the guide is designed to follow the osteotomy line; the cutting guide and the mandibular prosthesis share at least two screw hole positions (Fig. 3.52).

3.3.5 Case B. Surgical Procedure

- Preoperative laboratory tests: the same as described in Sect. 3.2.5, Preoperative Laboratory Tests.
- Preoperative Preparation: the same as described in Sect. 3.2.5, Preoperative Preparation.
- Steps of the surgical procedure
  1. Surgical approach: a modified preauricular-temporal incision and a small transbuccal incision was used.
  2. Subcondylar osteotomy: install the subcondylar cutting guide, use two screws to secure the guide plate (Fig. 3.53), plan the osteotomy according to the guide plate, perform the subcondylar osteotomy, and resect the diseased condyle (Fig. 3.54).
  3. Eminence osteotomy: the eminence cutting guide is positioned and secured with two screws; the osteotomy is performed (Fig. 3.55).
  4. Implantation of the prosthesis: implantation and fixation of the fossa prosthesis in accordance with the original two screw holes in the eminence cutting guide. The mandibular prosthesis is inserted through the preauricular incision and preliminarily fixed in place with screws placed in the original two screw holes made for the subcondylar cutting guide (Fig. 3.56).

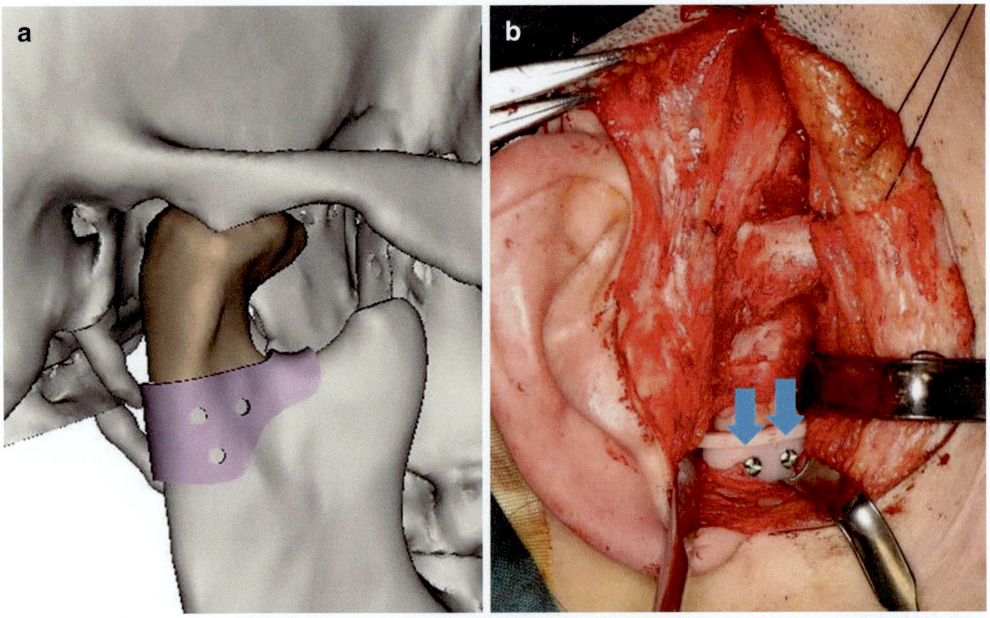

Fig. 3.53 Case B. Subcondylar osteotomy. (**a**) Design. (**b**) Actual, installation of the subcondylar cutting guide (pink) with two screws (blue arrows), which are also the preferred fixation holes for the mandibular prosthesis

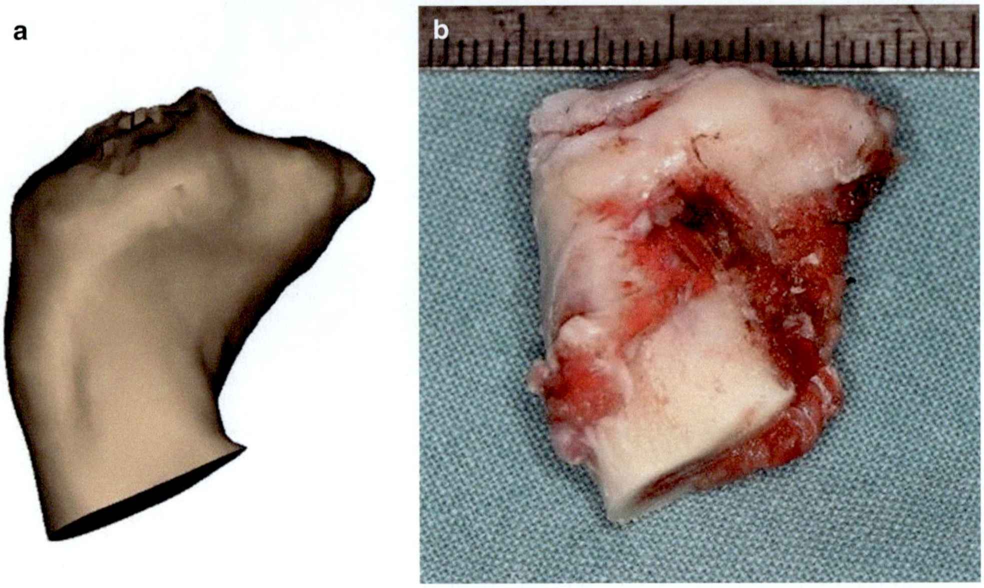

Fig. 3.54 Case B. Precise excision of the condyle. (**a**) Virtual plan. (**b**) Surgical specimen

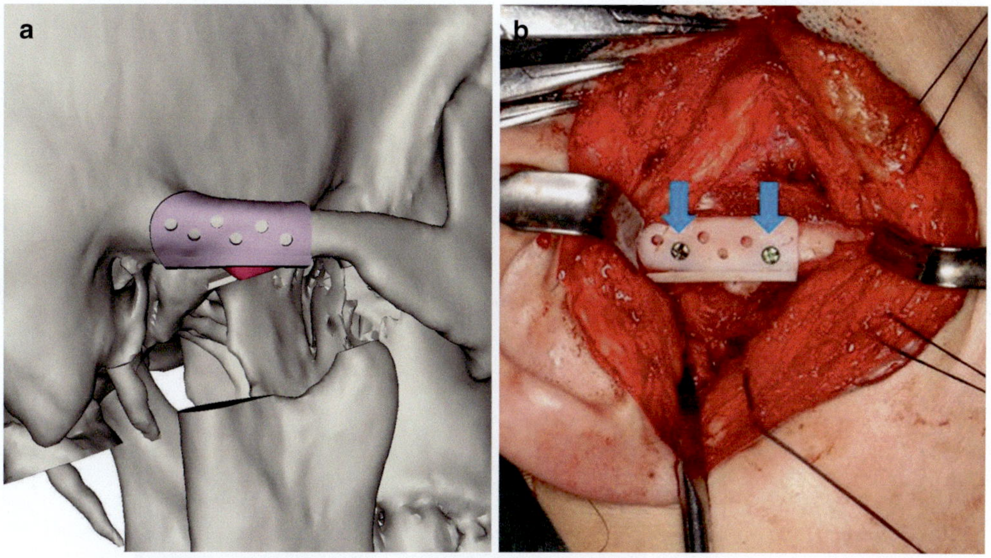

Fig. 3.55 Case B. Eminence osteotomy. The cutting guide (purple in virtual plan) was digitally designed to fit the zygomatic arch. It was stabilized with two screws (blue arrows in the operative view) while the osteotomy was performed according to the guide. (**a**) Design. (**b**) Actual

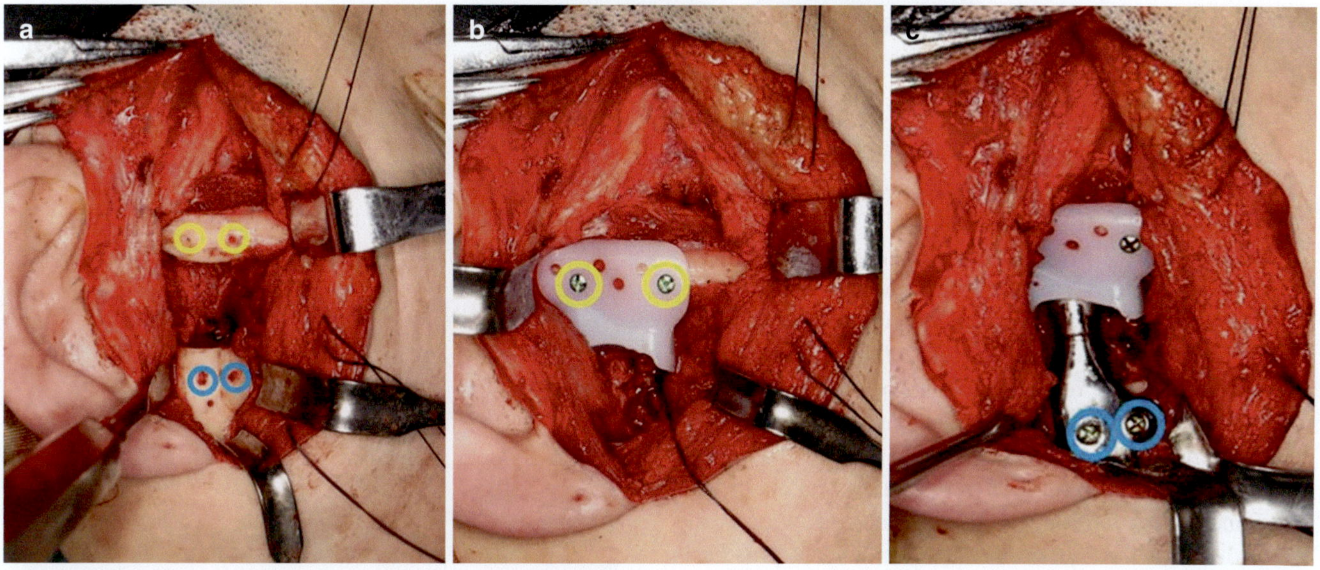

Fig. 3.56 Case B. Prosthesis implantation. The small yellow circles show the eminence cutting guide screw holes, while the small blue circles show the mandibular cutting guide screw hole sites. (**a**) Screw holes after the two cutting guides have been removed (small yellow and blue circles). (**b**) Fossa prosthesis fixation with two screws at first (large yellow circles). (**c**) Securing the mandibular prosthesis first with two screws in the two holes left by the cutting guide (large blue circles)

Fig. 3.57 Case B. Endoscopically assisted fixation of the mandibular prosthesis. (**a**) Actual. (**b**) Schematic

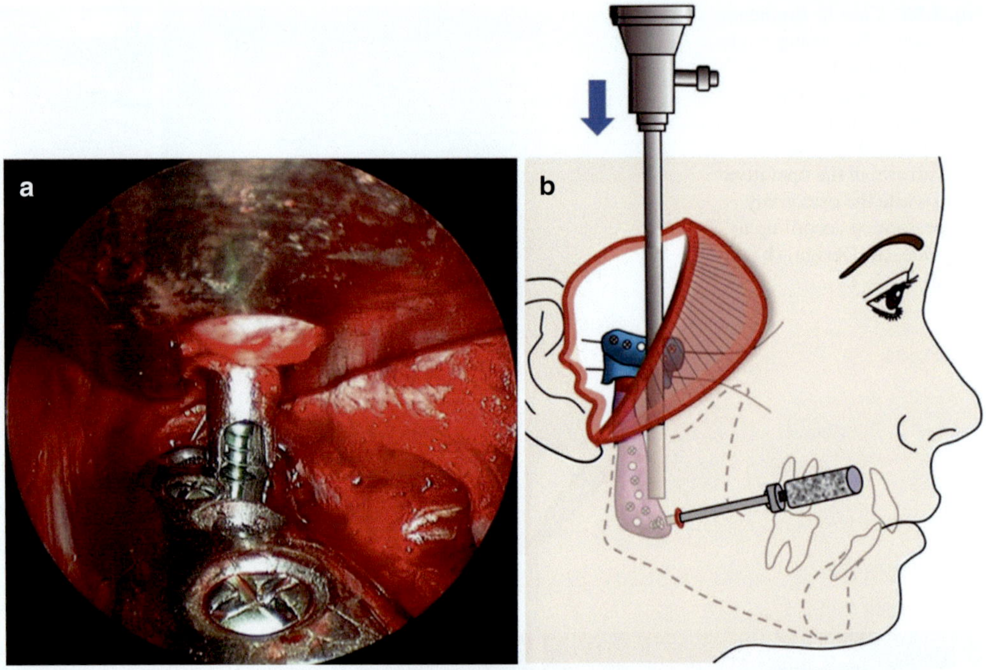

5. Endoscopic-assisted mandibular prosthesis fixation: using endoscopic-assisted manipulation, fix the mandibular prosthesis securely with several more screws in the planned holes of the mandibular prosthesis extension (Fig. 3.57). The mandibular prosthesis can be affixed without the need for a retromandibular incision, but through only the modified preauricular incision plus a small incision through the cheek. After fixation is complete, the occlusal relationship must be checked to ensure that the fossa prosthesis and condylar prosthesis are in a correct relationship (Fig. 3.58).
6. Treatment of the surgical area: take 1 cm × 3 cm of subcutaneous free fat from preauricular incision, wrap it, and fix around the neck of the mandibular prosthesis (Fig. 3.59).

- Postoperative orders and nursing care: see Sect. 3.2.5, Postoperative Orders and Nursing Care.
- Follow-up: see Sect. 3.2.5, Follow-Up.

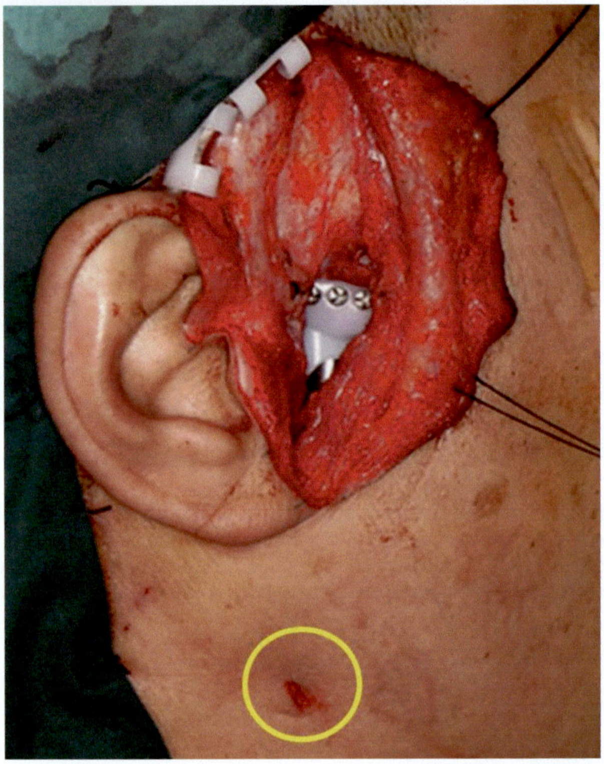

Fig. 3.58 Case B. The mandibular prosthesis can be screwed securely to the mandible using only a modified preauricular incision and a small incision through the cheek (yellow circle), with the assistance of an endoscope and transbuccal trocar

3.3.6 Case B. Postoperative Analysis of Prosthesis Implantation Precision

The cutting guides were accurately positioned during surgery, and the prosthesis was fitted smoothly (Fig. 3.60). The comparison between the preoperative design and the postoperative CT 3D scans showed that the prosthesis position was precise (Fig. 3.61). The analysis of the postoperative prosthesis fitting error showed that the error in the core compo-

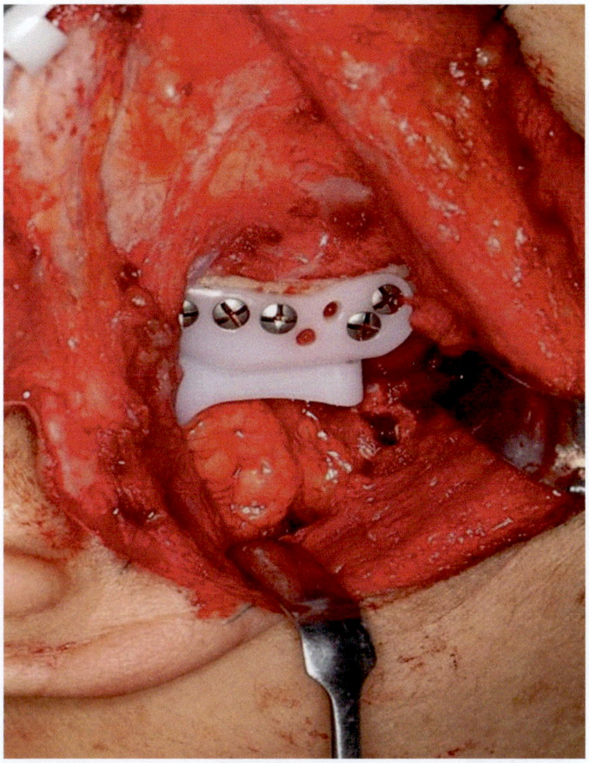

Fig. 3.59 A 1 × 3 cm subcutaneous fat graft was used to fill the dead space surrounding the condylar prosthesis

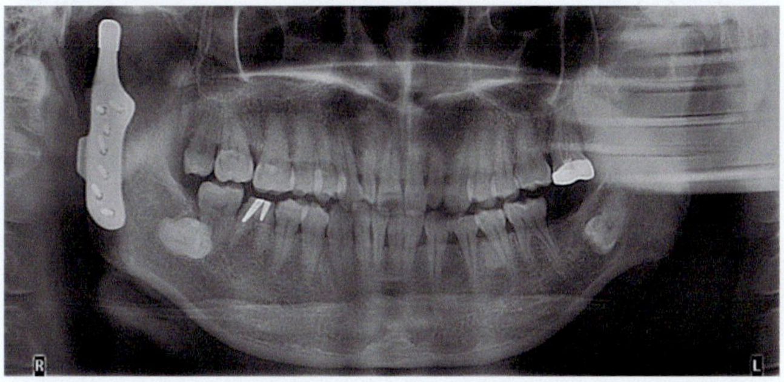

Fig. 3.60 Case B. Immediate postoperative panoramic film

nent was 0.54 mm, and the overall error in the prosthesis position was 1.07 mm (Figs. 3.62 and 3.63).

3.3.7 Case B. Long-Term Follow-Up and Prognosis

- One-year postoperative follow-up
  1. No complaints of discomfort, good facial appearance with no abnormalities, no redness or swelling in the operative area, or other reactions (Fig. 3.64).
  2. No obvious pain in front of the ear, VAS pain score improved to 1, joint-mandibular-occlusal-facial coordination, and stable occlusal relationship (Fig. 3.65).
  3. Mouth opening improved to 32 mm, with 6 mm lateral movement to the affected side and 6 mm lateral movement to the healthy side, although the mouth opening was deviated 5 mm to the affected side.
  4. Evaluation of prosthesis: the prosthesis was free from complications such as infection, rejection, loosening, displacement, fracture, ectopic osteogenesis, and allergy (Figs. 3.66 and 3.67).

- Three-year postoperative follow-up

The mouth opening improved to 38 mm, and the preauricular pain VAS score improved to 0 (no pain) (Figs. 3.68, 3.69, 3.70, and 3.71). The rest was the same as the 1-year postoperative follow-up.

3.3.8 Case B. Advantages and Disadvantages

- Advantages

The design goal of the innovation was achieved. The mandible prosthesis extension with self-positioning wings, an innovation over the standard design scheme, demonstrated that the digitally designed total TMJ prosthesis and cutting

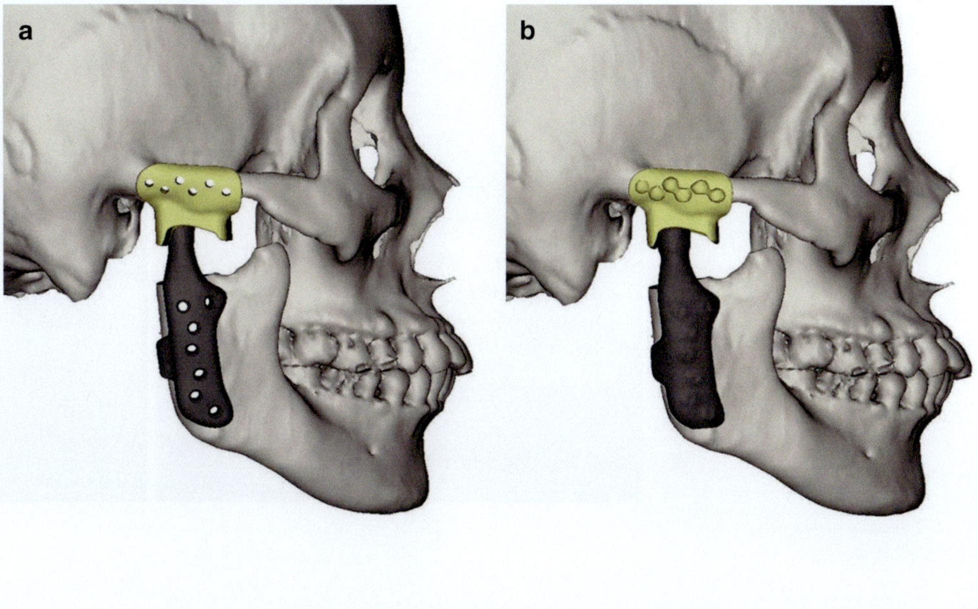

Fig. 3.61 Case B. Comparison of CT 3D scans showing precise prosthesis placement. (**a**) Preoperative design. (**b**) Immediate postoperative CT

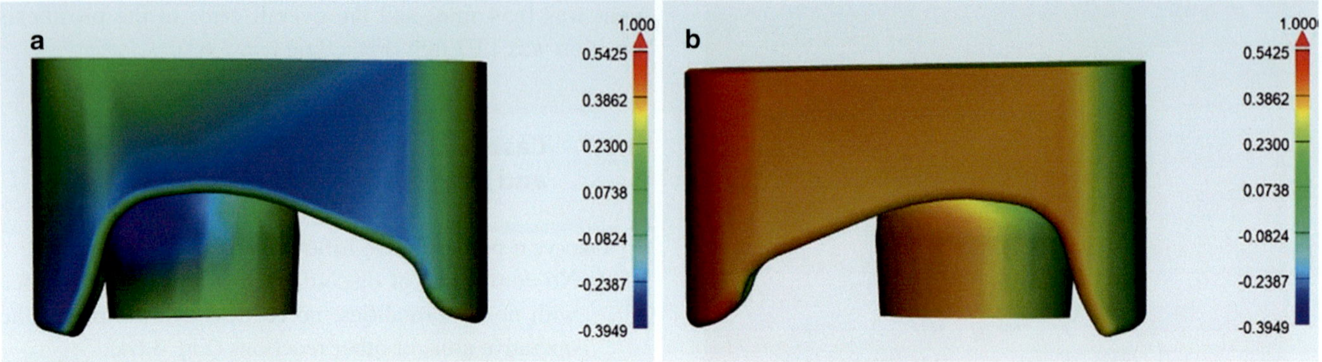

Fig. 3.62 Case B. Prosthetic core component error 0.54 mm. (**a**) Lateral error. (**b**) Medial error

Fig. 3.63 Case B. Overall prosthesis error of 1.07 mm. (**a**) Lateral error. (**b**) Medial error

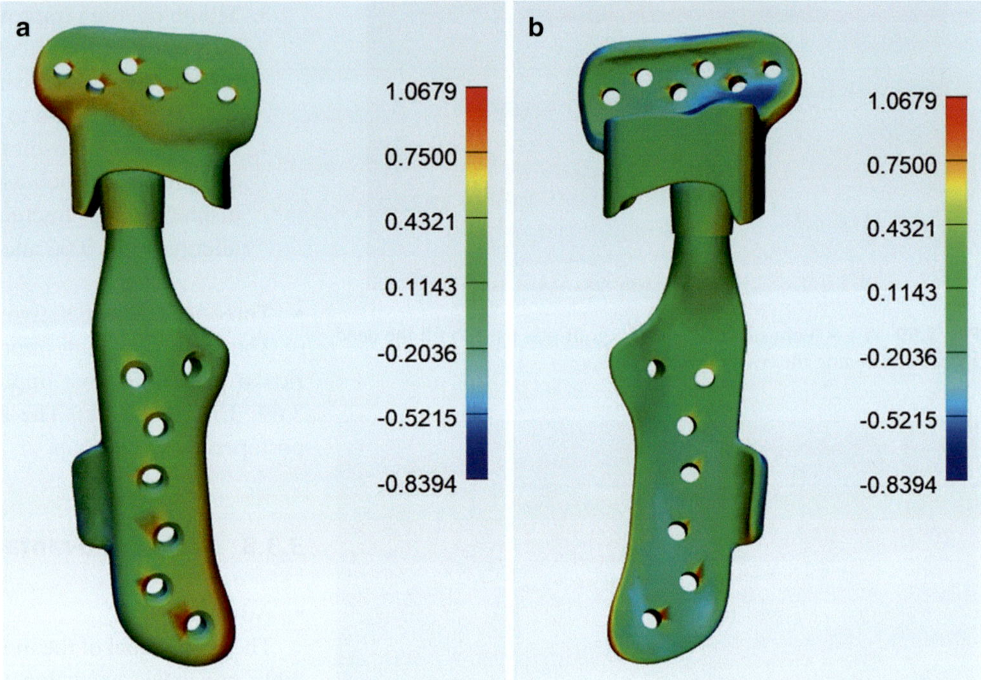

Fig. 3.64 Case B. Good facial shape at 1-year postoperative follow-up. (**a**) Frontal view. (**b**) Lateral view

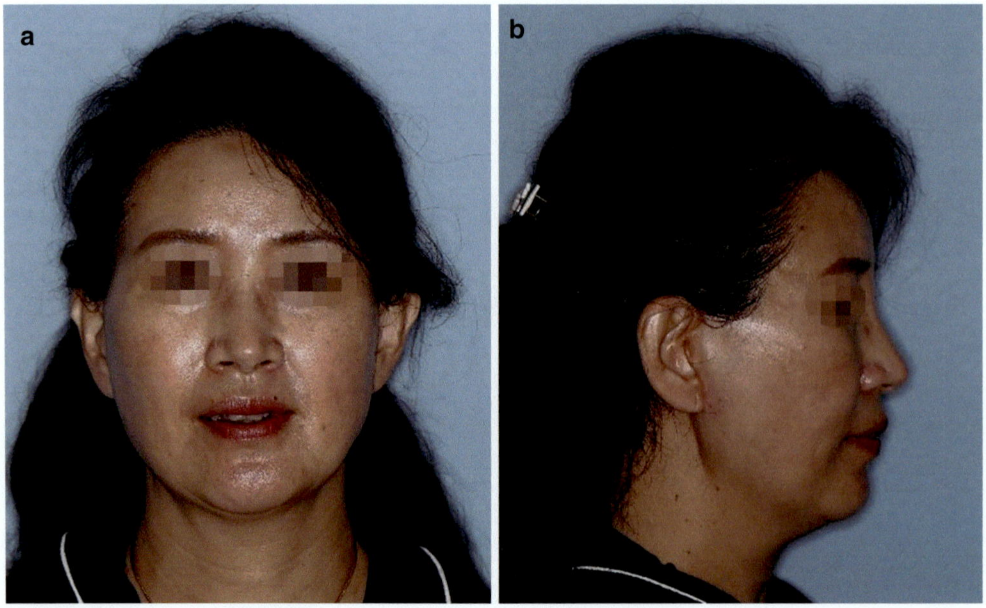

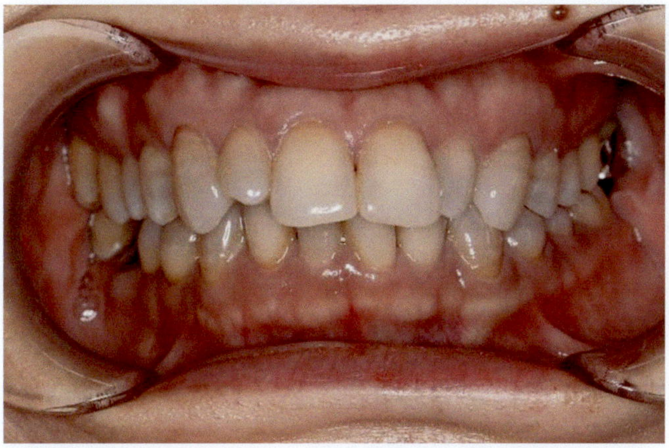

Fig. 3.65 Case B. Stable intraoral occlusal relationship at 1 year after surgery

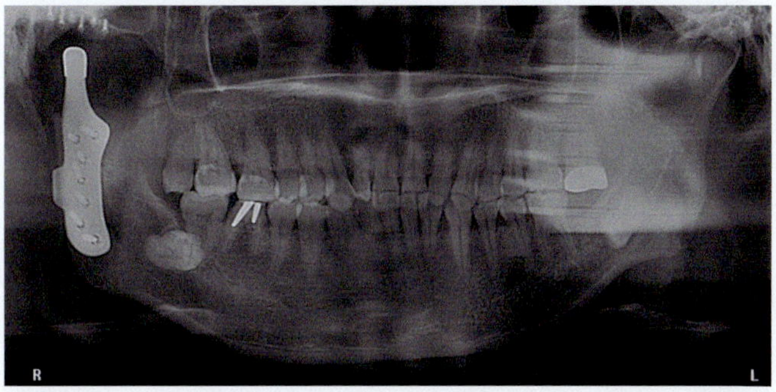

Fig. 3.66 Case B. 1-year postoperative panoramic view

guides can work together to realize the precise fitting of the prosthesis. This precise fitting can be obtained without the need for a retromandibular incision and intermaxillary ligation. Only a single incision through the cheek combined with endoscopy can accurately fix the position of the mandibular prosthesis. This can make the surgery minimally invasive, safer, and less time-consuming and reduce risk of postoperative infections.

- Disadvantages
  1. The problem of reattaching the lateral pterygoid muscle has not yet been solved. The result is insufficient forward gliding of the prosthetic condyle, manifested by poor recovery of protrusive and lateral movements, and deviation on mouth opening.
  2. The problem of lack of osseointegration of the articular fossa has not been solved.
  3. Customized design of core components has not yet been achieved.

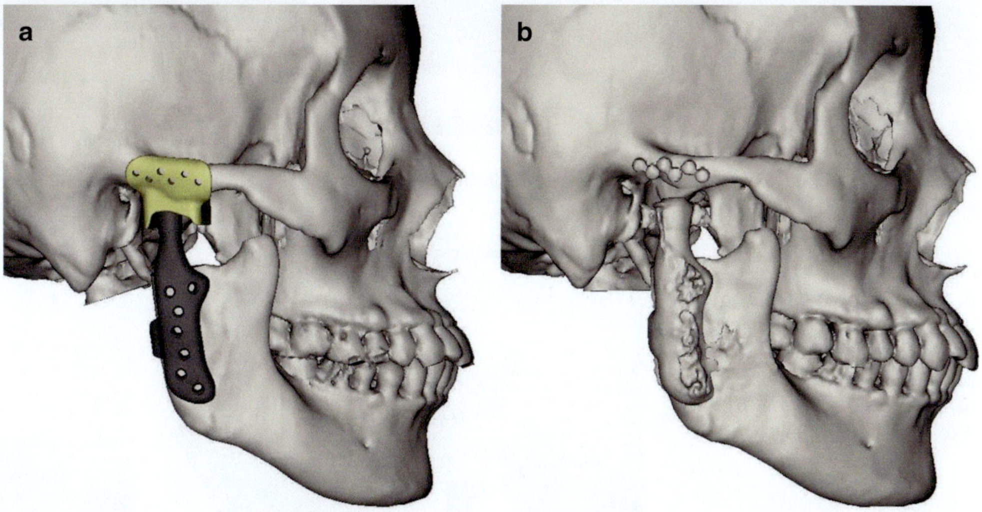

Fig. 3.67 Case B. Comparison of CT 3D scans at 1 year postoperatively showing precise placement of the prosthesis. (**a**) Preoperative design. (**b**) 1 year postoperatively

Fig. 3.68 Case B. Good facial shape at 3-year follow-up. (**a**) Frontal view. (**b**) Lateral view

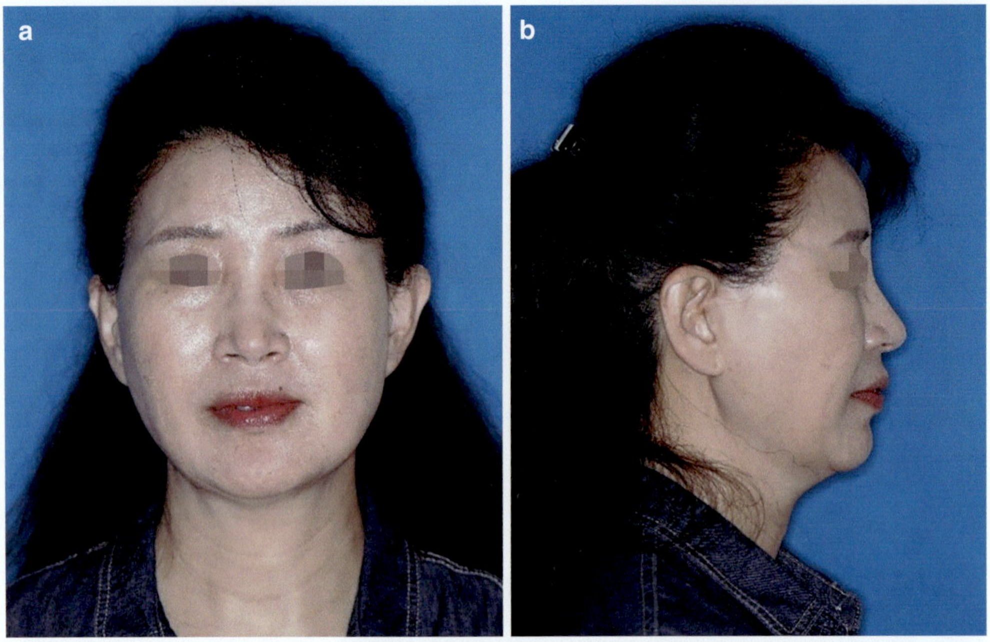

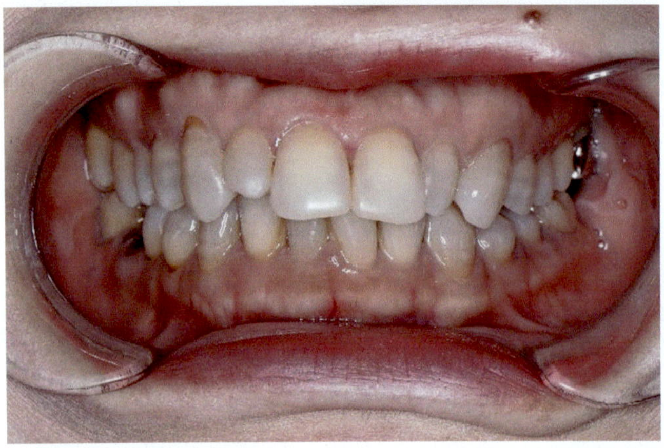

Fig. 3.69 Case B. Stable intraoral occlusal relationship at 3 years postoperatively

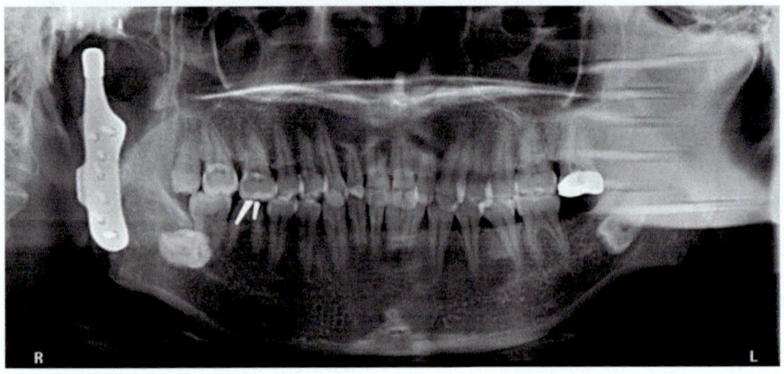

Fig. 3.70 Case B. 3-year postoperative panoramic view

Fig. 3.71 Case B. Comparison of CT 3D scans at 3 years postoperatively showing accurate prosthesis placement. (**a**) Preoperative design. (**b**) 3 years postoperatively

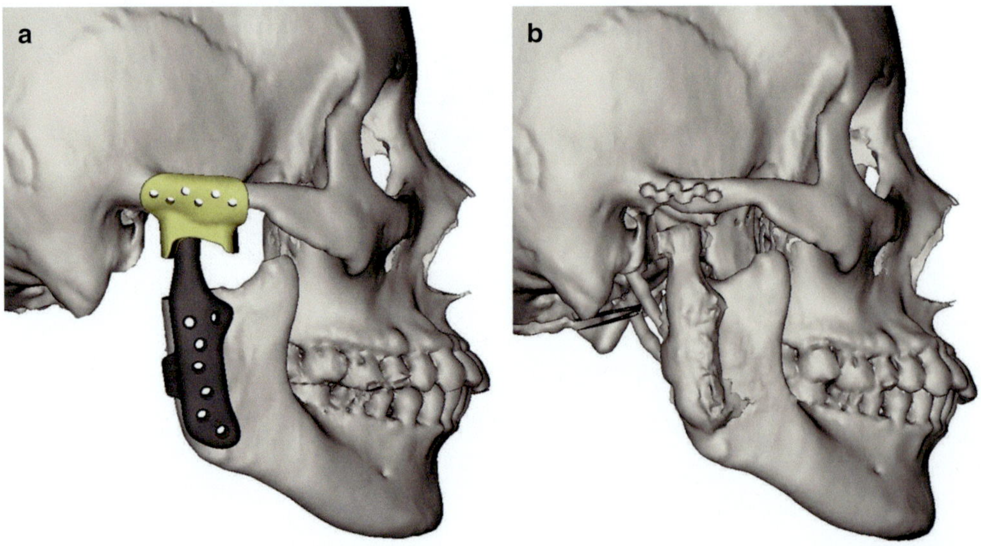

3.4 Materials Innovation: Metallic/Nonmetallic Fossa Prosthesis for Osteointegration of the TMJ Prosthesis

Chi Yang, Shanyong Zhang, and Jisi Zheng

3.4.1 Case C. Design and Application of a Metallic/Nonmetallic Articular Fossa for the Total TMJ Prosthesis

- Patient information: female, 56 years old.
- Complaint: right preauricular pain, crepitus, limited mouth opening for more than 1 year.
- History: the patient presented 1 year ago with right preauricular pain, crepitus, and with limited mouth opening; non-surgical treatment was ineffective over the past year.
- Past history: history of systemic disease was denied.
- Clinical examination: right preauricular region had marked tenderness, and pain VAS score of 6 out of 10. Crepitus is detectable, maximum mouth opening was only 17 mm. Intraoral occlusal relationship was stable (Figs. 3.72 and 3.73).
- Imaging examination: panoramic radiograph confirmed that the teeth left upper second molar and left lower first molar were missing (Fig. 3.74). An MRI of the TMJ showed severe bone destruction of the right condyle, with cystic changes, and anterior disc displacement and deformation, with perforation (Fig. 3.75). CT scan of the max-

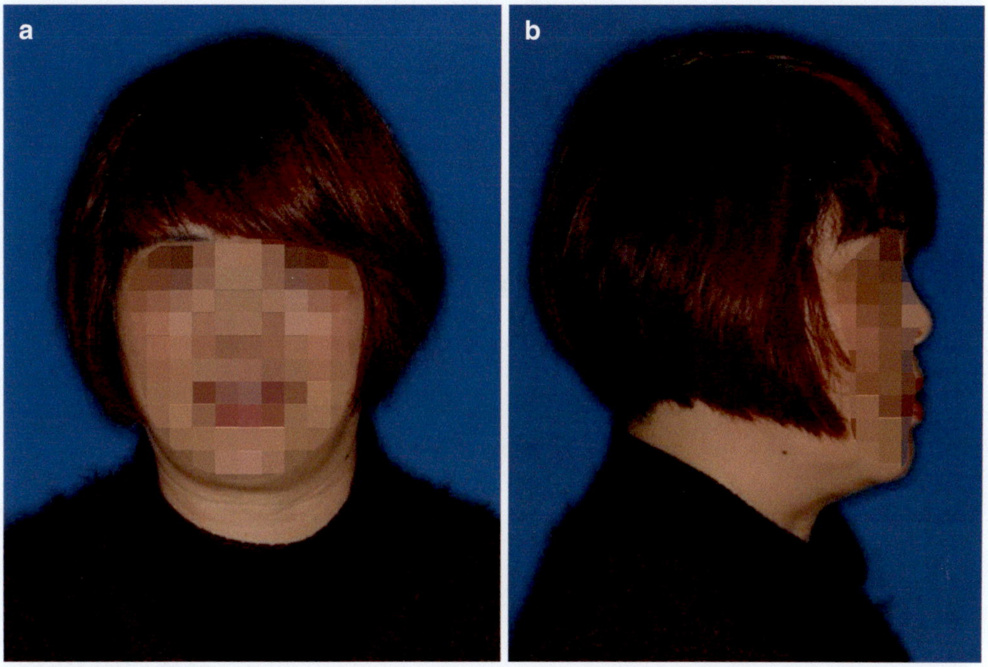

Fig. 3.72 Case C. Facial examination. The face was symmetrical. (**a**) Frontal view. (**b**) Lateral view

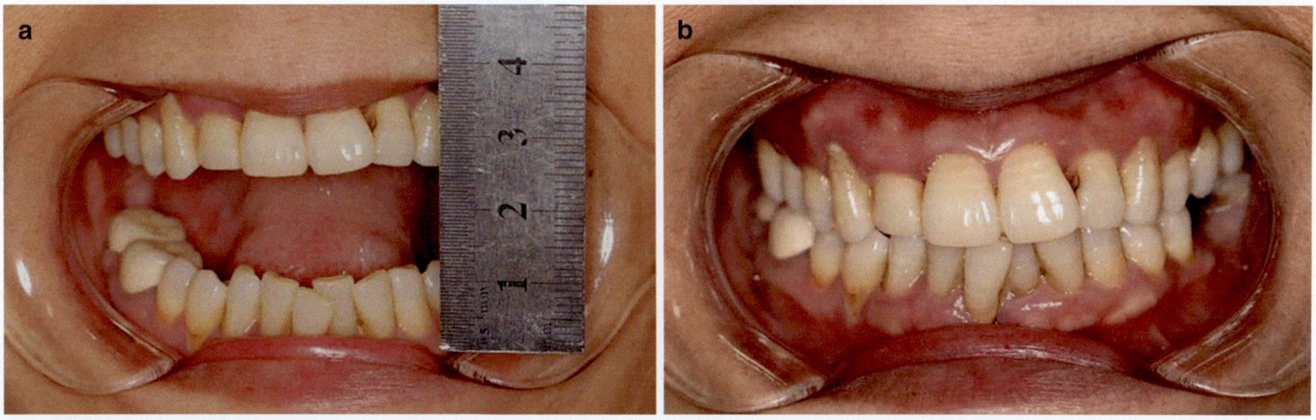

Fig. 3.73 Case C. Intraoral examination. (**a**) Maximum interincisal opening was 17 mm. (**b**) Occlusal relationship

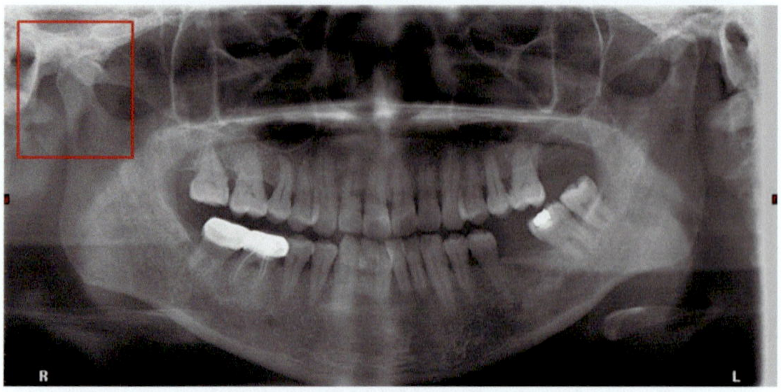

Fig. 3.74 Case C. Panoramic view. The red rectangle shows the condylar bony degeneration on the right side

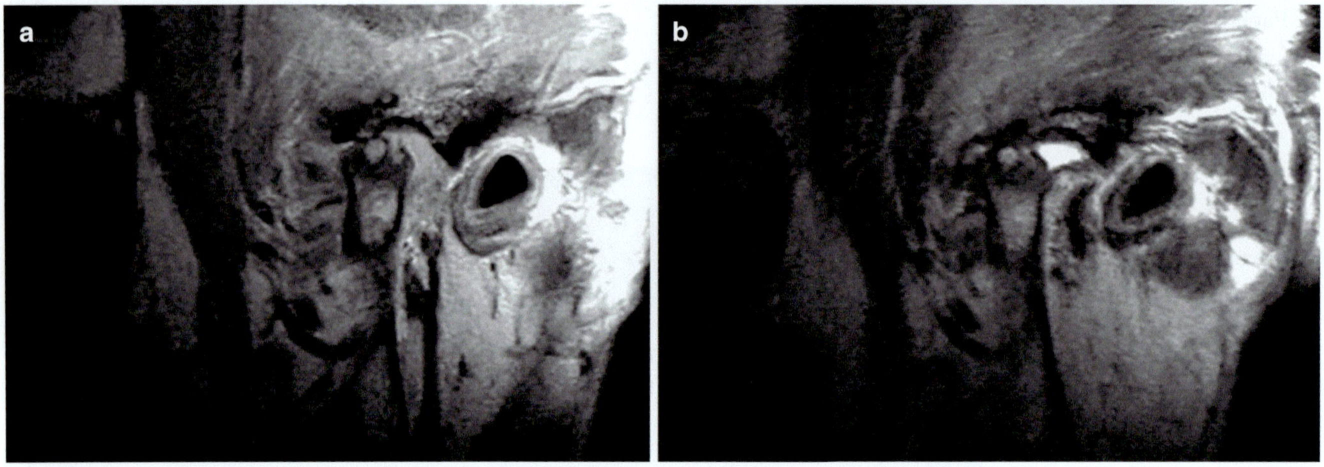

Fig. 3.75 Case C. MRI of the patient's right condyle. Severe bone resorption of the right condyle, with cystic degeneration; there is anterior disc displacement with deformation and perforation. (**a**) Closed position. (**b**) Open position

illofacial region showed bone quality deterioration in the right condyle (Fig. 3.76).
- Diagnosis: osteoarthritis of the right TMJ.

3.4.2 Case C. Diagnostic Imaging

3.4.3 Case C. Treatment Plan

- Overall treatment plan

Right-sided condyle resection, reconstruction with a customized total joint prosthesis utilizing a metallic/nonmetallic fossa prosthesis. The metallic/nonmetallic fossa is a technological innovation in the use of materials, using friction welding to combine an ultrahigh-molecular-weight polyethylene fossa prosthesis with a titanium alloy base, to achieve osseointegration of the fossa prosthesis with the fossa bone, which should prevent loosening of the prosthesis as well as to provide long-term stabilization.

- Surgical resection plan
  - Design of the resection scope: see Sect. 3.2.3.
  - Digital simulation of the surgery: see Sect. 3.2.3.

3.4.4 Case C. Design and Processing of the Prosthesis and the Cutting Guides

- Metallic/nonmetallic fossa prosthesis design, machining, and fitting
  1. Import and placement of core components: to ensure that there is enough space for the thickness of the metal base (1.5 mm) and the metallic/nonmetallic interface (1.5 mm), the metallic/nonmetallic-type fossa core is lowered by an additional 3 mm below the zygomatic arch, compared to that of a classical prosthesis (Fig. 3.77).

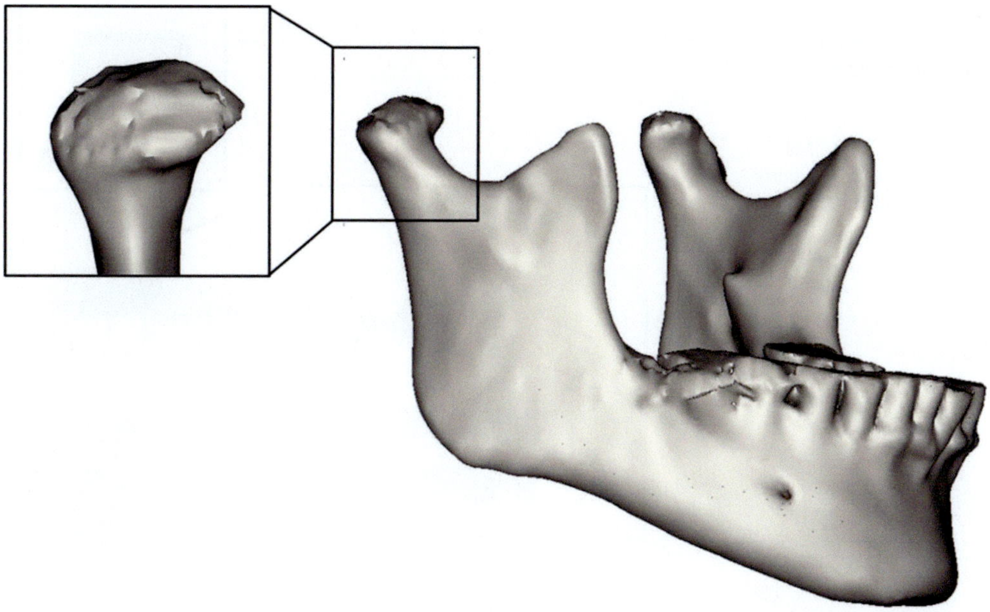

Fig. 3.76 Case C. 3D reconstruction of the maxillofacial CT. Degenerative changes in the right condyle

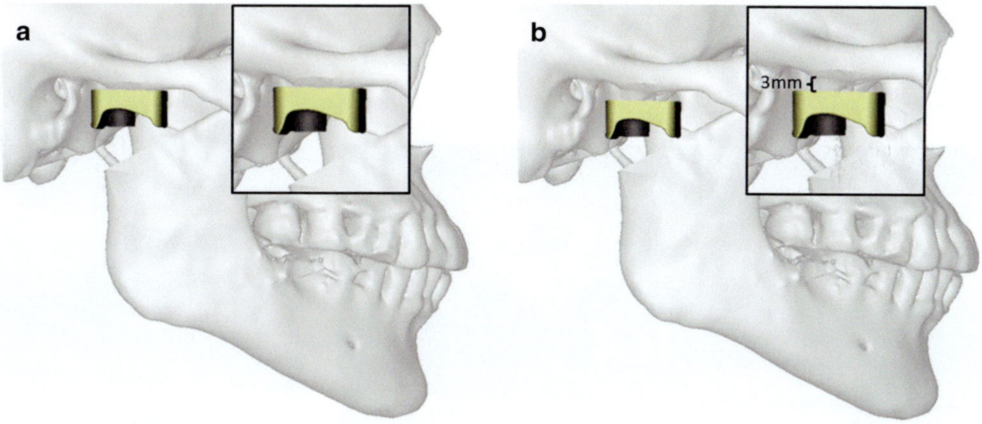

Fig. 3.77 Case C. (**a**) The placement for the core component of the articular fossa prosthesis, right below the eminence. (**b**) For the metallic/nonmetallic fossa-type prosthesis, the core component has been lowered by 3 mm

2. Fossa prosthesis design: metallic/nonmetallic design with 1.5 mm interface thickness and 900 μm porous titanium pore size (Fig. 3.78).
3. The metallic/nonmetallic connection of the fossa prosthesis component is accomplished by friction stir welding, which is mainly done by controlling the rotational speed, time, and temperature in joining the ultrahigh-molecular-weight polyethylene with the titanium alloy parts. The amount of polyethylene embedded in the porous titanium alloy structure results in a strong metallic and nonmetallic connection (Fig. 3.79).

- Fabrication and test fitting of the prosthesis: the same as described in Sect. 2.5 in Chap. 2 (Fig. 3.29) (Fig. 3.80).
- Design of the cutting guides: see Sect. 3.2.4.

3.4.5 Case C. Surgical Procedure

The fossa prosthesis was fixed using the screw holes identified by the cutting guide, followed by fixation with the remaining screw holes (Fig. 3.81). The implantation and fixation of the mandibular prosthesis and the rest of the surgical procedure are described in Sects. 3.2.5 and 3.3.5.

3.4.6 Case C. Postoperative Analysis of Prosthesis Implantation Precision

The postoperative period was followed up with an aesthetic evaluation of facial shape, a functional evaluation of mouth opening, and a prosthesis evaluation of safety and accuracy.

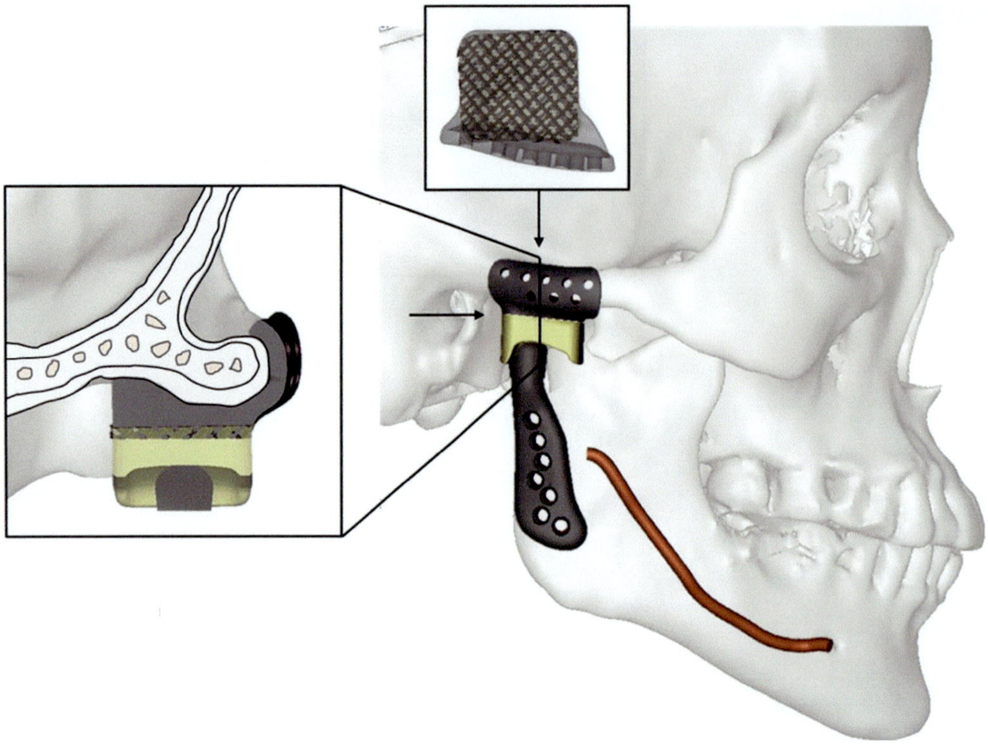

Fig. 3.78 Case C. Design of the fossa prosthesis component and the mandibular prosthesis component for the metallic/nonmetallic total TMJ prosthesis (titanium parts shown in black)

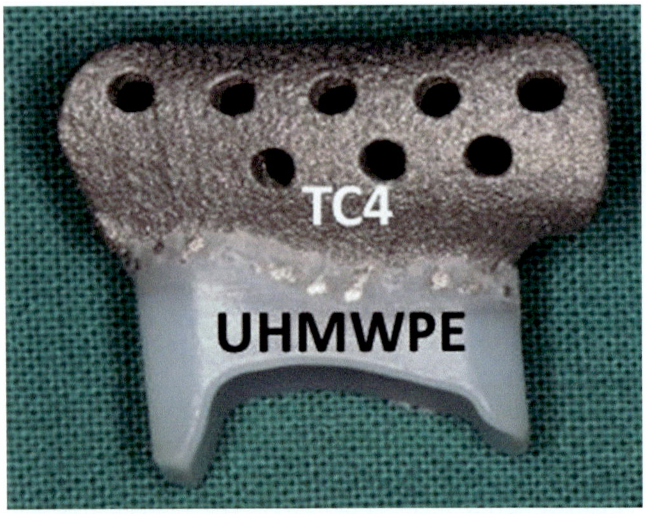

Fig. 3.79 Case C. Metallic/nonmetallic composite (titanium alloy and ultrahigh-molecular-weight polyethylene) fossa prosthesis produced with friction stir welding

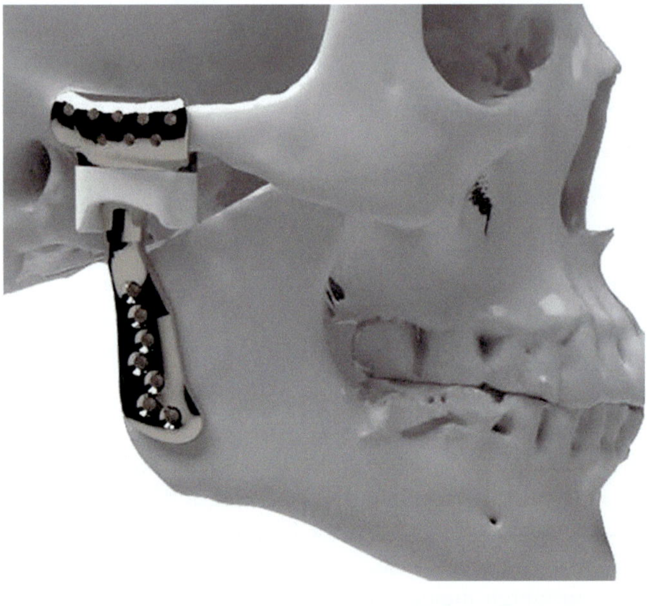

Fig. 3.80 Case C. Metallic/nonmetallic composite fossa prosthesis test fitting on the skull model

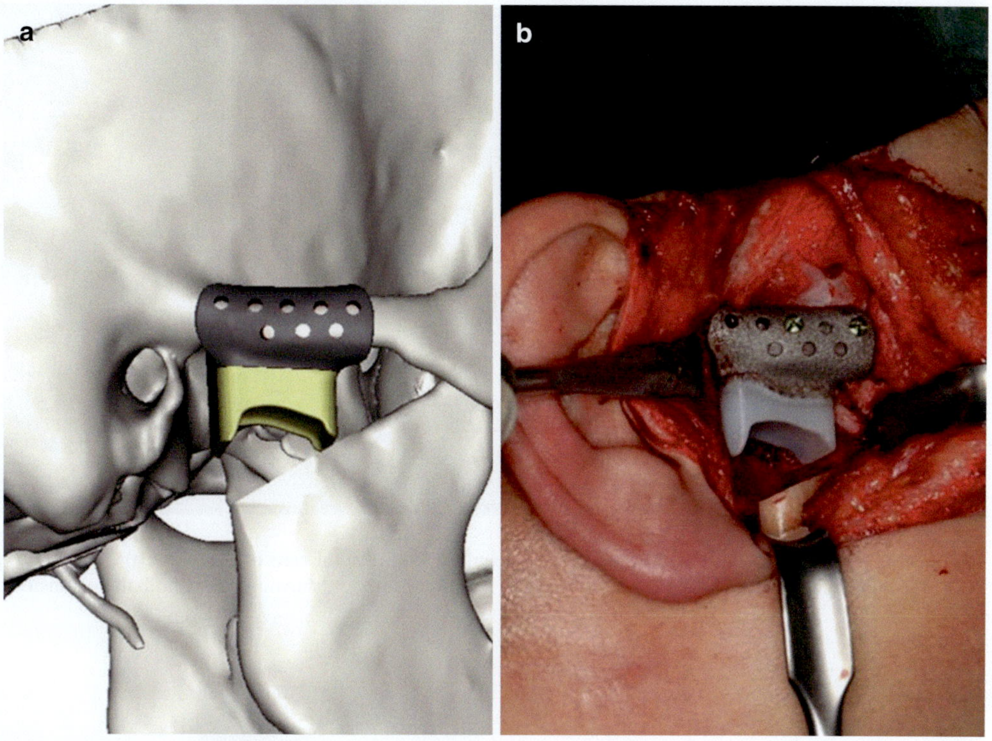

Fig. 3.81 Case C. Placement of the fossa prosthesis. (**a**) Design. (**b**) Actual

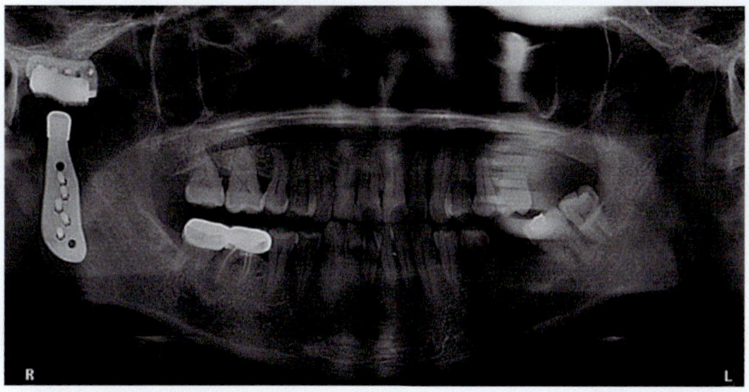

Fig. 3.82 Case C. Immediate postoperative panoramic film

The intraoperative cutting guides were accurately seated during surgery, and the prosthesis was fitted smoothly (Fig. 3.82). The comparison between the preoperative design and the postoperative panoramic representation showed that the prosthesis was accurately seated (Figs. 3.83 and 3.84). The analysis of the postoperative prosthesis fitting error showed that the core component error was 0.42 mm and the overall prosthesis error was 0.89 mm (Figs. 3.85 and 3.86).

3.4.7 Case C. Long-Term Follow-Up and Prognosis

- One-year postoperative follow-up
  1. No complaints of discomfort, good facial appearance with no abnormalities, and no redness, swelling, or other reactions in the operated area.
  2. Significant improvement in preauricular pain, VAS pain score improved to 1, negligible, and joint-mandibular-occlusal-facial shape harmonized and occlusal relationship stable.
  3. The mouth opening improved to 27 mm from 15 mm, with lateral movement of 5 mm to the affected side and 3 mm to the healthy side, although the mouth opening was deviated 3 mm to the affected side.
  4. Evaluation of the prosthesis: no complications such as infection, rejection, loosening, fracture, displacement, ectopic osteogenesis, and material allergy (Fig. 3.87).
  5. Prosthesis osseointegration: CT showed good osseointegration between the articular fossa prosthesis and the articular fossa bone (Fig. 3.88).

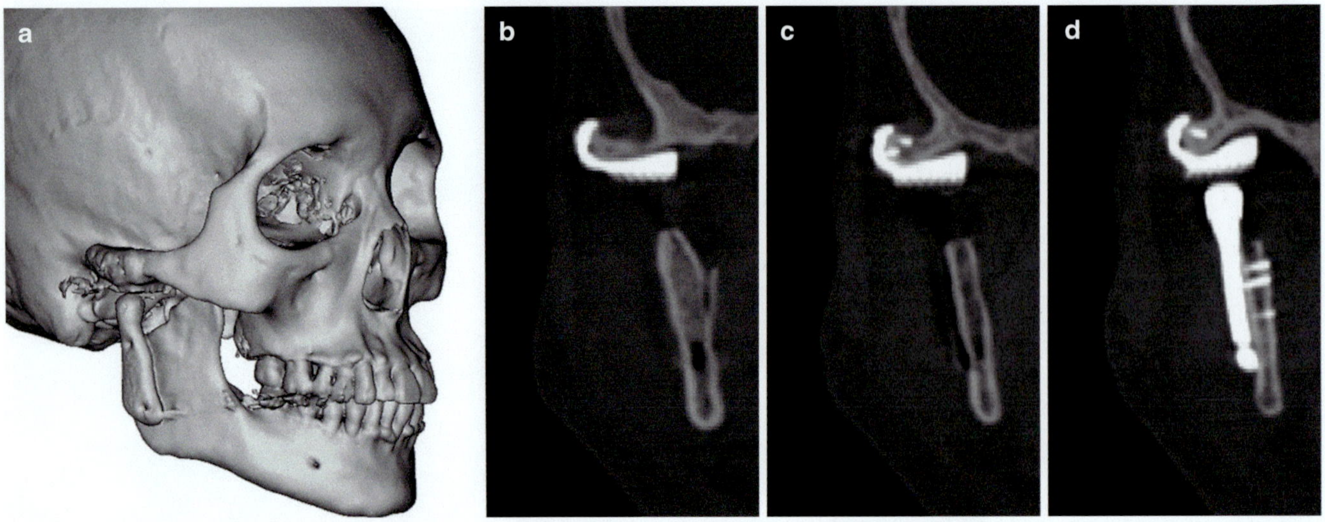

Fig. 3.83 Case C. Immediate postoperative CT 3D scan. (**a**) Right lateral view of cranium. (**b**) Coronal CT, position anterior through the prosthesis. (**c**) Coronal CT, position median. (**d**) Coronal CT, position posterior, showing the mandibular extension and screws

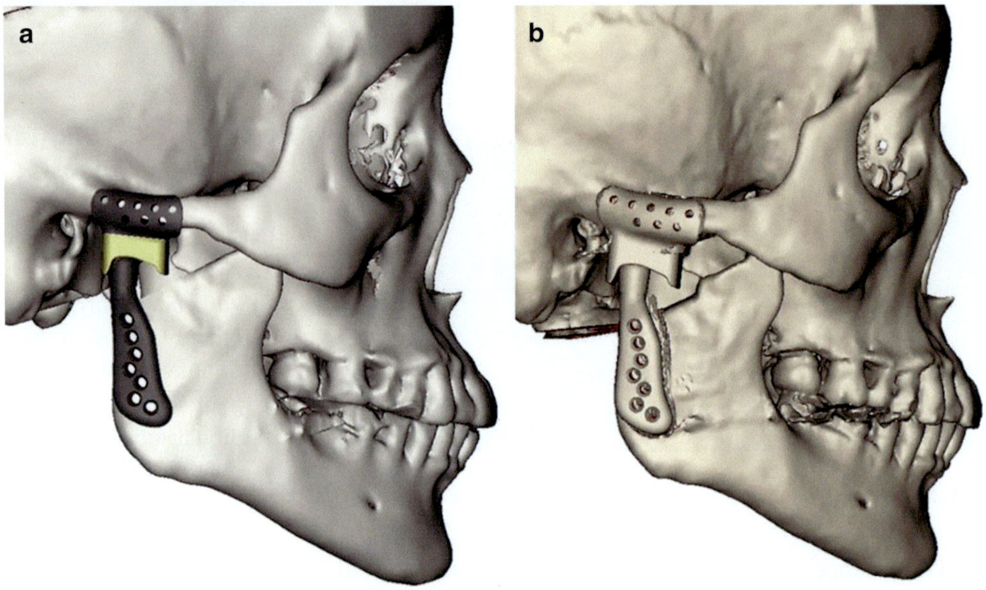

Fig. 3.84 Case C. Comparison of CT scans. (**a**) Preoperative design. (**b**) Immediate postoperative

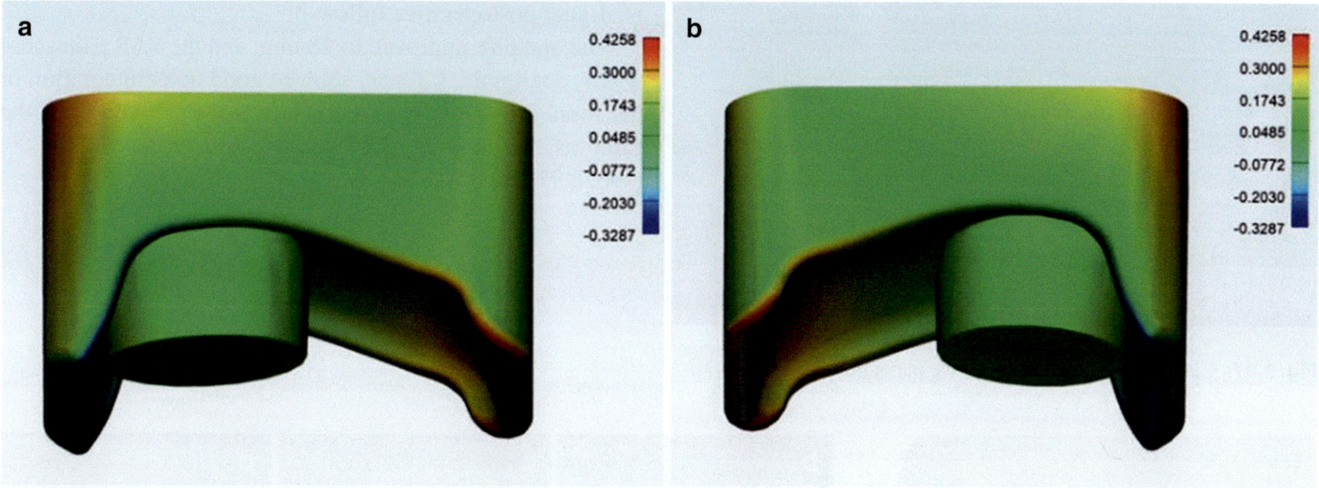

Fig. 3.85 Case C. Prosthetic core error of 0.42 mm. (**a**) Lateral error. (**b**) Medial error

Fig. 3.86 Case C. Overall error of 0.89 mm for metallic/nonmetallic fossa-type total joint prosthesis. (**a**) Lateral error. (**b**) Medial error

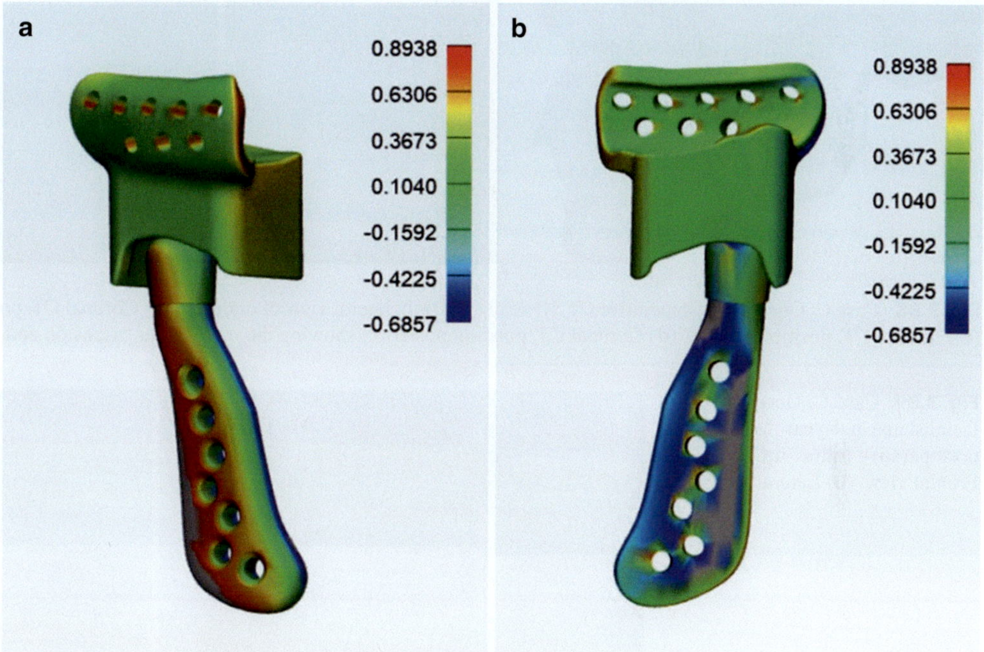

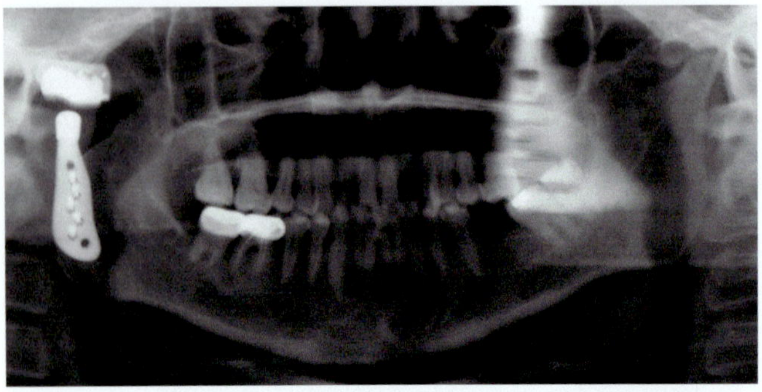

Fig. 3.87 Case C. One-year postoperative panoramic view

- 4-year postoperative follow-up

The opening improved to 28 mm, and the VAS pain score was 1, negligible. CT scan showed good osseointegration of the fossa prosthesis with the nearby bone. The rest was the same as the one-year postoperative follow-up (Figs. 3.89, 3.90, 3.91 and 3.92).

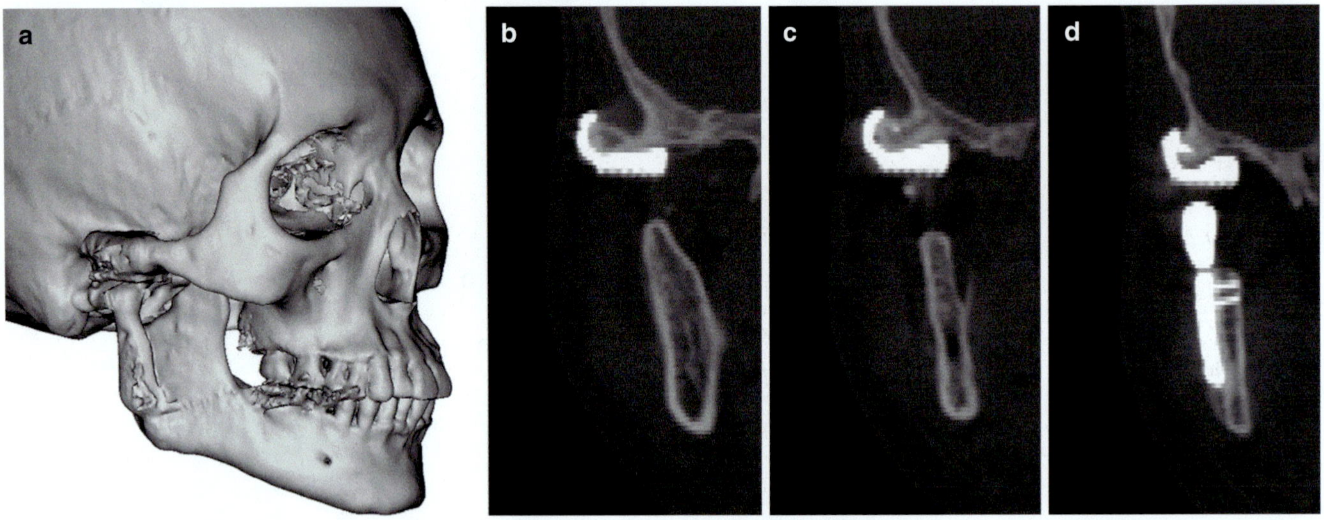

Fig. 3.88 Case C. One year postoperative CT 3D scan. (**a**) Right lateral view of cranium. (**b**) Coronal CT, position anterior through the prosthesis. (**c**) Coronal CT, position median. (**d**) Coronal CT, position posterior, showing the mandibular extension and screws

Fig. 3.89 Case C. Good facial shape at 4-year postoperative follow-up. (**a**) Frontal view. (**b**) Lateral view

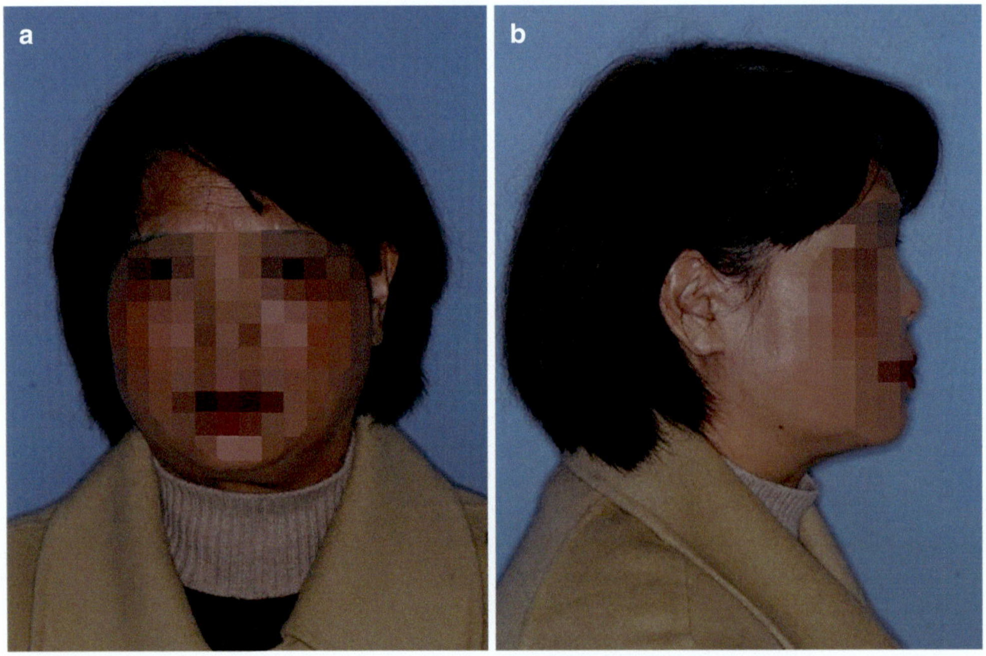

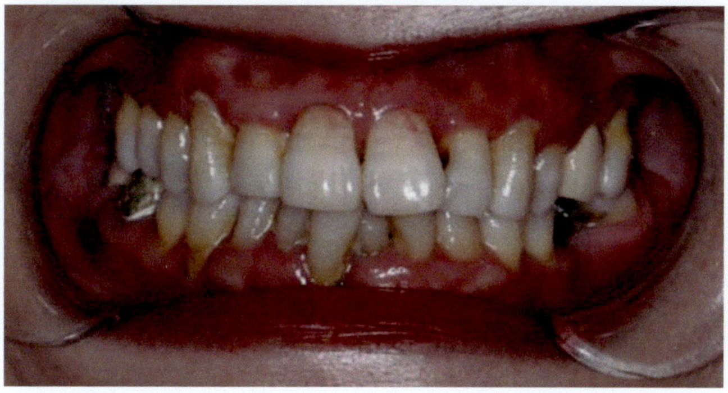

Fig. 3.90 Case C. Stable occlusal relationship at 4 years postoperatively

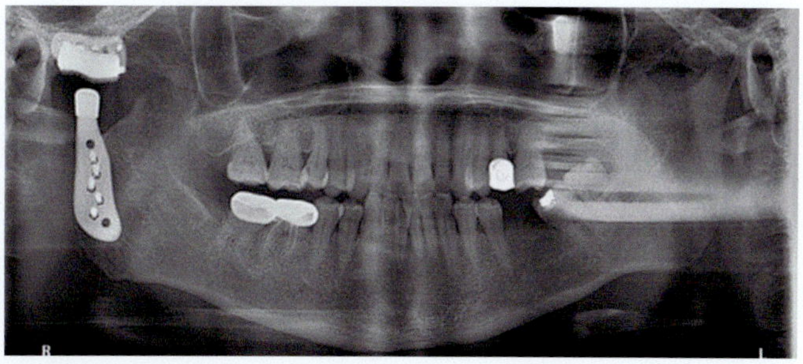

Fig. 3.91 Case C. 4-year postoperative panoramic view

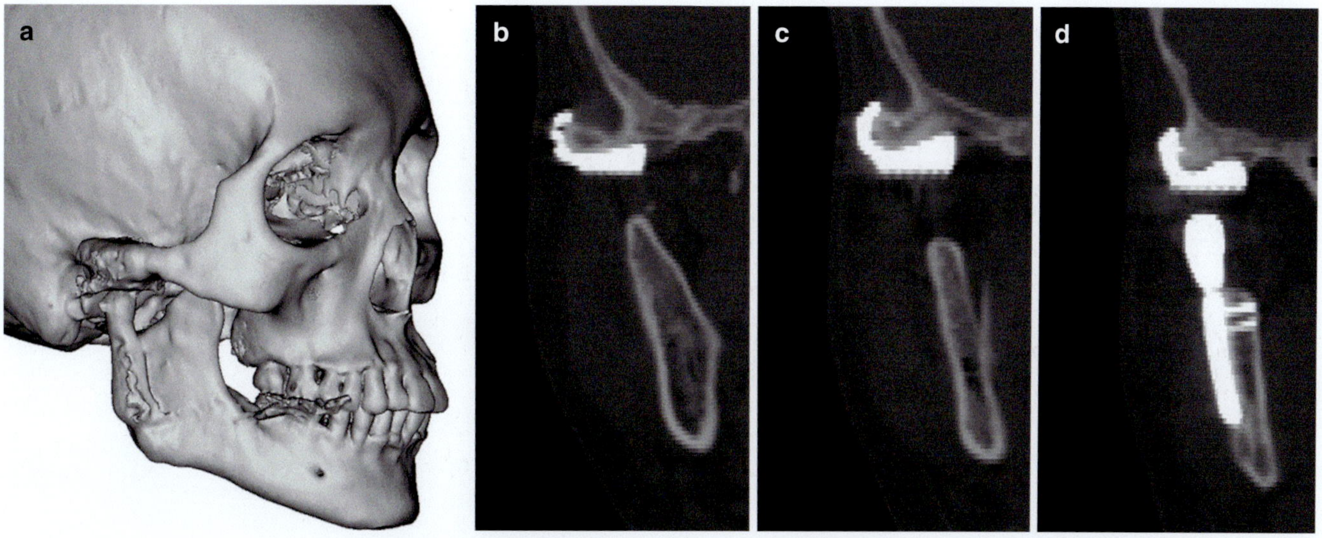

Fig. 3.92 Case C. 4-year postoperative CT 3D scan. (**a**) Right lateral view of cranium. (**b**) Coronal CT, position anterior through the prosthesis. (**c**) Coronal CT, position median. (**d**) Coronal CT, position posterior, showing the mandibular extension and screws

3.4.8 Case C. Advantages and Disadvantages

- Advantages

Compared to the classic fossa prosthesis, this new design not only retains its advantages but also incorporates osteointegration capabilities, resulting in enhanced stability. The success of this prosthesis will provide a viable option for prosthetic replacement in cases with insufficient fossa bone. More importantly, it offers a robust xenogeneic material connection solution for large-scale defects (fossa-skull base). Overall, the personalized prosthesis is straightforward to implant, delivers precise and controllable outcomes, and effectively addresses the challenges associated with standard prostheses, such as high surgical technical requirements, prolonged operative time, and a higher risk of complications.

- Disadvantages
  1. Currently, there is still uncertainty in the thickness of the interface between metallic/nonmetallic materials in the fossa. The filling and composition of the interface needs to be further improved, and the control of the internal consistency of the metal and the removal of debris from the metal need to be further investigated.
  2. The production cycle is relatively longer and more expensive.
  3. The prosthetic connection interface is relatively thick, increasing the overall thickness of the fossa prosthesis and requiring a lower osteotomy line on the condyle, which adds to the surgical complexity. More critically, the reduction in the core component lowers the rotational axis (center of rotation), placing it farther from the physiological position.

4 Total Joint Replacement with Simultaneous Orthognathic Surgery for Dentofacial Deformities Secondary to TMJ Diseases

Chi Yang, Qianyang Xie, Shanyong Zhang, and Zhigui Ma

This chapter addresses Class IIa of Yang's modified classification, i.e., Class II encompasses dentofacial deformities secondary to temporomandibular joint (TMJ) diseases, and within this, Class IIa covers only those cases where the condyle is non-salvageable. These cases require a combination of joint replacement, orthognathic surgery, and orthodontics for successful reconstruction.

In this chapter, we will first present an overview including following aspects. Firstly, we will discuss the definition of TMJ-Originated Dentofacial Deformities with non-salvageable temporomandibular joints and give a classification of types of such orthognathic surgery, as we have done in previous chapters. Then we will discuss the traditional methods of TMJ Replacement with Simultaneous orthognathic surgery and the various drawbacks in outcomes that have been recognized. Following this, we will focus on the innovative reconstruction methods that we have developed utilizing the digital design process of customized total joint prosthesis. More specifically, we have developed techniques for orthognathic surgery simultaneous with prosthesis and facial reconstruction.

Through six clinical cases, we will illustrate the whole process of customized total joint replacement surgery—from preoperative design to surgical application, through postoperative follow-up and evaluation—with the objective of improving the awareness and ability of joint surgeons and orthognathic and orthodontic specialists to deal with this kind of complex diseases.

4.1 Overview

Temporomandibular joint (TMJ) diseases are often accompanied by various degrees of maxillofacial deformities, such as idiopathic condylar resorption, joint ankylosis, and joint tumors that often lead to mandible retrognathia and/or deviation. Of these, 20–25% of cases experience severe jaw deformities that need to be relieved by orthognathic surgery; clinically, this group of patients tends to seek medical attention for the resolution of their dentofacial deformities as their chief complaint. But both joint replacement and orthognathic surgery are needed to resolve the jaw deformity for the long term, especially since mandible retrognathia is prone to recurrence.

However, whether the joints can be preserved or not is the primary issue in the treatment. In this section, we will introduce basic concepts such as, first, the definition of TMJ-originated dentofacial deformities with non-salvageable joint and, second, our classification of types of orthognathic surgery simultaneous with total joint replacement.

Following a summary of traditional surgical protocols and their most common complications, we will propose an innovative protocol of total joint prosthesis implantation with simultaneous orthognathic surgery, to achieve surgical precision, safety, and simplicity in operation, as well as long-term stability in the postoperative period. The procedure of simultaneous orthognathic surgery with total joint replacement is also standardized accordingly.

4.1.1 Definition of TMJ-Originated Dentofacial Deformities with Non-salvageable Joint

TMJ diseases where the articular disc and condylar morphology and quality indicate that the joint structure is no longer worth preserving—termed "non-salvageable joint"—and when accompanied by joint-derived dentofacial deformities (i.e., "TMJ-originated dentofacial deformities with non-salvageable joint"), a combined treatment approach involving joint replacement with or without orthognathic-orthodontic therapy may be adopted. This chapter focuses on such cases.

TMJ replacement with concurrent orthognathic surgery refers to performing joint reconstruction alongside orthognathic procedures, addressing both the joint pathology and secondary skeletal deformities while simultaneously correcting dental malocclusion and upper airway constriction, achieving

Chi Y. (✉) · Qianyang X. · Shanyong Z. · Zhigui M.
Shanghai Ninth People's Hospital, Shanghai Jiao Tong University School of Medicine, Shanghai, China

© People's Medical Publishing House, PR of China 2025
Chi Y. (ed.), *Atlas of Customized TMJ-Cranio-Jaw Prosthesis*, https://doi.org/10.1007/978-981-95-0611-8_4

multiple therapeutic goals in a single intervention. The two primary approaches for total joint replacement are autogenous bone grafting and total joint prosthesis. Since orthognathic surgery involves mandibular repositioning, which increases compressive stress on the reconstructed condyle, autogenous grafts are prone to resorption (see Clinical Case H in this chapter), making total joint prosthesis the more advantageous option. Furthermore, patient-specific total joint prosthesis offers greater convenience and precision compared to standardized prostheses.

4.1.2 Classification of Orthognathic Surgery Simultaneous with Total Joint Prosthesis

The classification of simultaneous orthognathic surgery for total joint prosthesis implantation can in general be divided into the following two categories (Fig. 4.1).

- Category I. Correction just through the prosthesis, i.e., the total joint prosthesis implantation itself can play an orthognathic role: it can be utilized to increase the height of the mandibular ramus, lengthen the mandibular body, and rotate the mandible (usually counterclockwise rotation) in order to correct the mandibular deformity. For example, lengthening the mandibular ramus through the prosthesis, while lengthening the mandibular ramus and mandibular body through bone grafting. This is especially suitable for the correction of a mandibular deformity.
- Category II. Correction with orthognathic surgery simultaneous with total joint prosthesis implantation: orthognathic surgery concomitant with total joint prosthesis implantation. There are several possible varieties of simultaneous orthognathic surgery: bilateral replacement with/without genioplasty, bilateral replacement with/without Le Fort I osteotomy with/without genioplasty, and unilateral replacement with sagittal split of the contralateral mandibular ramus with/without Le Fort I osteotomy with/without genioplasty, as illustrated below (Fig. 4.1). This is suitable for the correction of moderate and severe maxillary deformities in both jaws. Later sections of this chapter will illustrate the various types of surgeries utilizing a total joint prosthesis.

4.1.3 Traditional Reconstruction Methods for Temporomandibular Joint Replacement with Simultaneous Orthognathic Surgery

The history of orthognathic surgery simultaneous with joint surgery can be traced back to the 1970s. It started with arthroplasty and vertical osteotomy of the mandibular ramus for dentofacial deformity secondary to TMJ ankylosis (Fig. 4.2) and later emerged with simultaneous osteotomy of the healthy mandibular ramus, using reconstruction of the joint with CCG, to restore the facial shape and occlusal relationship. The earliest maxillary osteotomy was reported in 1980, when Dr. Ian R. Munro performed simultaneous autogenous osteoarthroplasty and Le Fort I osteotomy of the maxilla in 14 patients with hemifacial microsomia (Fig. 4.3); thereafter, he applied this surgical protocol to the treatment of joint ankylosis. In the 1980s and 1990s, simultaneous double jaw surgery with joint reconstruction was developed gradually.

In our experience, there are several problems associated with orthognathic surgery simultaneous with joint replacement:

1. The surgical interference problem: With two surgeries performed on the mandible at the same time, the process is prone to affecting the precision of the outcome of the position of the joints and the jaws. However, our sequential design of the surgery, cutting guides, and customized prostheses will effectively solve this problem.
2. The problem of maintaining asepsis: with simultaneous surgery inside and outside the mouth, special attention must be paid to aseptic operation. Our procedures address this concern.

The commonly used reconstruction method is a combination of autogenous bone graft and standardized total joint prosthesis. These two options do not address the common problems mentioned above and have the following shortcomings. Autogenous bone is commonly sourced from rib cartilage (see Case H in this chapter) and the mandibular coronoid process (Fig. 4.4), but aside from the issues of harvesting the bone, use of autogenous bone is prone to problems such as postoperative resorption of free bone grafts, leading to higher rates of recurrence of dentofacial deformities or pre-existing diseases (e.g., ankylosis). In the case of the standard-type prosthesis, it suffers from the risk of inaccurate positioning, large errors, and postoperative displacement problems (Fig. 4.5).

4.1.4 Innovative Reconstruction Methods for Orthognathic Surgery Simultaneous with Customized Total Joint Prosthesis

In order to achieve precision, stability, and ease of operation of the two surgeries, the author's team has innovatively developed and applied 3D-printed customized total joint prostheses to be used in the orthognathic surgery simultaneous with joint replacement; by combining digitally designed cutting guides, endoscopically assisted fixation and other key technologies, the accuracy of the prosthesis positioning

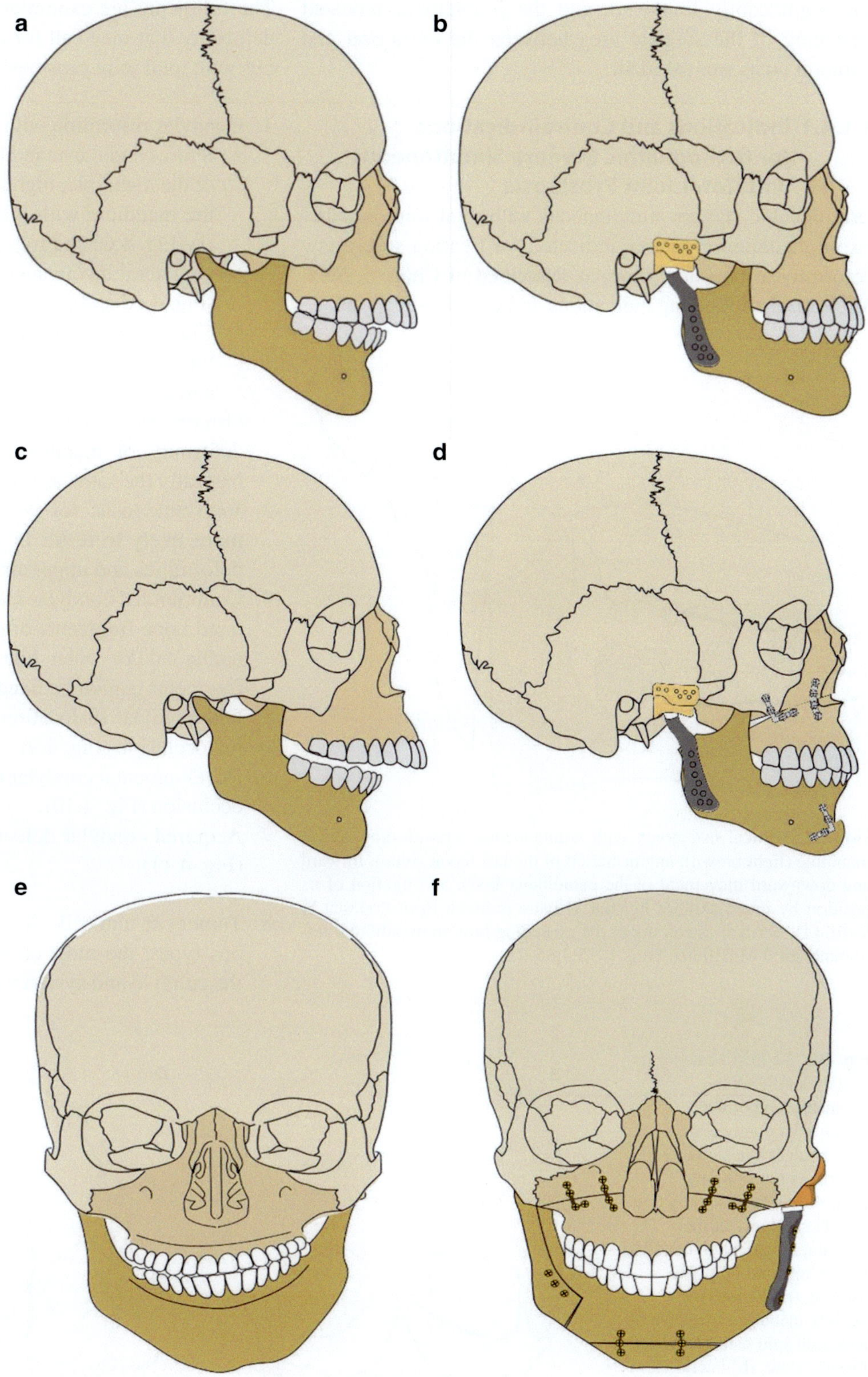

Fig. 4.1 Examples of procedures for total joint prosthesis implantation with simultaneous orthognathic surgery (**a**, **b**) (Category I) Orthognathic role of joint replacement with mandibular lengthening and simple arthroplasty (side view). (**c**, **d**) (Category II) For a more serious case of jaw retrognathia, bilateral arthroplasty with simultaneous Le Fort I osteotomy and genioplasty (side view). (**e**, **f**) (Category II) For a severe deviation of the jaw, Le Fort I osteotomy simultaneous with unilateral arthroplasty, sagittal split osteotomy of the contralateral mandibular ramus, and genioplasty (front view)

was significantly improved, and the problem of repeated switching of the surgical area between the extra-oral and intraoral areas was avoided.

4.1.4.1 Indications and Contraindications for Orthognathic Surgery Simultaneous with Total Joint Prosthesis

Orthognathic surgery simultaneous with total joint prosthesis implantation is mainly indicated for treating severe jaw deformity at the same time, as described in Chap. 3, Sect. 3.1, with the following indications and contraindications.

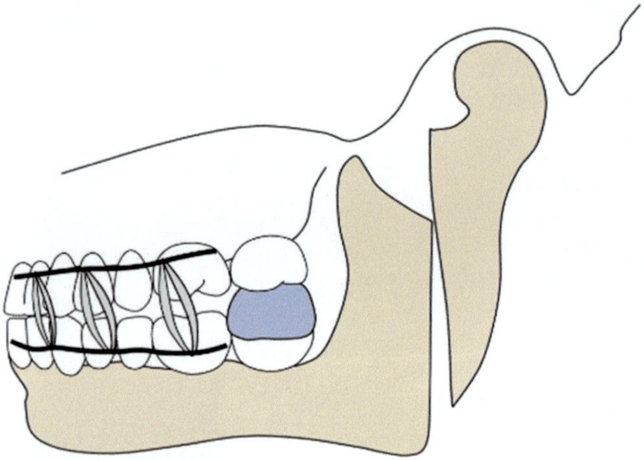

Fig. 4.2 Vertical osteotomy with simultaneous repositioning of the mandible (light brown): augmentation of the last molar (blue), forward and downward movement of the mandibular body, and fixation of its position by intermaxillary ligation. (Figure redrawn from Popescu V, Vasiliu D. Vertical osteotomy of the ascending rami in mandibular retrognathism. J Maxillofac Surg. 1975;3:65–73)

The following are examples of types of cases with serious deformity that may call for orthognathic surgery simultaneous with total joint prosthesis implantation.

1. Condylar resorption with anterior disc displacement:
   - Short condylar-mandibular ramus, clockwise rotation of the mandible, high angle, and posterior reduction of the mandible with bilateral involvement (bony Class II) (Fig. 4.6a and b).
   - Unilateral involvement of the mandible with deviation (Fig. 4.6d and e).
   - Class II malocclusion may be accompanied by open bite, as well as upper airway stenosis (Fig. 4.6a, b and c).
2. Osteoarthritis: advanced osteoarthritis can lead to the deformity of mandibular retrognathia, which behaves basically the same as condylar resorption.
3. Joint ankylosis: for youth with this problem, they are more likely to result in severe dental and maxillofacial deformities and upper airway narrowing (Fig. 4.7).
4. Comminuted condylar fracture: displacement of the shattered bone fragments often results in mandibular retrognathia and/or open bite; the fractured condylar bone fragments cannot be fixed in place (Fig. 4.8)
5. Old condylar dislocation: it resembles a bony Class III malocclusion (Fig. 4.9).
6. Developmental condylar hyperplasia: bony Class III malocclusion (Fig. 4.10).
7. Acquired condylar defects: surgical or osteolytic causes (Fig. 4.11).
8. Tumors or tumorlike lesions of the joints: there are various types, the most common being osteochondroma of the condyle and synovial chondromatosis (Fig. 4.12).

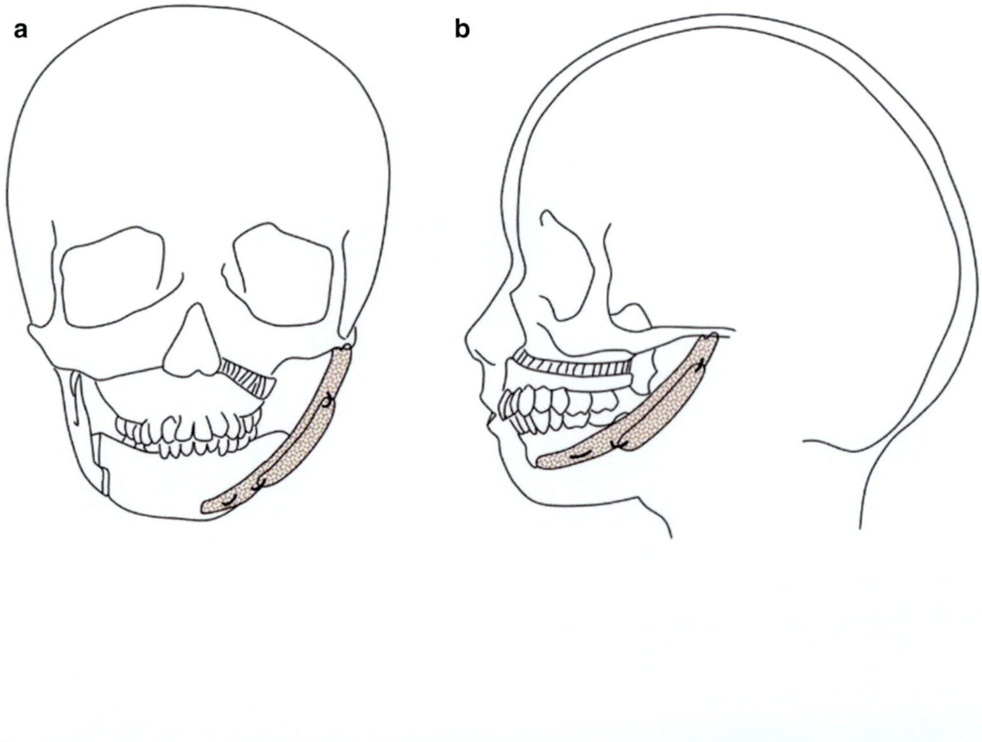

Fig. 4.3 Le Fort I osteotomy of the maxilla with reconstruction of the mandibular condyle and mandibular ramus: the maxilla is matched into position for occlusion by a Le Fort I osteotomy of the maxilla; the affected mandible is then lowered by bone grafting (pink), and the healthy mandible is rotated by a sagittal split osteotomy. (**a**) Frontal view; (**b**) lateral view. (Figure redrawn from Munro IR. One-stage reconstruction of the temporomandibular joint in hemifacial microsomia. Plast Reconstr Surg. 1980;66(5):699–710)

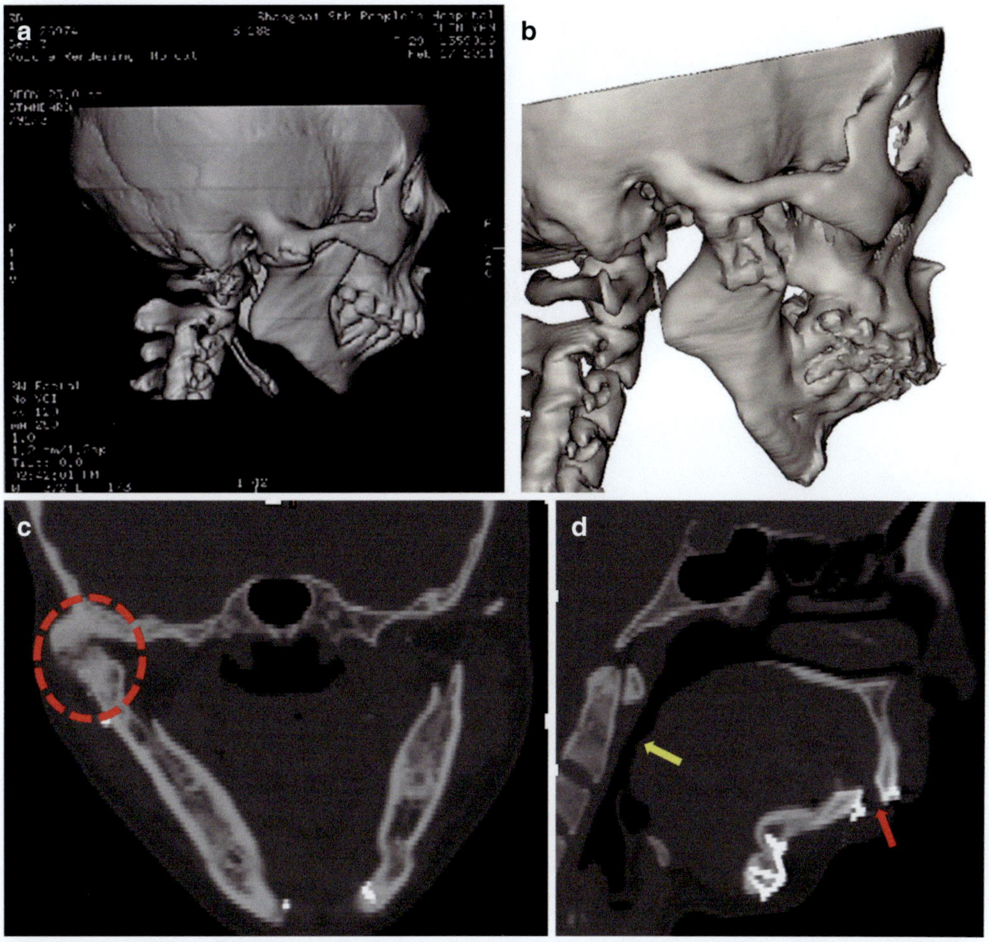

Fig. 4.4 Postoperative recurrence of ankylosis treated with a coronoid graft. (**a**) Right ankylosis and mandibular retrognathia before coronoid grafting. (**b**) Two years after coronoid grafting, recurrence of right ankylosis and resorption of grafted bone leading to the recurrence of mandibular retrognathia. (**c**) Recurrence of ankylosis, with fusion of the right head of the TMJ with the fossa in the red circle. (**d**) Recurrence leading to the mandibular retrognathia, horizontal opening of the anterior teeth (red arrow), and airway narrowing (yellow arrow)

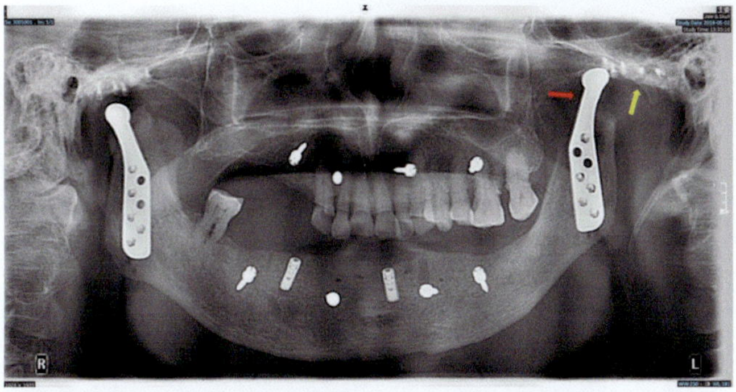

Fig. 4.5 Standard TMJ prosthesis complications after surgery, with the mandibular prosthesis component (red arrow) coming forward out of the fossa prosthesis component (yellow arrow), i.e., dislocation and malfunction

4.1.4.2 Contraindications to Simultaneous Orthognathic Surgery with Total Joint Prosthesis

See contraindications for application of the prosthesis in Sect. 3.1.4 of Chap. 3.

4.1.5 Preparation for Orthognathic Surgery Simultaneous with Customized Total Joint Prosthesis

Preoperative evaluation in orthognathic surgery requires comprehensive history taking and documentation, psychological assessment, treatment plan communication, as well as systemic and regional examinations. Systemic examination should focus on the functional status of major organs. Regional examination includes: TMJ assessment (joint function and morphology), facial examination (soft tissue and skeletal symmetry), intraoral and dental model analysis (occlusion, arch form, and dentition), and imaging examinations (radiographic evaluation of craniofacial structures). Specifically included are:

4.1.5.1 Surgical Plan

CT-based 3D reconstruction of the jaws is performed to simulate osteotomy, correct craniofacial deformities, and restore normal jaw positioning. Based on this analysis, the morphology and placement of the patient-specific total joint prosthesis are customized.

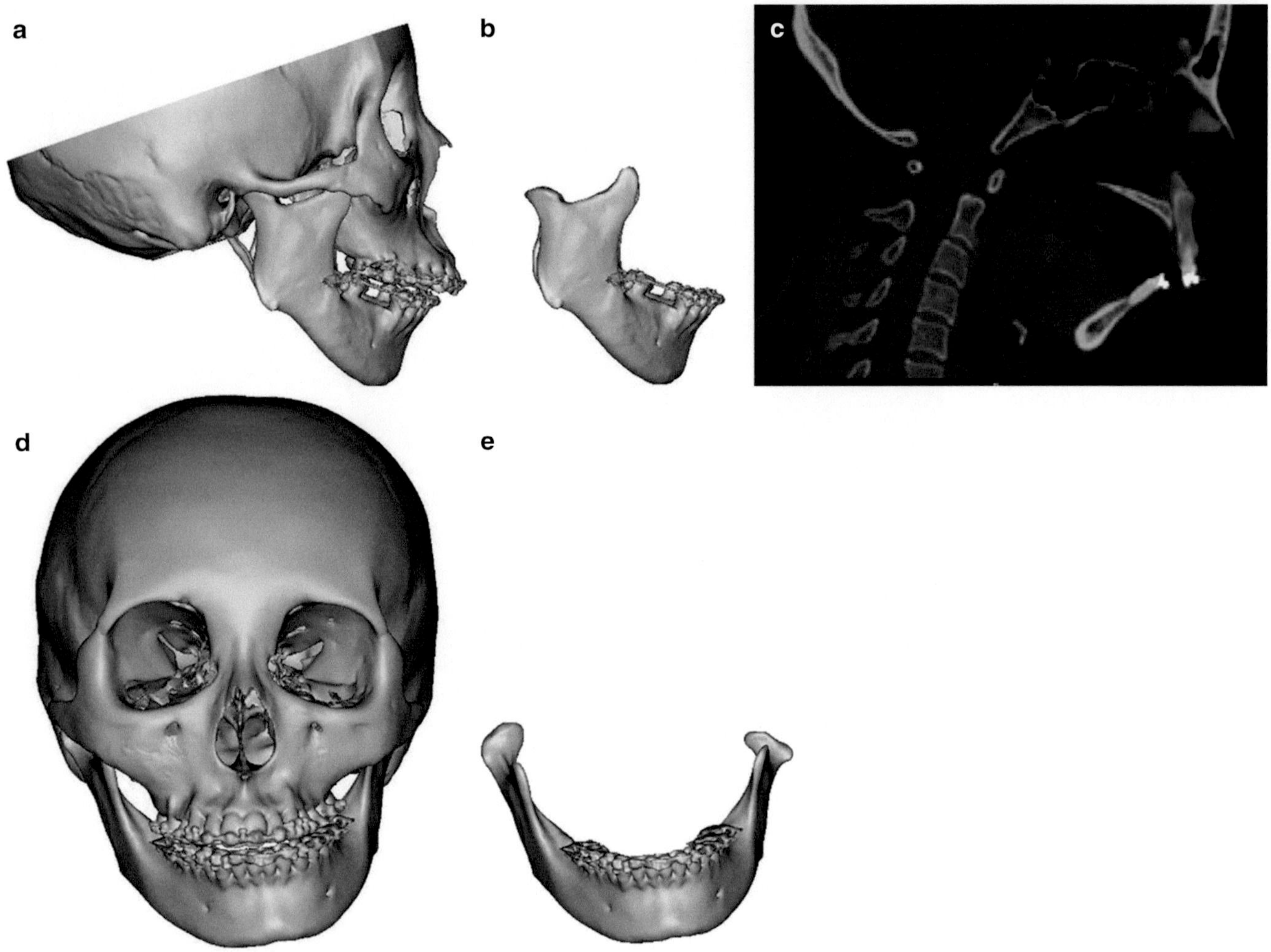

Fig. 4.6 Condylar resorption or osteoarthritis resulting in dentofacial deformity. (**a, b, c**) Bilateral condylar resorption with mandibular retrognathia and airway narrowing. (**d** and **e**) Left condylar resorption with mandibular deviation

Fig. 4.7 Joint ankylosis leading to dentofacial deformity. (**a**) Right joint ankylosis with mandibular retrognathia; (**b**) airway narrowing

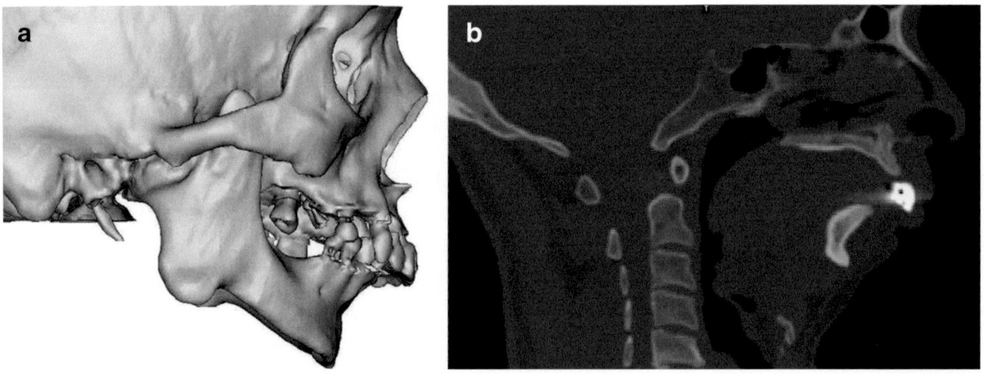

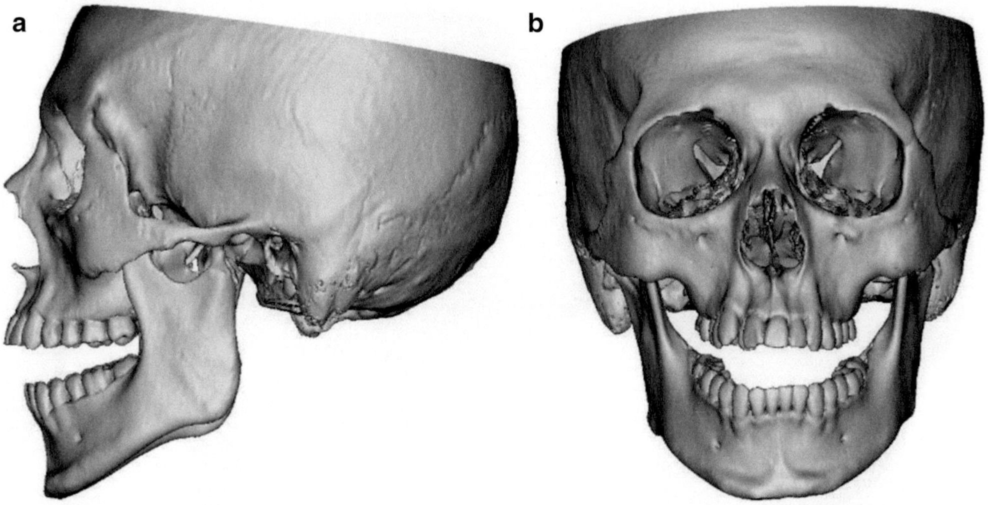

Fig. 4.8 Comminuted condylar fracture. (**a**) Lateral view: left comminuted condylar fracture with mandibular retrognathia. (**b**) Frontal view: mandibular deviation to the affected side

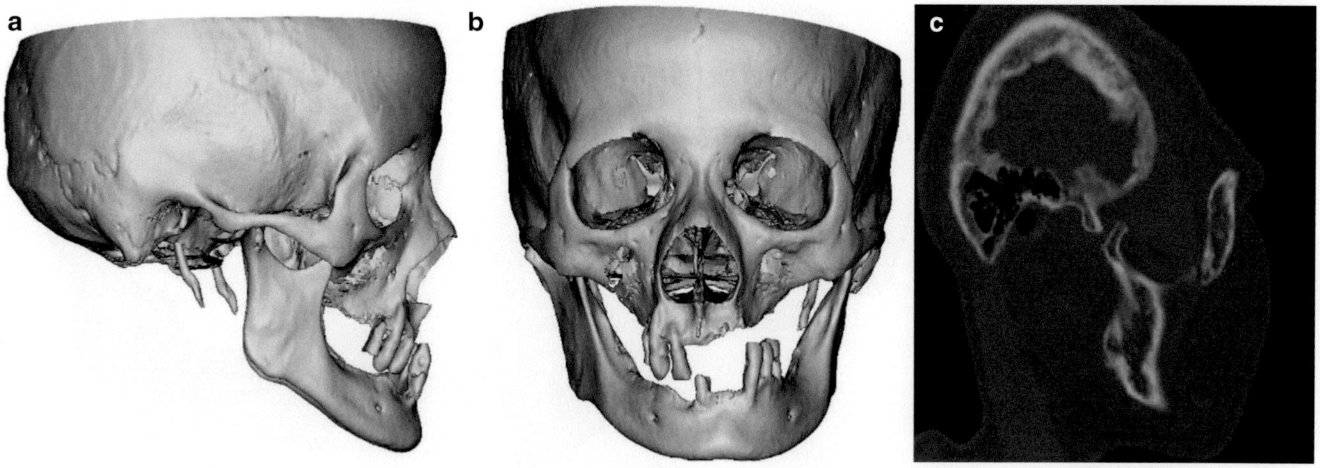

Fig. 4.9 Old dislocation. (**a**) Lateral view: dislocation of the right joint with anterior protrusion of the mandible. (**b**) Frontal view: deflection of the mandible toward the healthy side. (**c**) Dislocation of the condyle

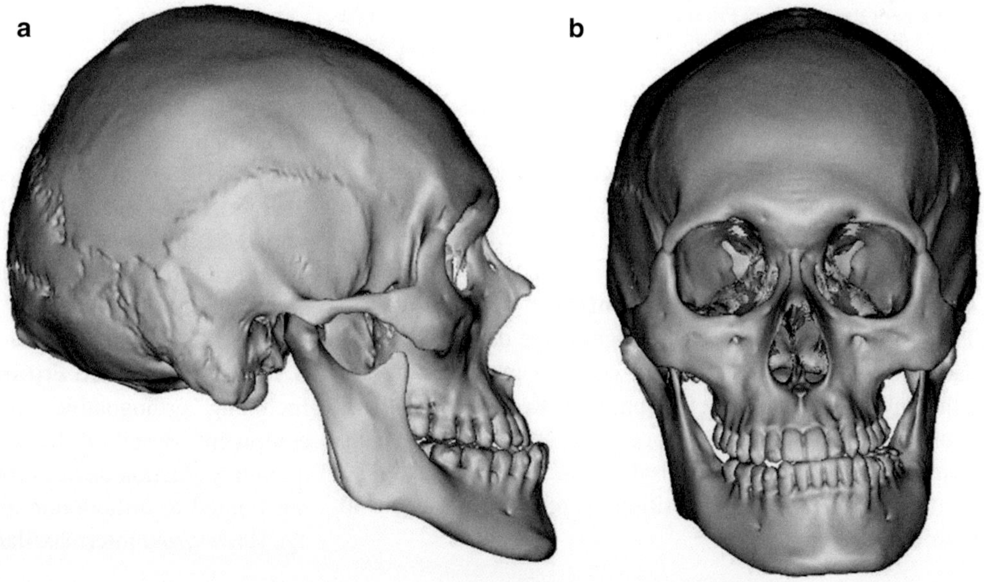

Fig. 4.10 Developmental condylar hyperplasia. (**a**) Lateral view, right condylar hyperplasia with mandibular protrusion. (**b**) Frontal view, mandibular deviation to the left

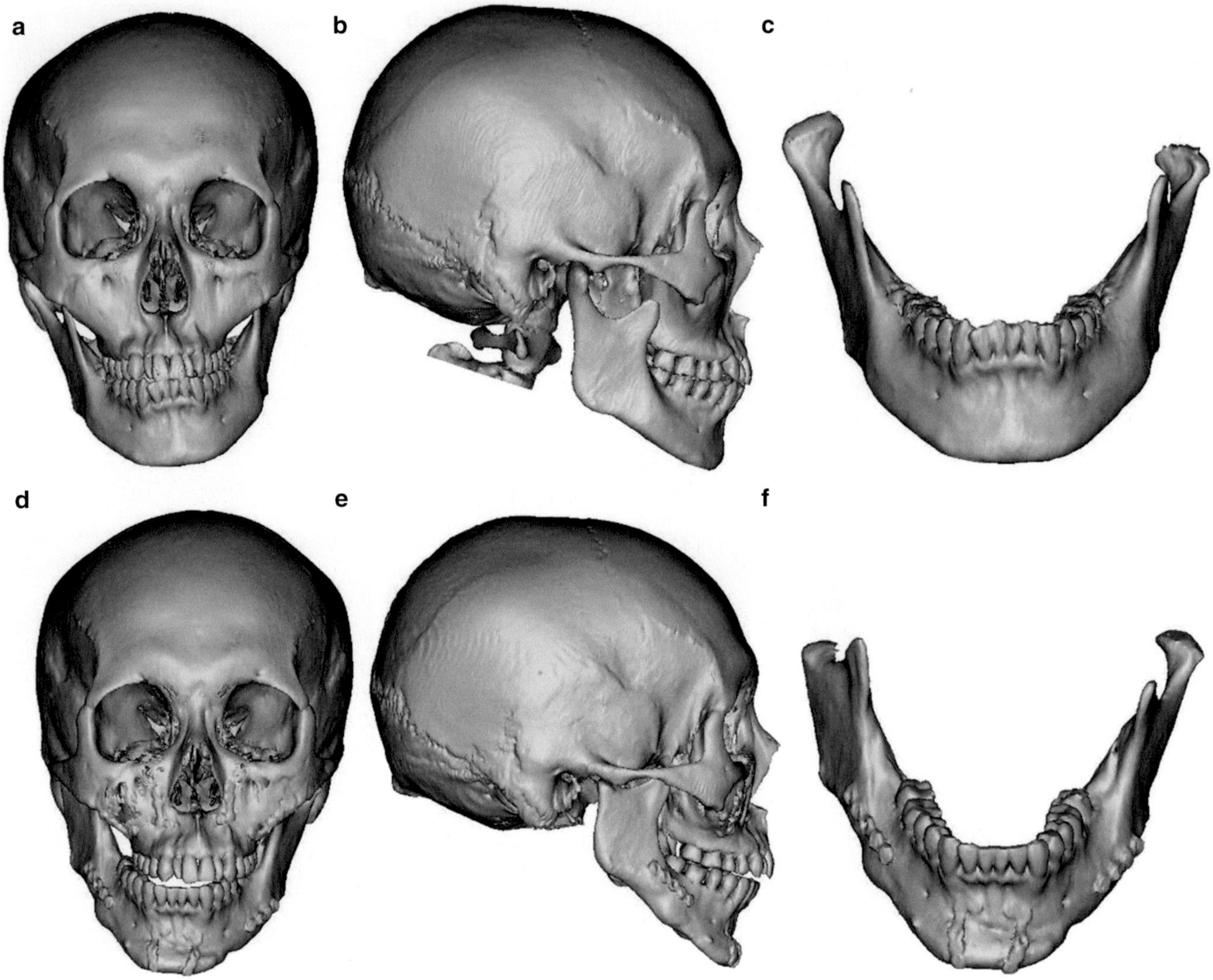

Fig. 4.11 The patient's right condylar hyperplasia resulted in postoperative condylar loss due to inappropriate surgical procedures and secondary deformities, leading to mandibular retrognathia, deviation, and open bite of the jaw. (**a–c**) Pre-orthognathic surgery (diagnosis of right condylar hyperplasia). (**d–f**) After orthognathic surgery (right condylar hyperplastic bone excised and double jaw surgery); 2 years later, right condylar resorption

Cutting guides, including osteotomy guides, positioning guides, and surgical splints, are designed and 3D printed. For selected cases, patient-specific titanium 3D-printed fixation plates may also be fabricated (see Chap. 5).

4.1.5.2 Preoperative Orthodontics

The primary objectives include aligning the dentition, eliminating dental compensation and occlusal interference, and adjusting the dental arch morphology to achieve optimal coordination between the upper and lower arches. This ensures broad, stable occlusal contacts during surgery, facilitating the precise repositioning of bone segments to their ideal locations.

4.1.5.3 Preoperative Implant Preparation

If conventional titanium plates for bone block fixation are to be applied to the patient, it is necessary to prepare suitable titanium plates and screws. The correct length of the screws should be measured by CT scan before surgery; the screws should be prepared adequately, and they should be packed and sterilized.

4.1.5.4 Specialized Equipment

Including orthognathic surgical instruments and power equipment. Based on the patient's specific condition, intermaxillary traction devices should be designed, including but not limited to orthodontic brackets, traction hooks, anchorage screws, and intermaxillary ligation screws.

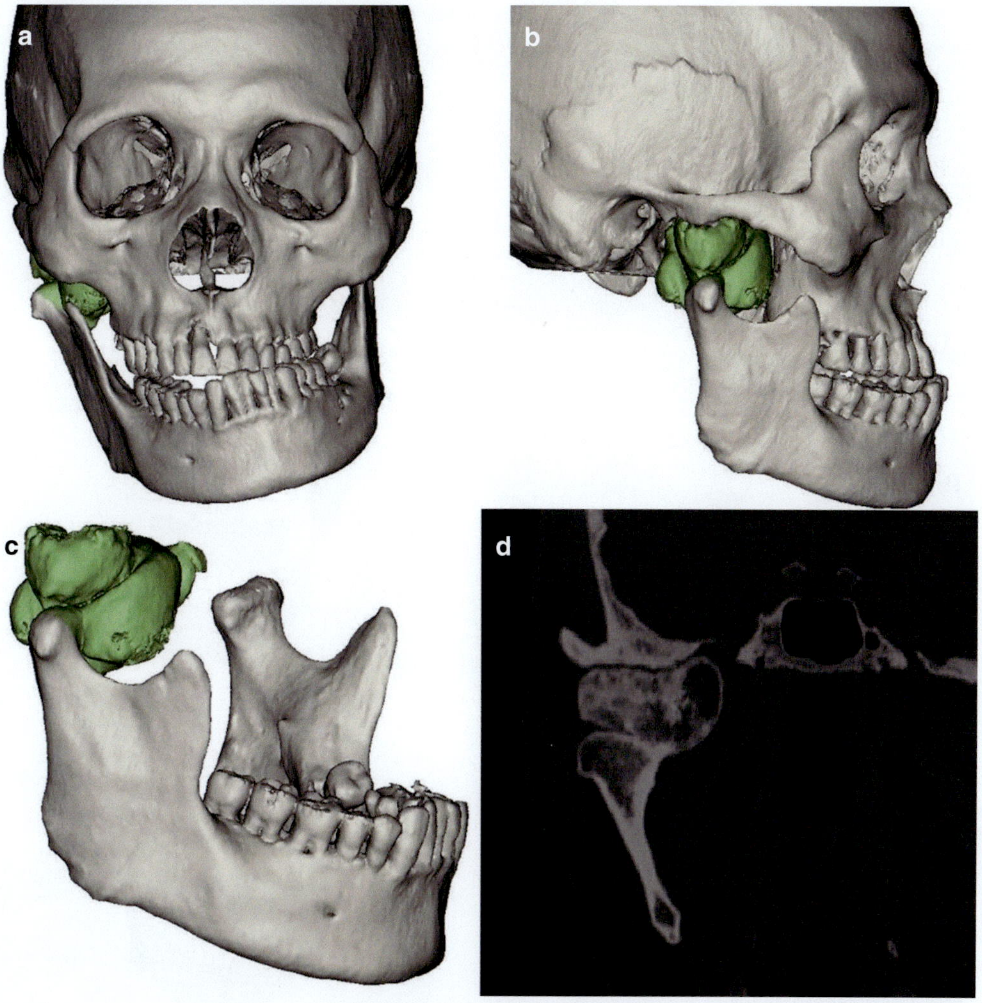

Fig. 4.12 Benign tumors of the condyle with dentofacial deformities. (**a**) Osteochondroma of the right condyle (green) with mandibular deviation. (**b**) Mandibular protrusion. (**c**) Tumor (green). (**d**) Coronal section of the tumor

4.1.6 General Digital Design Process for Orthognathic Surgery Simultaneous with Customized Total Joint Prosthesis

This chapter focuses on the design and practice of orthognathic surgery simultaneous with customized total joint prosthesis implantation. Its general process includes three aspects: orthognathic and lesion resection design, prosthesis and cutting guides design, and surgical procedure design (Fig. 4.13).

4.1.6.1 Design of Orthognathic and Lesion Resection

3D reconstruction of jaw deformities: perform 3D cephalometric analysis and simulate orthognathic osteotomies.

Determine final jaw positions and occlusion: based on measurement results and dental arch morphology, establish the final positions of the maxilla and mandible. Then design the condylar osteotomy range according to the required jaw positioning.

4.1.6.2 Design of Prosthesis and Cutting Guides

The total joint prosthesis is designed based on the final mandibular position and the residual mandibular stump morphology after condylar osteotomy.

Design the prosthesis, orthognathic, and TMJ cutting guides (see Chap. 3, 3.1.5).

4.1.6.3 Surgical Procedure Design

The procedure for performing orthognathic surgery simultaneous with total joint prosthesis implantation is of two types, either orthognathic surgery first or prosthesis implantation first.

A. Orthognathic-first procedure: maxillary surgery is performed first, and after precise fixation of the maxilla, the mandible position is restored according to the final occlusion, and then the prosthesis is fixed in place.
B. Total joint prosthesis-first procedure: the preauricular-temporal incision procedure is completed first, which

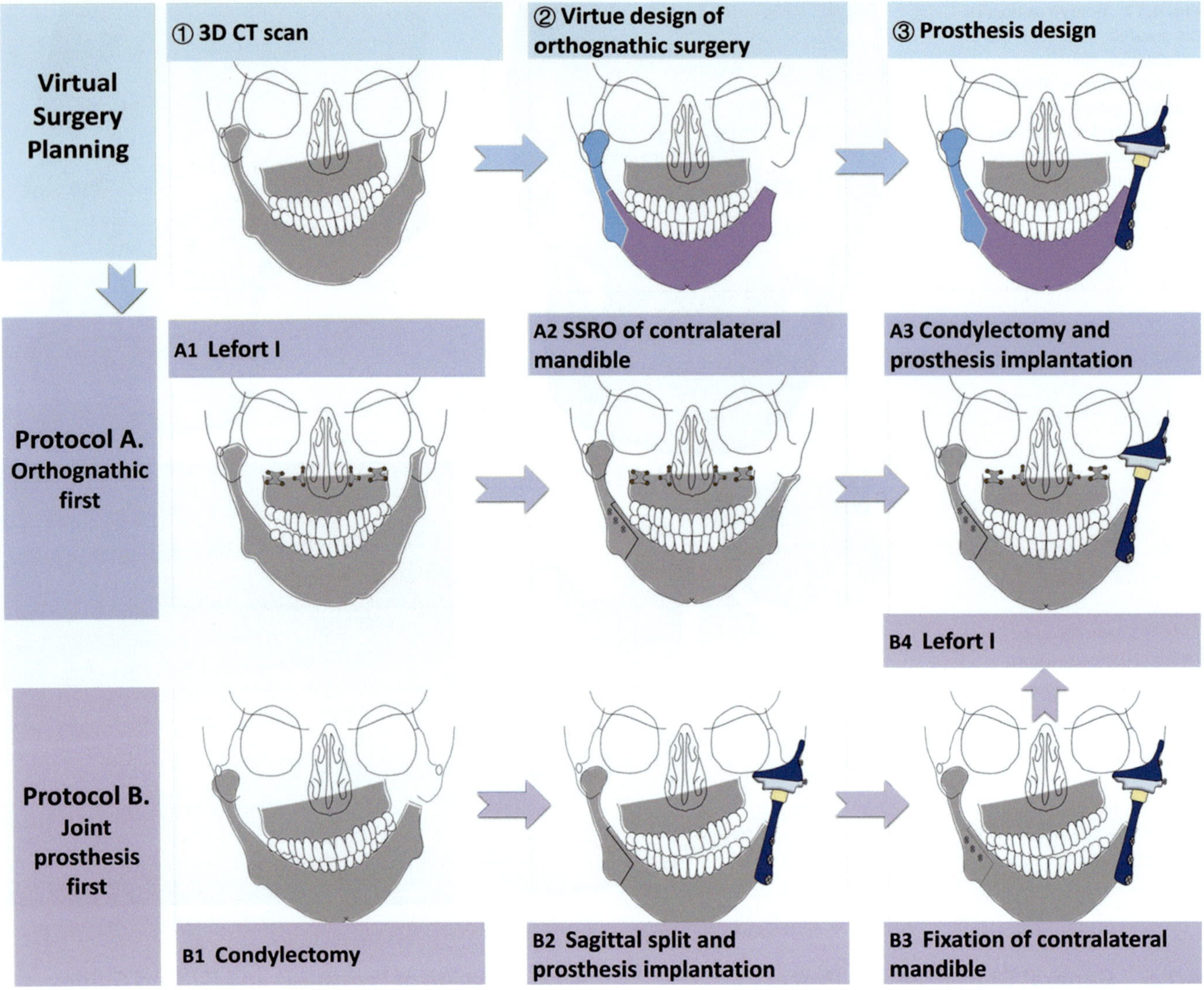

Fig. 4.13 General process of digital design for orthognathic surgery simultaneous with total joint prosthesis implantation. The gray area shows the maxilla and mandible, the pink area shows the digitally designed outcome for the mandibular position, and the blue area shows the digitally designed outcome for the healthy mandibular ramus. The total joint prosthesis designed for the left TMJ is shown in dark blue and yellow

consists of osteotomy of the condyle, resection of the lesion, prosthesis installation, and fat flap grafting and filling. After closure of the extraoral incision, orthognathic surgery is performed.

With the optimization of the prosthesis structure, the advantages of a prosthesis-first surgical procedure are becoming more and more apparent. Such a surgical process avoids switching between intraoral and extraoral surgery, i.e., completing the surgery related to the extraoral incision first and then carrying out the intraoral surgery after the incision is closed. This avoids the possibility of contaminating the operating area of the total joint prosthesis, and it reduces the risk of postoperative infection around the total joint prosthesis. At the same time, the use of the "H-" and "Y"-shaped orthognathic surgical bone fixation plate makes it possible to accurately position the maxilla during the surgery, and together with the customized total joint prosthesis, the overall accuracy is increased. This also has the advantages of simple installation and convenient operation, thus shortening the operation time and reducing bleeding and trauma.

These two options for the order of the surgery, A and B, are illustrated in Fig. 4.13. But in either case, all the components of the prosthesis and the cutting guides must be prepared in advance with the digitally precise customization techniques, as shown in the first line of the figure.

4.2 Reconstruction and Repair of Dentofacial Deformities Through Orthognathic Surgery Simultaneous with Bilateral Customized Total Temporomandibular Joint Prostheses Implantation

For patients with various types of dentofacial deformities secondary to TMJ diseases, concomitant orthognathic surgery is indicated to resolve the deformities, while replacement of the diseased TMJ with the total joint prosthesis restores the TMJ function and aids in facial reconstruction. In the following sections of this chapter, six clinical cases will be described in detail, covering:

- The orthognathic role of simple TMJ prosthesis implantation (Sect. 4.2 Case D)
- Treatment of condylar tumor with deviated jaw, with orthognathic surgery and simultaneous TMJ prosthesis implantation (Sect. 4.3 Case E)
- Treatment of ankylosis with deviated jaw, with orthognathic surgery and simultaneous TMJ prosthesis implantation (Sect. 4.4 Case F)
- Treatment of congenital malocclusion, with orthognathic surgery and simultaneous TMJ prosthesis implantation (Sect. 4.5 Case G)
- Treatment of resorption of autologous bone grafts, with orthognathic surgery and simultaneous TMJ prosthesis implantation (Sect. 4.6 Case H)
- Treatment of orthognathic malocclusion for failed orthognathic surgery, with orthognathic surgery and simultaneous TMJ prosthesis implantation (Sect. 4.7 Case I)

4.2.1 Case D: The Orthognathic Role of Bilateral Total Joint Prosthesis Implantation

- Patient information: male, 26 years old.
- Complaint: progressive mandibular retrognathia with bilateral preauricular noising and pain for more than 5 years.
- History: over the past 5 years, the patient presented with progressive aggravation of mandibular retrognathia, accompanied by bilateral preauricular noising and pain, 3 to 5 times per year, each time lasting from 1 week to 1 month.
- Past history: the patient reported that he was physically fit, denied any history of systemic diseases, and denied any history of drug or food allergy.
- Clinical examination: the facial shape was basically symmetrical, the height of the angle of the mouth was the same, the mandible was retracted, the chin muscle was tense, and the degree of opening of the mouth was 45 mm, without deviation. Bilateral posterior teeth were in complete distal relationship, classified as a characteristic of Angle's Class II division 2 malocclusion; anterior teeth were horizontally open bite but centered in the midline. #36 and #46 residual roots, #37 and #47 mesially tilted, and #21 non-vital tooth (Figs. 4.14, 4.15, 4.17 and 4.18); pain VAS score was 4 points.
- Imaging examinations: MRI showed bilateral condylar resorption and anterior disc displacement without reduction. CT scan showed disruption of cortical continuity at the top of the condyle, bone roughness, and irregular condylar morphology (Figs. 4.16 and 4.19).
- Diagnosis: bilateral anterior disc displacement without reduction, condylar resorption; bony Class II, mandibular retrognathia; malocclusion, anterior open bite, #36 and #46 residual roots.

4.2.2 Case D. Diagnostic Imaging

4.2.3 Case D. Treatment Plan

Preoperative orthodontics: after 13 months of preoperative orthodontics, a surgical plan was developed (Figs. 4.17, 4.18 and 4.19).

- Overall treatment plan: bilateral total joint prosthesis replacement. Resection of severely resorbed condyles and reconstruction with total joint prostheses, utilizing prosthetic lengthening of the mandible to replace sagittal split ramus osteotomy advancement.

4.2.4 Case D. Design and Processing of the Classic Total Joint Prosthesis Components and the Cutting Guides

The desired location of the mandible is the most critical element to be determined, and the parameters for this are illustrated in Fig. 4.20. Then the prosthesis and guides are routinely designed (Fig. 4.21). Prosthesis fabrication and fitting are described in Sect. 2.5 in Chap. 2.

4.2.5 Case D. Surgical Procedure

4.2.5.1 Preoperative Examination

The same as described in Sect. 3.2.5, Preoperative Laboratory Tests.

Preoperative preparation: prepare 400 ml of blood preoperatively. The others are same as described in Sect. 3.2.5, Preoperative Preparation.

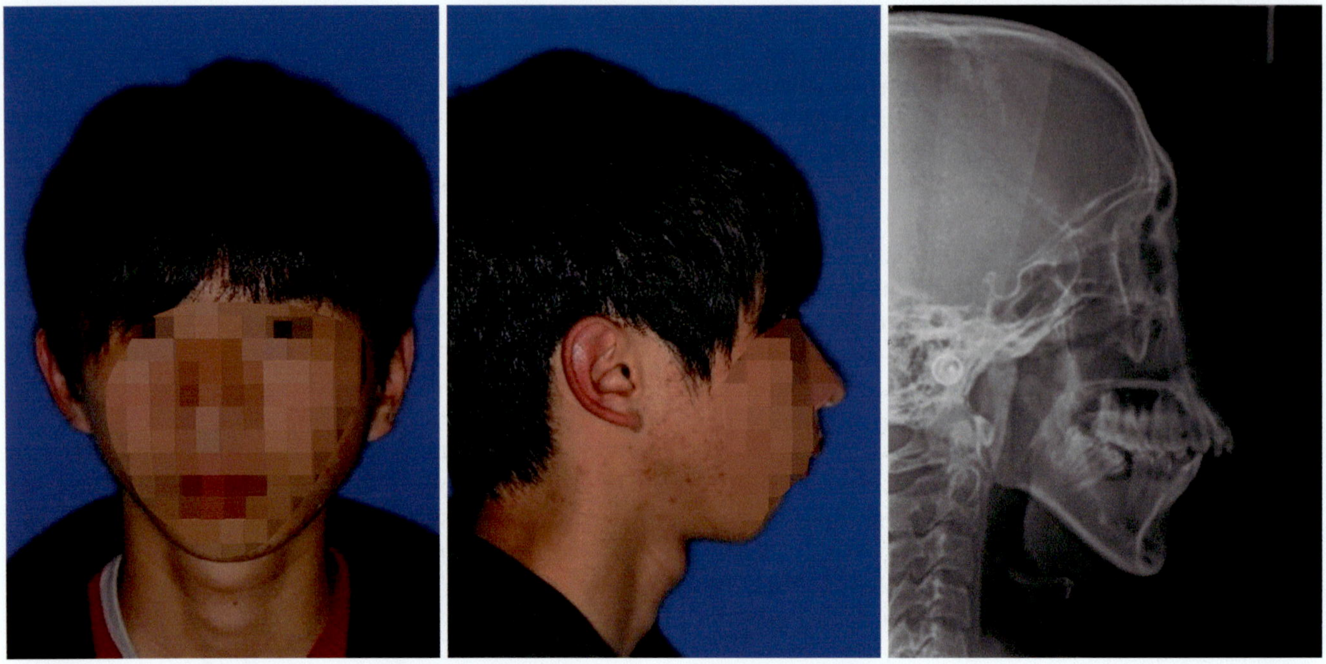

Fig. 4.14 Case D. Facial examination. The face was basically symmetrical, with consistent height of the corners of the mouth, but the mandibular retrognathia and tension of the chin muscles, and the lateral view showed serious mandibular retrognathia, with the overjet by 11 mm. The condition of the condylar process was unclear. The mouth opening was 45 mm and was centered

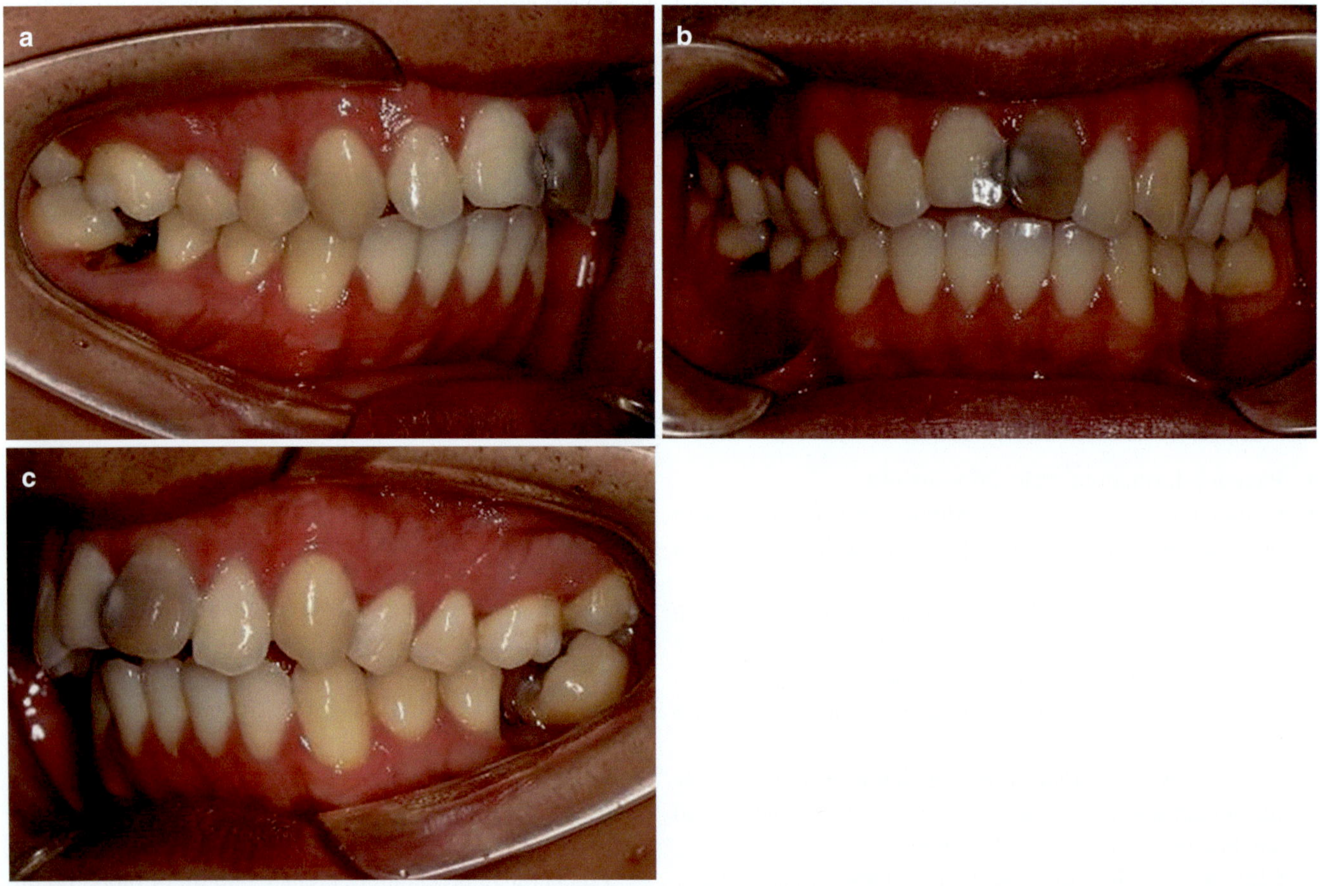

Fig. 4.15 Case D. Intraoral examination. (**a**) Right lateral view, (**b**) Frontal view. (**c**) Left lateral view

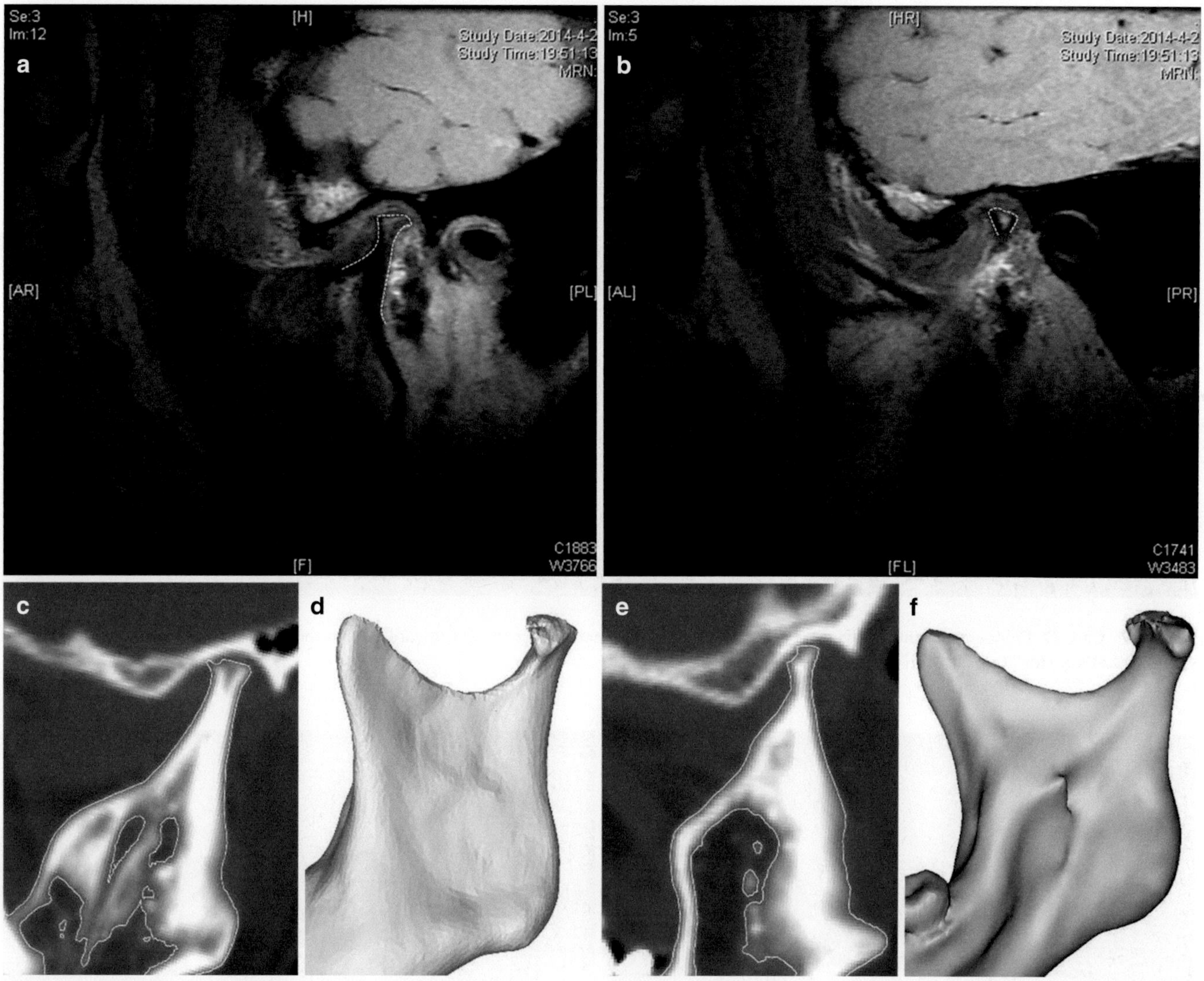

Fig. 4.16 Case D. Diagnostic imaging. Bilateral condylar resorption and anterior disc displacement without reduction. CT image shows disruption of cortical continuity at the top of the condyle, bone roughness, and irregular condylar morphology. (**a**) MRI of the left joint. (**b**) MRI of the right joint. (**c**) Sagittal section of the left condyle. (**d**) CT reconstruction of the left condyle. (**e**) CT sagittal section of the right condyle. (**f**) CT reconstruction of the right condyle

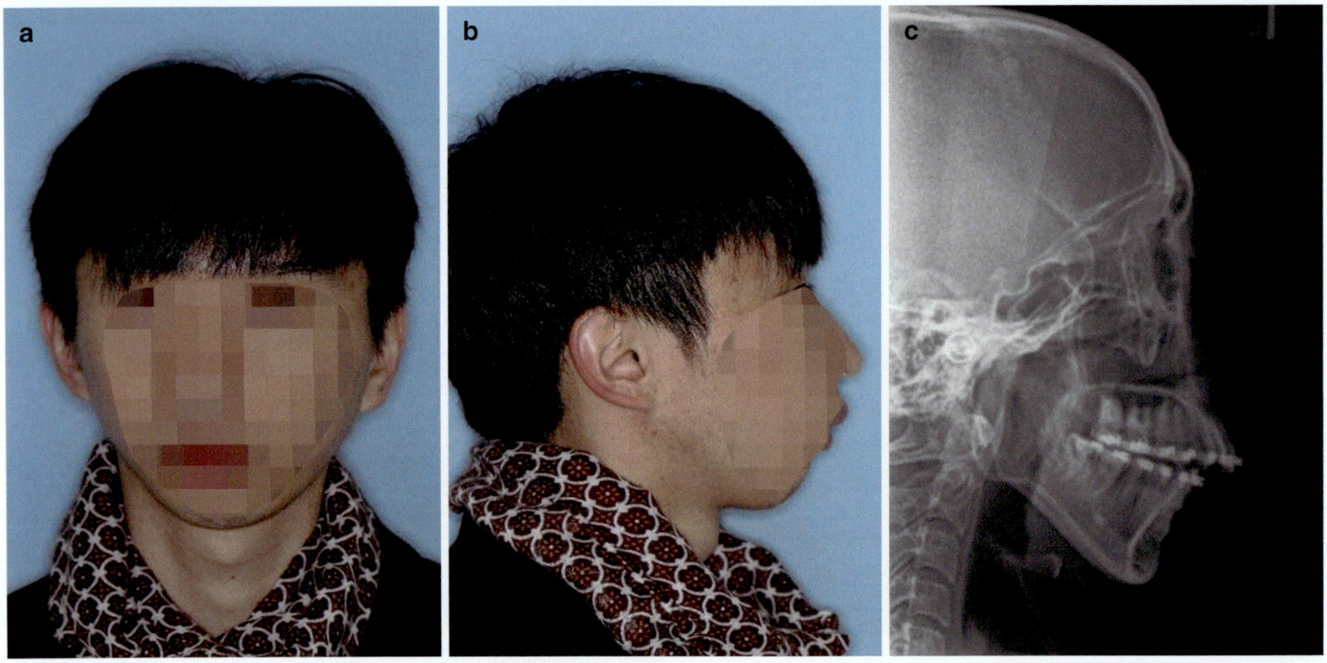

Fig. 4.17 Case D. Preoperative anterior view. The lower front teeth were further moved inward after orthodontic decompensation. (**a**) Frontal view. (**b**) Lateral view. (**c**) Lateral film

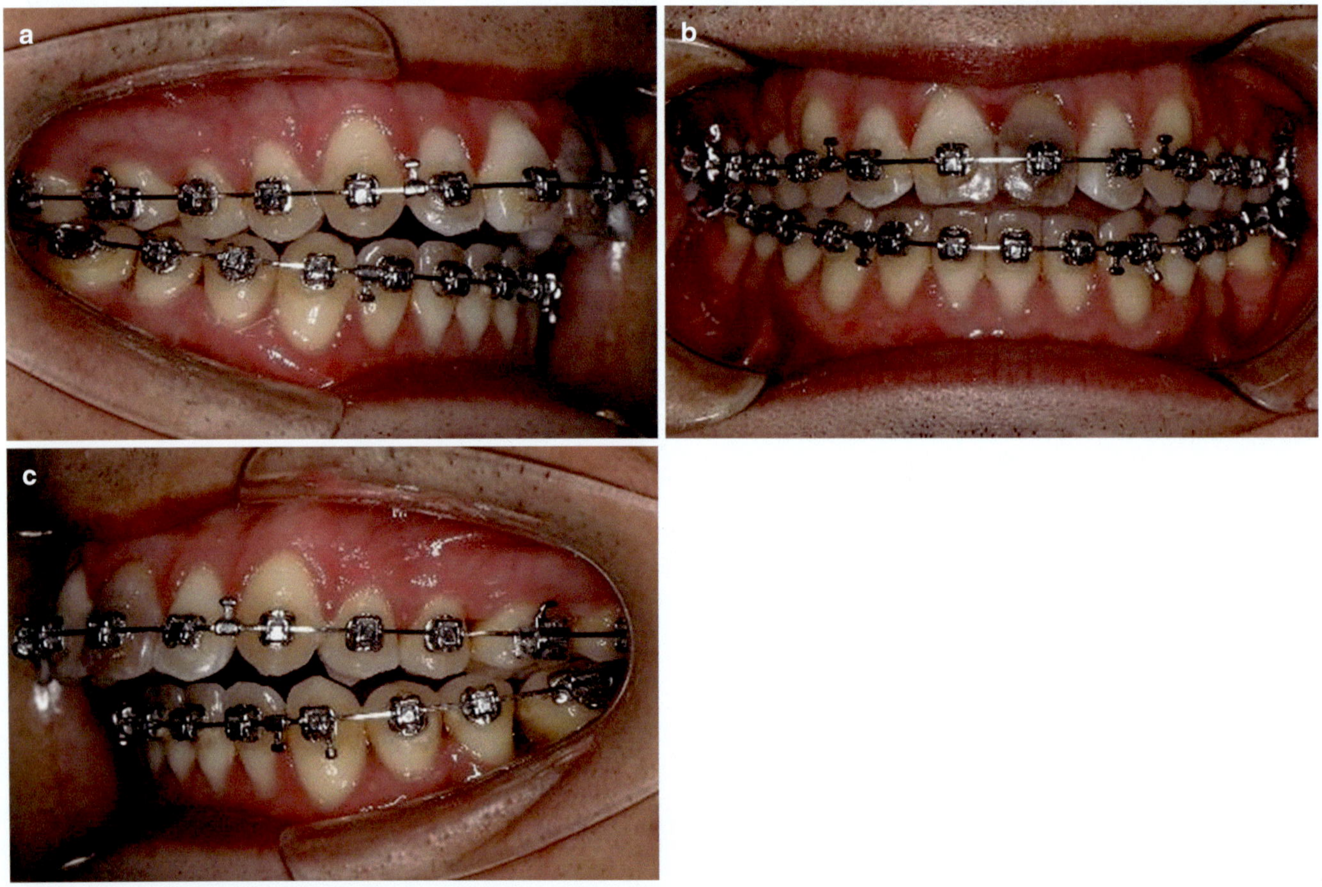

Fig. 4.18 Case D. Intraoral examination. After orthodontic decompensation, closure of the mandibular tooth gap and inward movement of the lower front teeth. (**a**) Right occlusion. (**b**) Frontal occlusion. (**c**) Left occlusion

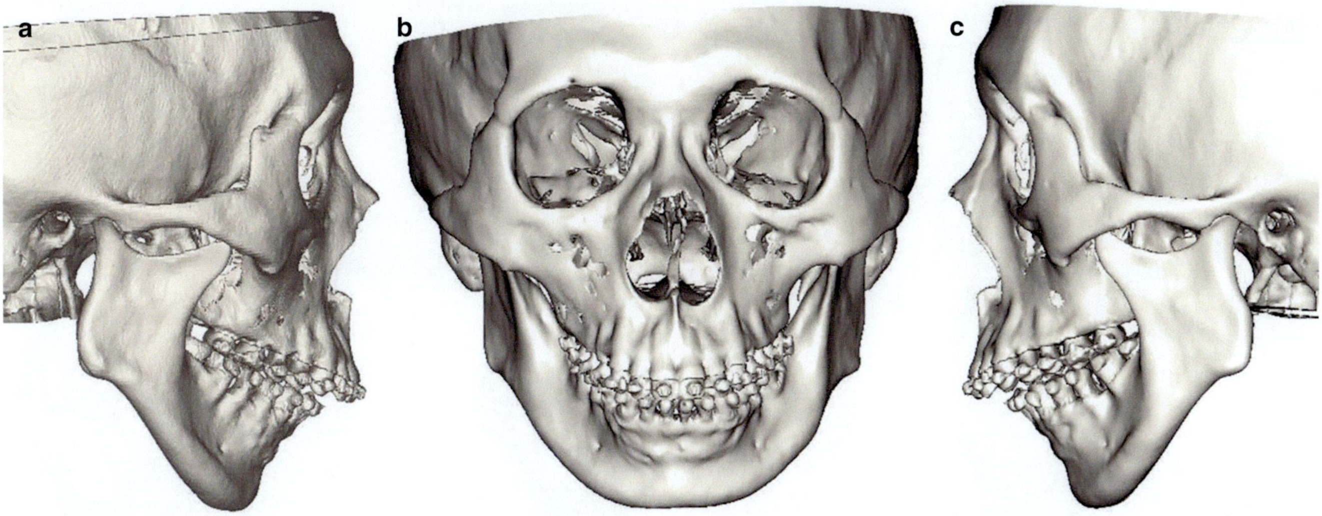

Fig. 4.19 Case D. Preoperative CT 3D reconstruction. Bony Class II deformity with serious bilateral mandibular retrognathia. (**a**) Right view; (**b**) Frontal view; (**c**) Left view

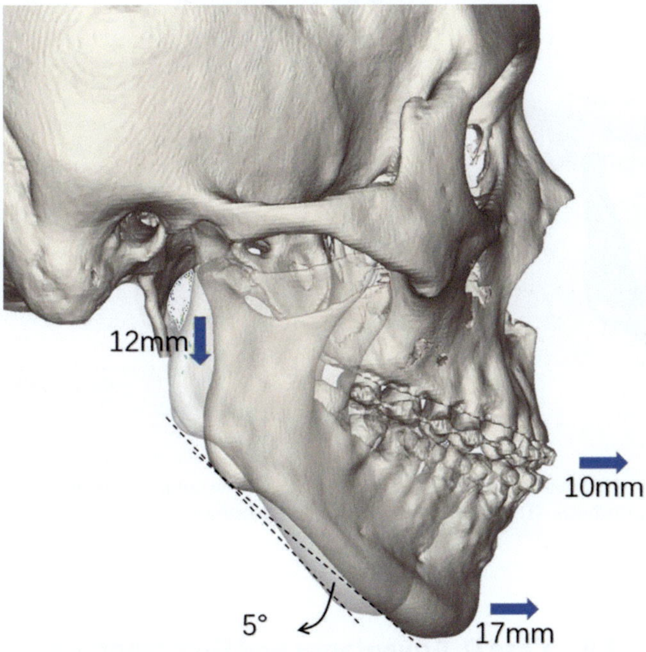

Fig. 4.20 Virtual postoperative position of the mandible. The mandible was brought down and forward to achieve the final occlusion. The ramus was lengthened vertically 12 mm. The lower incisors moved forward 10 mm. Pogonion moved forward 17 mm. The mandibular plane rotated counterclockwise by 5°

4.2.5.2 Steps of the Surgical Procedure

1. Surgical approach: preauriculotemporal incision and a small through-buccal incision were used.
2. Prosthesis implant bed management: subcondylar osteotomy and articular eminence osteotomy to prepare the implant bed.
3. Implantation of the total joint prosthesis. See Sect. 3.2.5, Prosthesis Implantation.
4. Postoperative advice and care: see Sect. 3.2.5, Postoperative Orders and Nursing Care.

4.2.6 Case D. Postoperative Analysis of Prothesis Implantation Precision

Regular postoperative follow-ups were performed for appearance (facial shape), function (mouth opening, mouth shape), and prosthesis evaluation (safety, accuracy).

Immediately after surgery: intraoperative prosthesis installation was smooth, occlusal relationship was stable, bleeding volume was 300 mL, and surgical time was 3 h and 30 min.

Preoperative design and postoperative CT image reconstruction were matched. The maximum error of the core components was 0.46 mm, and the maximum error of the whole component was 1.31 mm (Figs. 4.22 and 4.23).

For the patient, the postoperative appearance and occlusal relationship improved significantly. The mouth opening was 40 mm (Figs. 4.24 and 4.25).

4.2.7 Case D. Long-Term Follow-Up and Prognosis

3-Year Postoperative Follow-Up

There were no complaints of discomfort, the face was well shaped, and there was no redness, swelling, or other reactions in the operative area.

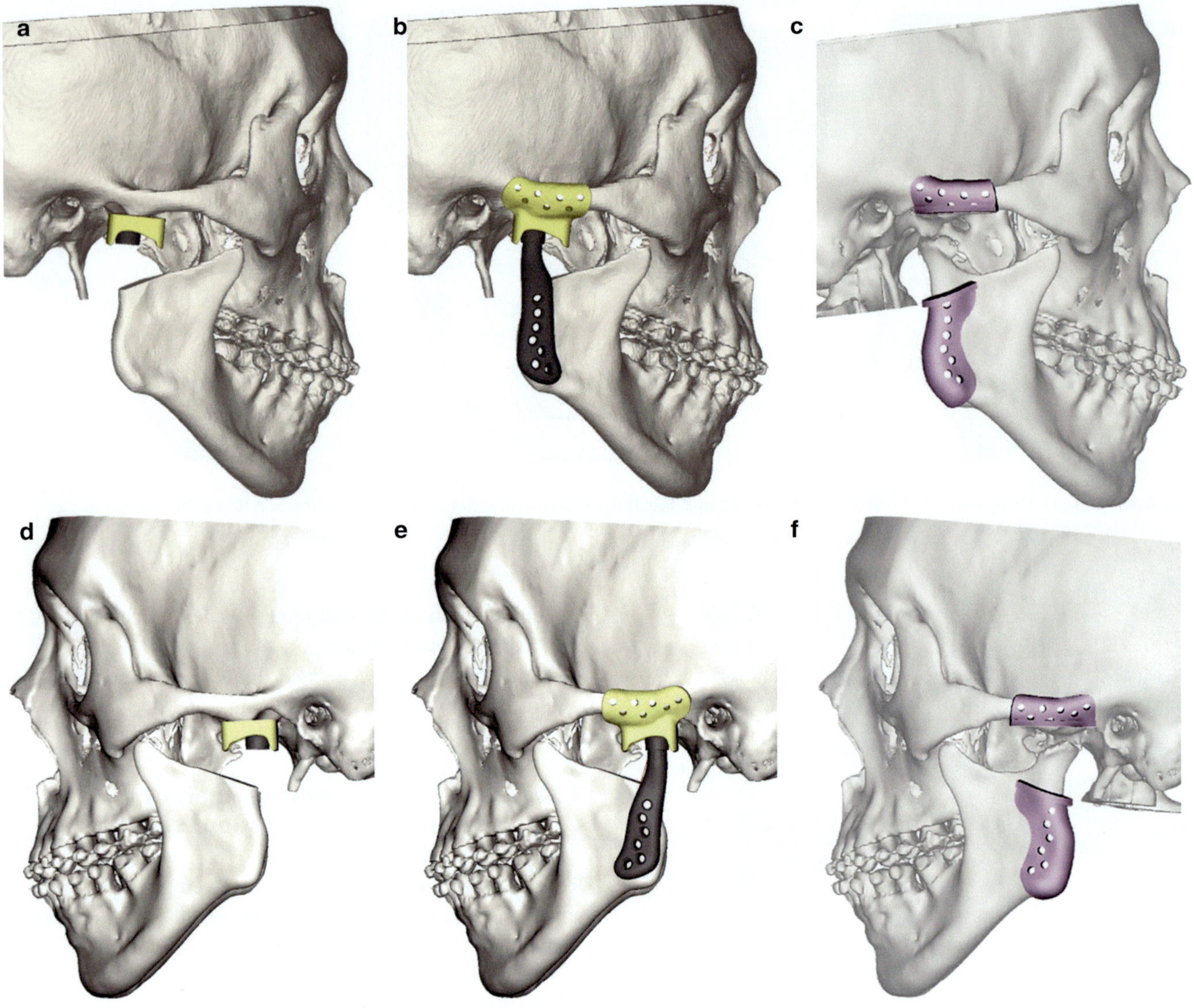

Fig. 4.21 Case D. Design of prostheses and cutting guides. (**a**) Core components of the right prosthesis. (**b**) Extension components of the right prosthesis. (**c**) Cutting guides for the right prosthesis. (**d**) Core components of the left prosthesis. (**e**) Extension components of the left prosthesis. (**f**) Cutting guides for the left prosthesis

The preauricular pain improved significantly, and the VAS pain score was 1 out of a maximum of 10.

The mouth opening was 37 mm, with 3 mm lateral movement to the right and 4 mm lateral movement to the left.

Masticatory function: normal feeding.

Facial shape and occlusal relationship: improved facial shape without visible scarring; good occlusal relationship (Figs. 4.26 and 4.27).

Evaluation of the prosthesis: the 3-year postoperative panoramic radiographs showed no complications such as infection and rejection, loosening, fracture, and material allergy, and the prosthesis was well integrated with the bone (Fig. 4.28).

4.2.8 Case D. Advantages and Disadvantages

4.2.8.1 Advantages

After 3 years of follow-up, there were no adverse reactions or complications, and the occlusal relationship was stable.

Reduced surgical trauma: although the TMJ prosthesis implantation was performed through a preauriculotemporal incision, the postoperative scar was not obvious due to the cosmetic incision design with endoscopic fixation. There was less surgical bleeding and no surgical incision within the mouth.

Ease of lengthening and angle adjustment of the mandible: the mandibular lengthening and restoration of occlusal

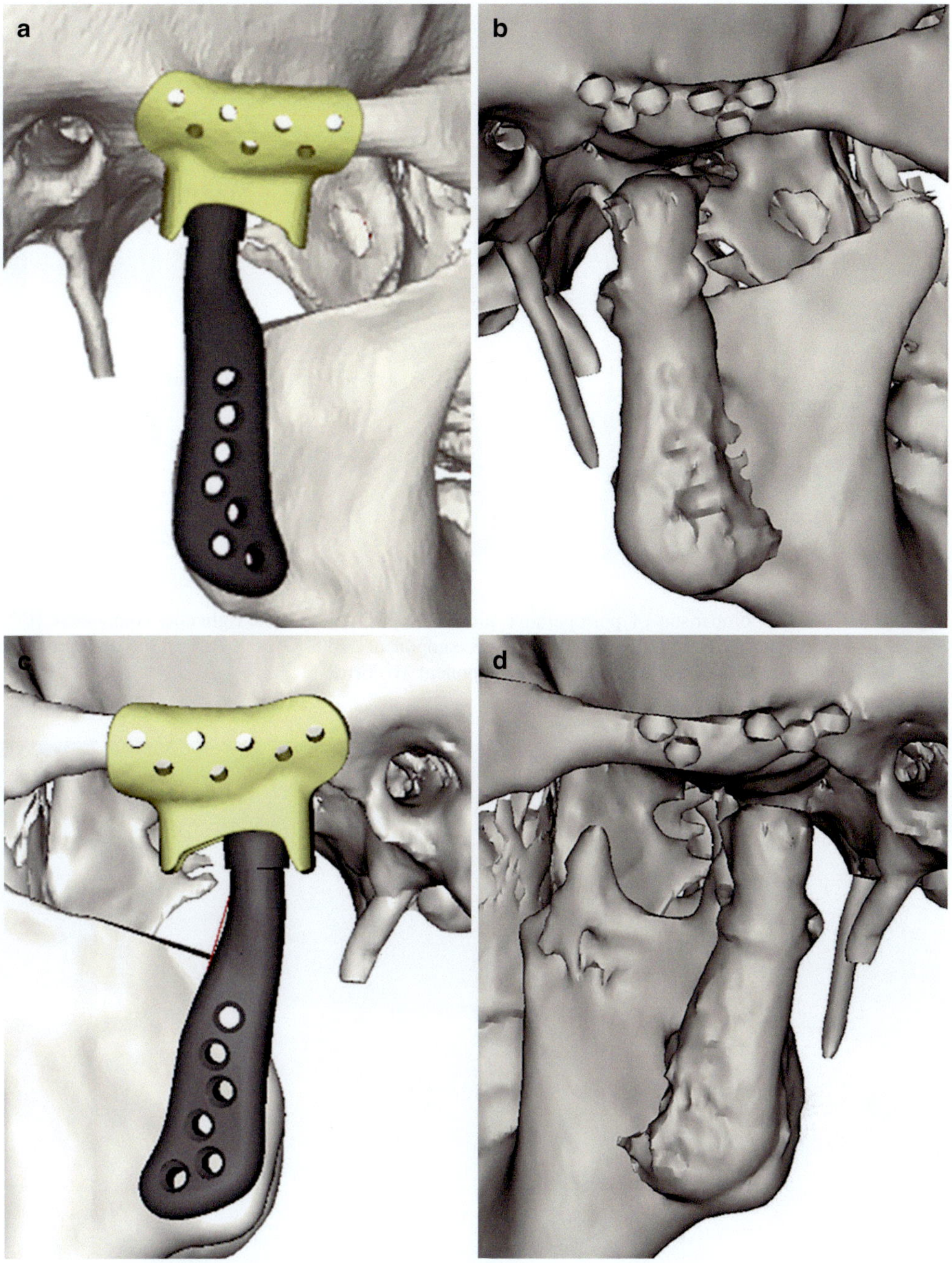

Fig. 4.22 Case D. 3D CT reconstruction of postoperative prosthesis position. For accurate analysis of positioning error, the preoperative digital model of the prosthesis needs to be matched with the CT reconstruction according to the screw holes. (**a**) Right prosthesis design plan. (**b**) Right prosthesis postoperative reconstruction. (**c**) Left prosthesis design plan. (**d**) Left prosthesis postoperative reconstruction

relationship that routinely requires sagittal splitting of the bilateral mandibular ramus can be achieved in this case by total joint implantation alone.

Due to the change in the angle of the posterior edge of the patient's mandibular ramus, it is difficult for a standard prosthesis to be adequately and stably fixed in place. Customized prostheses that are digitally designed and fabricated allow for excellent mechanical stability of position.

4.2.8.2 Disadvantages

This surgical procedure is suitable for patients with mandibular retrognathia but with maxillary position that is basically within the normal range; in this case, only a small forward rotation of the mandibular plane can solve the problem of a gap between the upper and lower incisors. But most patients with more obvious or extreme maxillary deformity also need maxillary surgery, as will be described in cases in the following sections of this chapter.

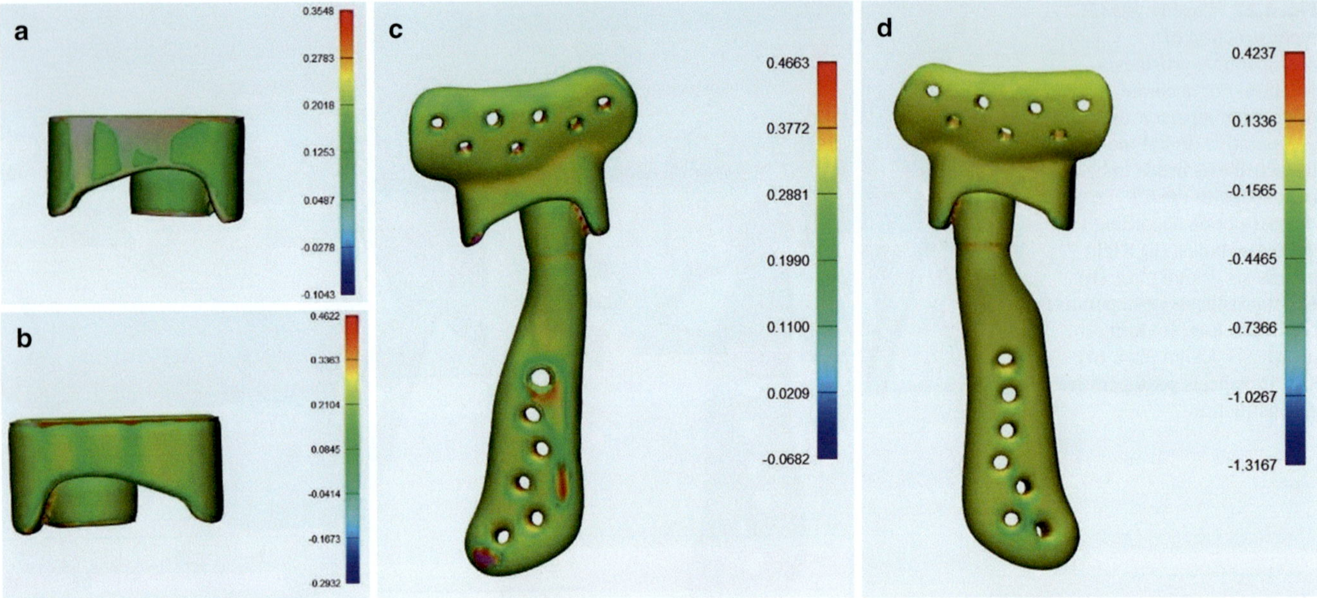

Fig. 4.23 Case D. Comparison of postoperative prosthesis position and design. Maximum error of 0.46 mm for the core component and 1.31 mm for the whole. (**a**) Error of the left core component. (**b**) Error of the right core component. (**c**) Overall error of the left prosthesis. (**d**) Overall error of the right prosthesis

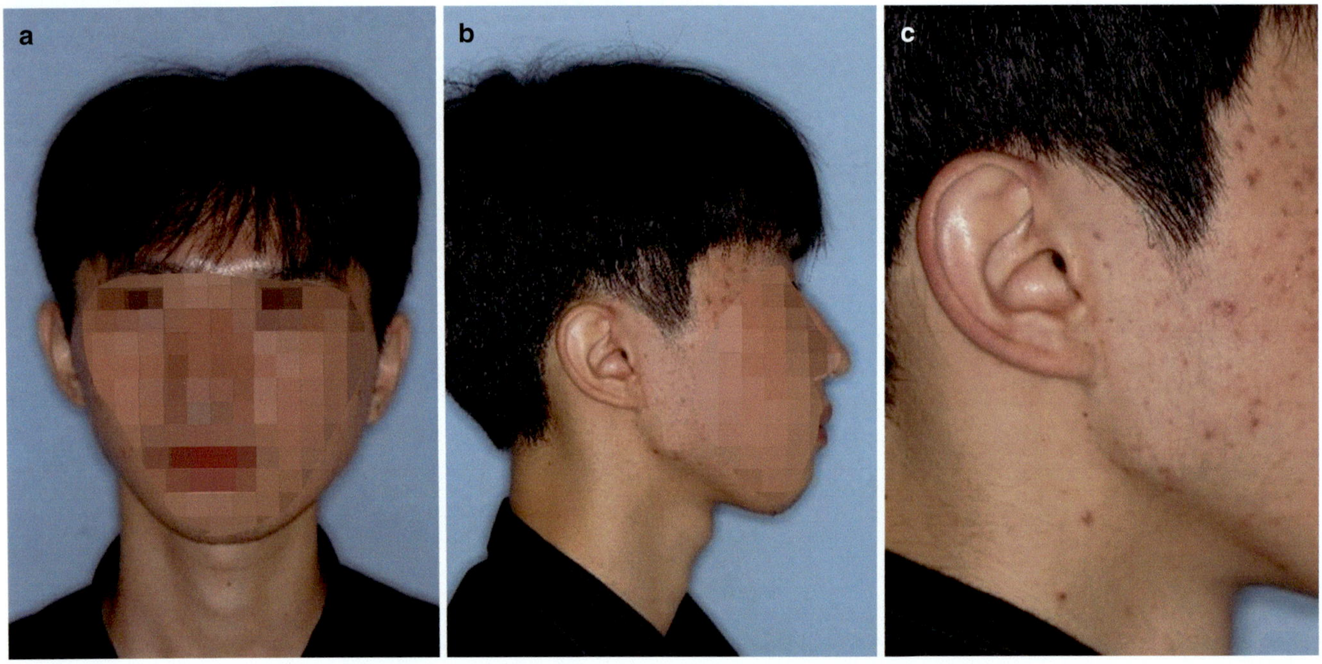

Fig. 4.24 Case D. 3-month postoperative facial examination. The chin is centered, the jaw position is improved, and the surgical scar is not obvious. (**a**) Frontal view. (**b**) Lateral view. (**c**) Close-up of the right preauricular region

In Case D, due to the simultaneous resection of the condyle and the lateral pterygoid muscle, the patient's postoperative mouth opening was slightly less than before the operation, and the ability of the patient to stretch his mouth for lateral and anterior extension was not ideal in postoperative outcome. We will try to deal with this shortcoming in the future.

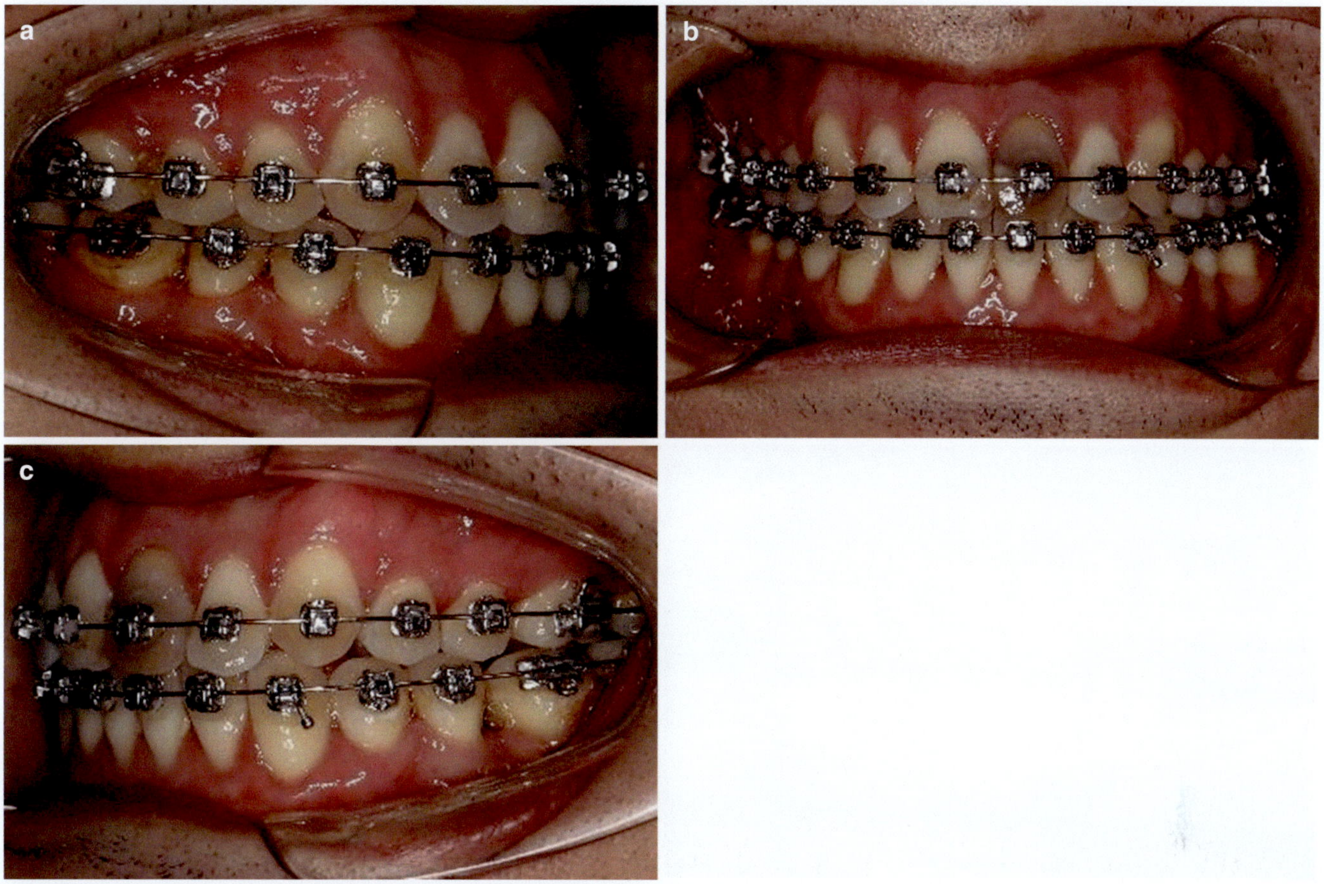

Fig. 4.25 Case D. Intraoral examination at 3 months postoperatively. Class I occlusal relationship with good occlusion relationship. (**a**) Right occlusion. (**b**) Frontal occlusion. (**c**) Left occlusion

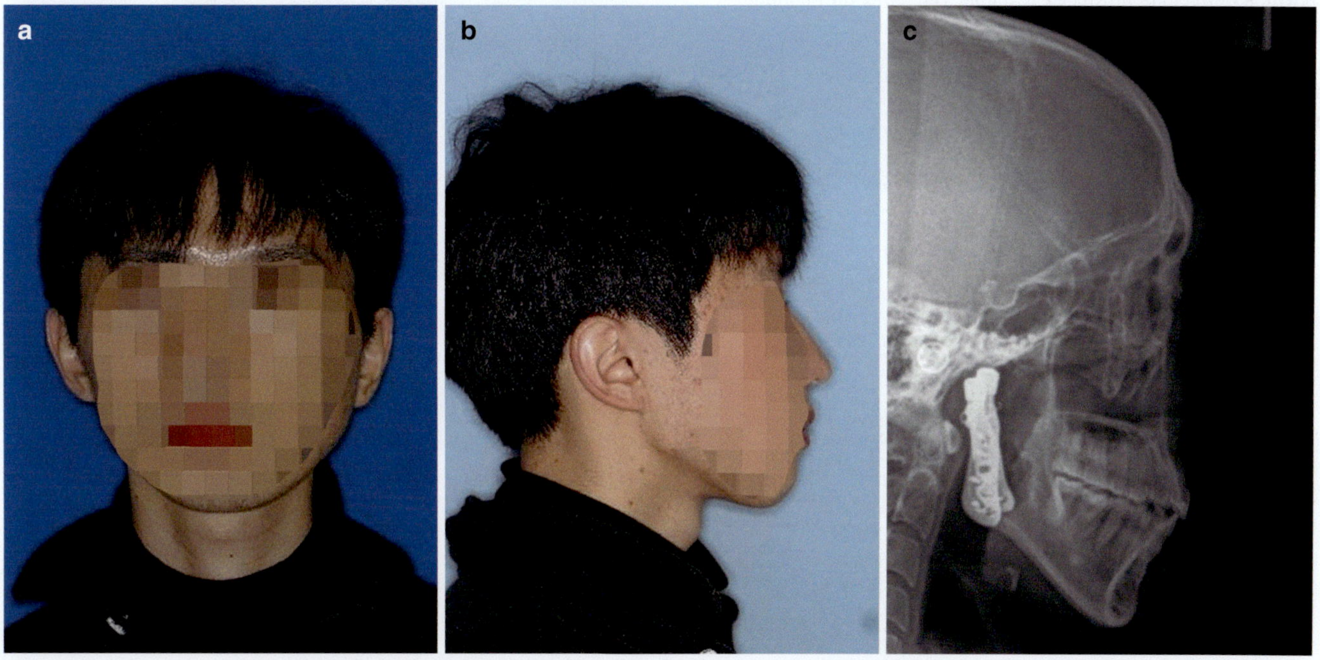

Fig. 4.26 Case D. Stabilization of the facial shape 3 years after surgery. (**a**) Frontal view. (**b**) Right lateral view. (**c**) Cephalometric X-ray

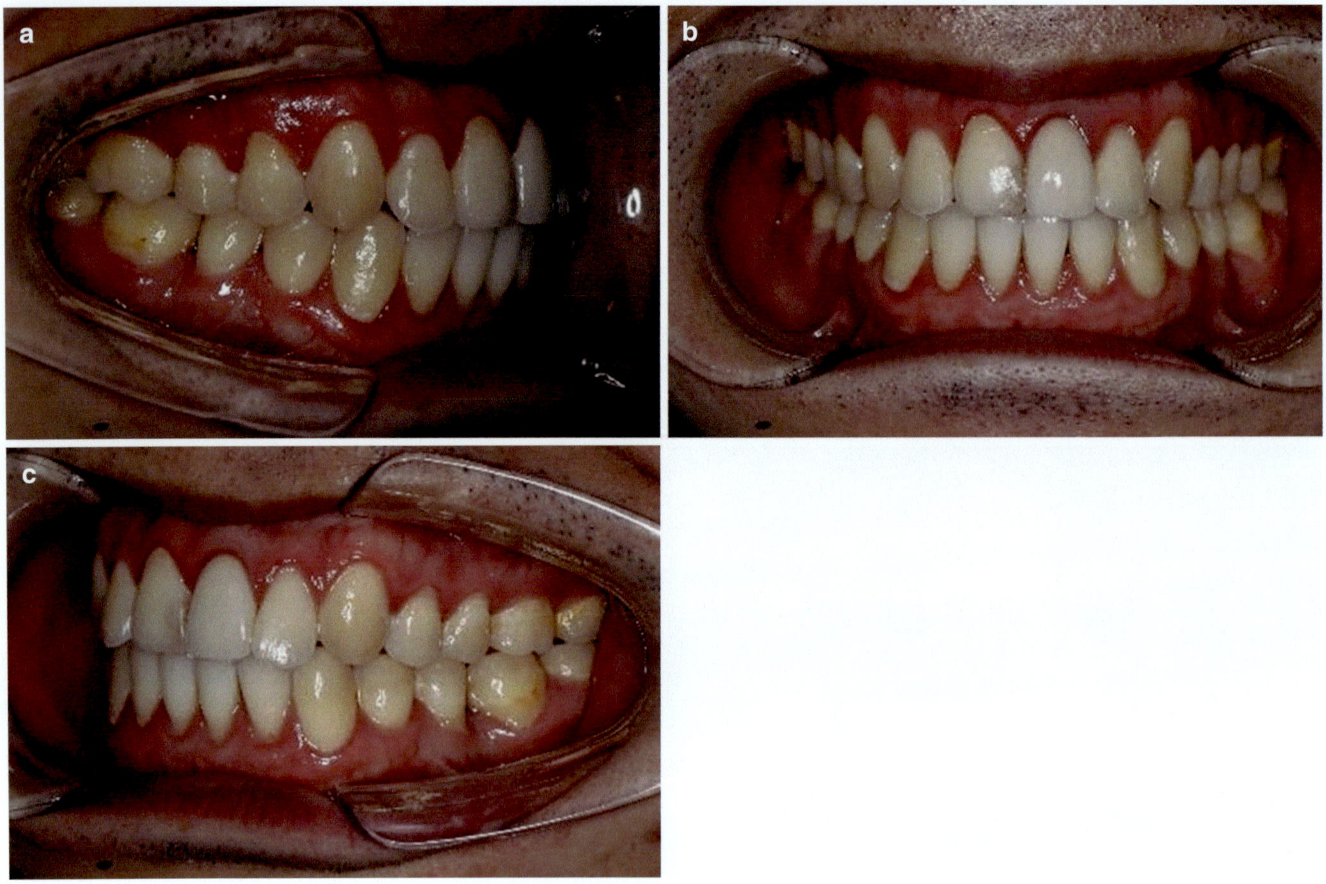

Fig. 4.27 Case D. Stable occlusal relationship 3 years after surgery. (**a**) Right occlusion. (**b**) Front occlusion. (**c**) Left occlusion

Fig. 4.28 Case D. Panoramic film 3 years after surgery. The position of the joint prosthesis is stable. The wires surrounding the condylar prostheses are connected to the bone blocks attached to the lateral pterygoid muscles

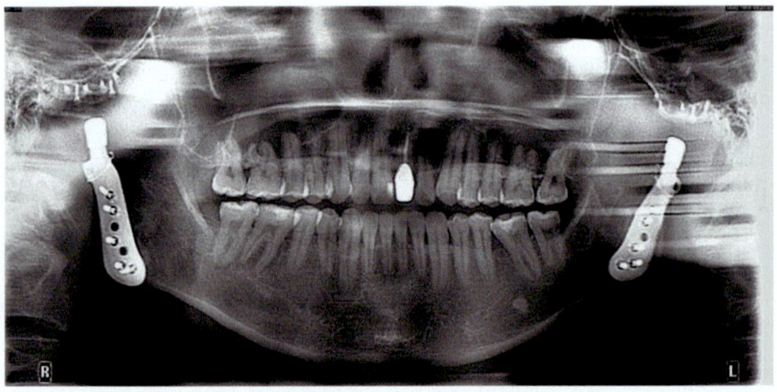

4.3 Reconstruction and Repair of Condylar Tumor with Deviated Jaw Deformity Through Orthognathic Surgery Simultaneous with Customized Total Temporomandibular Joint Prosthesis Implantation

4.3.1 Case E. Condylar Tumor with Deviated Jaw Deformity

- Patient information: male, 27 years old.
- Complaint: progressive left-sided mandibular deviation with right-sided preauricular pain for more than 5 years.
- History: the patient's jaw had been gradually deviated to the left side for 5 years, and he had frequent paroxysms of pain in the right preauricular region in the last year.
- Past history: the patient reported that he was physically fit and denied any history of systemic diseases and drug or food allergies.
- Clinical examination: the mandible is deviated 25 mm to the left, with the upper lip midline shifted to the left and the oral commissures showing left-sided elevation. The mouth opening measures 40 mm, with a left-deviated opening pattern. The right first molar exhibits a Class III full mesial relationship (Angle's classification), accompanied by an anterior crossbite and a left-deviated midline of the lower dentition. The left first molar demonstrates a Class I occlusal relationship (Angle's classification), with teeth #35 to #37 lingually inclined (Figs. 4.29, 4.30, 4.33, and 4.34). The pain VAS score is 6.
- Imaging examination: X-ray showed left deviation of the mandible, increased length of the right mandibular ramus compared with the opposite side, increased volume of the condyle, anterior protrusion of the mandible, and anterior crossbite of the teeth. CT showed that the cartilage of the right condylar process was hyperplastic and hypertrophied, with unclear boundaries, and that the swelling of the mass protruded medially, pushed anteriorly, and sclerotized the bone to the top of the foramen of the mandible (Figs. 4.31, 4.32, and 4.35).
- Diagnosis: possible osteochondroma of the right condyle; deviated jaw deformity.

4.3.2 Case E. Diagnostic Imaging (Figs. 4.31 and 4.32)

4.3.3 Case E. Treatment Plan

Preoperative orthodontics: after 13 months of preoperative orthodontics, a surgical plan was developed (Figs. 4.33, 4.34 and 4.35).

After orthodontic decompensation, there was no significant change in the facial shape. As a result of the decompensation, the right posterior teeth were separated by a gap, and the lower dentition deviated 9 mm to the left of the midline.

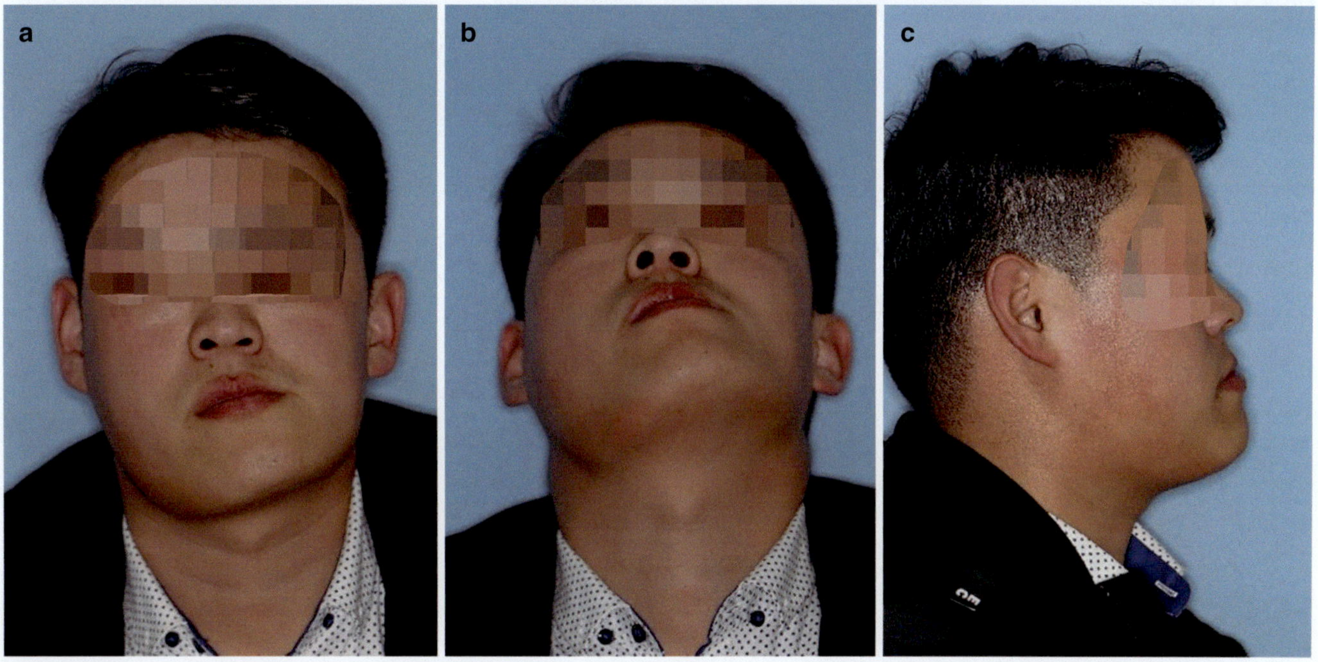

Fig. 4.29 Case E. Facial examination. (**a**) Frontal view. (**b**) View from below. (**c**) Lateral view

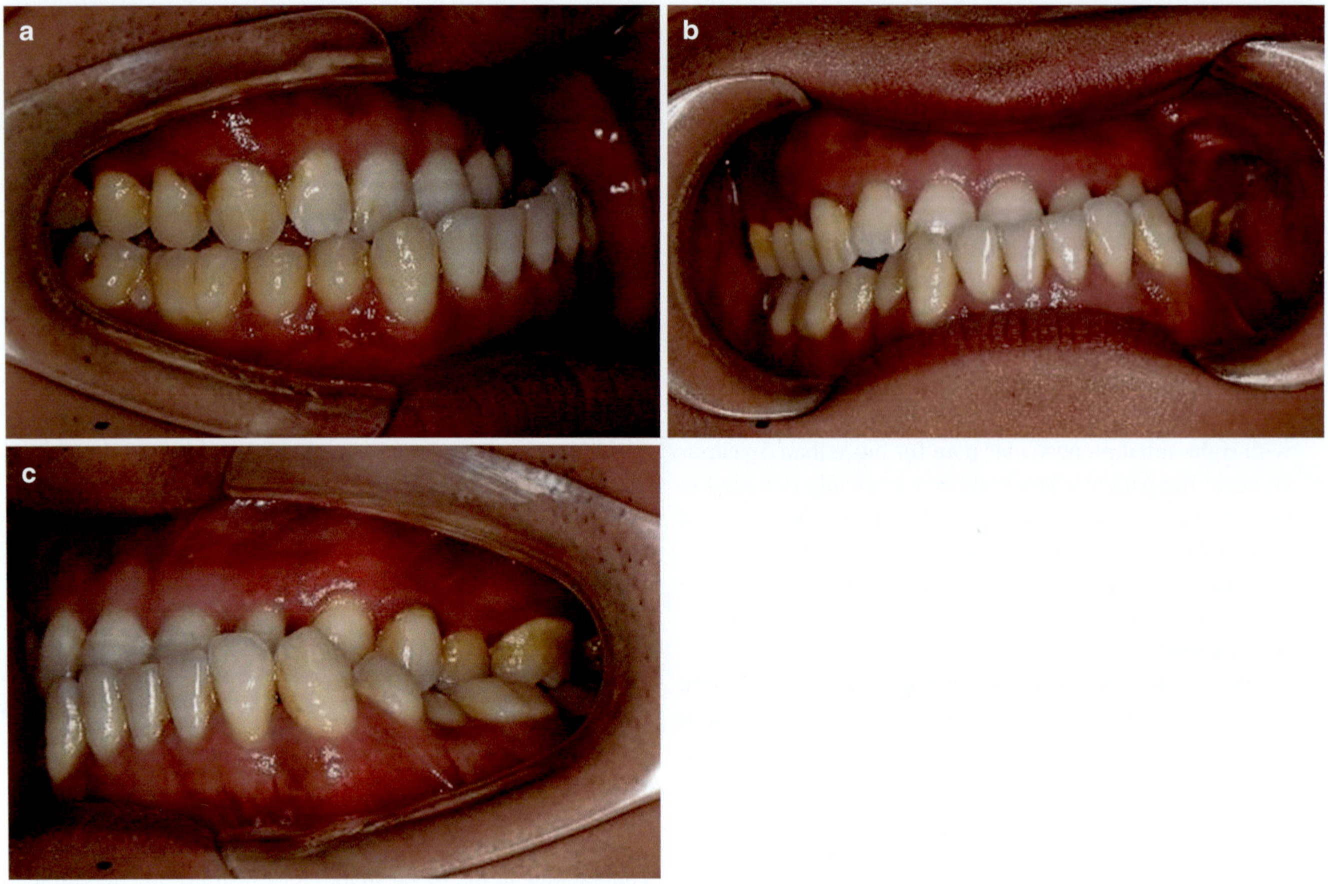

Fig. 4.30 Case E. Intraoral examination, showing abnormal protrusion of the lower teeth. (**a**) Right occlusion. (**b**) Frontal occlusion (**c**) Left occlusion

Fig. 4.31 Case E. Cephalometric X-rays. The mandible is deviated to the left, with the length of the right ramus greater than that of the left. The volume of the right condyle is far greater than that of the left. The mandible is protrusive, with the anterior teeth in crossbite. (**a**) Frontal view. (**b**) Lateral view

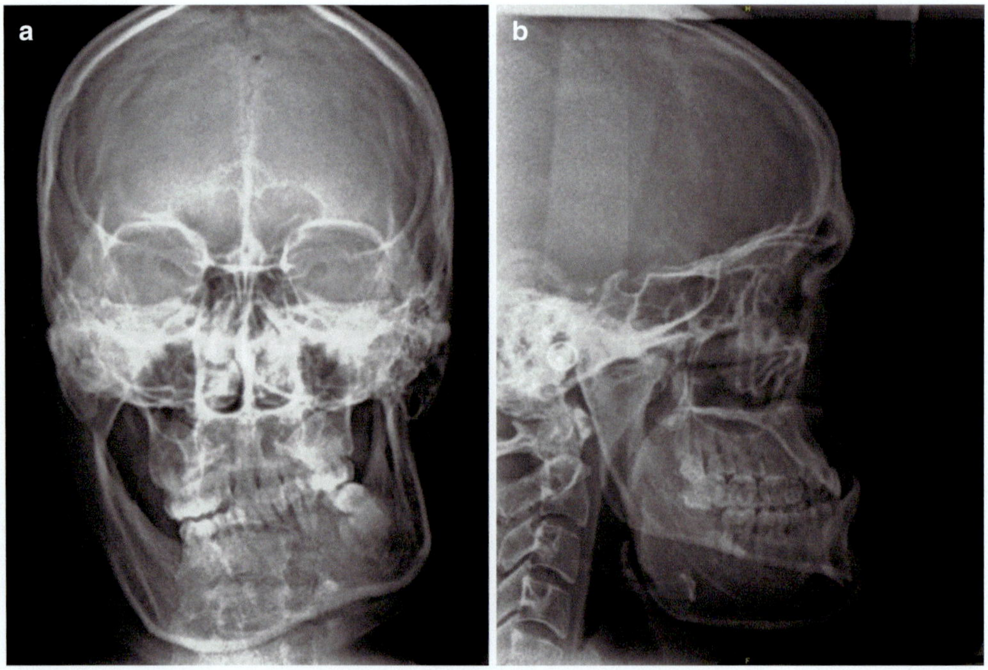

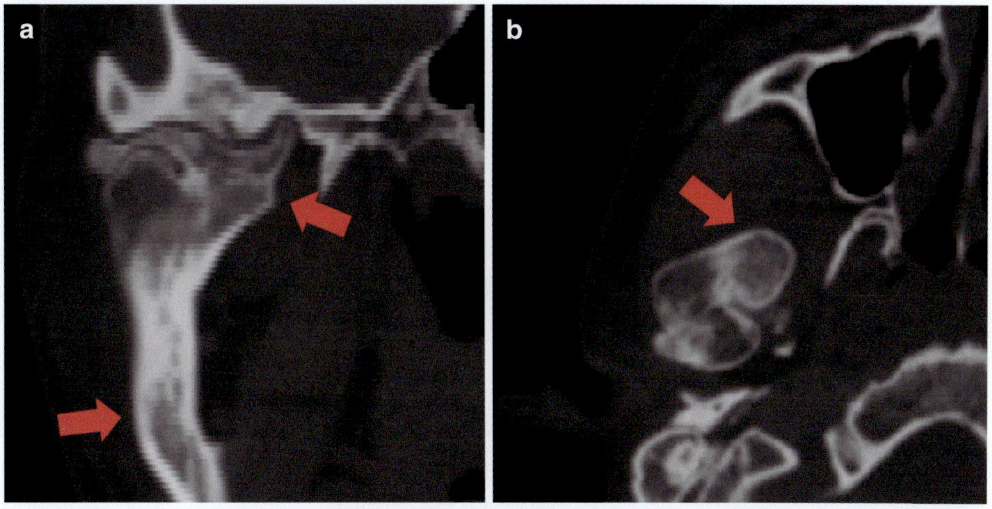

Fig. 4.32 Case E. TMJ CT. A tumor of the right condyle is consistent with osteochondroma. It is bulging both medially and anteriorly (upper red arrows). The inferior tumor margin is not clear; however, osteosclerosis reaches just above the lingula of the mandible (lower left red arrow). (**a**) Coronal view. (**b**) Axial view

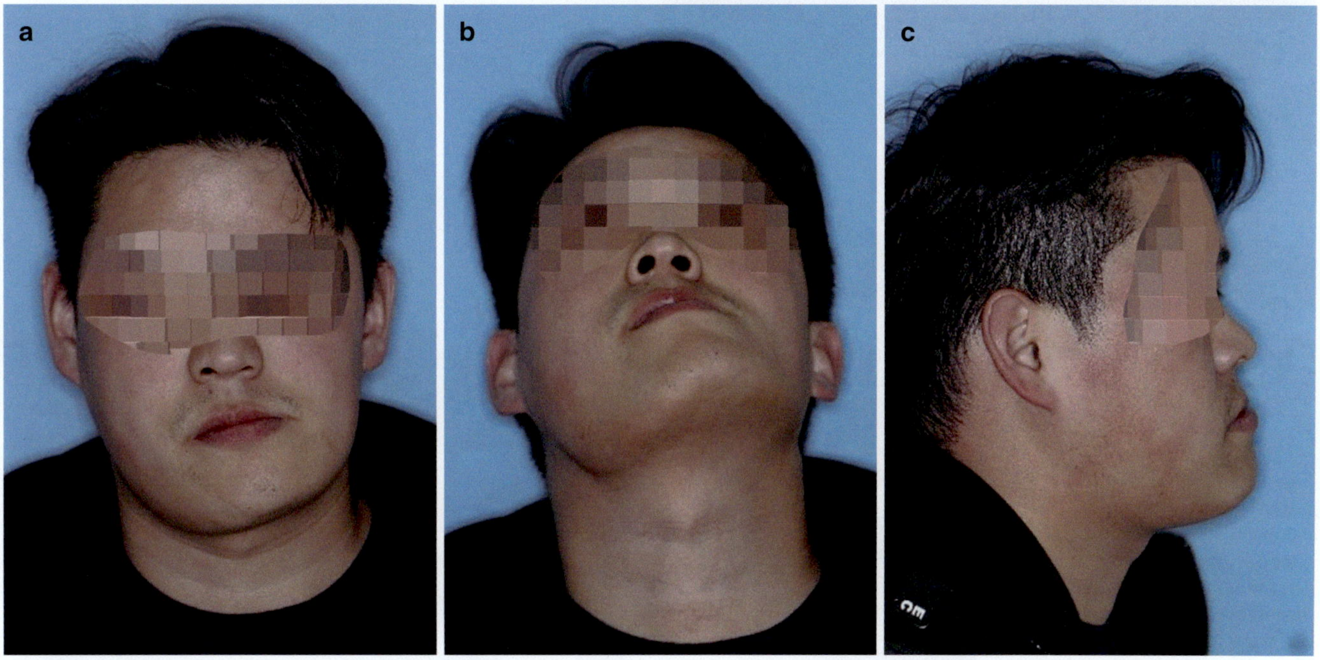

Fig. 4.33 Case E. Preoperative anterior view after orthodontic treatment. (**a**) Frontal view. (**b**) View from below. (**c**) Lateral view

- Overall treatment plan: orthognathic surgery simultaneous with right total joint prosthesis implantation. After resection of the abnormal condylar mass, the total joint prosthesis is to be implanted, and orthognathic surgery performed to correct the dentofacial deformities.
- Surgical resection design: resection of the condylar mass with space reserved for prosthesis.
- Reconstruction plan: customized total joint prosthesis implantation.
- Orthognathic plan: sagittal split osteotomy of the left mandibular ramus and Le Fort I osteotomy of the maxilla; due to the severe facial deformity, a second phase of genioplasty and contouring were to be designed after the surgery depending on the recovery of soft tissues. Due to the large osteochondroma of the right condylar eminence, which caused a severe tilting of the plane of the jaw (high left and low right), it was difficult to carry out the prosthesis implantation first plan, so the orthognathic surgery first plan was adopted. According to this plan, the right maxillary posterior teeth were first elevated, to obtain the appropriate vertical space for the subsequent implantation of the total joint prosthesis.

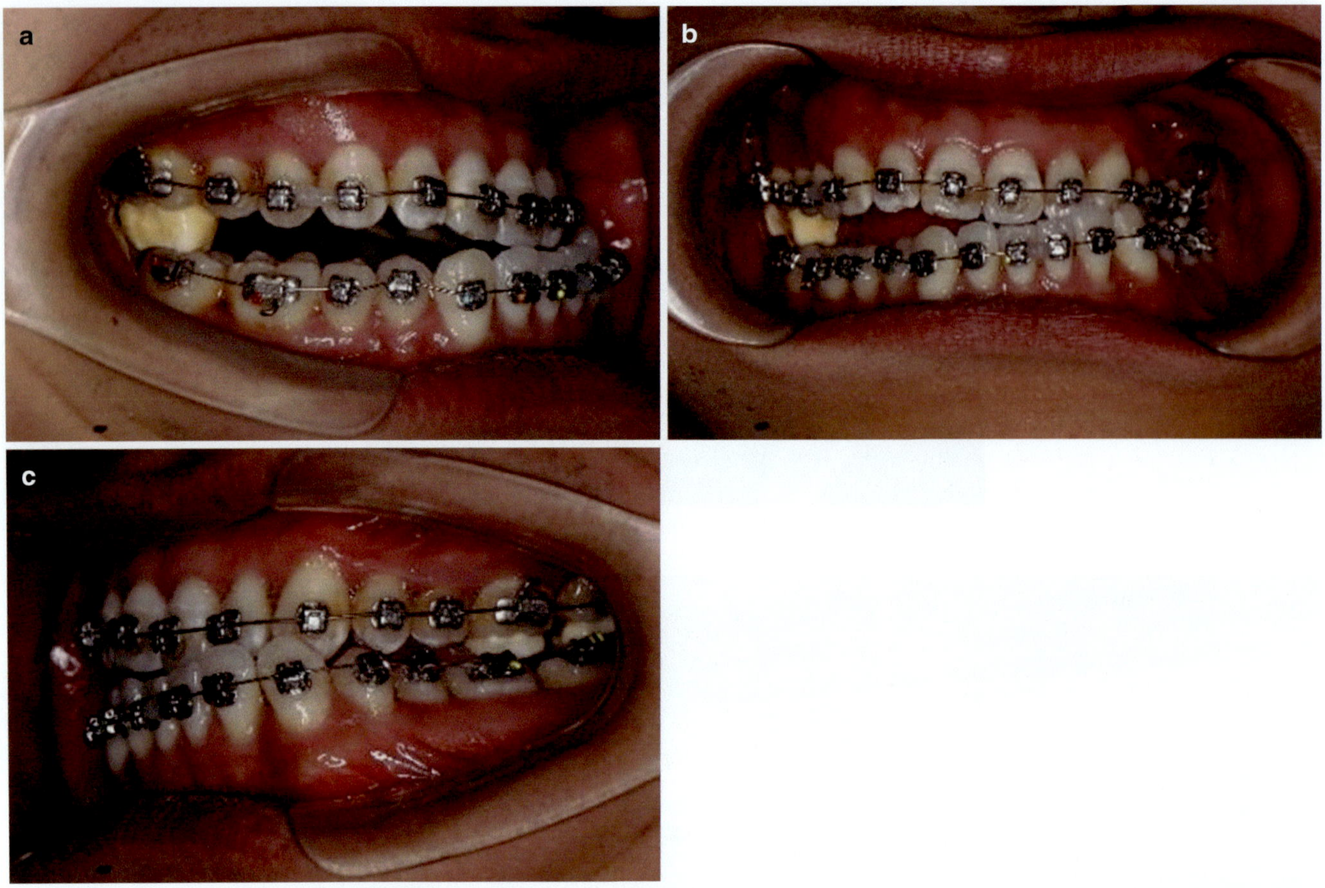

Fig. 4.34 Case E. Post-orthodontic intraoral examination, showing an increased gap between the right posterior teeth due to orthodontic decompensation. (**a**) Right occlusion. (**b**) Frontal occlusion. (**c**) Left occlusion

Fig. 4.35 Case E. 3D reconstruction of the preoperative maxillofacial CT after orthodontic treatment. The mandible is deviated to the left and protrudes because of a mass in the right condyle. There is an anterior crossbite and right posterior open bite. Both dental midlines are deviated to the left. (**a**) Frontal view. (**b**) Lateral view

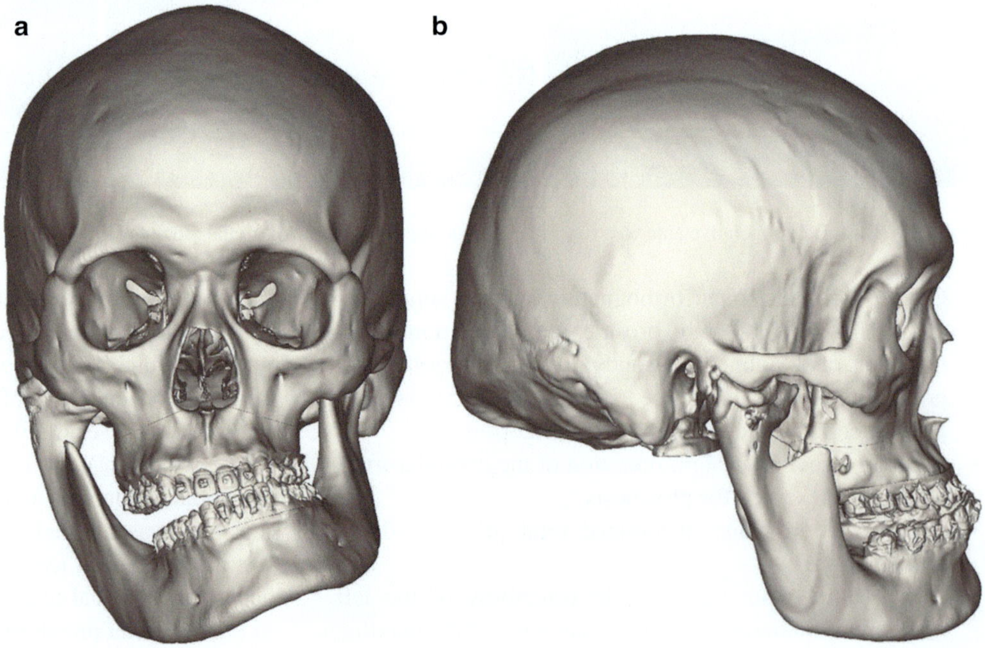

4.3.4 Case E. Orthognathic Plan and Design and Processing of Total Joint Prosthesis and Cutting Guides

- Surgical simulation and prosthesis design (Figs. 4.36, 4.37 and 4.38): The maxilla (blue) is first positioned to restore the angle suitable for a level jaw; the mandible is then repositioned according to the occlusal relationship to restore symmetry of the chin and the lower edge of the mandible. Then the condylar mass protruding upward into the skull can be seen and resected. The core component of the prosthesis is positioned, and the osteotomy line of the mandibular ramus is designed according to the following principles: First, the lower edge of the fixation plate at the front of the articular fossa component is to be placed at least 3 mm away from the anterior and inferior osteotomy lines. Second, the positions of the articular fossa and mandibular components of the prosthesis are designed according to the morphology of the zygomatic arch and the mandibular stump of the affected side.

4.3.4.1 The Design of the Cutting Guide (Figs. 4.39 and 4.40)

In accordance with the orthognathic surgical plan, the upper and lower jaw cutting guides were designed to mark the osteotomy lines while taking account of the extent of orthodontic decompensation.

- Prosthesis fabrication and fitting: the fabrication process is described in Sect. 2.5 in Chap. 2.

4.3.5 Case E. Surgical Procedure

Preoperative laboratory tests: the same as described in Sect. 3.2.5, Preoperative Laboratory Tests.

Preoperative preparation: prepare 400 ml of blood preoperatively. The others are the same as described in Sect. 3.2.5, Preoperative Preparation.

4.3.5.1 Steps of the Surgical Procedure

1. Surgical approach: preauriculotemporal incision, submandibular incision, and intraoral incision were used.
2. Prosthesis implant bed management: right subcondylar osteotomy and articular eminence osteotomy were performed to prepare the implant bed.
3. Orthognathic surgery: guide-assisted Le Fort I osteotomy of the maxilla, sagittal split osteotomy of the left mandibular ramus.
4. Intermaxillary ligation.
5. Total joint prosthesis installation.
6. Prosthesis mandible neck surrounded with abdominal fat.
    - Postoperative instructions and care: see Sect. 3.2.5, Postoperative Orders and Nursing Care. In addition, intermaxillary elastic traction was performed, and daily oral care was administered.

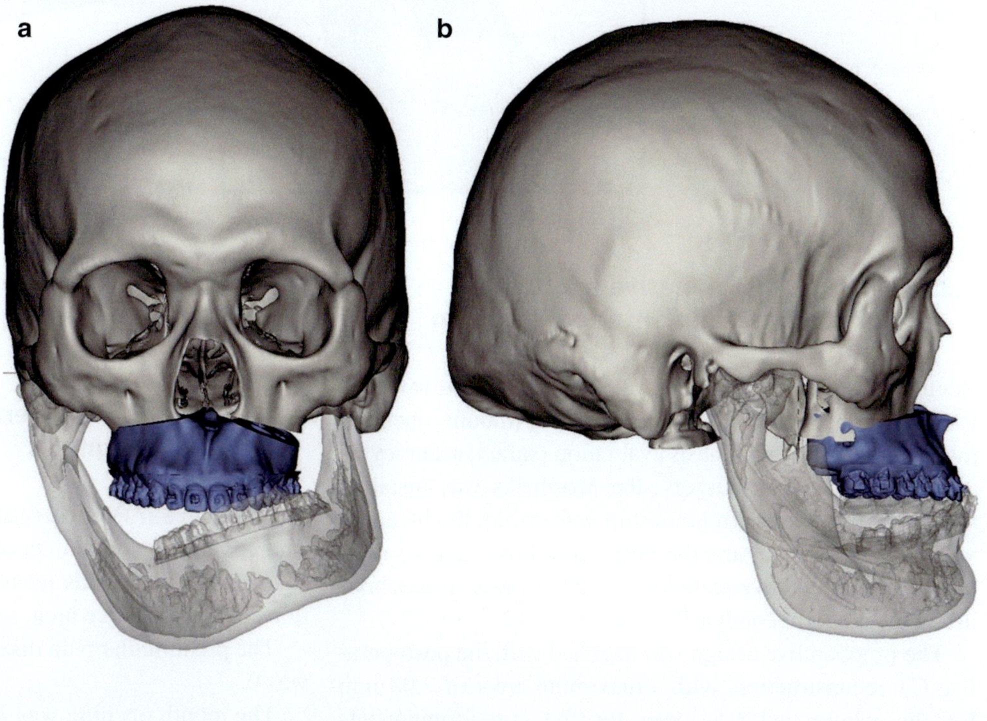

Fig. 4.36 Case E. Virtual Le Fort I osteotomy to level the maxillary occlusal plane and correct the dental midline. (**a**) Front view. (**b**) Lateral view

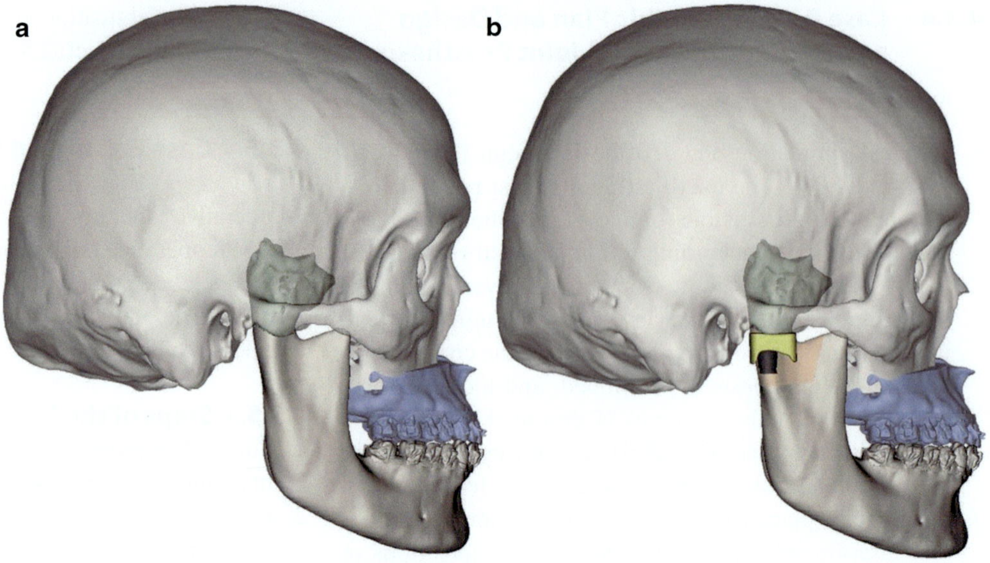

Fig. 4.37 Case E. Virtual TMJ surgery and prosthesis design. (**a**) The mandible was repositioned so that the occlusion was corrected, and the symmetry of the chin and the lower borders was restored. (**b**) At this time, the tumor (green) can be seen projecting upward into the skull. The core components are positioned, and the mandibular ramus osteotomies are planned. The distance from the lower edge of the fossa prosthesis to the resection margin should be at least 3 mm

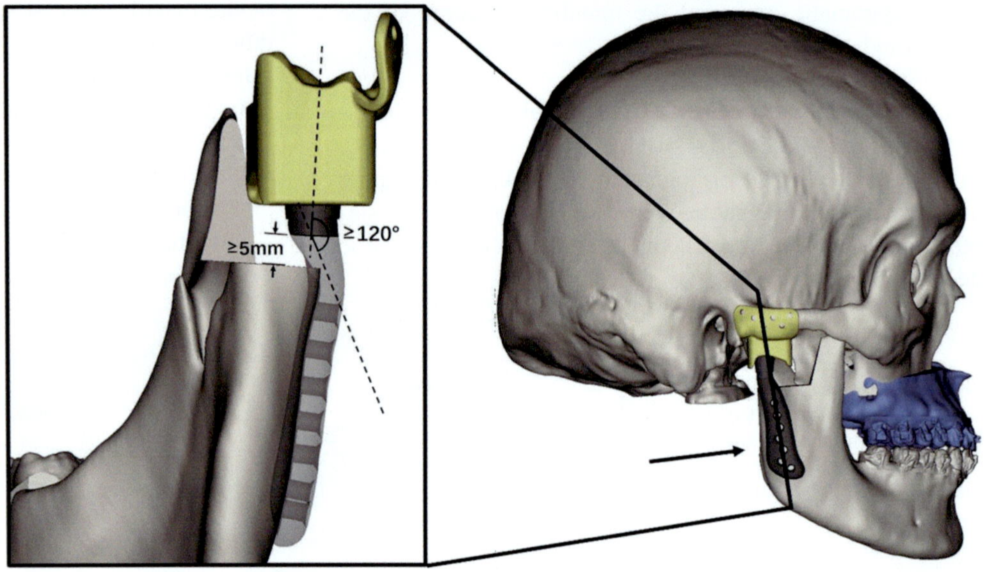

Fig. 4.38 Case E. Design of the mandibular fixation component. The distance from the lower edge of the condylar component to the horizontal ramus osteotomy is ≥5 mm. The angle on the coronal plane between the mandibular fixation component and the condylar component is ≥120°

4.3.6 Case E. Postoperative Analysis of Prothesis Implantation Precision

Regular postoperative follow-ups were performed to check for appearance (facial shape), function (mouth opening, mouth shape), and prosthesis evaluation (safety, accuracy).

Immediately after surgery: the prosthesis was installed smoothly, the occlusal relationship was stable, the bleeding volume was 600 mL, and the time was 6 hours and 45 minutes; the postoperative pathology diagnosis was "osteochondroma of the right condyle."

The preoperative design was matched with the postoperative CT reconstruction, with a maximum error of 2.08 mm for the whole and 0.81 mm for the core components (Fig. 4.41). Postoperative pain and diet were improved, and postoperative appearance and occlusal relationship were much improved. Postoperative mouth opening was 38 mm (Figs. 4.42, 4.43 and 4.44).

4.3.7 Case E. Long-Term Follow-Up and Prognosis

4.3.7.1 1-Year Postoperative Follow-Up

There were no complaints of discomfort, the face was well shaped, and there was no redness, swelling, or other reactions in the operative area.

The preauricular pain disappeared and the VAS pain score was 0.

The mouth opening was 37 mm with 5 mm lateral movement to the right and 2 mm lateral movement to the left.

Masticatory function: normal eating.

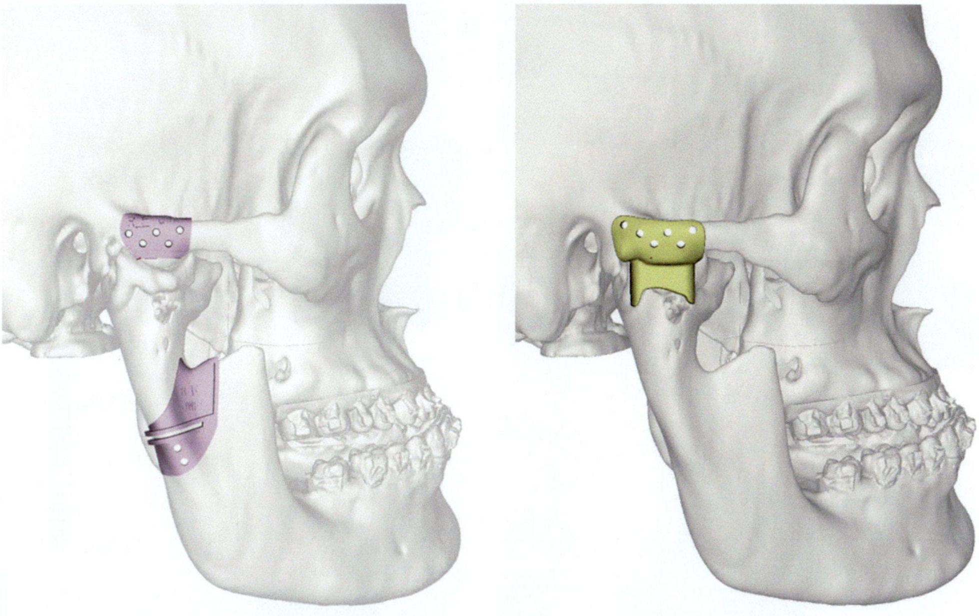

Fig. 4.39 Case E. Cutting guides design. (**a**) Virtual design of cutting guides (in purple) for the articular eminence and the condylar resection. (**b**) Holes placed to stabilize the guides will be used later for positioning the TMJ prosthesis

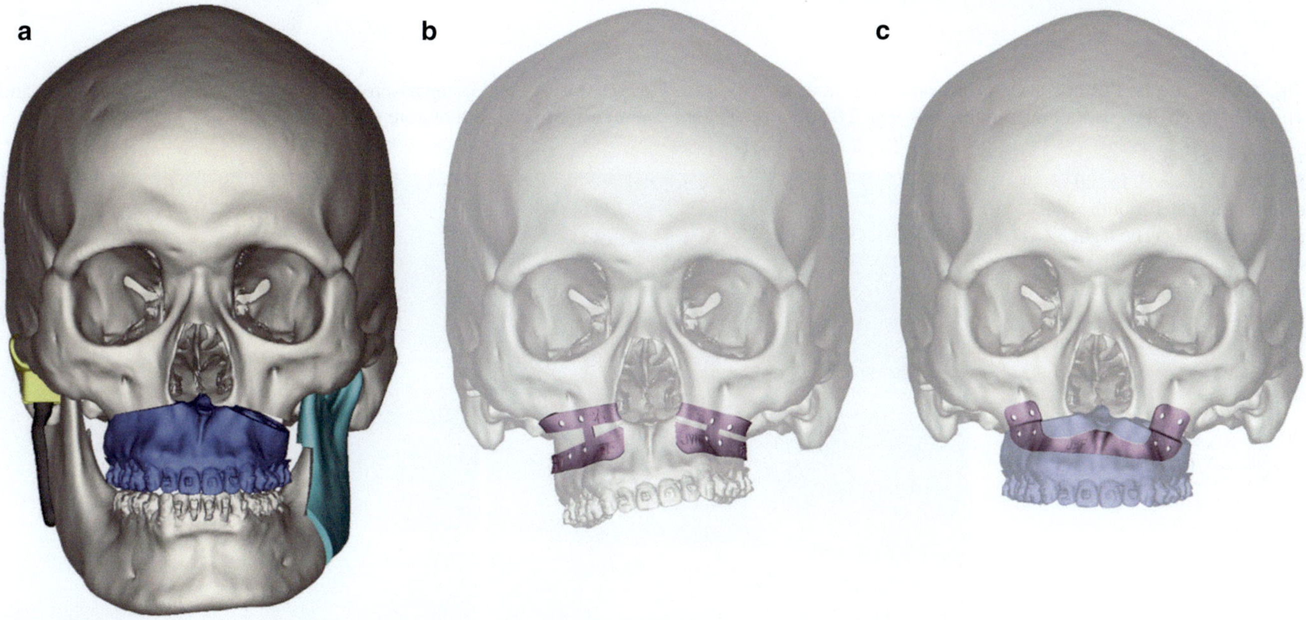

Fig. 4.40 Case E. Virtual orthognathic plan, Le Fort I cutting guides, and custom fixation plate. The screw holes in the cutting guides coincide with those of the fixation plate, for precise final positioning of the maxilla. (**a**) Overall orthognathic design result. (**b**) Maxillary osteotomy guide. (**c**) Maxillary positioning guide

Joint-mandibular-occlusal-facial coordination, stable occlusal relationship (Figs. 4.45, 4.46 and 4.47).

Prosthesis evaluation: 1 year after surgery, the prosthesis had no complications such as infection, rejection, loosening, displacement, fracture, ectopic osteogenesis, and allergy (Fig. 4.48).

4.3.7.2 3-Year Postoperative Follow-Up

The degree of mouth opening was 38 mm, and the rest was the same as the one-year postoperative follow-up (Figs. 4.49 and 4.50).

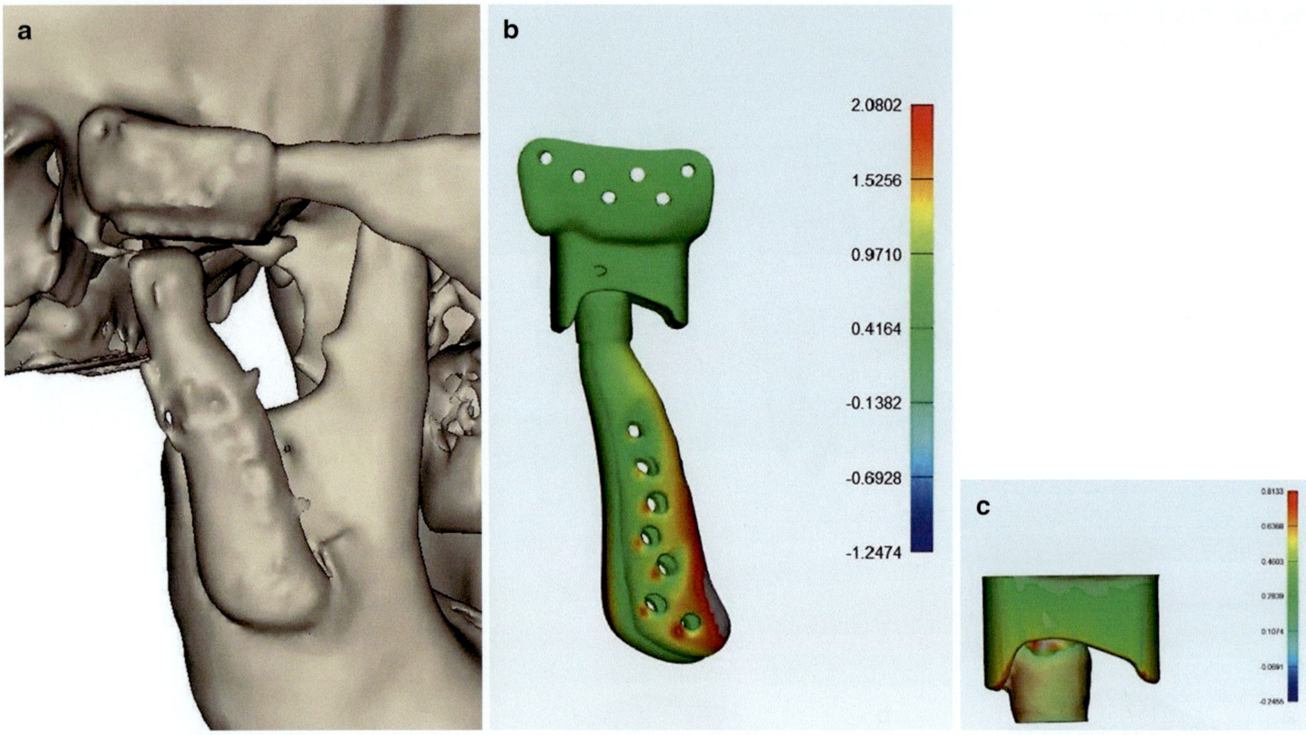

Fig. 4.41 Case E. Postoperative prosthesis error analysis. (**a**) 3D CT reconstruction and comparison of postoperative prosthesis position and virtual plan. (**b**) The overall maximum error was 2.08 mm. (**c**) The maximum error in position of core components was 0.81 mm

Fig. 4.42 Case E. Facial examination at 1 month postoperatively. The right occlusal area is slightly swollen, but the facial shape is basically symmetrical. (**a**) Frontal view. (**b**) Lateral view

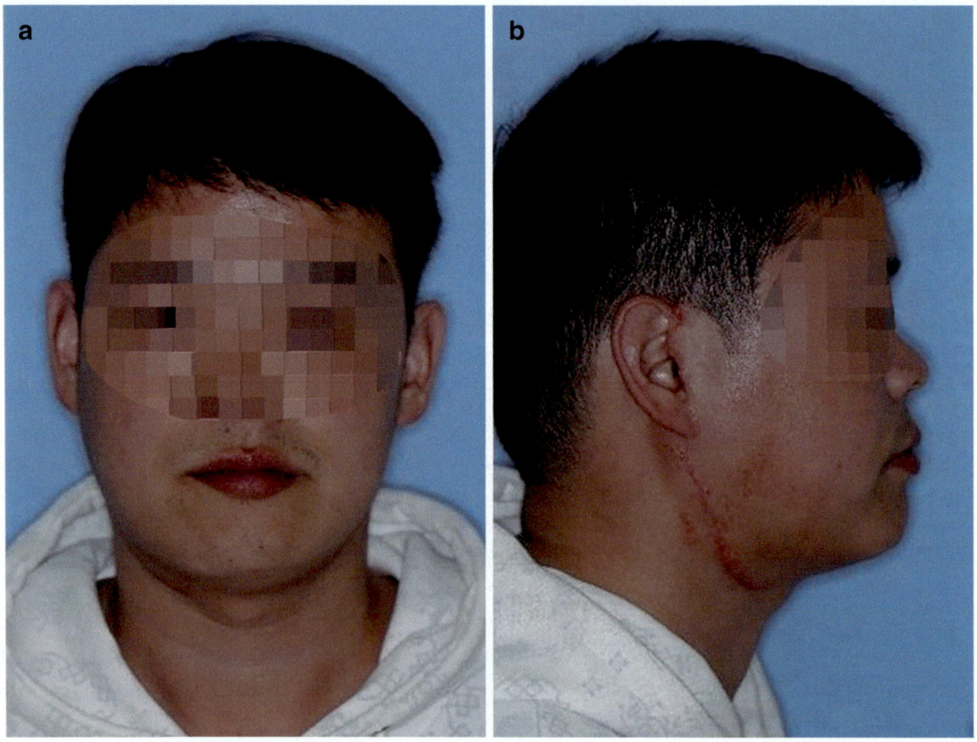

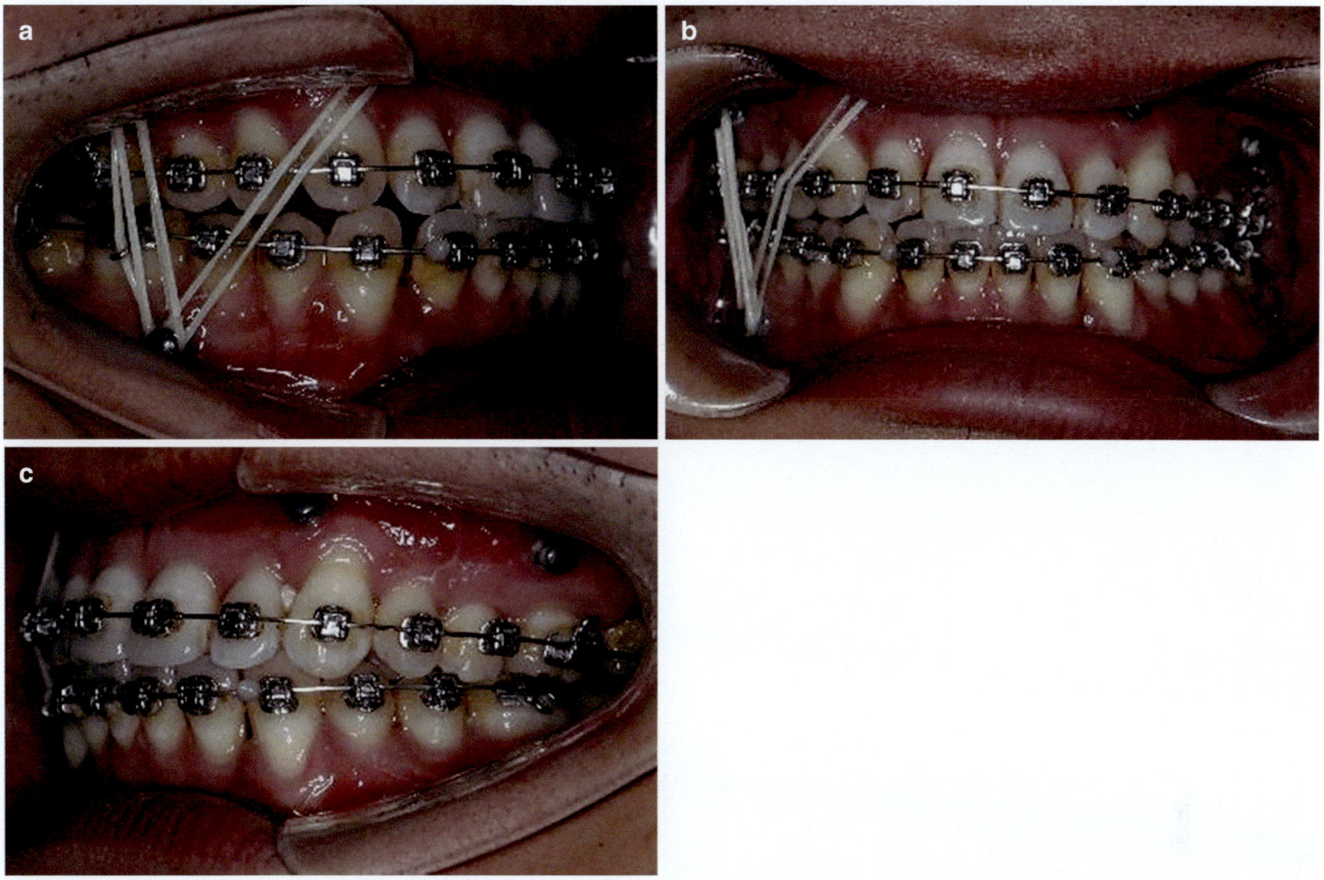

Fig. 4.43 Case E. Intraoral examination 1 month after surgery. Elastic traction is being used to stabilize the mandibular position. The interdental relationship is good. (**a**) Right occlusion. (**b**) Frontal occlusion. (**c**) Left occlusion

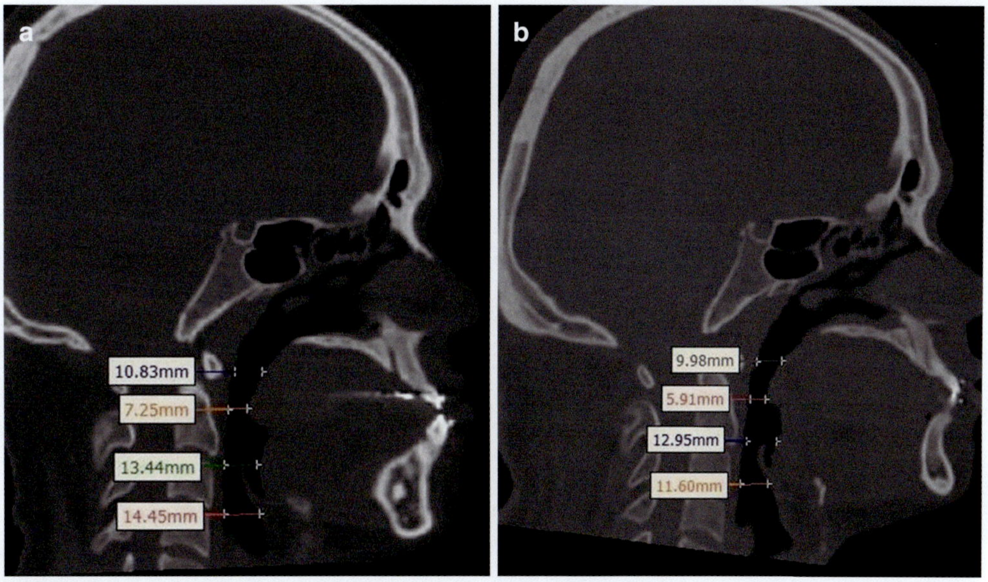

Fig. 4.44 Case E. The 2D posterior airway space is slightly narrowed after surgery. The smallest AP distance is still almost 6 mm. (**a**) Preoperative airway measurement. (**b**) Postoperative airway measurement

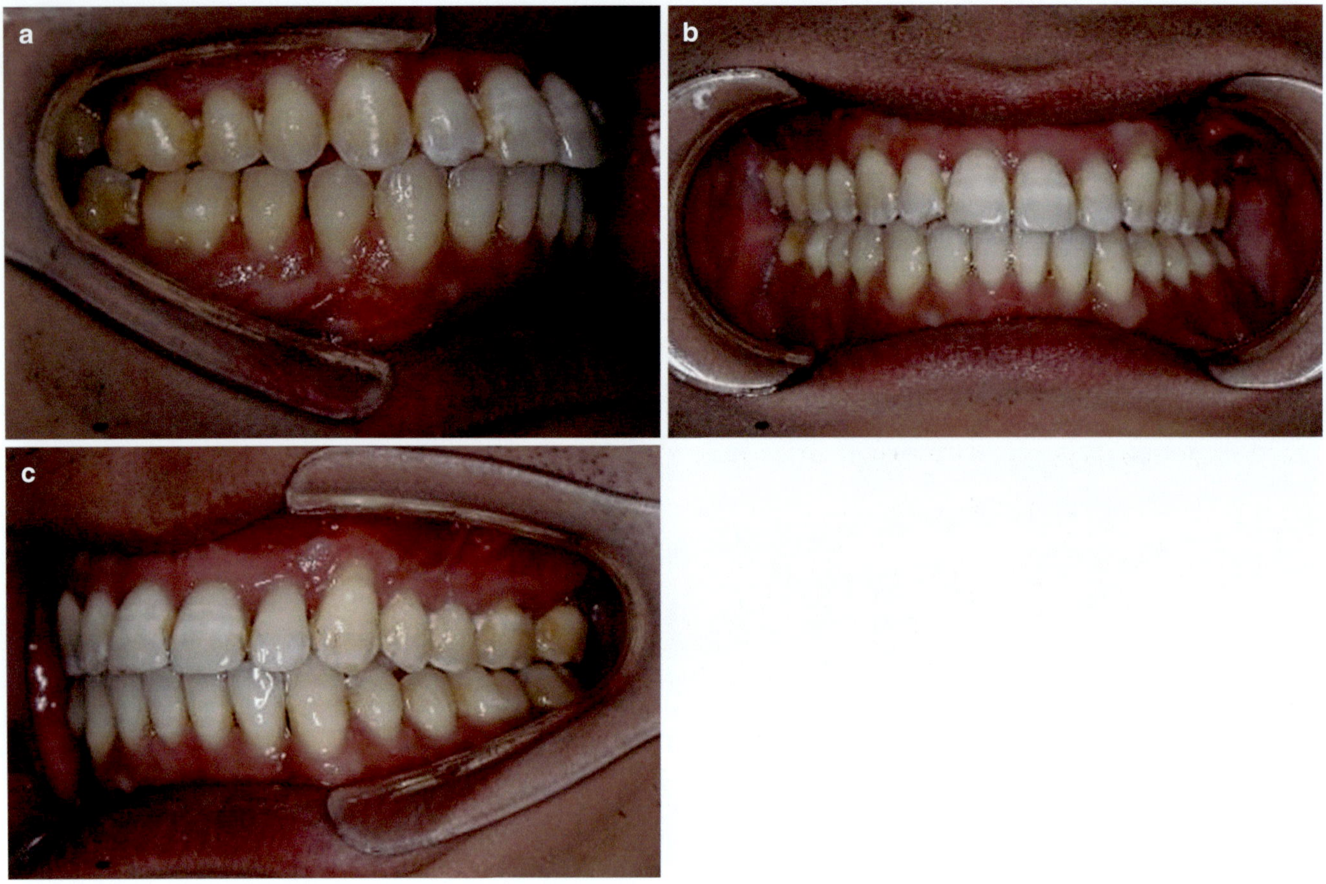

Fig. 4.45 Case E. Intraoral examination 1 year after surgery. There is a Class I occlusal relationship. (**a**) Right occlusion. (**b**) Frontal occlusion. (**c**) Left occlusion

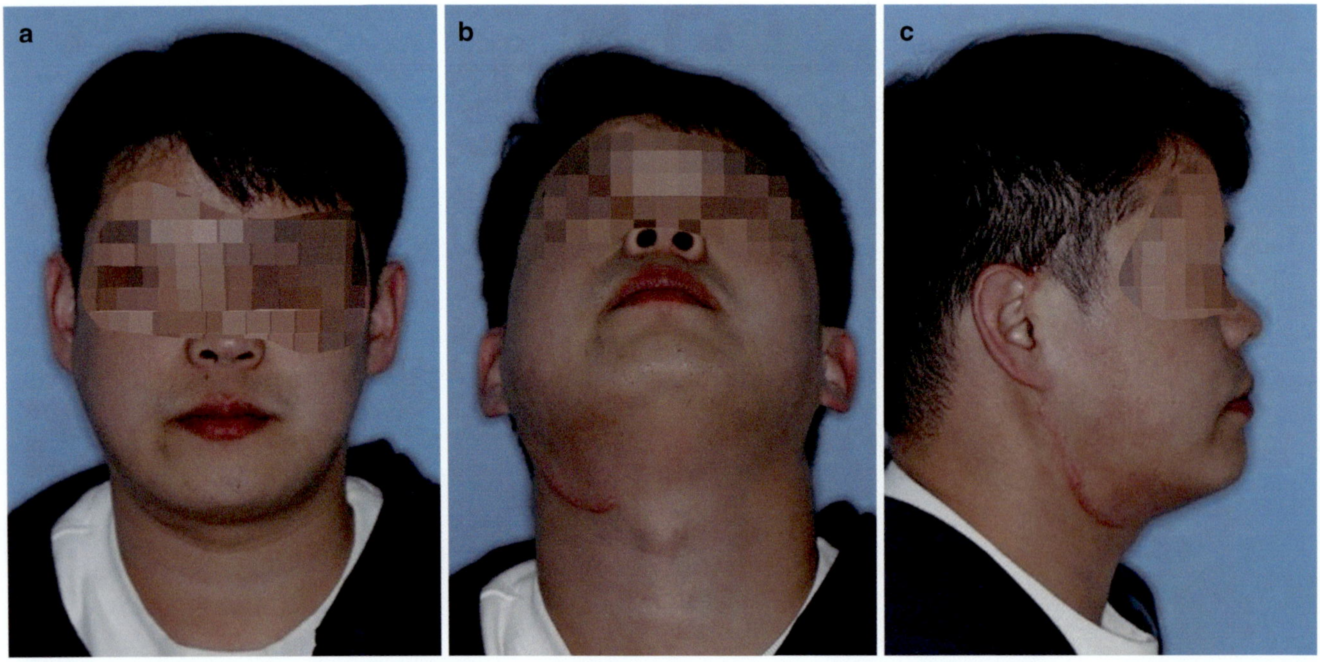

Fig. 4.46 Case E. Facial examination 1 year after surgery. (**a**) Frontal view. (**b**) View from below. (**c**) Lateral view

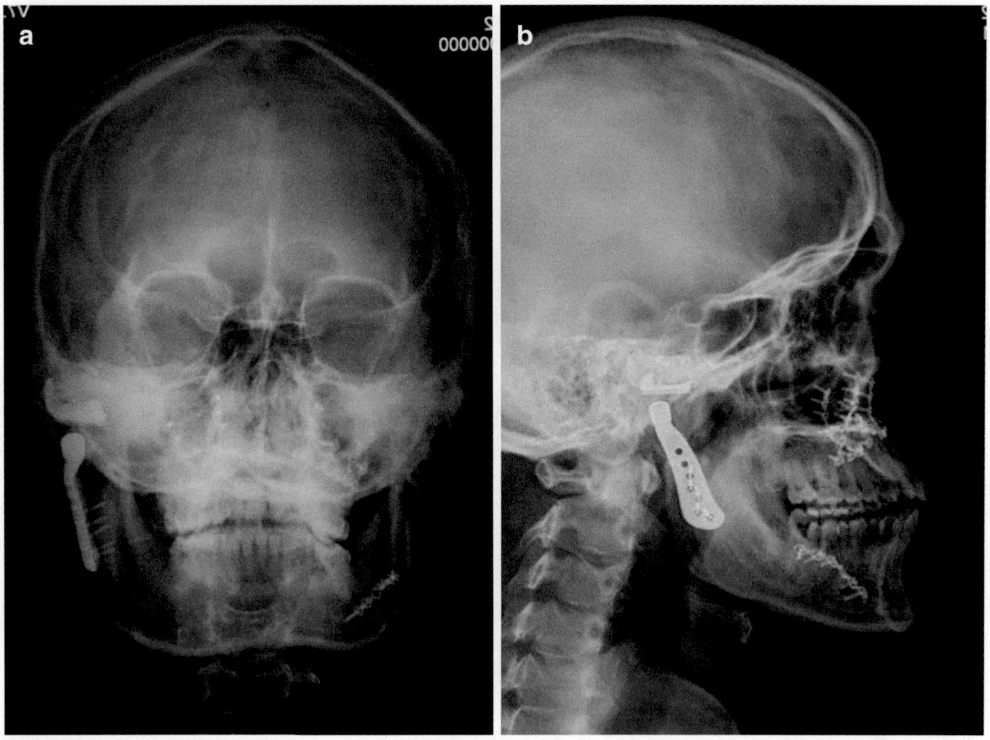

Fig. 4.47 Case E. Cephalometric examination 1 year after surgery. There is good mandibular symmetry. The position of the TMJ prosthesis is consistent with the plan. The relationship between the maxilla and mandible is skeletal Class I. (**a**) Frontal image. (**b**) Lateral image

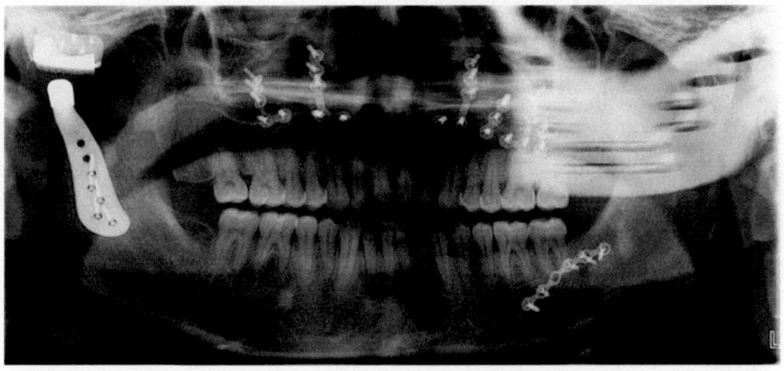

Fig. 4.48 Case E. One-year postoperative panoramic view. There was no loosening, displacement, dislocation, or fracture of the prosthesis

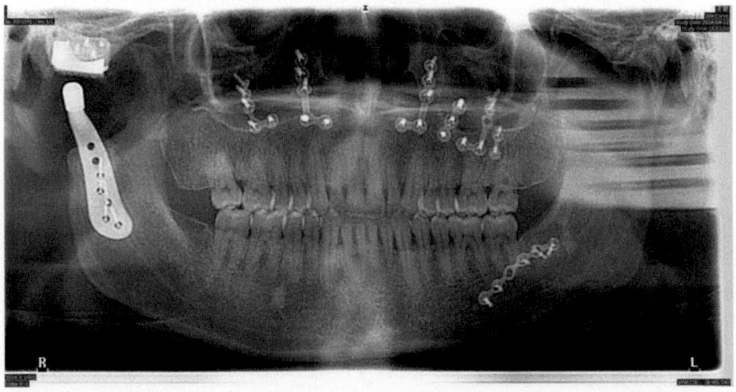

Fig. 4.49 Case E. Panoramic view 3 years after surgery. There was no loosening, displacement, dislocation, or fracture of the prosthesis

4.3.8 Case E. Advantages and Disadvantages

4.3.8.1 Advantages

The patient's occlusal relationship, facial shape, and joint function were restored, while the abnormal joint mass was removed.

After removal of the mass in this group of patients, severe occlusal disorders and secondary deformities can occur if simultaneous correction of the occlusion and facial shape is not carried through, and then the treatment period is extended, and the long process traumatizes the patient with multiple surgeries.

4.3.8.2 Disadvantages

The error between the position of the prosthesis and the design was large, which was mainly due to the severe deformity of the jaws in this case. The prosthesis fitting was the last surgical step, so the error accumulated gradually and was finally reflected in the position of the prosthesis. Due to the simultaneous resection of the condylar and lateral pterygoid muscle, the patient's postoperative mouth opening decreased slightly (from 40 to 38 mm) compared with the preoperative period.

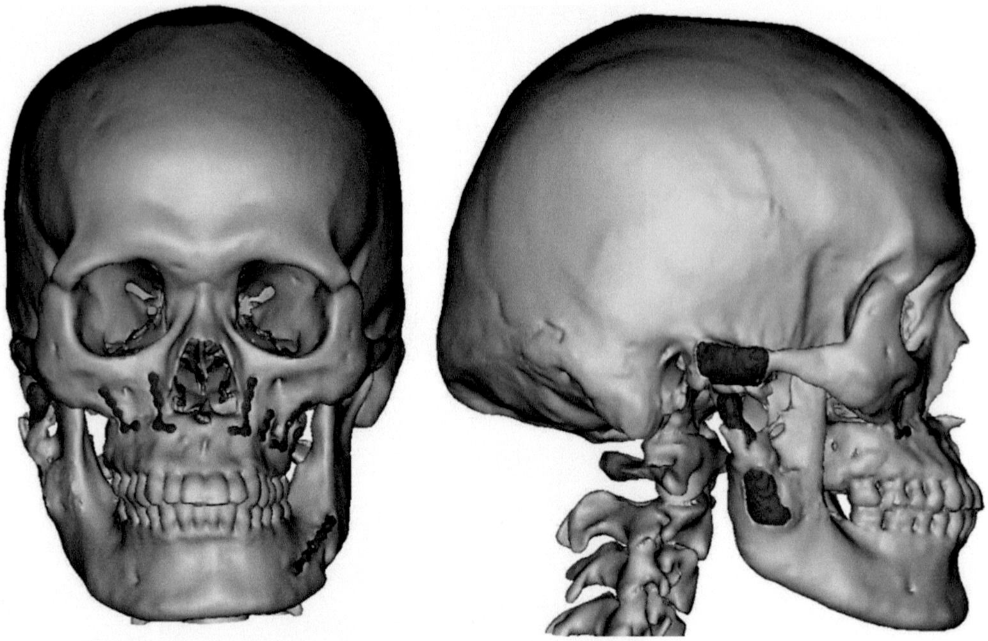

Fig. 4.50 Case E. 3-year postoperative CT review. The prosthesis (dark gray) is not loose, displaced, dislocated, or fractured

4.4 Reconstruction of Joint Ankylosis with Deviated Jaw Deformity Through Orthognathic Surgery Simultaneous with Customized Total Temporomandibular Joint Prosthesis Implantation

4.4.1 Case F. Joint Ankylosis with Deviated Jaw Deformity

- Patient information: female, 39 years old.
- Complaint: inability to open the mouth, with mandibular deviation and retrognathia for more than 30 years.
- History: the patient has been unable to open her mouth wide since childhood and was diagnosed as "right joint ankylosis" at local hospital, so she came to our hospital for treatment. She reported a history of nocturnal snoring.
- Past history: the patient reported that she was healthy and denied any history of systemic diseases and drug or food allergies.
- Clinical examination: the mandible is deviated to the right and retruded, with a mouth opening of 0 mm. The right first molar exhibits a Class II full mesial relationship (Angle's classification), while the left first molar shows a Class I occlusal relationship (Angle's classification). Tooth 21 is missing, and tooth 22 is a residual root (Figs. 4.51 and 4.52).
- Imaging examination: panoramic film showed bone fusion in the right TMJ region with loss of joint space. The imaging examination showed mandibular retrognathia, bony Class II, right deviation of the mandible, and shortness of the right mandibular ramus. CT examination showed bony ankylosis of the right TMJ region, narrowing of the airway, and deformity of the jaws (Figs. 4.53, 4.54, 4.55 and 4.56).
- Diagnosis: right joint ankylosis, skeletal Class II with right mandibular deviation, and obstructive sleep apnea.

4.4.2 Case F. Diagnostic Imaging

4.4.3 Case F. Treatment Plan

- Overall treatment plan: right total joint prosthesis implantation with simultaneous orthognathic surgery. The ankylosis will be resolved, and the affected joint replaced with a total joint prosthesis. The upper and lower jaw positions and occlusion will be restored at the same time, with re-angling the upper teeth towards the left (centered), lengthening the jaw on both sides, and resolving the facial deformity of severe jaw retrognathia.
- Surgical resection design: resection of the ankylosed bony fusion with space reserved for the total joint prosthesis.
- Reconstruction plan: customized total joint prosthesis implantation.
- Orthognathic plan: Le Fort I osteotomy of the maxilla and sagittal split osteotomy of the left mandibular ramus; due to the severe facial deformity, a phase II genioplasty and contouring will be planned depending on the recovery of the soft tissues after surgery. To secure the position of the prosthesis and the mandible, and to lengthen the height of

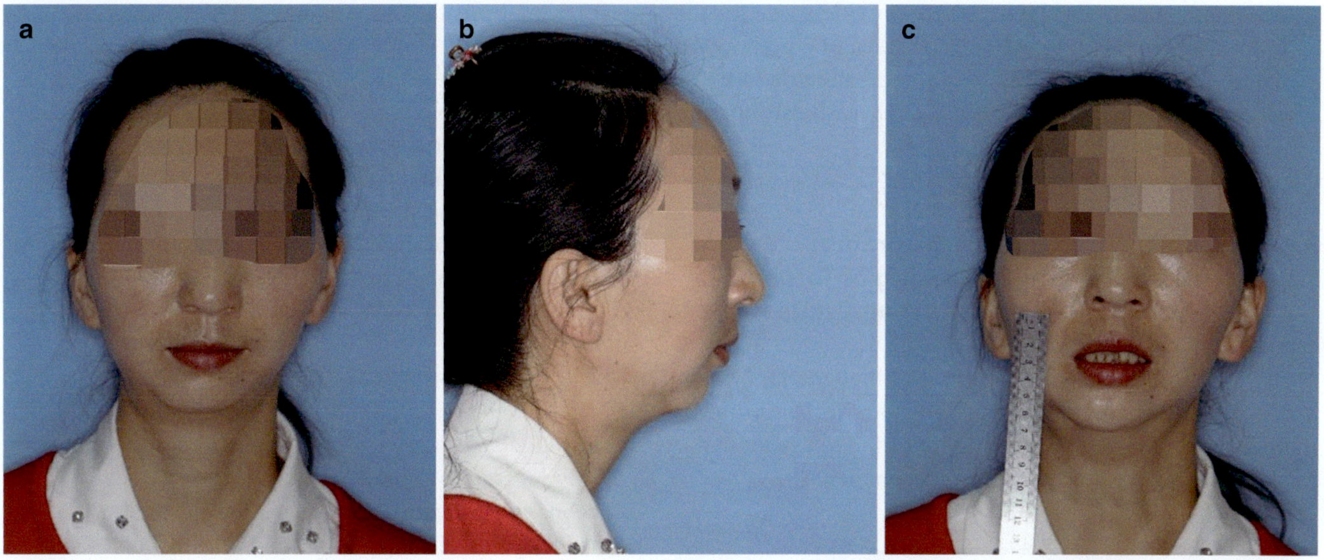

Fig. 4.51 Case F. Facial examination. The mandible is deviated to the right and the mouth opening is 0 mm. (**a**) Frontal view. (**b**) Lateral view. (**c**) Mouth opening

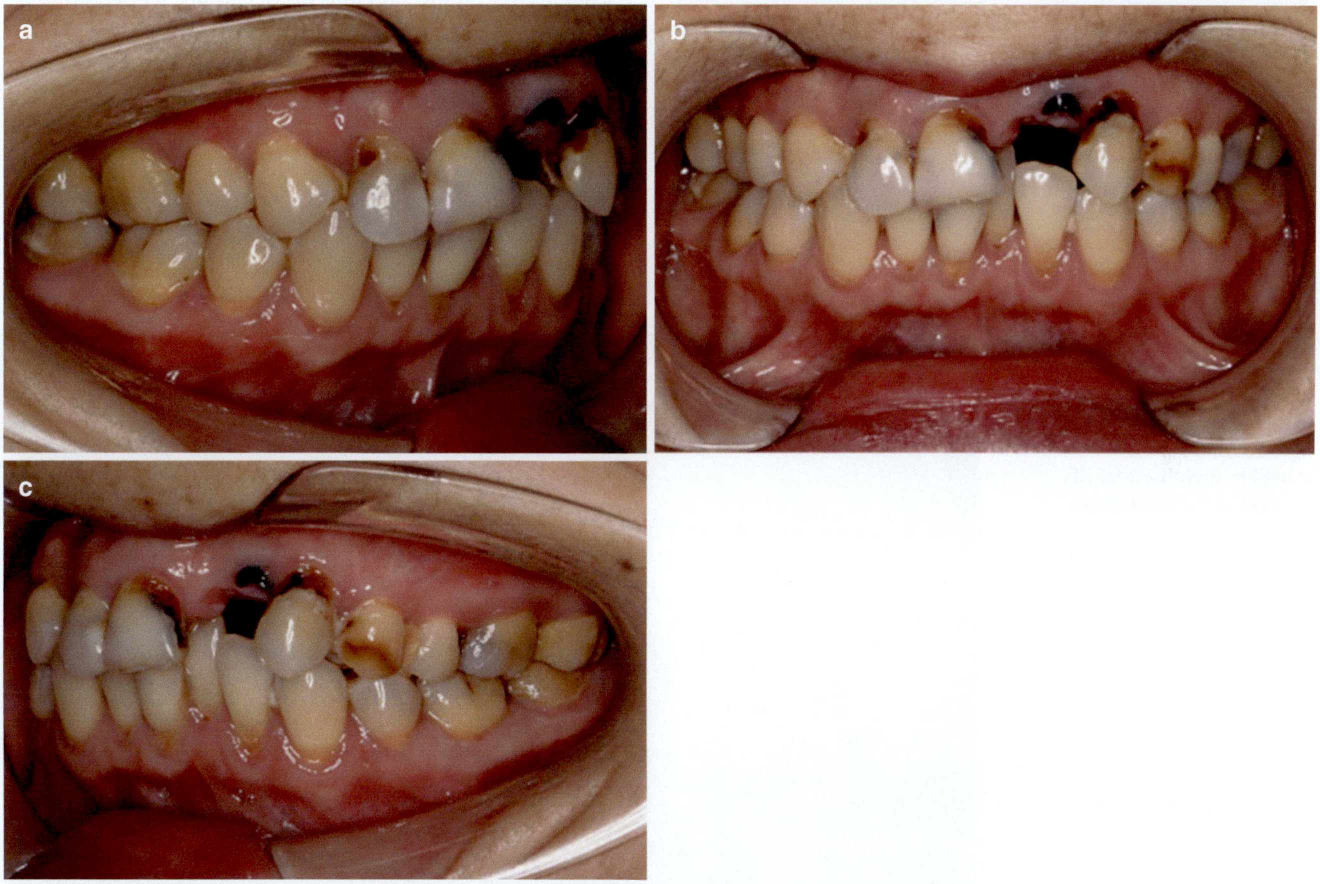

Fig. 4.52 Case F. Intraoral examination. (**a**) Right occlusion. (**b**) Frontal occlusion. (**c**) Left occlusion

the mandibular ramus bilaterally to provide space for the descent of the posterior maxillary teeth and correction of the angle of the maxillary plane, the patient was to be treated with a plan of surgery with TMJ prosthesis implantation first.

4.4.4 Case F. Orthognathic Program and Design and Processing of Total Joint Prosthesis and Cutting Guides

Total joint prosthesis implantation with simultaneous orthognathic surgery program design: right total joint prosthesis implantation, sagittal split osteotomy of the left mandibular ramus, and Le Fort I osteotomy of the maxilla.

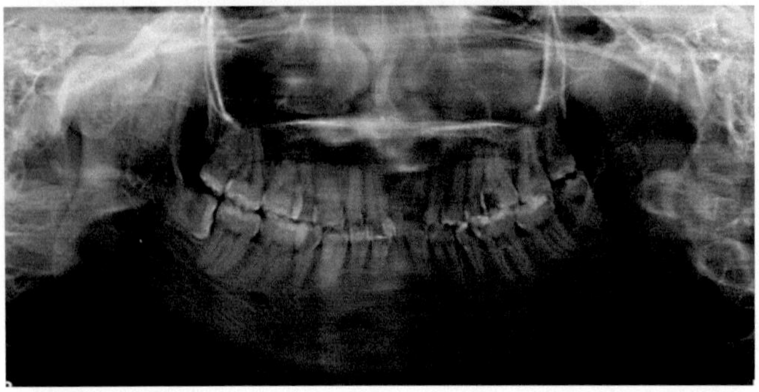

Fig. 4.53 Case F. Panoramic view. Bone fusion in the right TMJ region with loss of joint space

Total joint prosthesis and surgical guide design and processing (Fig. 4.57). This is basically the same as in Case A in Chap. 3.

4.4.4.1 Design and Processing of Prosthesis and Cutting Guides

- Classic total joint prosthesis design.
- Prosthesis manufacturing and fitting: the manufacturing process is described in Sect. 2.5 in Chap. 2.

4.4.5 Case F. Surgical Procedure

Preoperative laboratory tests: the same as described in Sect. 3.2.5, Preoperative Laboratory Tests.

Preoperative preparation: the same as described in Sect. 3.2.5, Preoperative Preparation, and 400 mL of blood was prepared preoperatively.

- Steps of surgical procedure: the steps of resection of ankylosis, prosthesis implantation, sagittal splitting of the mandibular ramus, and maxillary surgery were completed in the order shown (Fig. 4.58).
  1. Surgical approach: a preauriculotemporal incision, a small transbuccal incision, and an intraoral incision were used.
  2. Prosthesis implant bed management: right subcondylar osteotomy and articular eminence osteotomy were performed to prepare the implant bed.

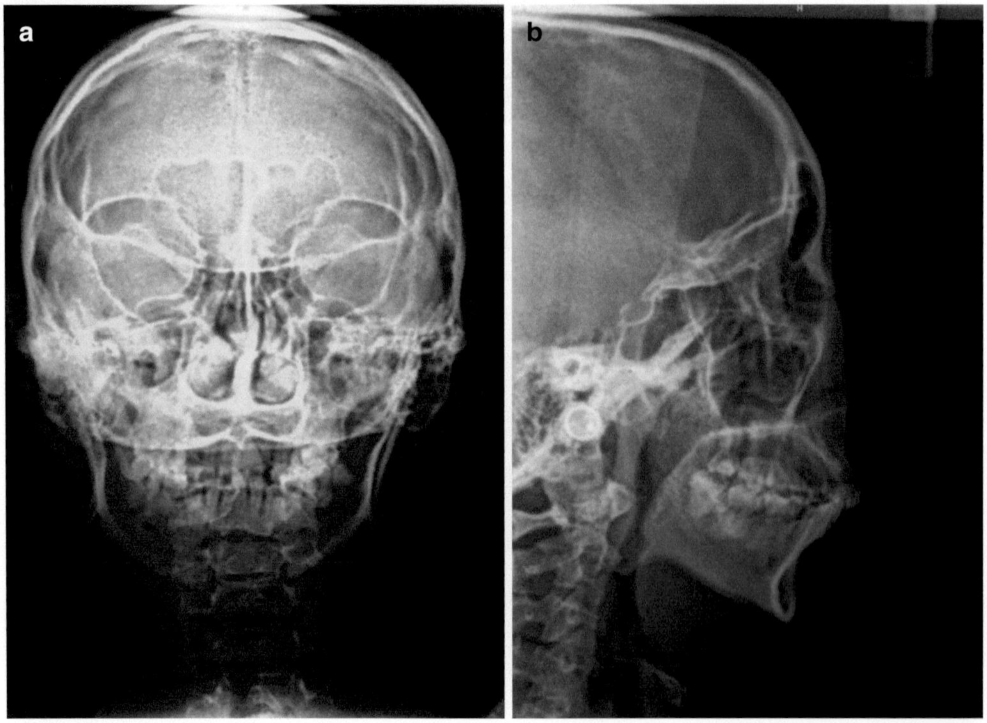

Fig. 4.54 Case F. Cephalometric X-rays showing mandibular retrognathia, bony Class II, right deviation of the mandible, and shortness of the right mandibular ramus. (**a**) Frontal view. (**b**) Lateral view

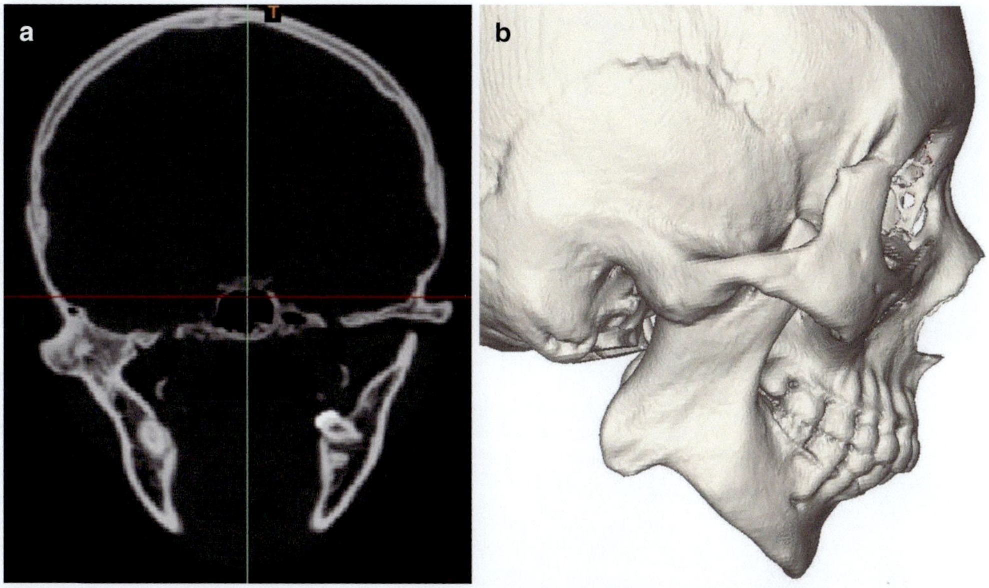

Fig. 4.55 Case F. CT scan examination. Diagnosis, bony ankylosis of the right joint. (**a**) Coronal view. (**b**) 3D reconstruction

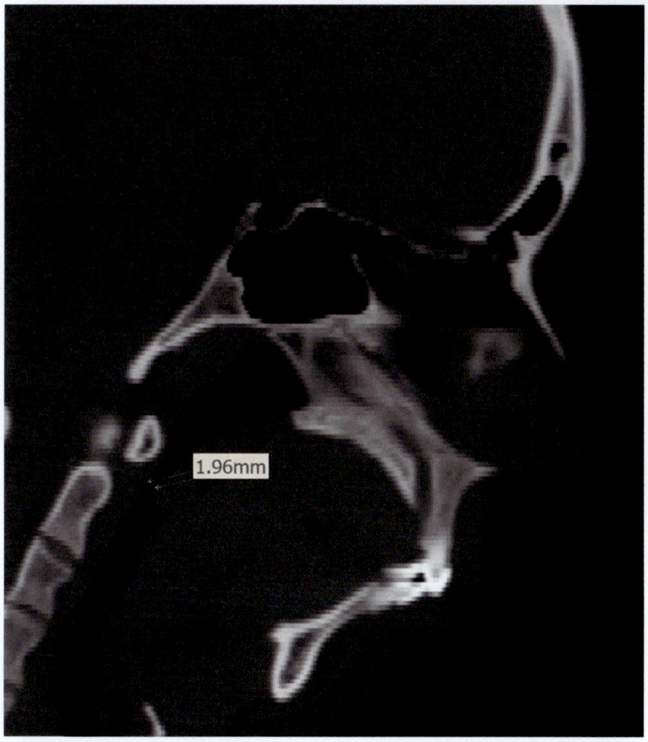

Fig. 4.56 Case F. CT sagittal view. The airway is narrow, with the narrowest point being the palatopharyngeal airway, which is less than 2 mm wide front to back

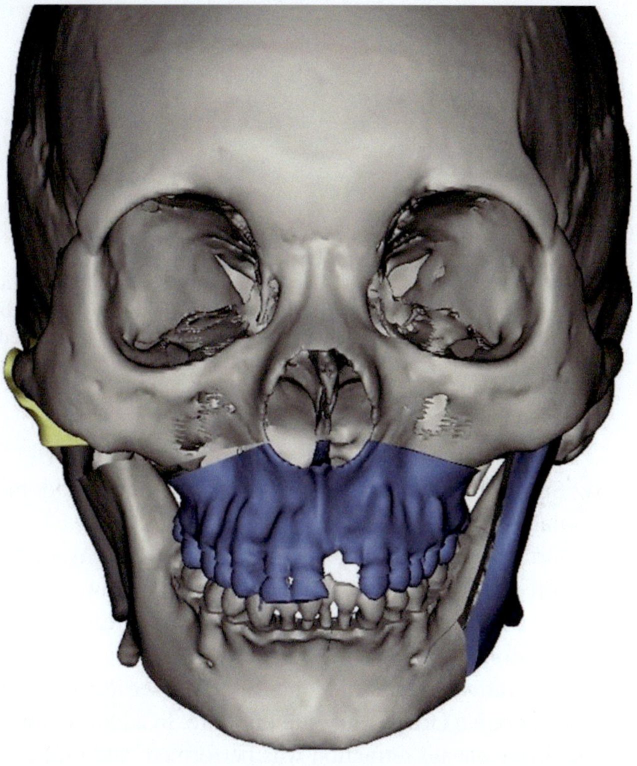

Fig. 4.57 Case F. Virtual surgical plan of the final postoperative position. The ankylotic bone has been removed, orthognathic surgery has been completed (blue), and the custom right TMJ prosthesis (yellow and gray) has been implanted

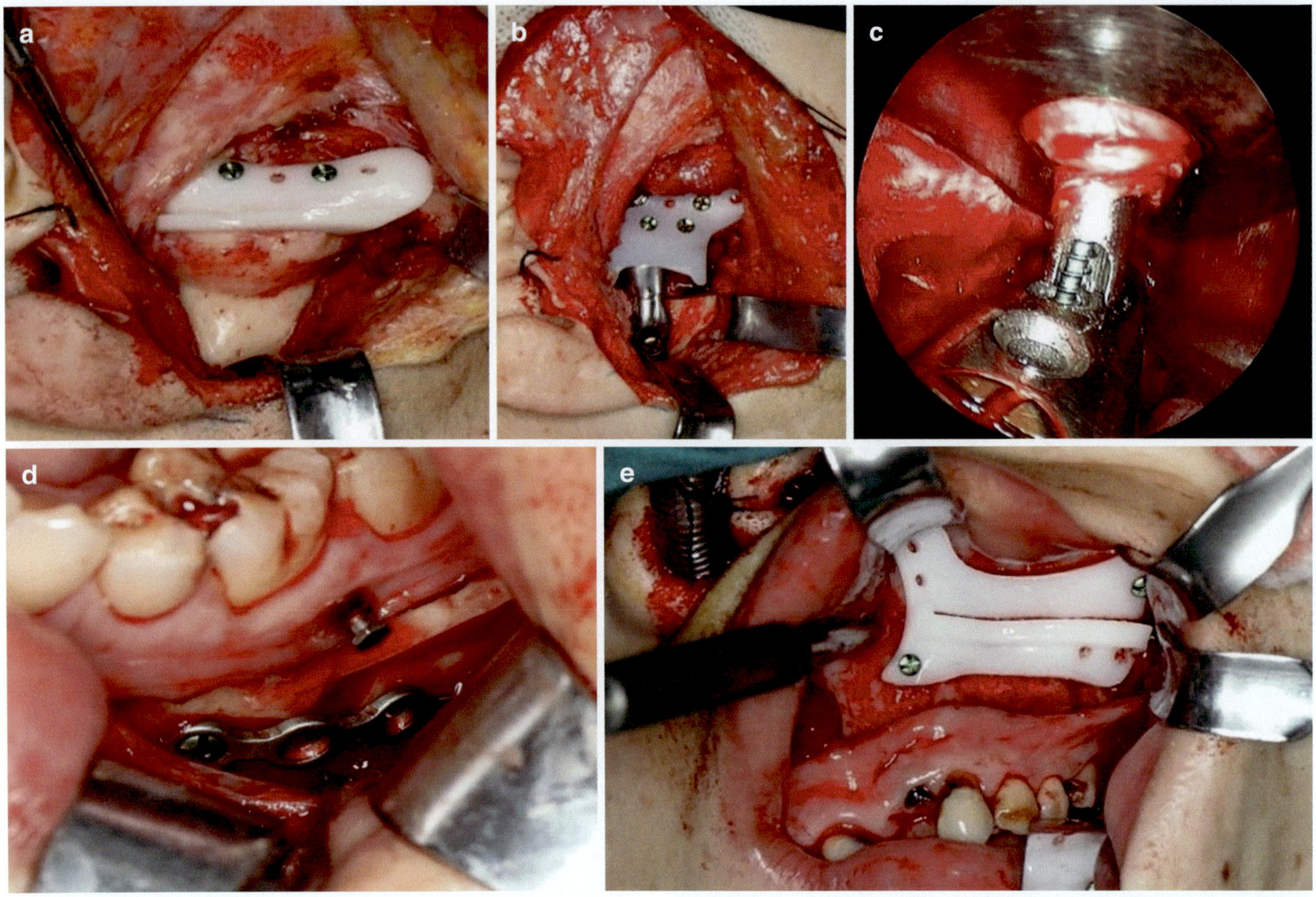

Fig. 4.58 Case F. Overview of the surgery. (**a**) A cutting guide was used for precise removal of bone from the ankylosed right TMJ. (**b**) After sagittal osteotomy of the left ramus, the mandible was mobilized, and the joint prosthesis was implanted. (**c**) Fixation of the condylar prosthesis was assisted with an endoscope to avoid a retromandibular incision. (**d**) Plating of the left mandibular ramus osteotomy was performed after fixation of the joint prosthesis. (**e**) A cutting guide was used to create a precise Le Fort I osteotomy

3. Total joint prosthesis was implanted.
4. Space around the prosthesis was filled in with abdominal fat.
5. Orthognathic surgery: sagittal split osteotomy of the left mandibular ramus to lengthen the left jaw, Le Fort I osteotomy of the maxilla, and intermaxillary ligation.

- Postoperative orders and nursing care: see Sect. 3.2.5, Postoperative Orders and Nursing Care. In addition, intermaxillary elastic retraction was performed, and oral care was provided daily.

4.4.6 Case F. Postoperative Analysis of Prothesis Implantation Precision

Regular postoperative follow-ups were performed to check on appearance (facial shape), function (mouth opening, mouth shape), and prosthesis evaluation (safety, accuracy).

Immediately after surgery: intraoperative prosthesis installation was smooth, occlusal relationship was stable, bleeding volume was 700 mL, and operation time was 4 hours and 30 minutes. Preoperative design and postoperative CT reconstruction were matched with a maximum error of 0.47 mm for the core component and 1.35 mm for the overall maximum error (Figs. 4.59 and 4.60). The mandibular motor functions such as mouth opening and chewing were significantly improved at 1 month after surgery. The mouth opening was 30 mm, the mandible was adjusted forward, and the facial shape was basically symmetrical (Figs. 4.61, 4.62, 4.63 and 4.64). The narrowest part of the palatopharyngeal airway was enlarged from 1.96 mm to 4.38 mm (Fig. 4.64).

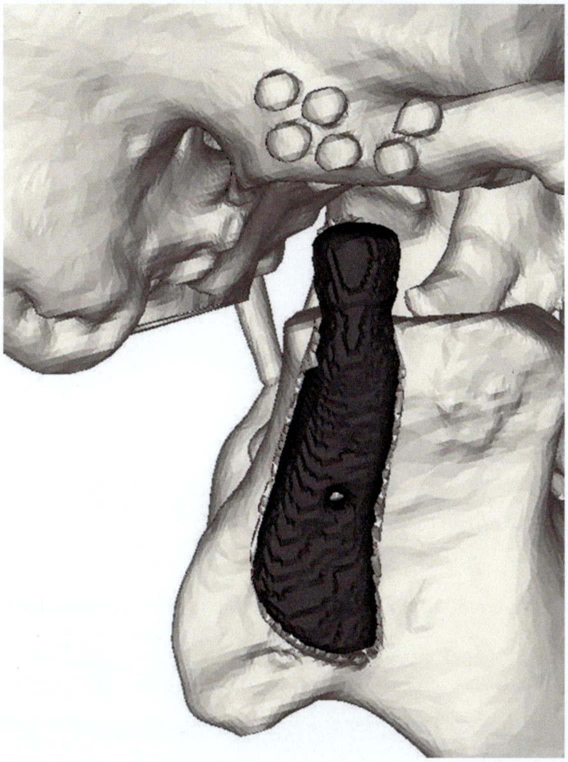

Fig. 4.59 Case F. Immediate postoperative CT reconstruction of the prosthesis position

4.4.7 Case F. Long-Term Follow-Up and Prognosis

4.4.7.1 One Month Postoperatively

4.4.7.2 5-Year Postoperative Follow-Up

There were no complaints of discomfort, the face was well shaped, and there was no redness, swelling, or other reactions in the operative area.

The joint-mandibular-occlusal-facial shape was harmonious, and the occlusal relationship was stable (Fig. 4.65). Nocturnal snoring symptoms improved significantly.

The mouth opening was 37 mm, with 5 mm lateral movement to the right and 3 mm lateral movement to the left.

Chewing function: normal diet.

Evaluation of the prosthesis: 5 years after the operation, there were no complications such as infection, rejection, loosening, fracture, displacement, ectopic bone formation, material allergy, and the prosthesis was in good position with the bone (Figs. 4.66 and 4.67).

4.4.8 Case F. Advantages and Disadvantages

4.4.8.1 Advantages

In cases of joint ankylosis, especially old ankylosis with rough and irregular bone surfaces in the joint area and the mandibular ramus, it is appropriate that the customized total

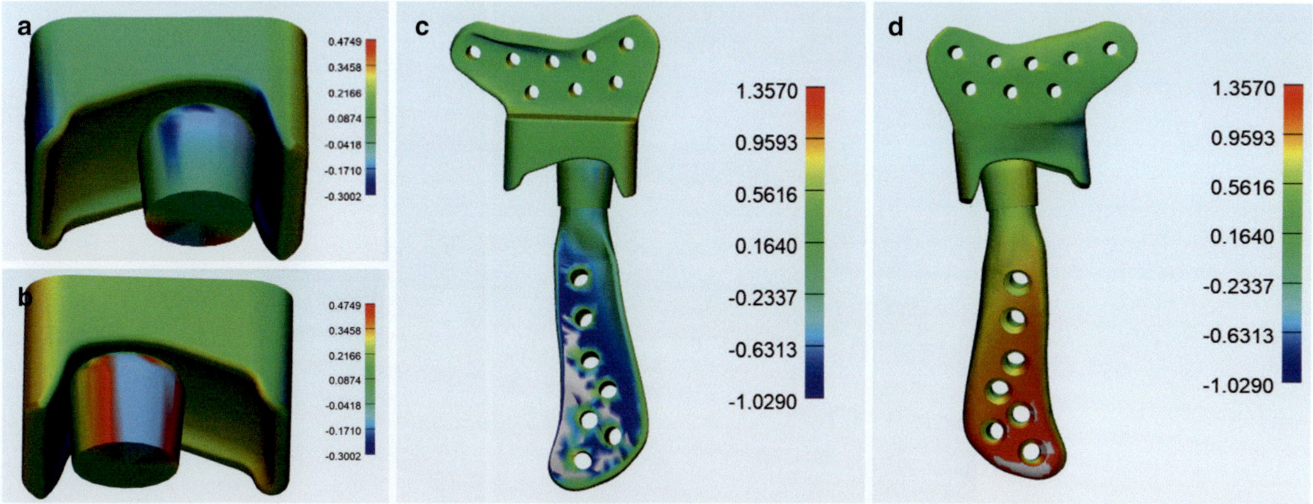

Fig. 4.60 Case F. Postoperative prosthesis position compared to design. The maximum error was 0.47 mm for the core and 1.35 mm for the whole. (**a**) Core component medial error. (**b**) Core component lateral error. (**c**) Overall medial error. (**d**) Overall lateral error

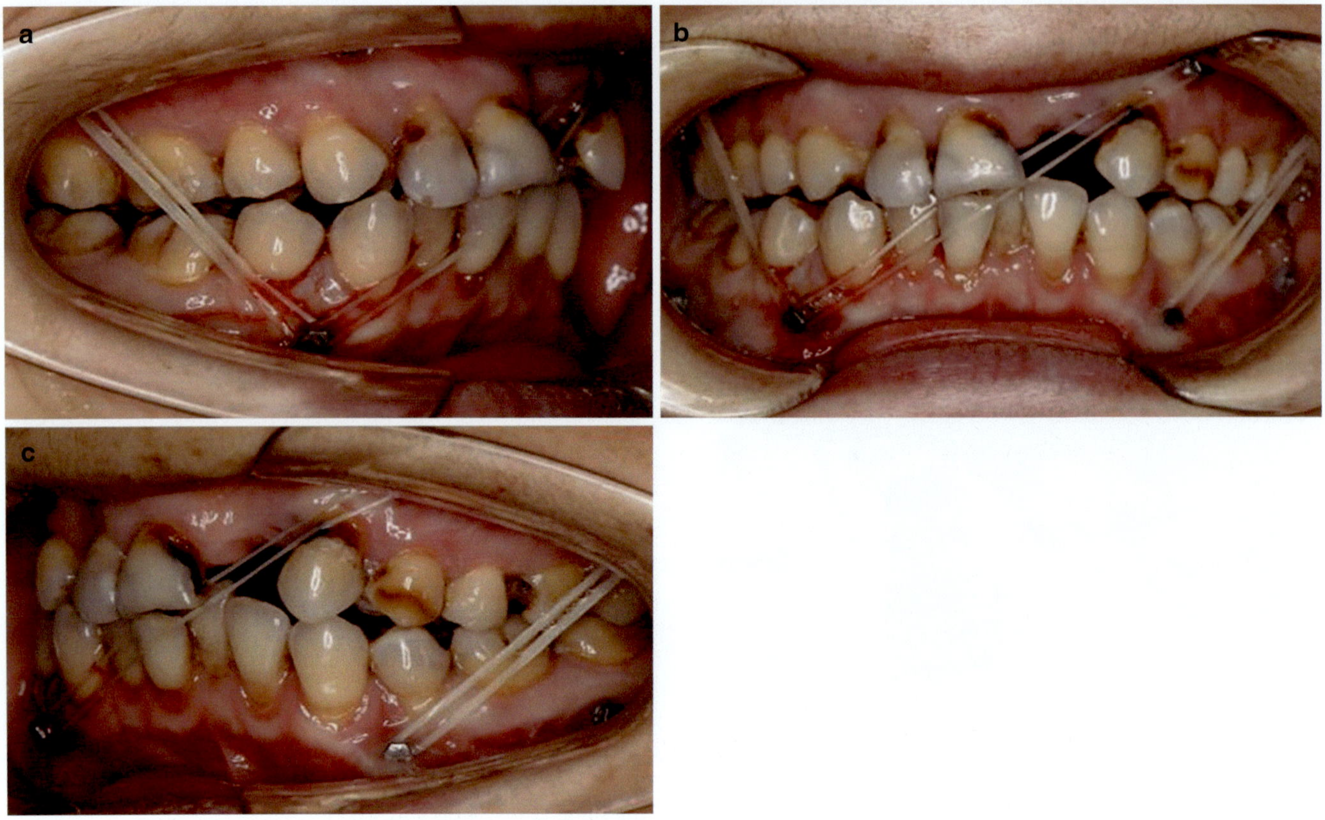

Fig. 4.61 Case F. Intraoral examination at 1 month postoperatively. Intermaxillary traction stabilized the mandible in good position. (**a**) Right occlusion. (**b**) Frontal occlusion. (**c**) Left occlusion

Fig. 4.62 Case F. Facial examination at 1 month postoperatively. The facial shape is basically symmetrical and pleasing. (**a**) Frontal view. (**b**) Lateral view

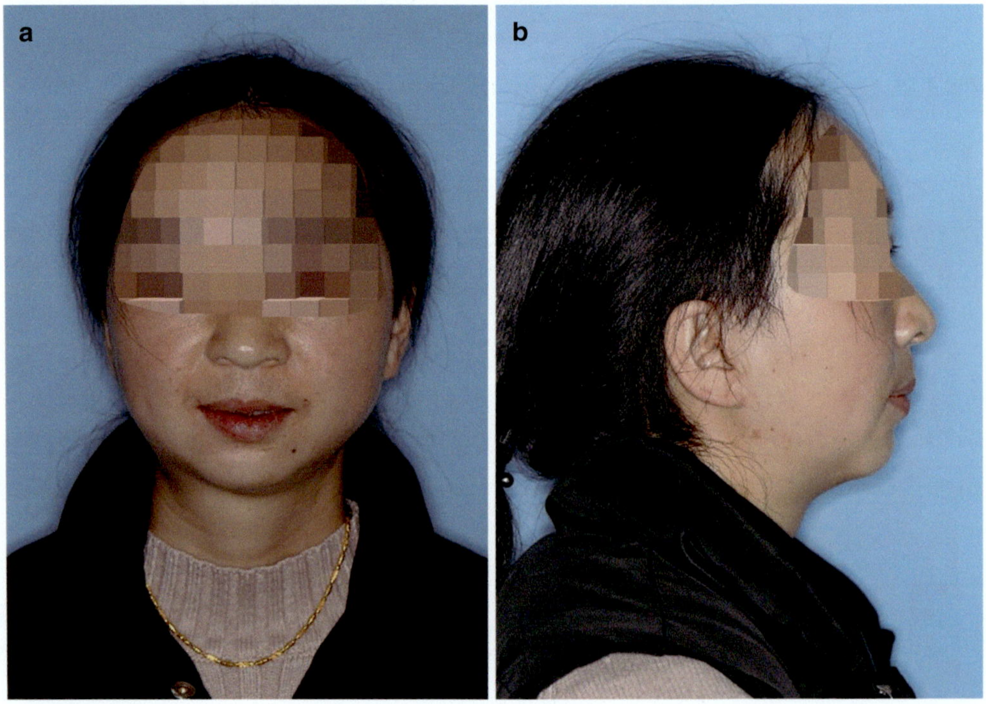

joint prosthesis is designed to match the bone contours and so it can be put into place without grinding or adjustments, thus achieving quick and easy joint replacement.

Because of the original jaw deformity, the height of the right mandibular ramus had to be extended while the joint was replaced. If an autologous CCG was used, it would likely be resorbed over time due to the high impact of mastication. But the joint prosthesis has a strong load-bearing capacity and durability, which can effectively avoid this adverse outcome.

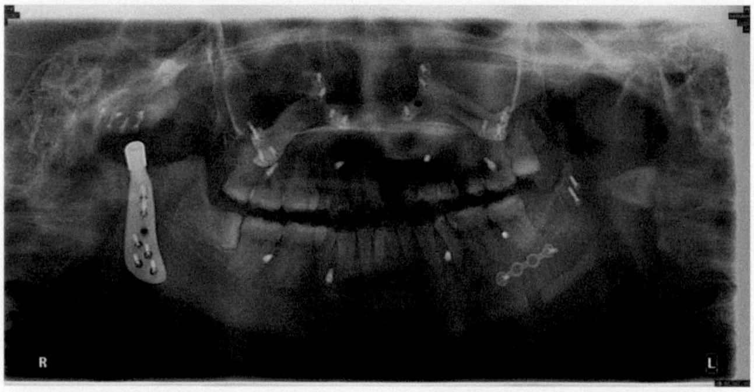

Fig. 4.63 Case F. One-month postoperative panoramic view. The positions of the maxilla, mandible, and joint prosthesis are acceptable

In this case, for the precision of the prosthesis implantation with simultaneous orthognathic surgery, all procedures were digitally controlled, with the total joint prosthesis and the maxillary Le Fort I osteotomy cutting guide customized to minimize errors.

4.4.8.2 Disadvantages

Joint ankylosis without much jaw movement for a long period of time results in stiffness and very limited possibility for manipulation of the musculoskeletal system during the operation, and techniques for how to completely loosen the joint and soft tissues need to be further explored. In addition, the maxillary Le Fort I bone grafting fixation plate in this case was too thick, and so there is room for improvement.

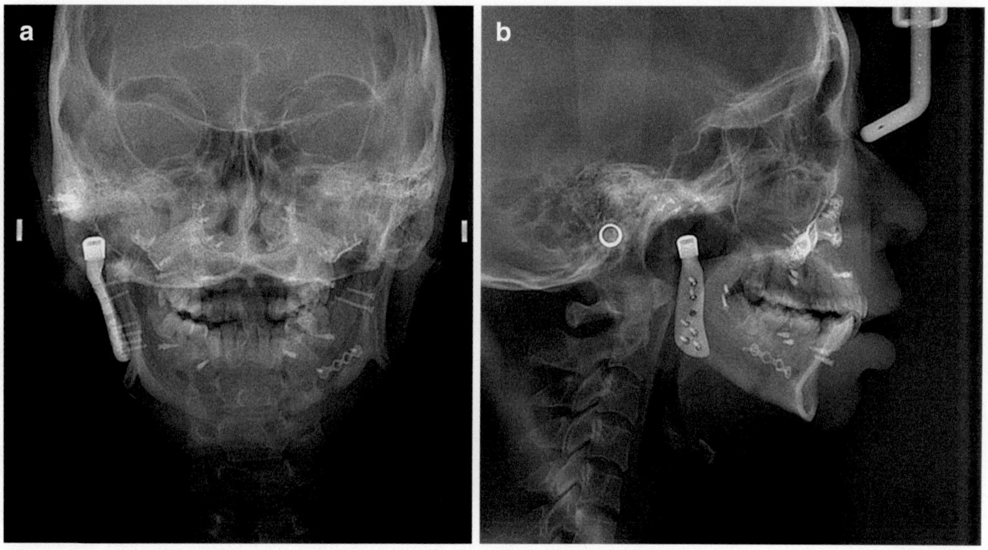

Fig. 4.64 Case F. Cephalometric X-rays 1 month after surgery. The facial shape is basically symmetrical, and the mandible is obviously shifted forward. (**a**) Frontal view. (**b**) Lateral view

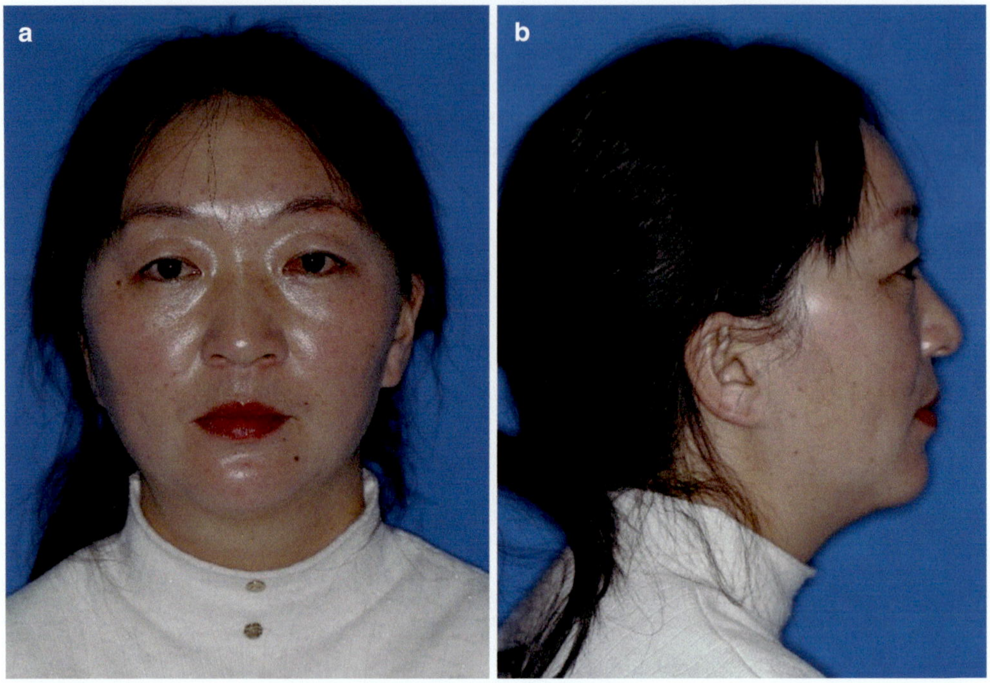

Fig. 4.65 Case F. Examination of the facial shape 5 years after surgery, a genioplasty has been performed. The facial shape was basically symmetrical. The shape of the chin was significantly improved. (**a**) Frontal view. (**b**) Lateral view, no visible scarring in the preauricular region

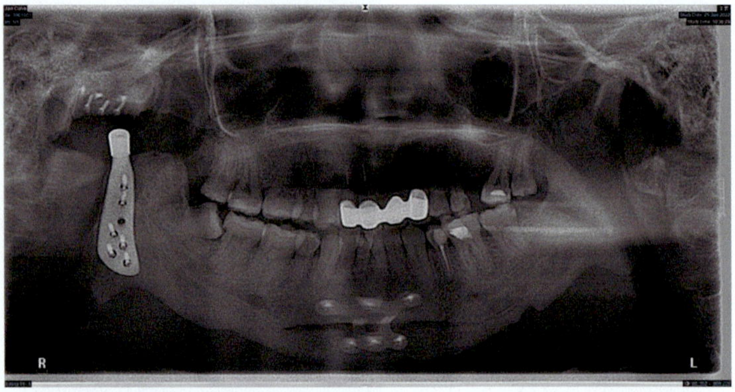

Fig. 4.66 Case F. 5-year postoperative panoramic view. The position of joint prosthesis is stable. The titanium plates were removed from the maxilla and left mandible when the genioplasty was performed

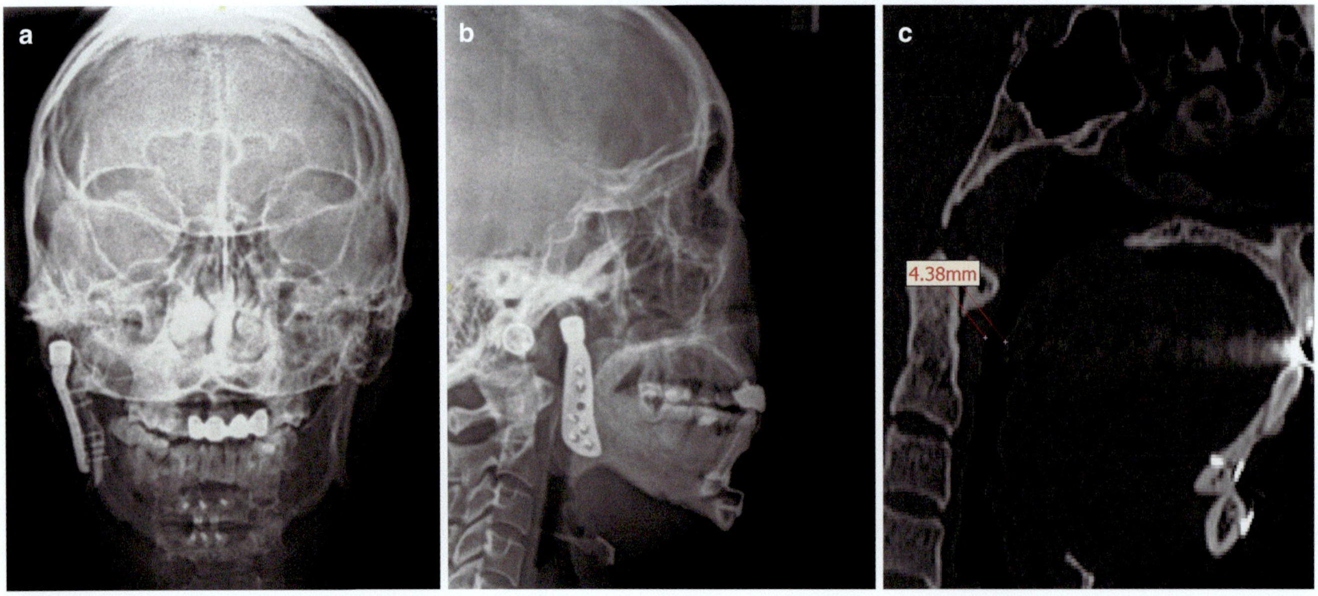

Fig. 4.67 Case F. Cephalometric X-rays 5 years after surgery. Facial symmetry, with significant improvement in profile. (**a**) Frontal view. (**b**) Lateral view. (**c**) CT sagittal view, showing much wider airway

4.5 Reconstruction of Congenital Dentofacial Deformity Through Orthognathic Surgery Simultaneous with Customized Total Temporomandibular Joint Prosthesis Implantation

4.5.1 Case G. Congenital Dentofacial Deformity (Figs. 4.68 and 4.69)

- Patient information: female, 20 years old.
- Complaint: left maxillofacial thinning deformity for more than 20 years.
- History: the patient was diagnosed with first and second branchial arch syndrome after being born with a left maxillofacial thinning deformity, accompanied by left orofacial dehiscence, and she underwent "left transverse facial deformity correction" in a local hospital at the age of 3 years. With growth and development, the left facial thinning deformity gradually worsened.
- Previous history: the patient reported being in good health and denied a history of systemic disease and drug and food allergies.
- Clinical examination: the mandible is retruded and deviated to the left, with scarring on the left cheek and mentalis muscle strain upon lip closure. Intraoral examination (under orthodontic decompensation): the midlines of both upper and lower dental arches are deviated from the facial midline. Anterior deep overjet (3.8 mm) is present. The left first molar exhibits a mesial relationship, while the right first molar shows a distal relationship.
- Imaging examinations: X-ray showed abnormal development of the left mandible (Figs. 4.70 and 4.71), and 3D CT reconstruction showed the absence of the normal structure of the left TMJ, with the chin retracted and tilted to the left (Fig. 4.72).
- Diagnosis: congenital left first and second branchial arch syndrome; deviated mandible deformity.

4.5.2 Case G. Diagnostic Imaging

4.5.3 Case G. Treatment Plan

- Overall treatment plan: left total joint prosthesis implantation simultaneous with orthognathic surgery. Customized total joint prosthesis to reconstruct the left joint and simultaneous orthognathic surgery to restore the position of the upper and lower jaws.
- Reconstruction plan: customized total joint prosthesis implantation.
- Orthognathic plan: Le Fort I osteotomy of the maxilla and sagittal split osteotomy of the right mandibular ramus to shorten it. Due to the severe facial deformity, a phase II genioplasty with facial fat filling was designed for the postoperative period, depending on the recovery of the soft tissues.

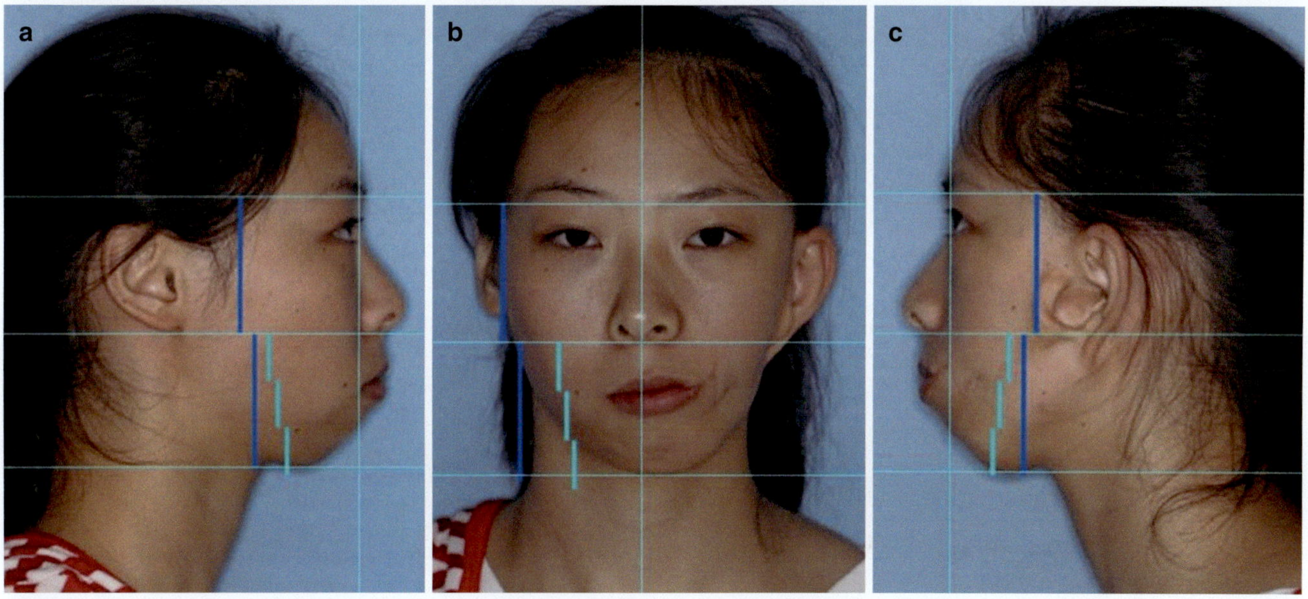

Fig. 4.68 Case G. Facial examination. The ratio of mid-face to lower face is slightly greater than 1:1. The ratio of upper lip length to chin-lip length is greater than 1:2. The mandible is retrusive and deviated to the left. There is a Z-plasty scar on the left face from the macrostomia repair. The left external ear is deformed. (**a**) Right face view. (**b**) Frontal view. (**c**) Left face view

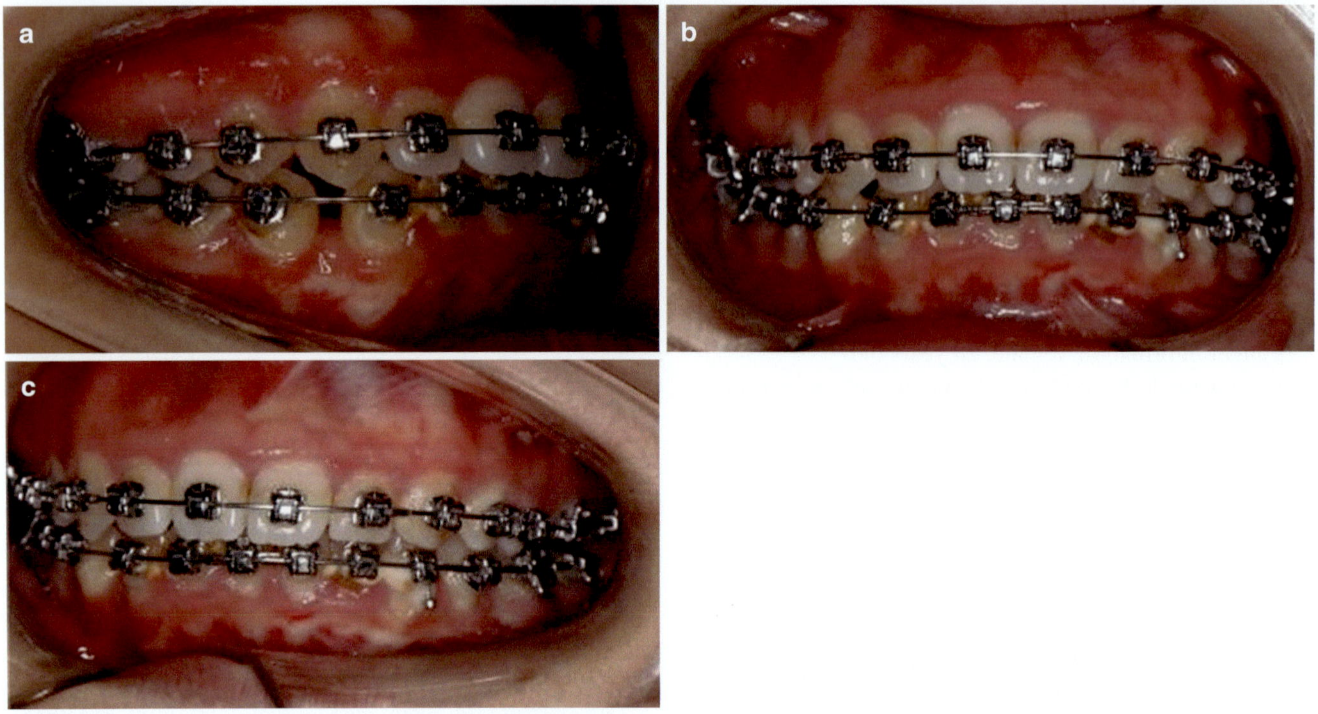

Fig. 4.69 Case G. Intraoral examination after 18 months of orthodontic decompensation. Both upper and lower dental midlines are deviated to the left of the facial midline. There is a 3.8 mm overjet of the anterior teeth. The left molars are Class III. The right molars are Class II. A surgical treatment plan can now be proposed. (**a**) Right occlusion. (**b**) Front occlusion. (**c**) Left occlusion

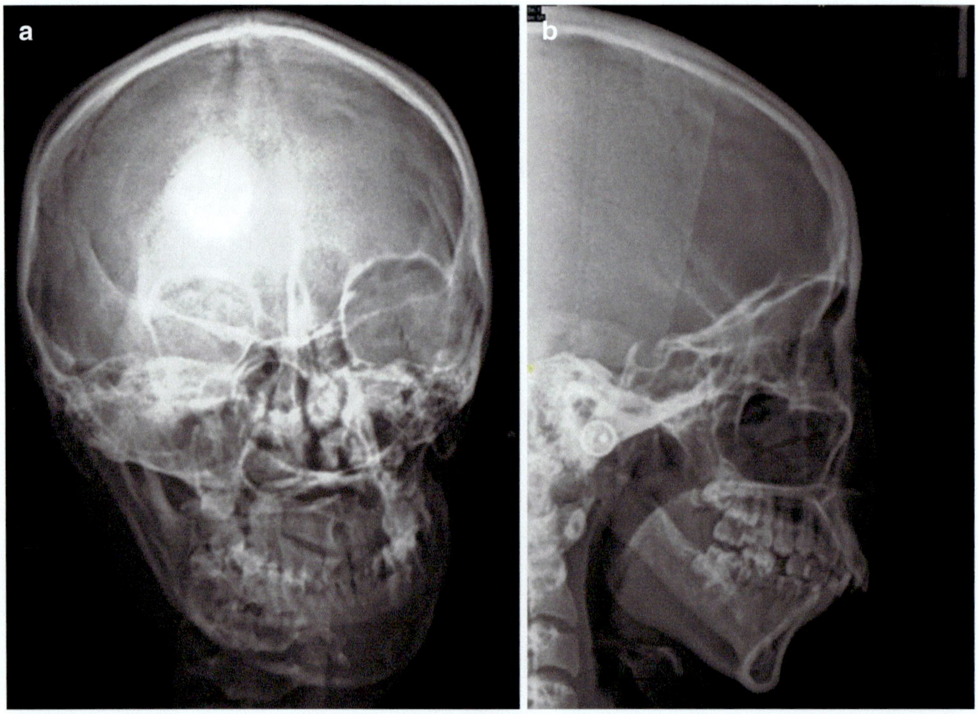

Fig. 4.70 Case G. Cephalometric X-rays. The mandible is deviated to the left and is retruded. (**a**) Frontal view. (**b**) Lateral view

4.5.4 Case G. Orthognathic Plan and Design and Processing of Total Joint Prosthesis and Cutting Guides

Surgical simulation and prosthesis design (Figs. 4.73 and 4.74): firstly, the maxillary plane is to be corrected (blue) and the angle of the plane restored; then the mandible will be reset according to the occlusal relationship to restore the symmetry of the chin and the lower edge of the mandible. Then the sagittal split of the right healthy side mandible (bright blue) is designed to shorten and reposition the body of the mandible toward the right; and then the affected side is implanted with the core components of the prosthesis. Below, the fossa prosthesis component is shown in yellow, and the condylar head component is shown in dark grey. Finally, the zygomatic arch attachment to the fossa component and the mandibular components of the prosthesis are designed according to the morphology of the zygomatic arch and the mandibular stump on the affected side.

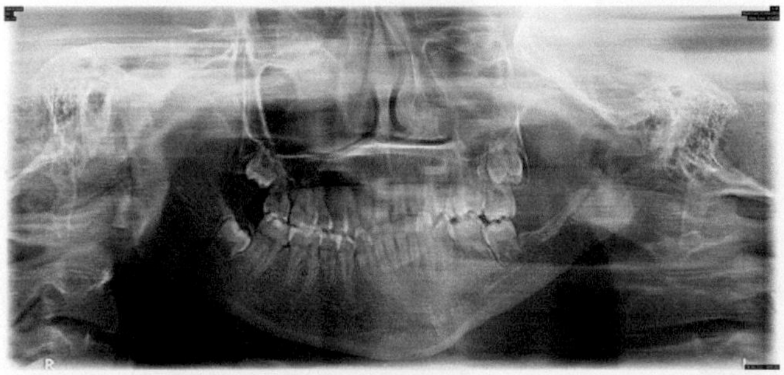

Fig. 4.71 Case G. Panoramic X-ray before treatment. There is hypoplasia of the left mandible, with no TMJ

4.5.4.1 Design and Processing of Digital Guides

According to the orthognathic surgical plan, design the maxillary and mandibular cutting guides, mark the osteotomy line and the range of decompensation, and design a personalized bone grafting plate according to the final position of the jaws (Figs. 4.75 and 4.76).

- Prosthesis fabrication and fitting: the fabrication process is described in Sect. 2.5 in Chap. 2.

4.5.5 Case G. Surgical Procedure

Preoperative laboratory tests: the same as described in Sect. 3.2.5, Preoperative Laboratory Tests.

Preoperative preparation: the same as described in Sect. 3.2.5, Preoperative Preparation, and preparation of 400 mL of blood.

Surgical approach: preauriculotemporal incision, mandibular incision, and intraoral incision were used.

First stage: priority is given to fitting the TMJ prosthesis (Fig. 4.77).

Orthognathic surgery followed the implantation of the prosthesis. The contralateral mandibular ramus was first split sagittally and fixed by intermaxillary ligation. A maxillary Le Fort I osteotomy was then performed, utilizing the cutting guides to assist in the osteotomy, and fixation with customized plates was accomplished after complete release of the maxilla (Fig. 4.78).

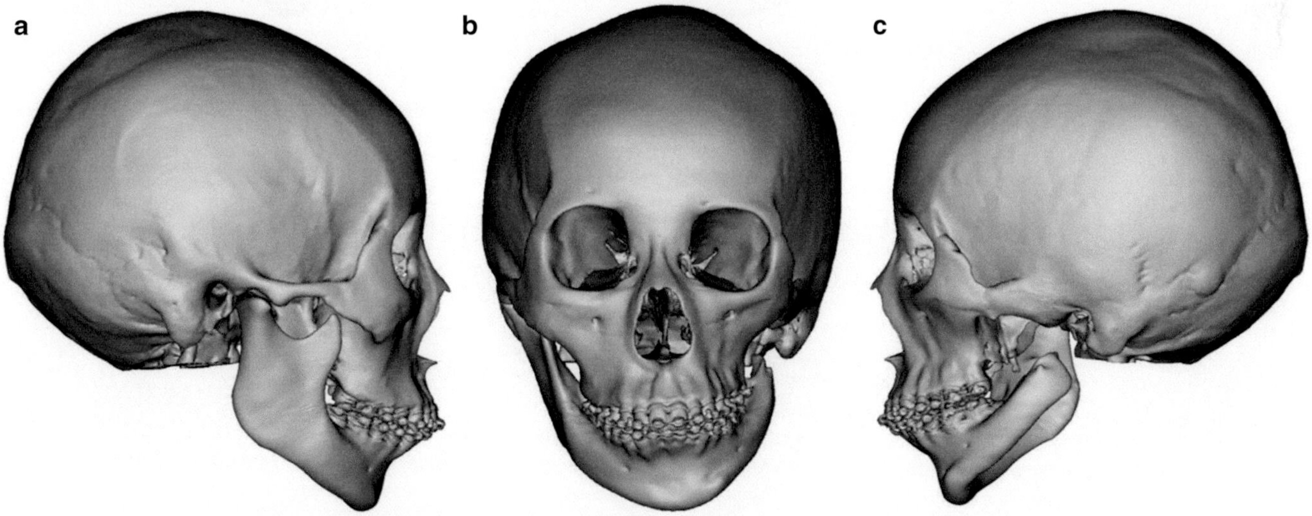

Fig. 4.72 Case G. 3D CT reconstruction showing absence of normal structures in the left joint, with the chin retracted and deviated to the left. (**a**) Right view. (**b**) Frontal view. (**c**) Left view

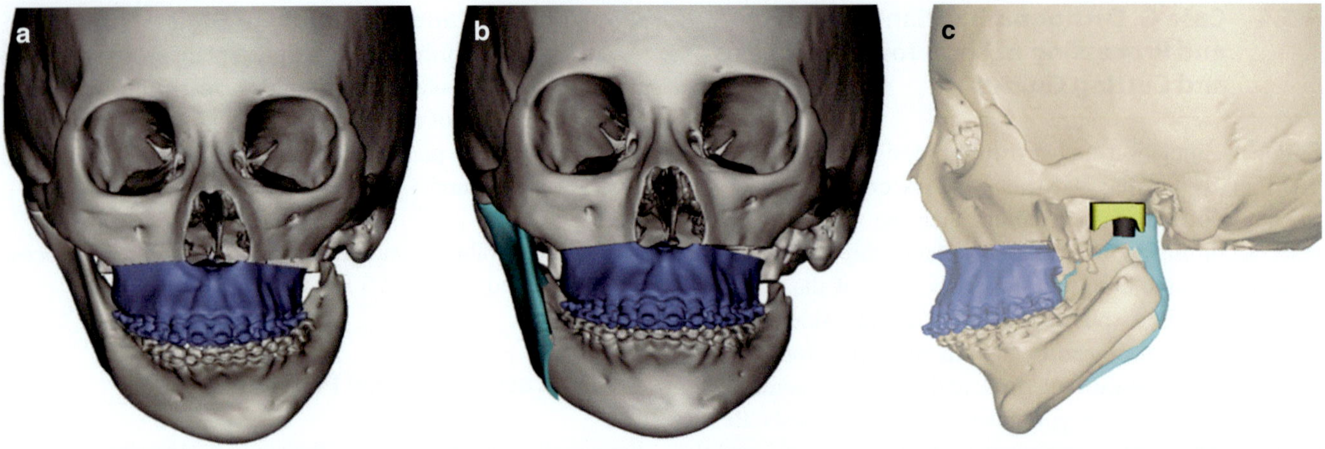

Fig. 4.73 Case G. Virtual osteotomies and placement of the core components of the prosthesis. (**a**) The maxillary occlusal plane is leveled, and the midline is corrected. (**b**) The mandible is repositioned to correct the occlusion and improve the symmetry of the chin and the lower border of the mandible. (**c**) Core components of the left TMJ prosthesis are positioned

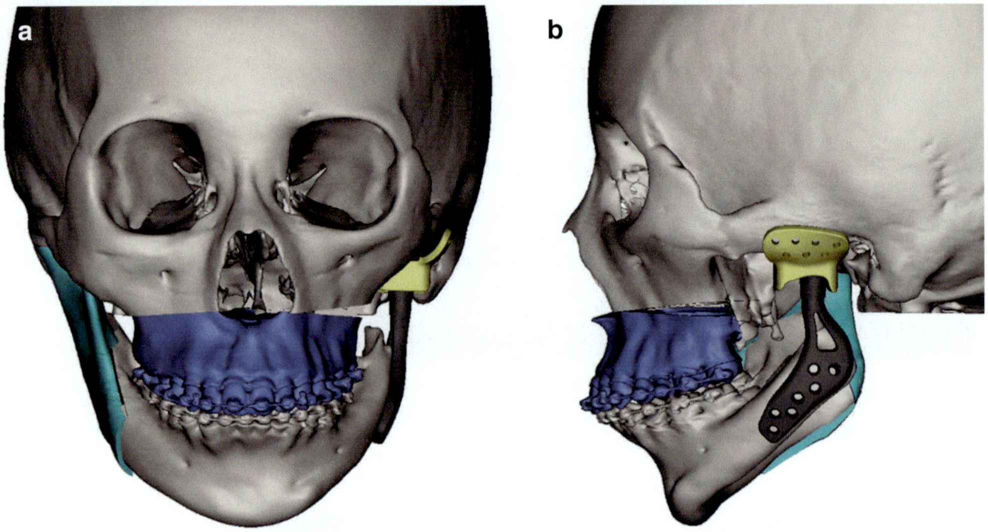

Fig. 4.74 Case G. Prosthesis design with fossa prosthesis component in yellow and mandibular prosthesis component in dark gray. (**a**) Frontal view. (**b**) Lateral view

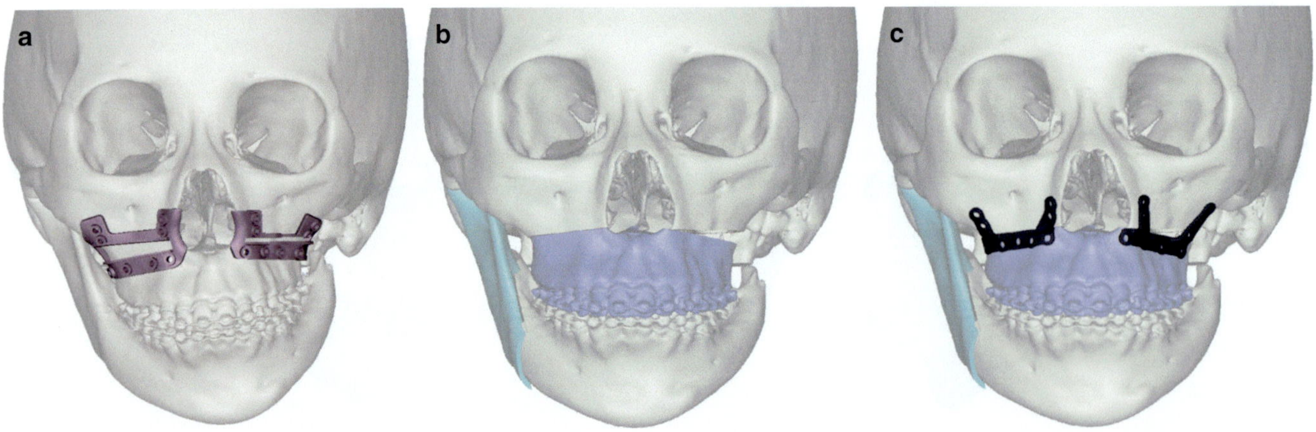

Fig. 4.75 Case G. Virtual design of the maxillary osteotomy. (**a**) The customized cutting guides are designed. (**b**) The postoperative position of the jaws is planned. (**c**) Customized fixation plates are designed

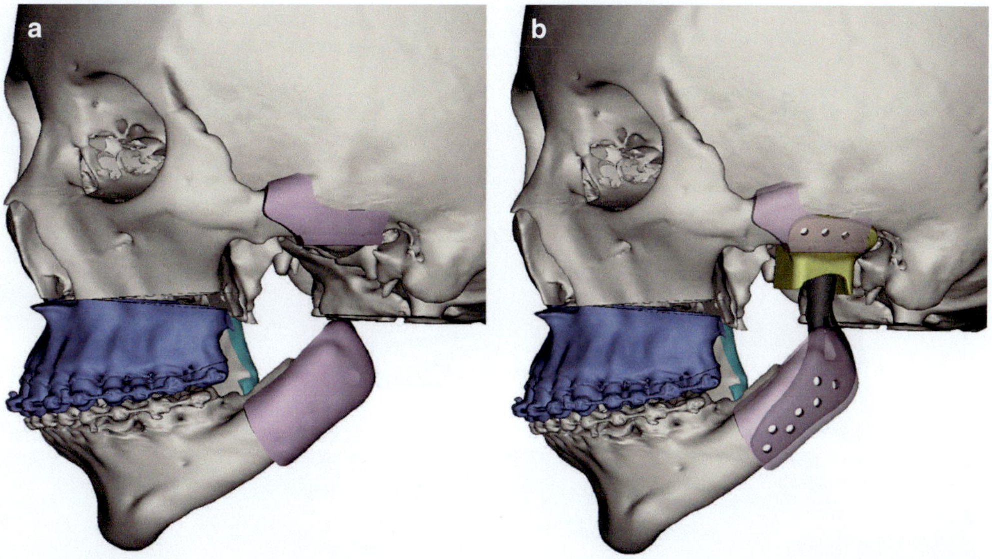

Fig. 4.76 Case G. Designing the articular eminence and mandibular cutting guides (pink). (**a**) Cutting guides design. (**b**) Screw-hole placement for the positioning guides based on the planned prosthesis screw holes

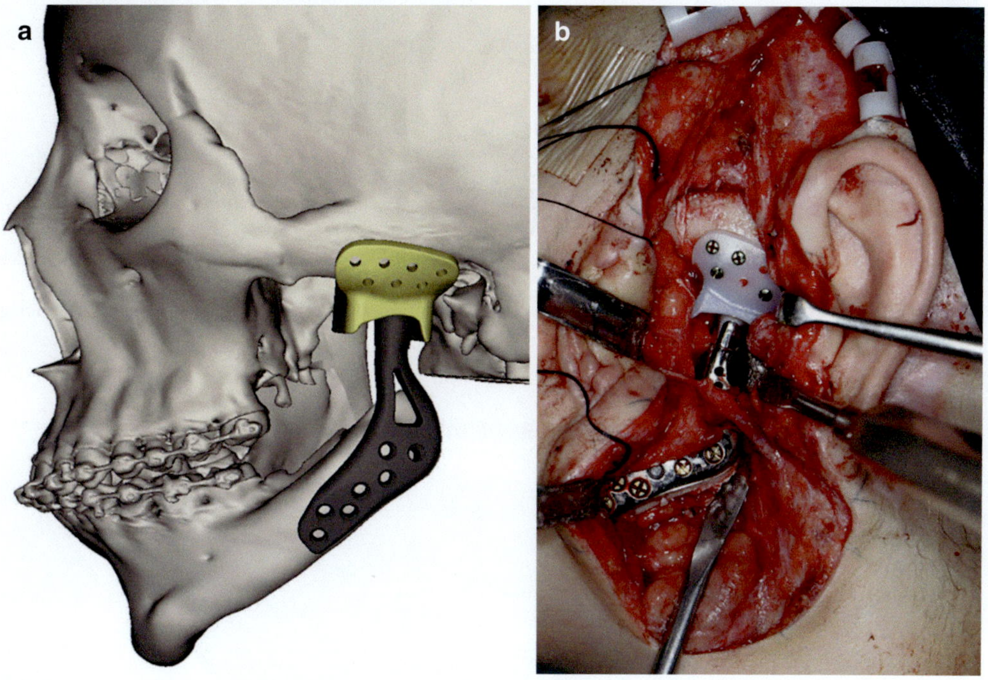

Fig. 4.77 Case G. Preferred option for surgical procedure, joint replacement first. (**a**) Design of prosthesis placement with fossa prosthesis component (yellow) and mandibular prosthesis component (dark gray). (**b**) Actual prosthesis implantation

- Postoperative orders and nursing care: see Sect. 3.2.5, Postoperative Orders and Nursing Care. In addition, intermaxillary elastic traction was performed, and daily oral care was administered.

4.5.6 Case G. Postoperative Analysis of Prothesis Implantation Precision

Regular postoperative follow-ups were performed for appearance (facial shape), function (mouth opening, mouth shape), and prosthesis evaluation (safety, accuracy).

Immediately after surgery: the prosthesis was fitted smoothly, the final occlusion was stable, and the bleeding volume was 620 mL for the 5 hours and 45 minutes of the surgery; the preoperative design was matched to the postoperative CT reconstruction, with a maximum error of 0.47 mm for the core components and an overall maximum error of 1.47 mm (Figs. 4.79 and 4.80).

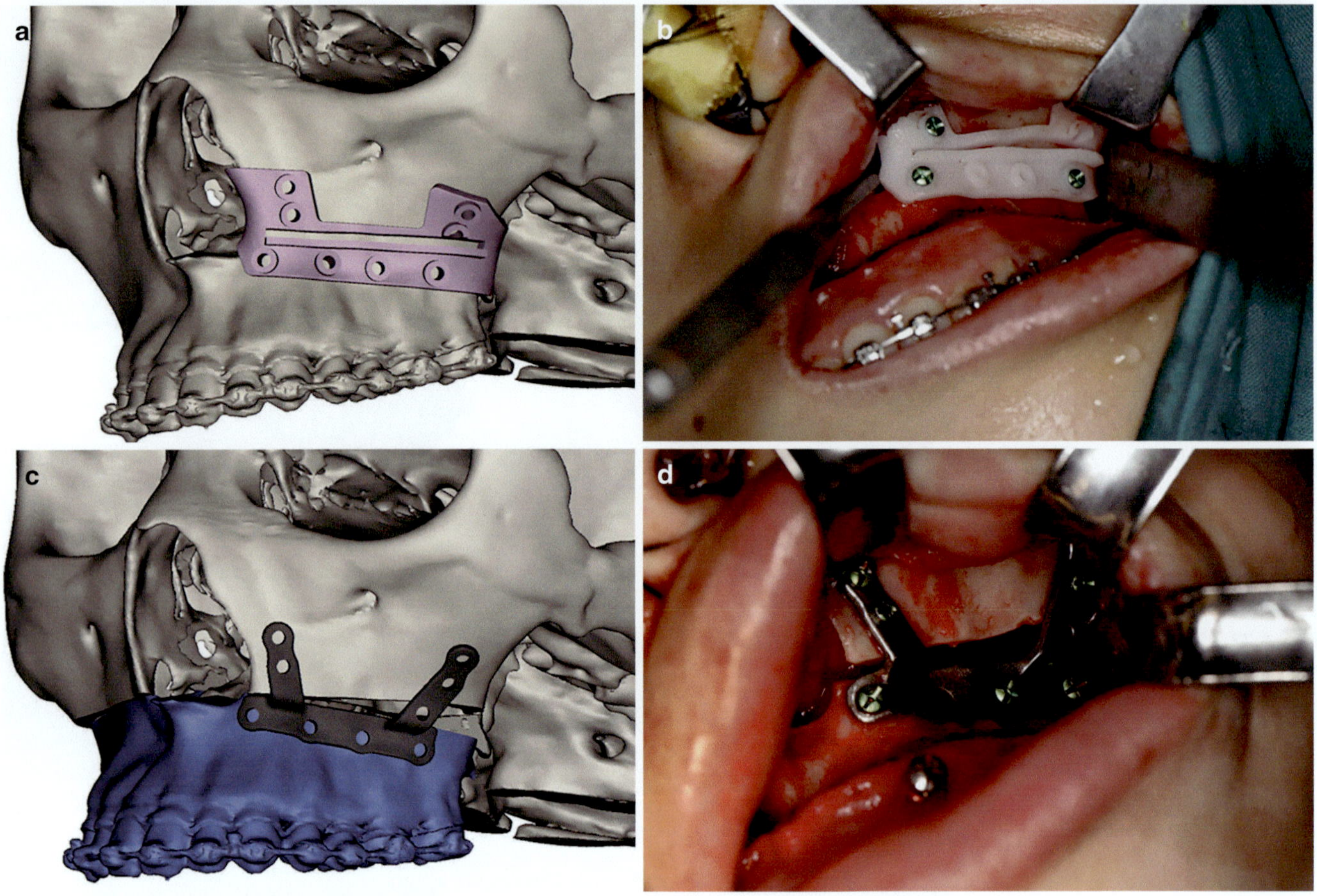

Fig. 4.78 Case G. Orthognathic surgical osteotomy and fixation after repositioning. (**a**) Osteotomy design. (**b**) Cutting guides placement. (**c**) Fixation plate design. (**d**) Fixation plate in place

Fig. 4.79 Case G. Immediate postoperative CT reconstruction. The left total joint prosthesis was well seated, and the maxillary plate was accurately positioned. (**a**) Frontal view. (**b**) Left view

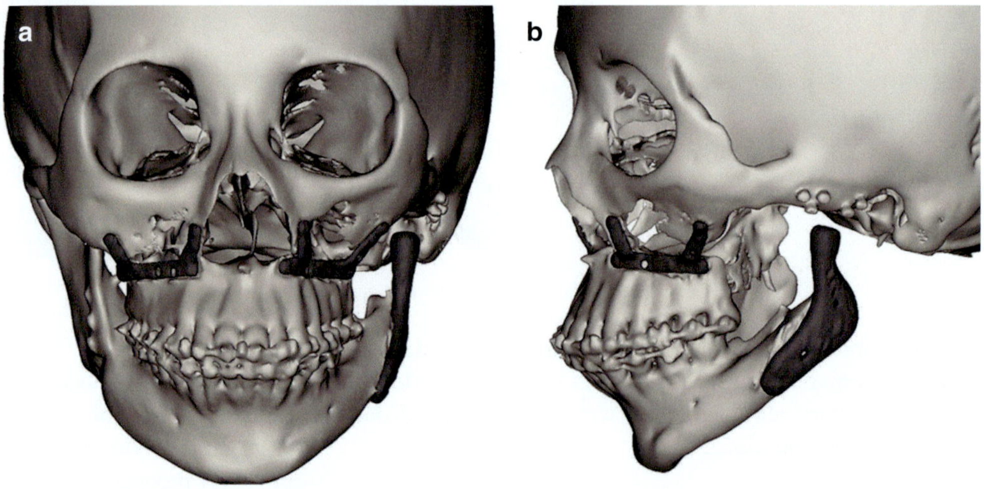

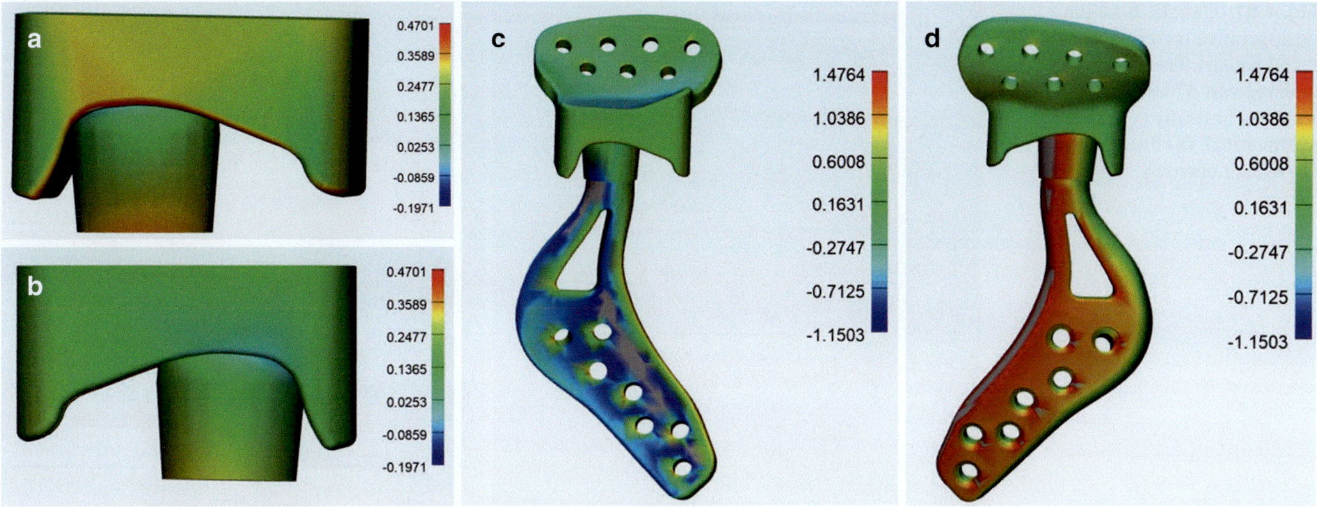

Fig. 4.80 Case G. Comparison of postoperative prosthesis position with design. Maximum error of 0.47 mm for the core and 1.47 mm for the whole. (**a**) Medial error of the core component. (**b**) Lateral error of the core component. (**c**) Medial error of the whole prosthesis. (**d**) Lateral error of the whole prosthesis

4.5.7 Case G. Long-Term Follow-Up and Prognosis

4.5.7.1 6-Month Postoperative Follow-Up

There were no complaints of discomfort, the face was well shaped, and there was no redness, swelling, or other reactions in the operative area (Fig. 4.81).

The joint-mandibular-occlusal-facial pattern was harmonized, and the occlusal relationship was stable (Fig. 4.82).

The mouth opening was 37 mm, with 3 mm lateral movement to the right and 6 mm lateral movement to the left.

Chewing function: normal diet.

Evaluation of the prosthesis: 6 months after the operation, and the prosthesis had no complications such as infection, rejection, loosening, displacement, fracture, ectopic osteogenesis, and allergy.

4.5.7.2 2-Year Postoperative Follow-Up

The prosthesis had no complications such as infection and rejection, loosening, fracture, ectopic osteogenesis, or material allergy, and the prosthesis was well integrated with the bone (Fig. 4.83). To further improve the facial appearance, the patient had the left maxillary titanium fixation plate removed and a customized PEEK prosthesis implanted in the left maxilla region.

4.5.8 Case G. Advantages and Disadvantages

4.5.8.1 Advantages

For severe maxillofacial deformities such as the first and second branchial arch syndrome, conventional standard prostheses cannot meet the requirements of repair and reconstruction; at this time, the advantages of prostheses personalized to custom fit for the individual are obvious. In this case, the normal structure of the joint on the affected side disappeared, and the customized prosthesis was used to correct the facial shape while restoring the joint function, to realize the comprehensive treatment of the joint-mandible-occlusion trinity.

4.5.8.2 Disadvantages

Poor postoperative soft tissue morphology was an unresolved issue in this case, and multiple surgeries are often required for such complex and severe dentofacial deformities.

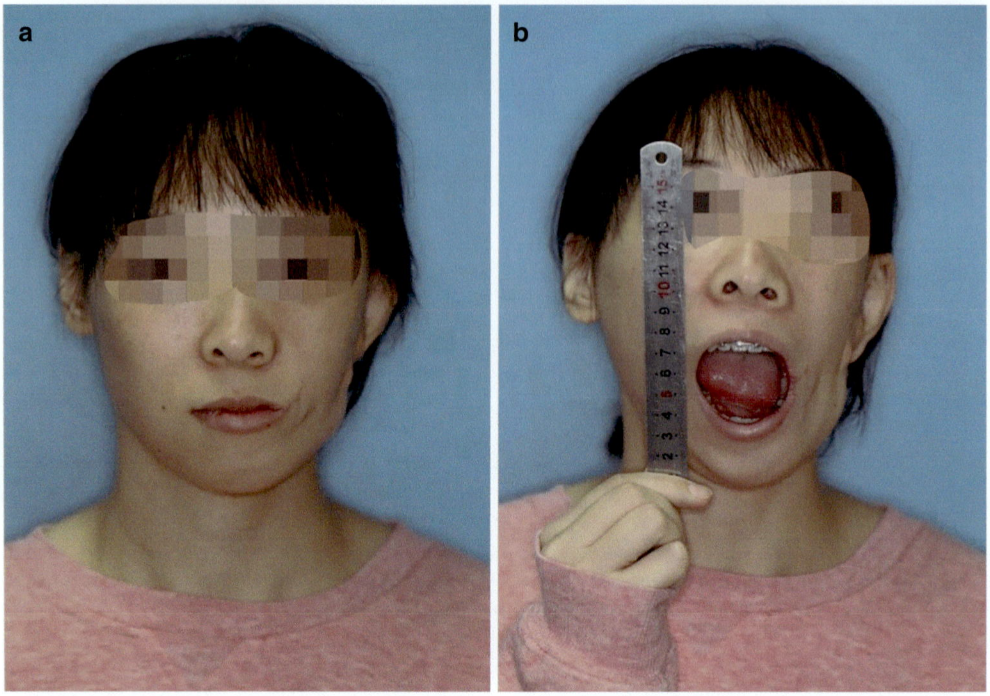

Fig. 4.81 Case G. 6-month postoperative review of the facial pattern. The mouth opening was 37 mm, and the face was basically symmetrical. (**a**) Front view. (**b**) Mouth opening

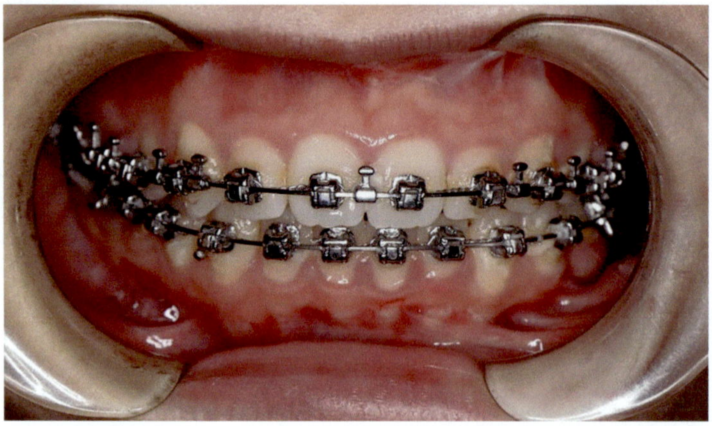

Fig. 4.82 Case G. Review of intraoral condition 6 months after surgery. The intraoral occlusal relationship was stable, with a shallow space between upper and lower anterior teeth, and the upper and lower teeth were aligned in the midline

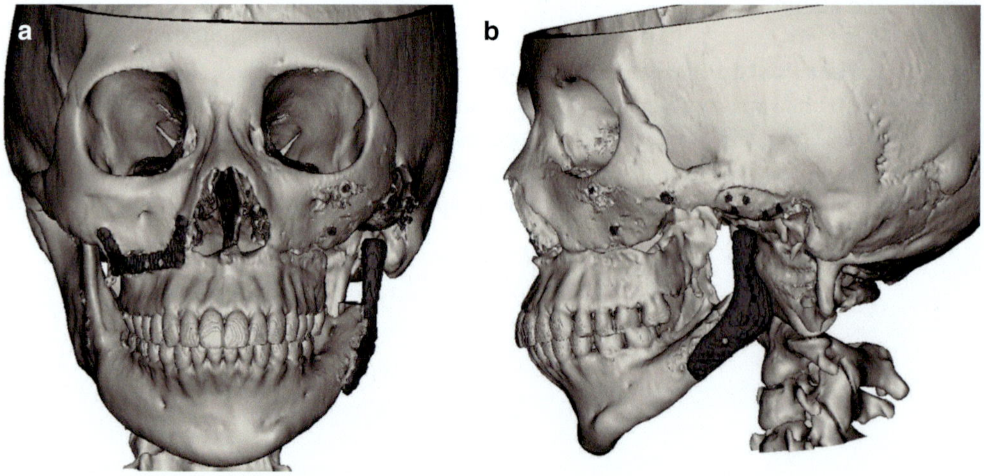

Fig. 4.83 Case G. 2-year postoperative CT follow-up (left maxillary titanium plate was removed, followed by replacement with PEEK prosthesis)

4.6 Reconstruction of Autologous Bone Graft Resorption Through Orthognathic Surgery Simultaneous with Customized Total Temporomandibular Joint Prosthesis Implantation

4.6.1 Case H. Autologous Bone Graft Resorption

- Patient information: female, 25 years old.
- Complaint: occlusal disorder with severe mandibular retrognathia after orthognathic surgery more than 2 years.
- History: 6 years ago, she was admitted to our hospital for mandibular retrognathia and was diagnosed with bilateral idiopathic condylar resorption. She underwent bilateral CCG and Le Fort I osteotomy of the maxilla. 2 years after the surgery, she developed progressive mandibular retrognathia and occlusal disorders. She reported a history of nocturnal snoring.
- Previous history: the patient reported being in good health and denied history of systemic disease or drug and food allergies.
- Clinical examination: mandibular retrognathia and maxillary protrusion. Bilateral Angle's Class II molar relationship with mandibular retrognathia and deep overbite (Figs. 4.84, 4.86, 4.88, 4.89, 4.90 and 4.91).
- Imaging examination: cephalometric X-ray and maxillofacial CT showed mandibular retrognathia and airway narrowing (Fig. 4.85, 4.87, 4.92 and 4.93, Table 4.1).
- Diagnosis: resorption of CCG after orthognathic surgery; bony Class II deformity with mandibular retrognathia; open-bite anterior teeth; obstructive sleep apnea (Figs. 4.85, 4.86, 4.87, 4.88, 4.89, 4.90 and 4.91).

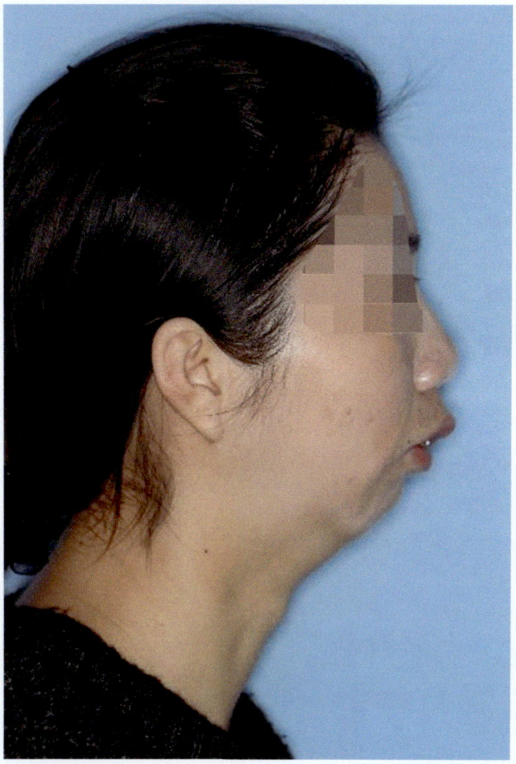

Fig. 4.84 Case H. Facial examination. There were mandibular retrusion, microgenia, and maxillary protrusion

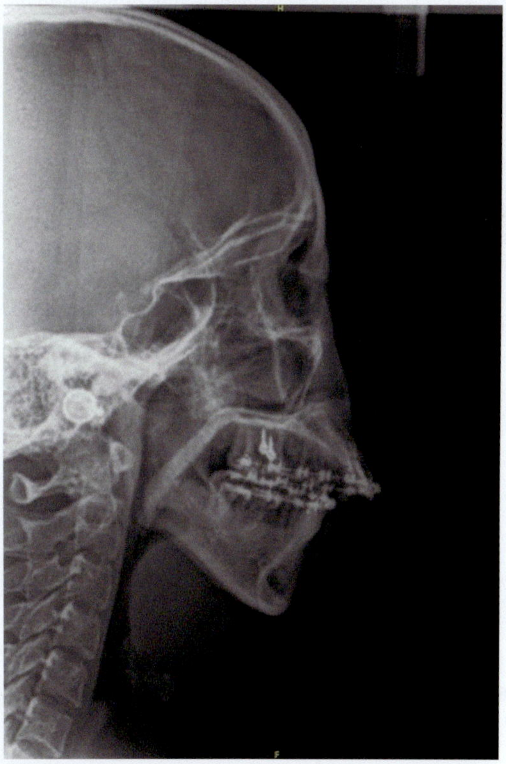

Fig. 4.85 Case H. Lateral cephalometric X-ray. There was mandibular retrusion and a narrow posterior airway space

4.6.2 Case H. Diagnostic Imaging 1.5 Years After CCG Surgery and Subsequent Bone Graft Resorption (Figs. 4.92 and 4.93)

4.6.3 Case H. Treatment Plan

- Overall treatment plan: removal of grafted bone and preparation of space for prosthesis implantation, and bilateral customized total joint prosthesis implantation with simultaneous correction of jaw deformity
- Surgical resection design: removal of the rib graft and related titanium plates, trimming of the lateral bone surface of the mandibular ramus, and preparation of the prosthesis implantation space
- Reconstruction plan: bilateral customized total joint prosthesis implantation

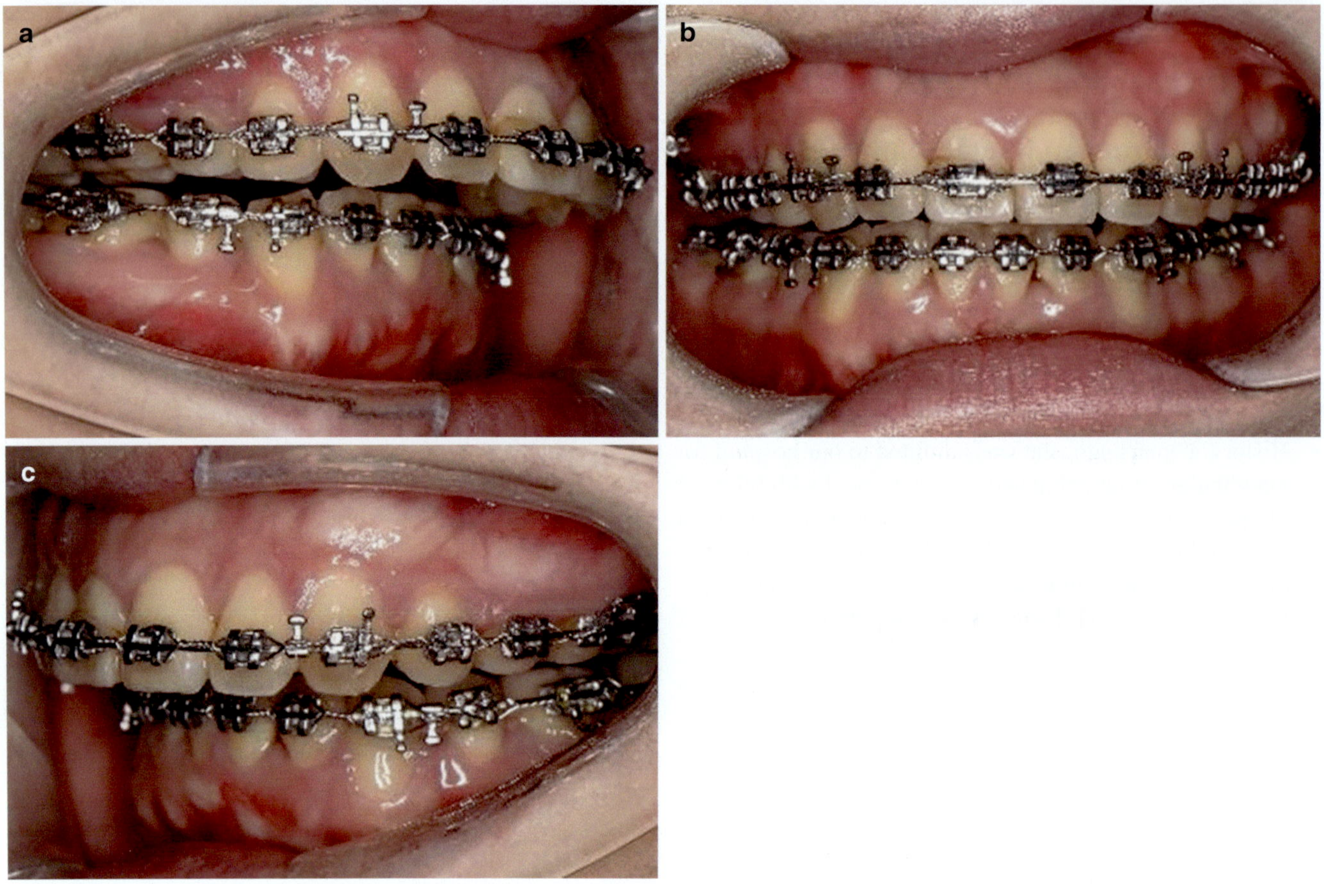

Fig. 4.86 Case H. Intraoral examination after orthodontic decompensation. There was a bilateral Class II molar relationship, mandibular retrusion, and a large overjet. The mandibular midline was deviated to the right. (**a**) Right occlusion. (**b**) Frontal occlusion. (**c**) Left occlusion

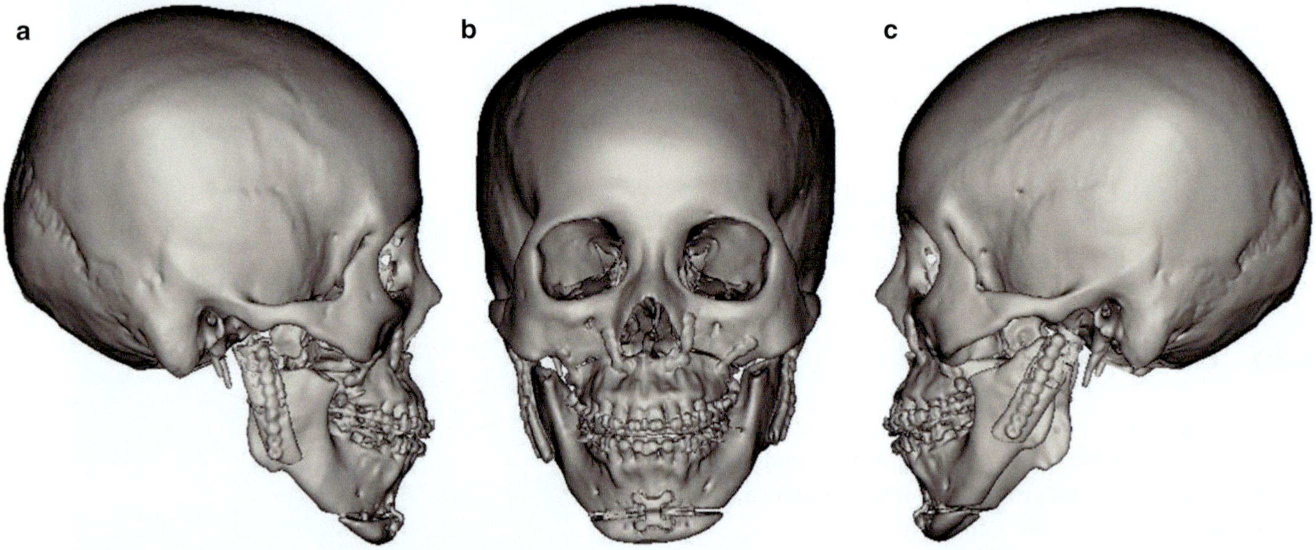

Fig. 4.87 Case H. CT reconstruction of the CCG, maxillary Le Fort type I osteotomy, and genioplasty 1 month after surgery. (**a**) Right view. (**b**) Frontal view. (**c**) Left view

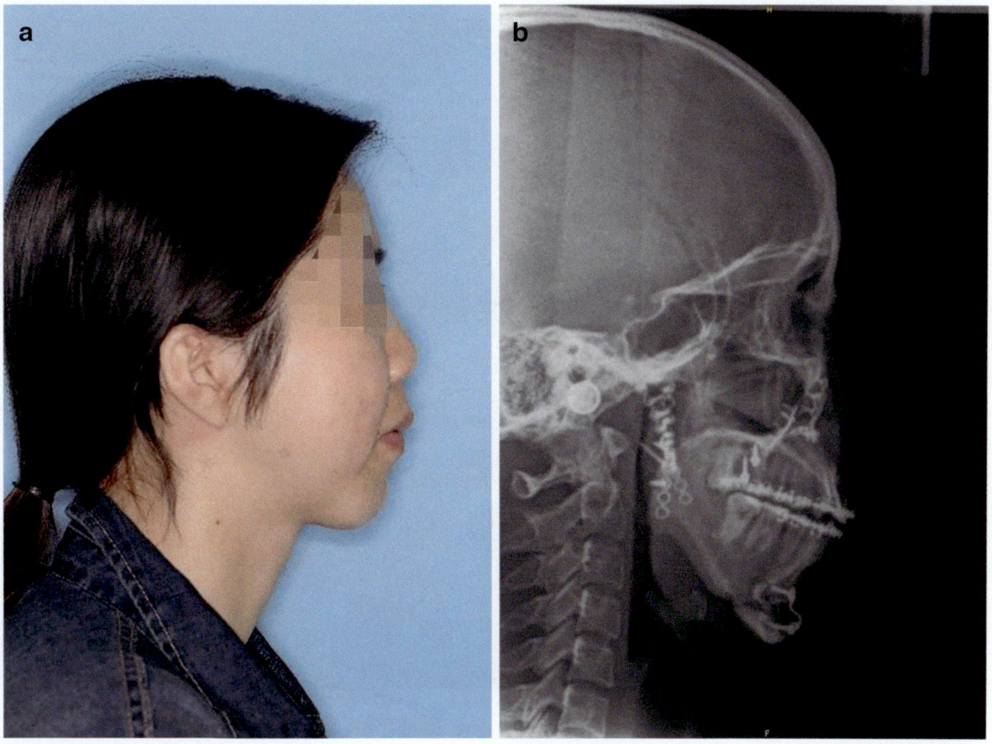

Fig. 4.88 Case H. Facial examination 3 months after CCG surgery. Significant improvement in mandibular retrognathia and narrow airway width increased compared with preoperative width. (**a**) Lateral facial profile. (**b**) Lateral cephalometric X-ray view

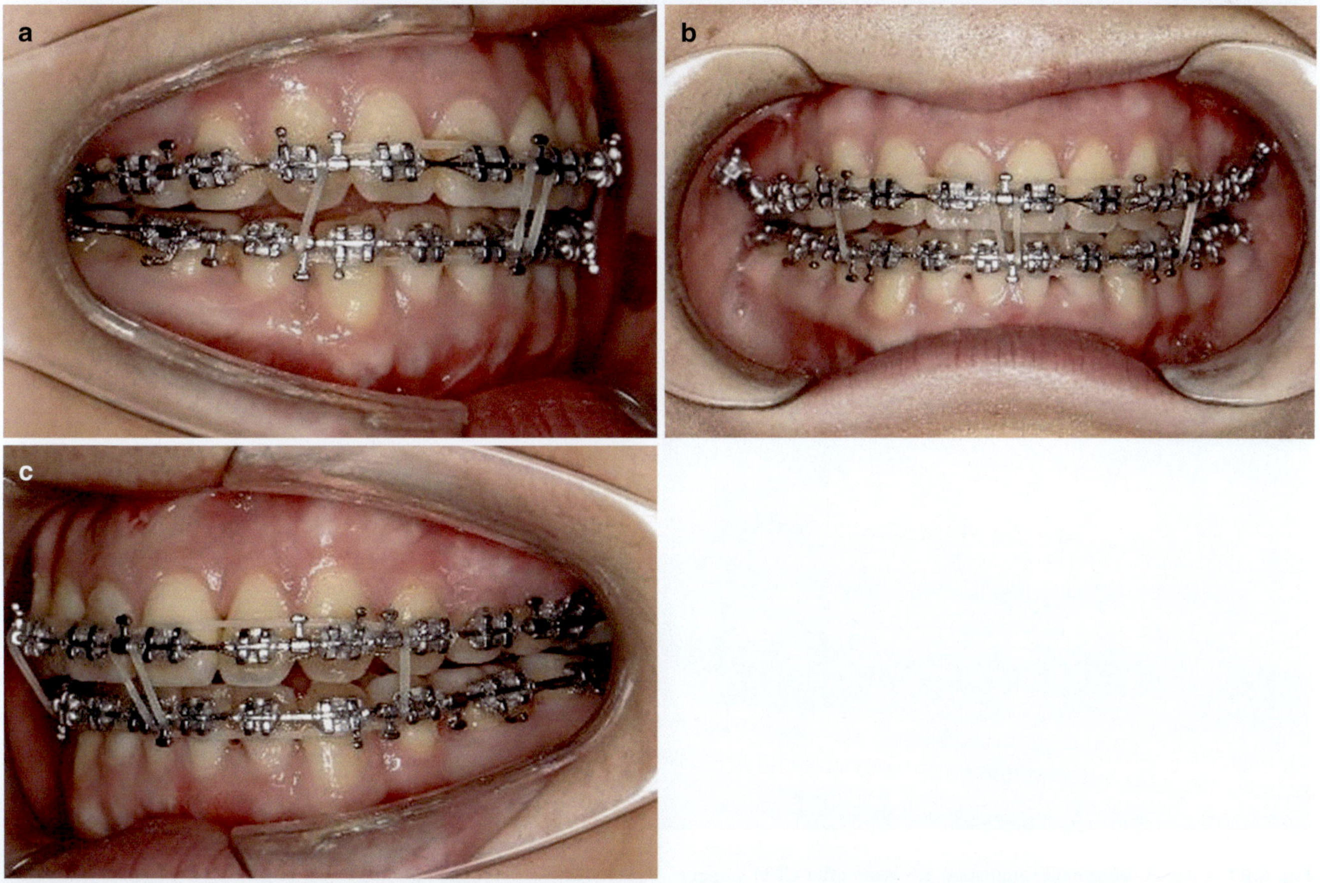

Fig. 4.89 Case H. Intraoral examination 3 months after CCG surgery. In light traction, the occlusal relationship is essentially stable. (**a**) Right occlusion. (**b**) Frontal occlusion. (**c**) Left occlusion

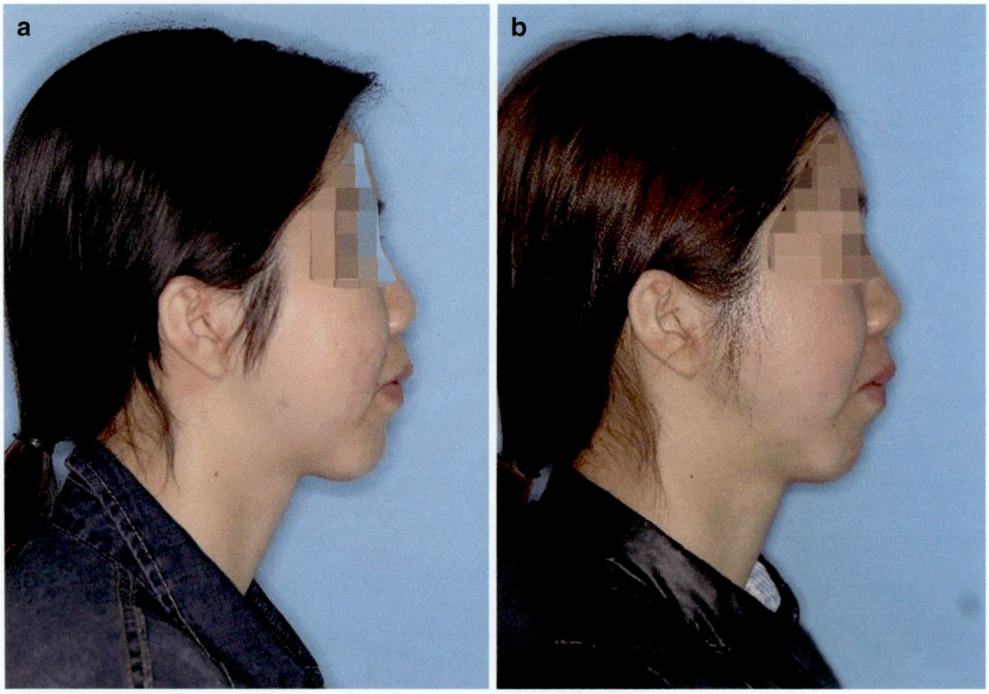

Fig. 4.90 Case H. Facial examination 1.5 years after the first surgery. As compared to the 3-month profile, mandibular retrusion has recurred. (**a**) 3 months after CCG surgery. (**b**) 1.5 years after CCG surgery with recurrence of mandibular retrognathia

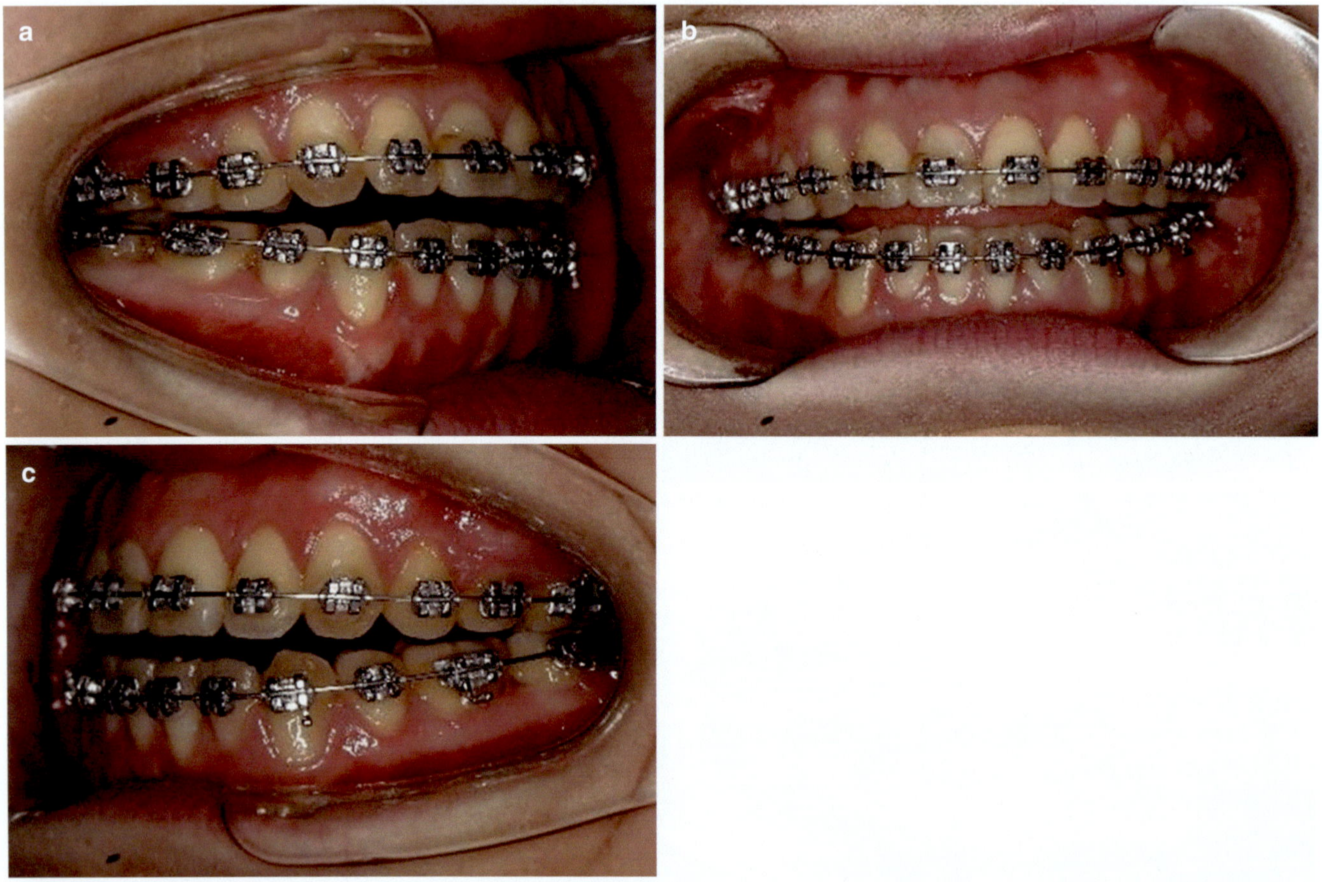

Fig. 4.91 Case H. Intraoral examination 1.5 years after CCG surgery. A recurrence of mandibular retrognathia was accompanied by the development of open-bite anterior teeth, which did not respond well to prolonged Class II traction. (**a**) Right occlusion. (**b**) Frontal occlusion. (**c**) Left occlusion

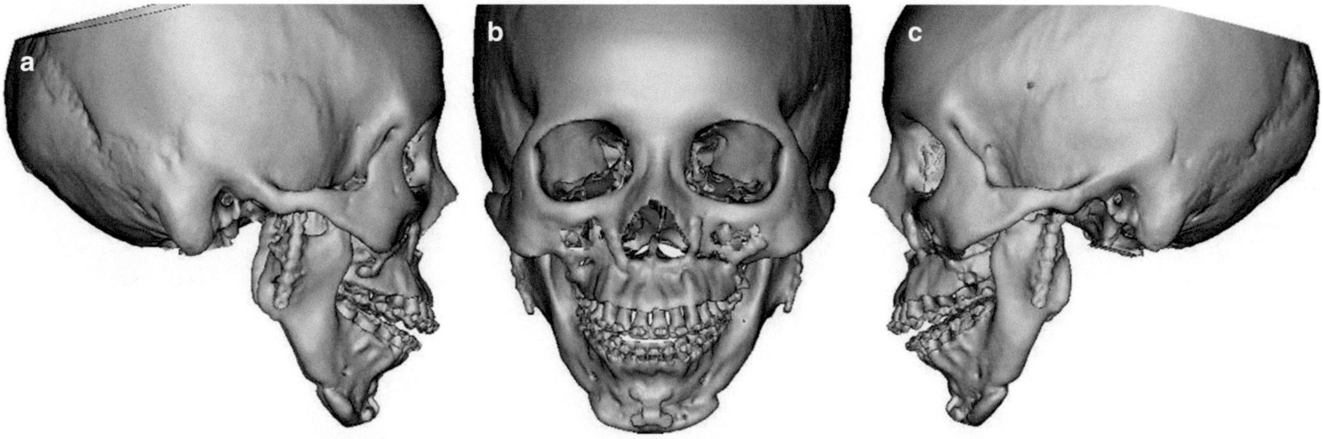

Fig. 4.92 Case H. 3D CT reconstruction of CCG 1.5 years after surgery. Recurrent mandibular retrognathia with open-bite anterior teeth. Bone graft resorption, leading to the titanium plate stump contacting the articular eminence on both sides. (**a**) Right view. (**b**) Front view. (**c**) Left view

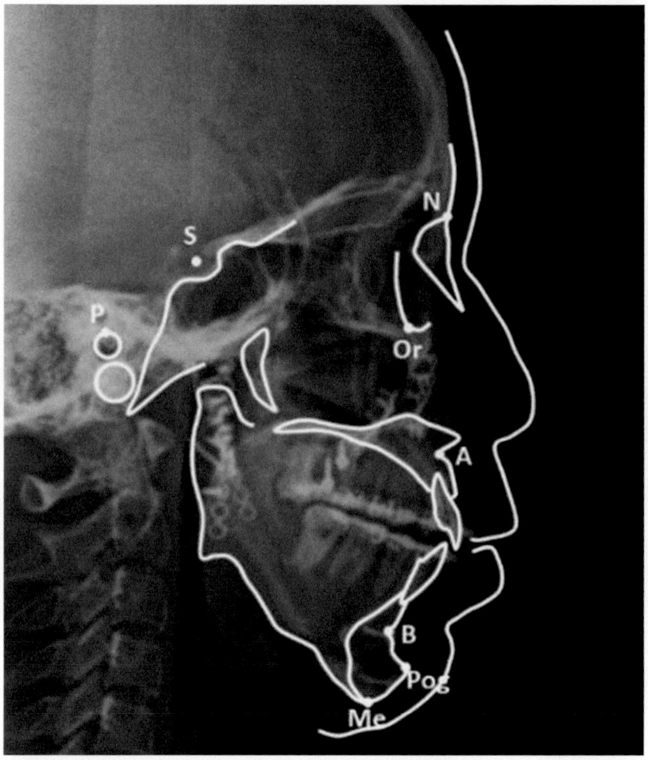

Fig. 4.93 Case H. Cephalometric X-ray measurement after rib cartilage flap reconstruction

4.6.4 Case H. Design and Processing of Total Joint Prostheses and Cutting Guides

- Surgical simulation and prosthesis design (Figs. 4.94, 4.95 and 4.96)
- Prosthesis fabrication and fitting: The fabrication process is described in Sect. 2.5 in Chap. 2.

Table 4.1 Case H. Cephalometric X-ray measurement data

	Measured value
Measurement indicators	Preoperative
ANB	7.3°
SNA	83.2°
SNB	75.9°
GOGN-SN	49.6°
OP-SN	25.5°
U1-L1	128.1°

4.6.5 Case H. Surgical Procedure

Preoperative laboratory tests: the same as described in Sect. 3.2.5, Preoperative Laboratory Tests.

Preoperative preparation: the same as described in Sect. 3.2.5, Preoperative Preparation, and preparation of 400 mL of blood

4.6.5.1 Steps of the Surgical Procedure

1. Surgical approach: preauriculotemporal incision and submandibular incision were used.
2. Preparation of the joint prosthesis implant bed: removal of the graft bone and titanium plates, osteotomy of the articular eminence, and preparation of the prosthesis implantation bed.
3. Intermaxillary ligation.
4. Total joint prosthesis installation.
5. The mandibular prosthesis neck is filled with abdominal fat.
    - Postoperative orders and nursing care: see Sect. 3.2.5, Postoperative Orders and Nursing Care.

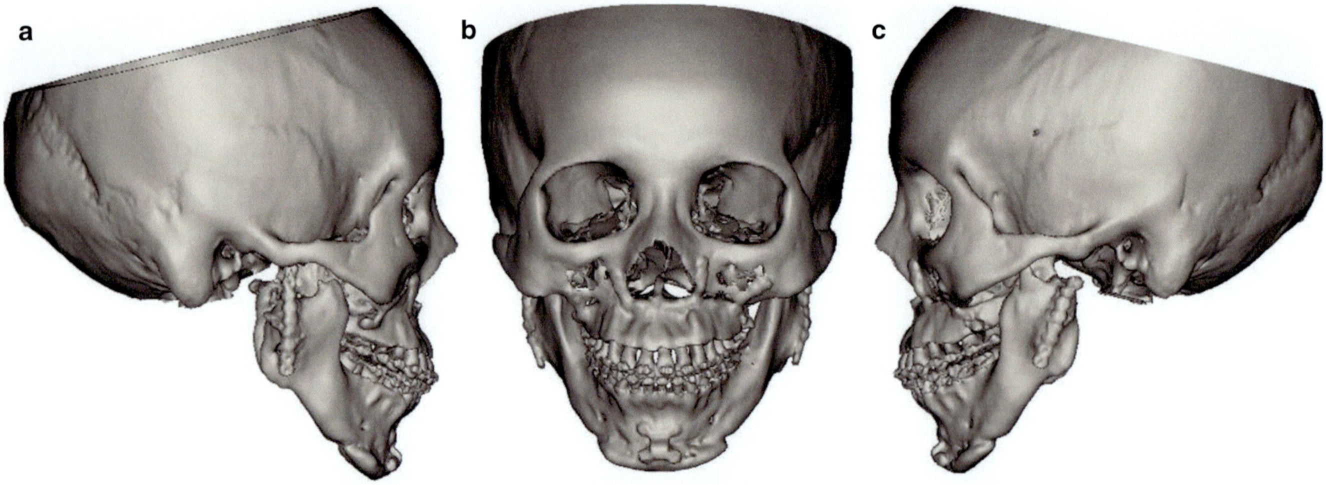

Fig. 4.94 Case H. Plan for repositioning the mandible according to the occlusal relationship, so mandibular ramus stumps are to be repositioned far from the articular fossa. (**a**) Right view. (**b**) Frontal view. (**c**) Left view

Fig. 4.95 Case H. Determining the desired positions of the fossa prosthetic core components. (**a**) Right view. (**b**) Left view

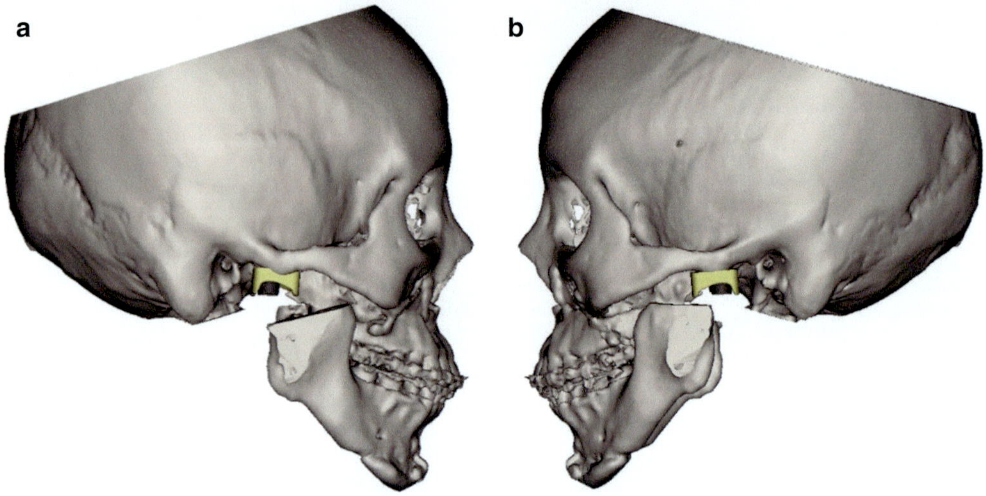

Fig. 4.96 Case H. Design of zygomatic arch articular fossa prosthetic core components and mandibular components. (**a**) Right view. (**b**) Left view

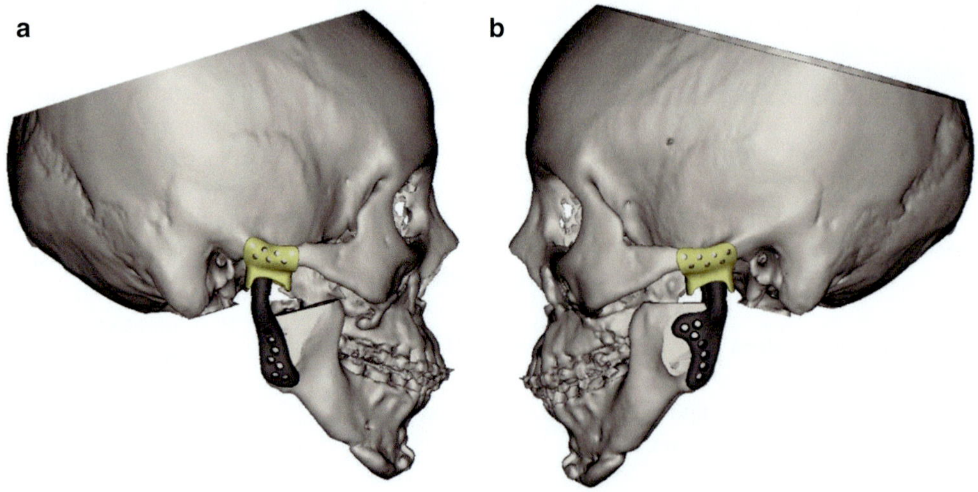

4.6.6 Case H. Postoperative Analysis of Prosthesis Implantation Precision

Regular postoperative follow-ups were performed to check for appearance (facial shape), function (mouth opening, mouth shape), and prosthesis evaluation (safety, accuracy).

Immediately after surgery: the intraoperative guides were accurately seated, the prosthesis was fitted smoothly, and a comparison between the preoperative design and the postoperative reconstruction showed that the prosthesis was accurately seated. Postoperative prosthesis installation error analysis showed a maximum error of 1.78 mm for the core component and 1.86 mm for the prosthesis (Fig. 4.97).

4.6.7 Case H. Long-Term Follow-Up and Prognosis

4.6.7.1 1-Year Postoperative Follow-Up

There were no complaints of discomfort, the face was well shaped, and there was no redness, swelling, or other reactions in the operative area (Fig. 4.98).

The joint-mandibular-occlusal-facial shape was harmonious, and the occlusal relationship was stabilized at the end of orthodontic treatment (Fig. 4.99). The symptoms of nighttime snoring improved significantly.

Mouth opening 35 mm, range of 3 mm lateral movement to the right, and 3 mm lateral movement to the left.

Evaluation of the prosthesis: 1 year after the second surgery, the prosthesis had no complications such as infection, rejection, loosening, displacement, fracture, ectopic osteogenesis, and allergy, and there was a significant improvement in the mandibular position after surgery compared with the preoperative position, and the surgical results were stable (Fig. 4.100, Table 4.2).

4.6.7.2 Follow-Up 2.5 Years After Surgery

The degree of mouth opening was 38 mm, and the rest was the same as the one-year postoperative follow-up (Figs. 4.101, 4.102, 4.103 and 4.104, Table 4.3).

4.6.8 Case H. Advantages and Disadvantages

4.6.8.1 Advantages

Joint prosthesis implantation is an effective treatment for autologous bone graft resorption.

In this case, the left mandibular ramus was short, and the unconventional design of the customized prosthesis was compensated for the lack of bone mass.

Mandibular anterior extension + mandibular ramus growth + substantial counterclockwise rotation increases the stress on the reconstructed joint, and the prosthesis has better stability than autogenous bone grafts.

4.6.8.2 Disadvantages

The reasons for failure of the first orthognathic surgery +/− arthroplasty are so varied that it will take time to summarize and generalize and find the most reasonable remedy. The large prosthesis fitting error in this case calls for further improvement in the digital measurements and design and surgical processes.

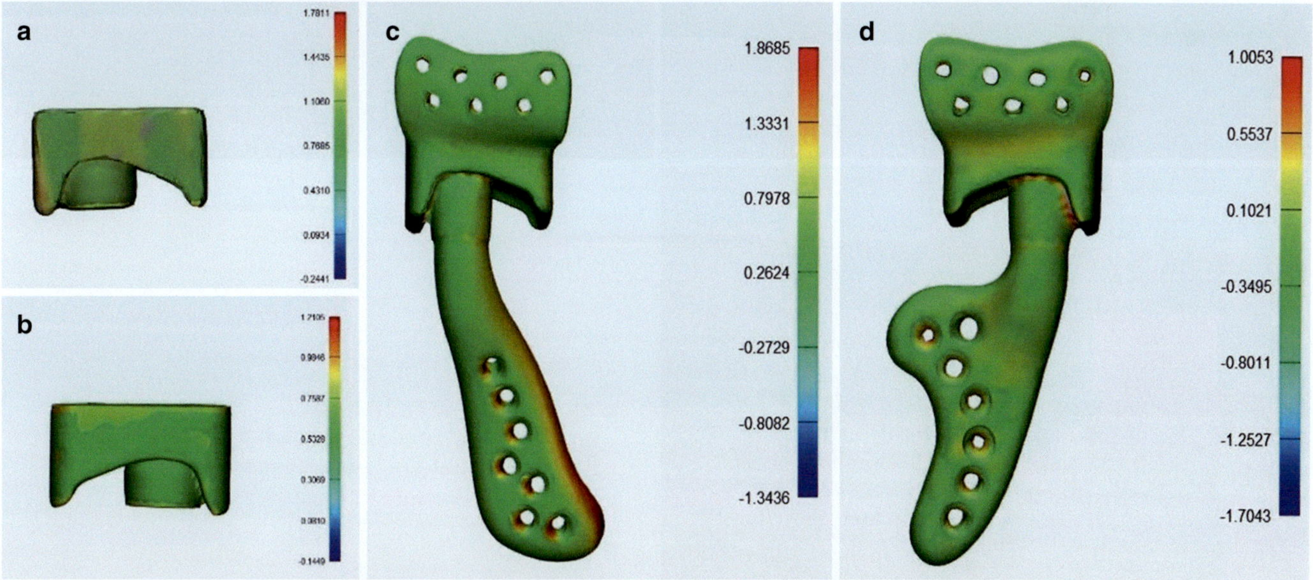

Fig. 4.97 Case H. Postoperative prosthesis position compared to design. Errors less than 2 mm. (**a**) Right core component error. (**b**) Left core component error. (**c**) Right overall error. (**d**) Left overall error

Fig. 4.98 Case H. One-year postoperative facial examination. Lateral view in cephalometric X-ray after removal of brackets. (**a**) Lateral photograph of the patient. (**b**) Lateral X-ray

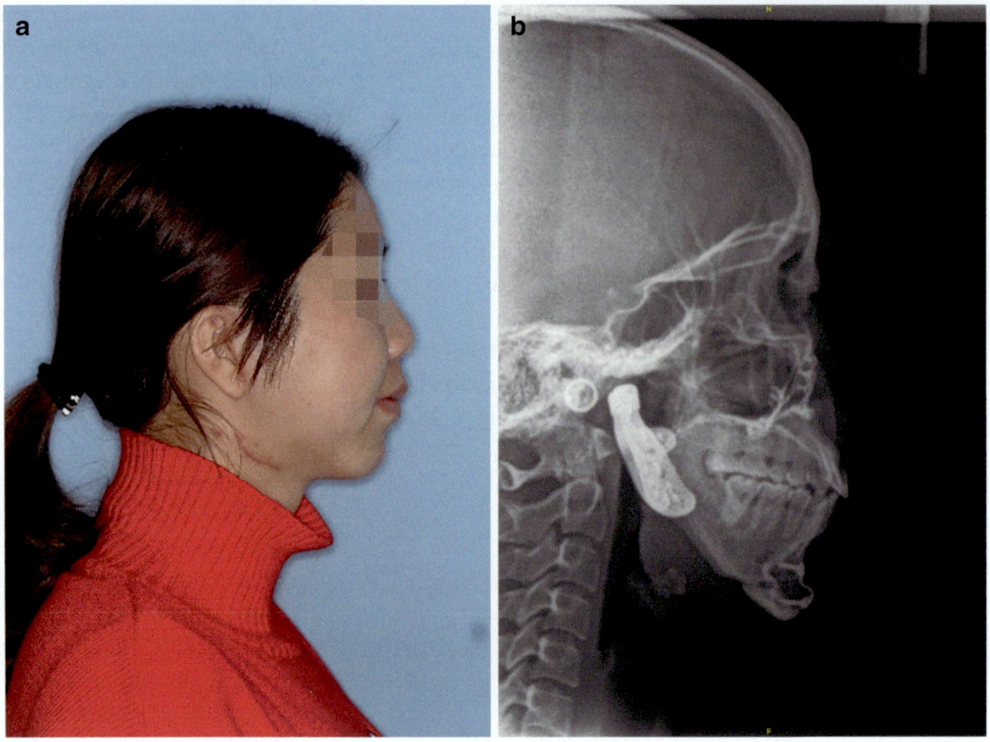

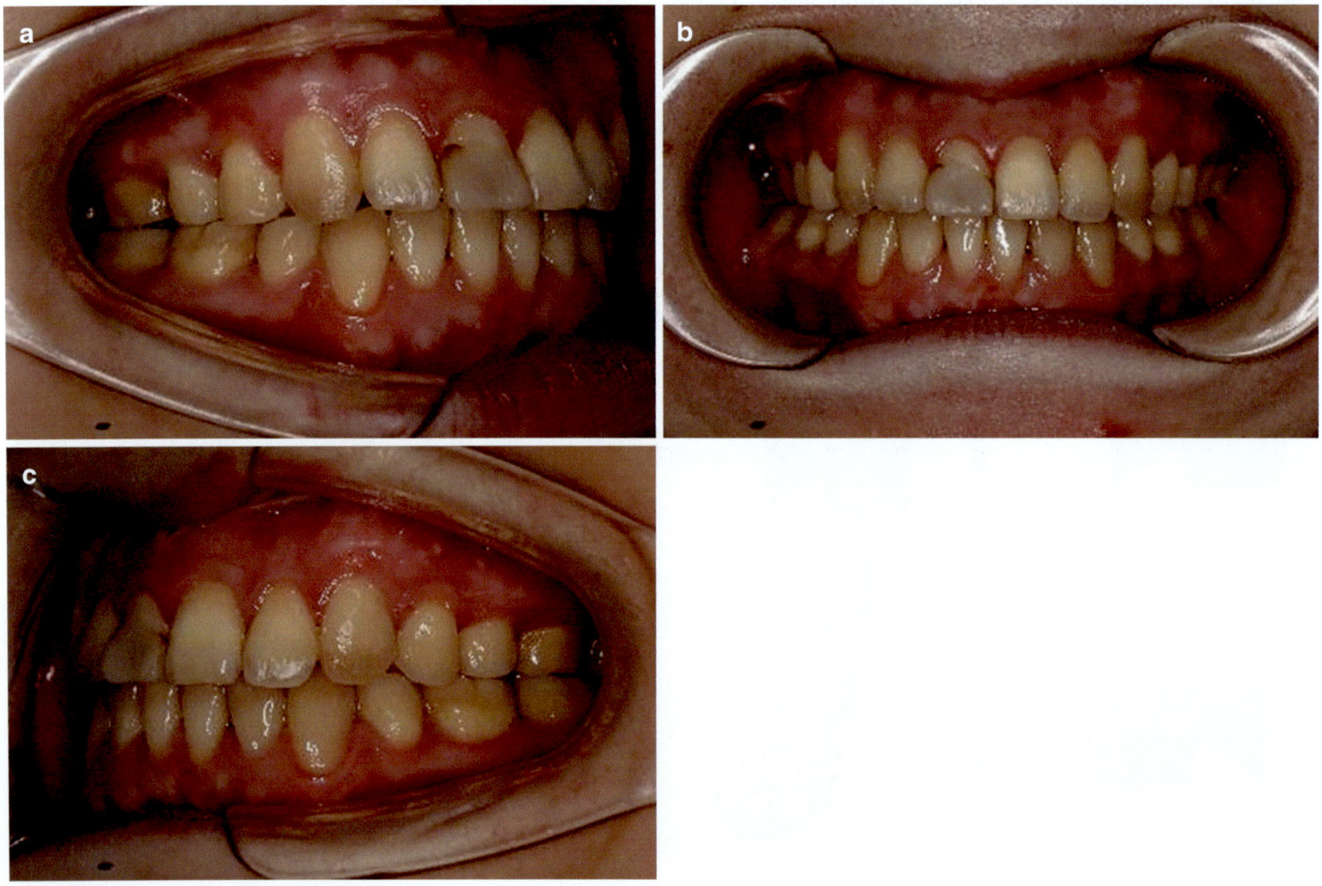

Fig. 4.99 Case H. Intraoral examination 1 year after surgery. Orthodontic treatment was completed, and the occlusion was stabilized. (**a**) Right occlusion. (**b**) Frontal occlusion. (**c**) Left occlusion

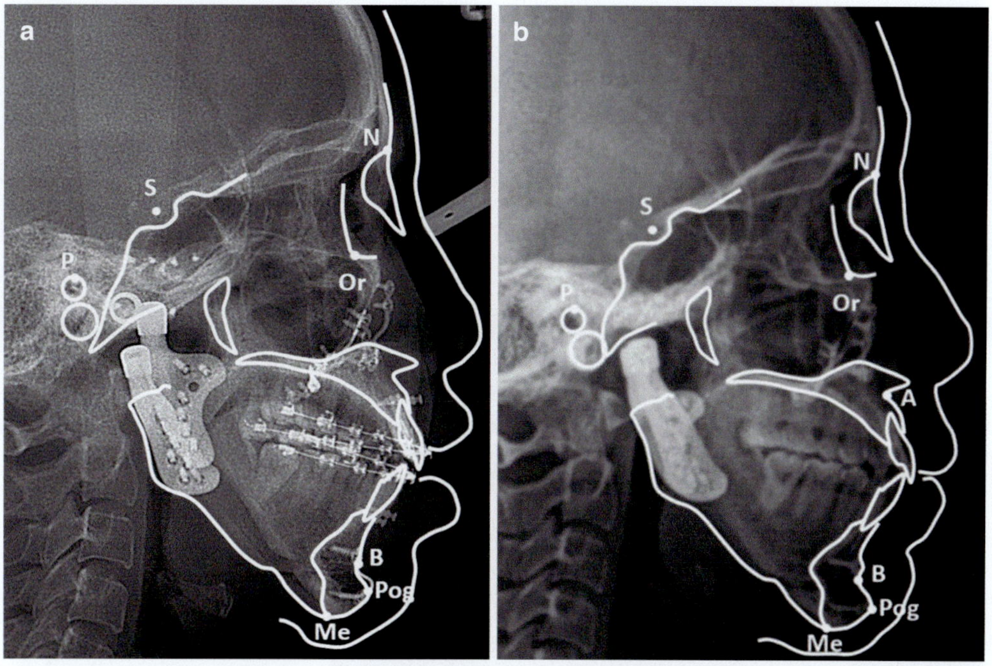

Fig. 4.100 Case H. Comparison of immediate postoperative and one-year postoperative cephalometric X-ray measurements. Significant improvement in mandibular position after surgery compared with preoperative position and stable surgical results. (**a**) Immediate postoperative lateral view. (**b**) One-year postoperative lateral view

Table 4.2 Case H. Comparison of preoperative, immediate postoperative, and one-year postoperative cephalometric X-ray measurements

	Follow-up time		
Measurement indicators	Preoperative	Immediately after surgery	One year after surgery
ANB	7.3°	6.5°	5.9°
SNA	83.2°	82.8°	83.0°
SNB	75.9°	76.3°	77.1°
GoGn-SN	49.6°	43.2°	46.1°
OP-SN	25.5°	19.9°	22.9°
U1-L1	128.1°	120.9°	120.1°

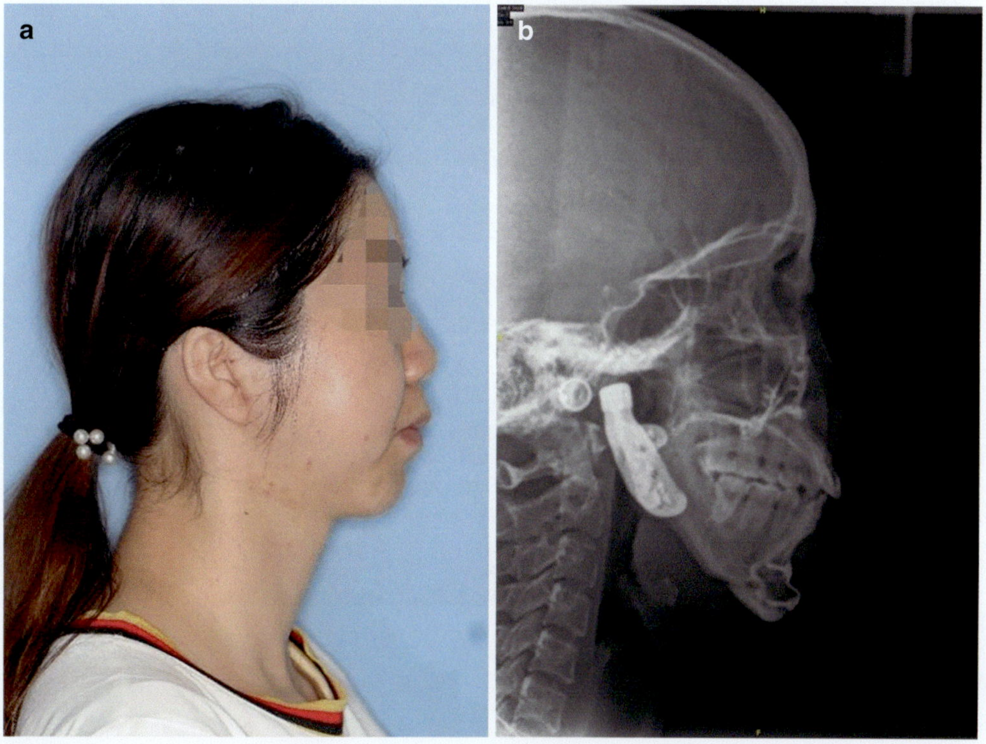

Fig. 4.101 Case H. Facial examination 2.5 years postoperative. Stabilization of the facial shape. (**a**) Lateral view. (**b**) Lateral cephalometric X-ray

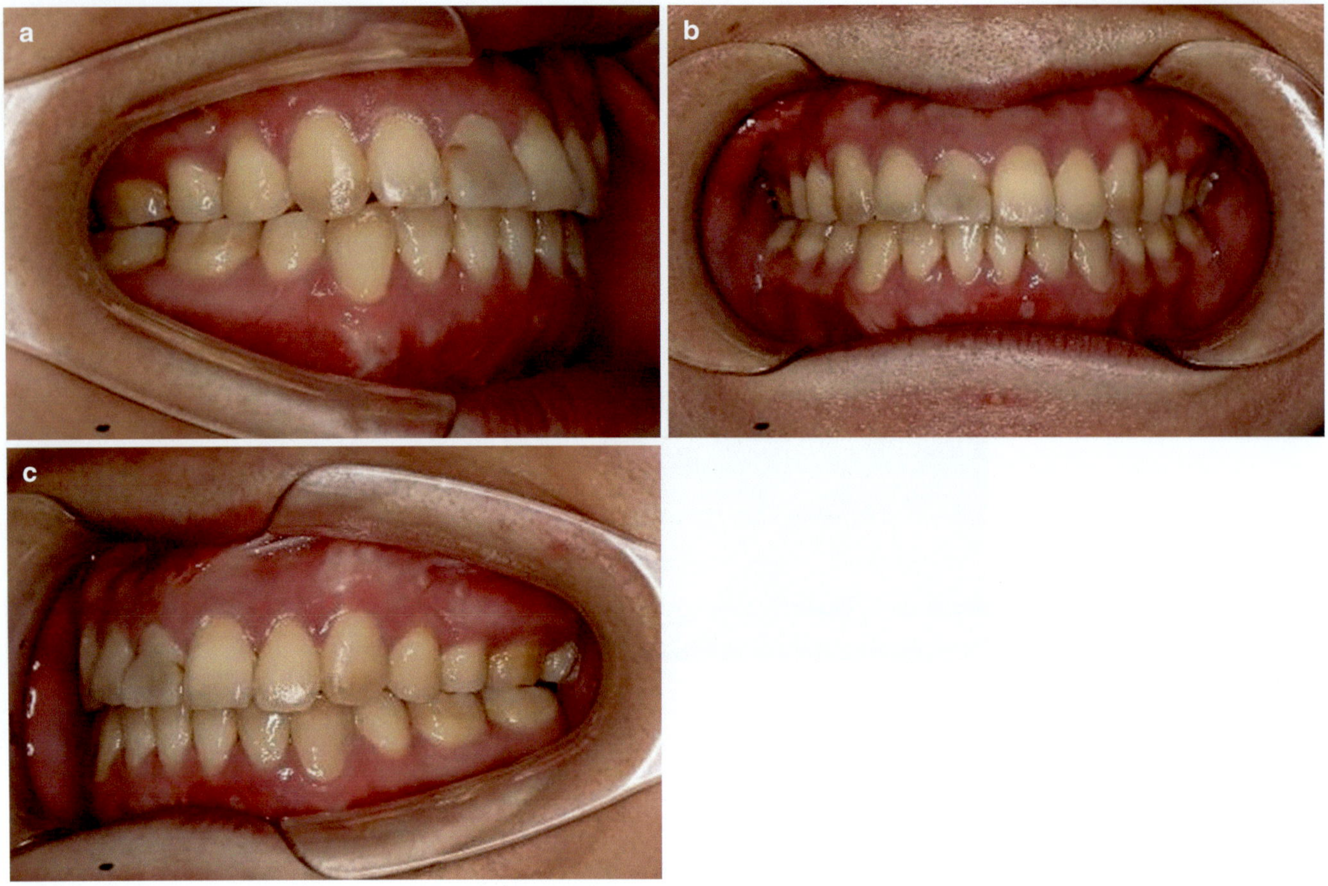

Fig. 4.102 Case H. Intraoral examination 2.5 years after surgery. Stable occlusion, no recurrence of open-bite occlusion. (**a**) Right occlusion. (**b**) Frontal occlusion. (**c**) Left occlusion

Fig. 4.103 Case H. Comparison of one-year postoperative and 2.5-year postoperative cephalometric X-ray measurements for examining long-term stabilization of the postoperative mandibular position. (**a**) One-year postoperative lateral view. (**b**) 2.5-year postoperative lateral view

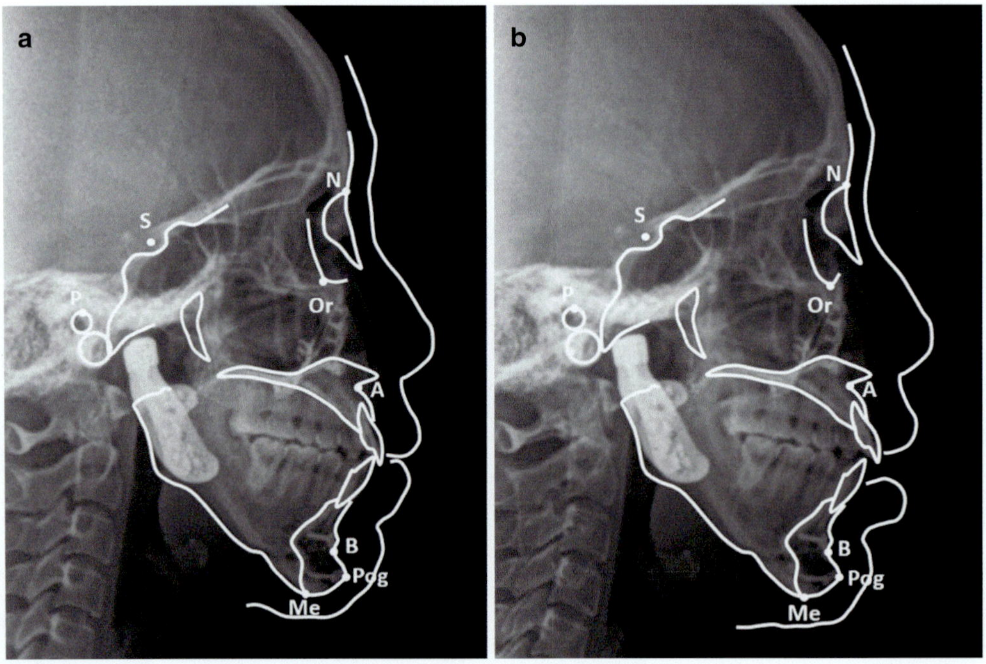

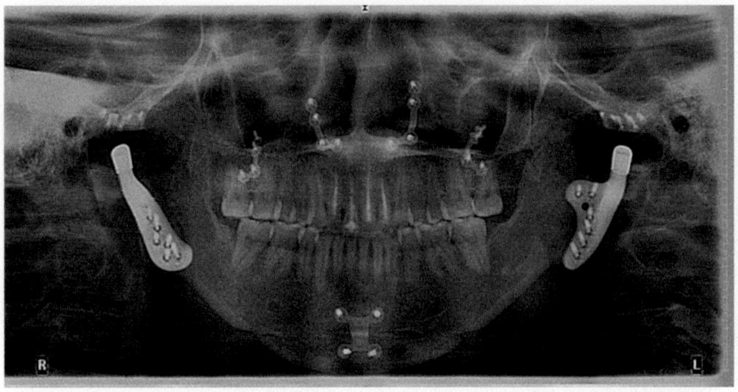

Fig. 4.104 Case H. Panoramic view 2.5 years after surgery. The bilateral TMJ prostheses were stable, and the genioplasty was healing well

Table 4.3 Case H. Comparison of cephalometric X-ray measurements in the immediate postoperative period, one-year postoperative period, and 2.5-year postoperative period

	Follow-up time		
Measurement indicators	Immediately after surgery	One year after surgery	2.5 years after surgery
ANB	6.5°	5.9°	5.8°
SNA	82.8°	83.0°	82.3°
SNB	76.3°	77.1°	76.4°
GoGn-SN	43.2°	46.1°	44.0°
OP-SN	19.9°	22.9°	21.4°
U1-L1	120.9°	120.1°	121.8°

4.7 Reconstruction of Orthognathic Surgery Failure Through Orthognathic Surgery Simultaneous with Customized Total Temporomandibular Joint Prosthesis Implantation

4.7.1 Case I. Orthognathic Surgery Failure

- Patient information: female, 38 years old.
- Complaint: left deviation of the lower jaw for 1 year after orthognathic surgery.
- History: 1 year ago, the patient underwent resection of left condylar osteochondroma, Le Fort I osteotomy of the maxilla, and bilateral sagittal split ramus osteotomy of the mandible at an external hospital. Postoperatively, anterior open bite developed, prompting the patient to seek treatment at our institution.
- Past history: the patient reported being in good health and denied a history of systemic disease or drug and food allergies.
- Clinical examination: oral commissures, left side elevated compared to the right. Mouth opening: 35 mm, with left-deviated opening pattern. Occlusion: anterior open bite. Bilateral first molars in Angle's Class III relationship. Upper dental midline deviated 2 mm to the right and lower dental midline deviated 1 mm to the left (Figs. 4.105 and 4.106).
- Imaging examination: panoramic radiograph (preoperative, external hospital), left condylar osteochondroma with associated jaw deformity. Missing teeth #32 and #42. CT 3D reconstruction of maxillofacial region (post-orthognathic surgery), post-surgical jaw deformity (anterior open bite, mandibular retrusion) (Figs. 4.107, 4.108, 4.109 and 4.110).
- Diagnosis: jaw deformity (mandibular deviation, mandibular retrognathia), post-orthognathic surgery, open bite of anterior teeth.

4.7.2 Case I. Diagnostic Imaging

4.7.3 Case I. Treatment Plan

4.7.3.1 Treatment Options

The fact that the patient's condylar tumor was previously removed without simultaneous repair of the joint resulted in the development of mandibular deviation and occlusal disorder. The following reconstructive and orthognathic options were offered to the patient:

- Option 1. Mandibular surgical plan: Customized total joint prosthesis implantation (metal/nonmetal articulating fossa prosthesis) and sagittal split osteotomy of the right mandibular ramus. The disadvantage of this plan is that it cannot correct the upper anterior teeth midline.
- Option 2. Double jaw surgical plan: Le Fort I osteotomy of the maxilla, customized total joint prosthesis implantation on the left side (metal/non-metal joint fossa prosthesis), and sagittal split osteotomy of the right mandibular ramus. This option has the advantage of correcting the upper anterior midline.

Ultimately, the patient chose option 1, and she refused maxillary surgery; she was fully informed preoperatively of the limitations of the plan.

- Reconstruction plan: customized total joint prosthesis implantation on the left side.
- Orthognathic plan: sagittal split osteotomy of the right mandibular ramus.

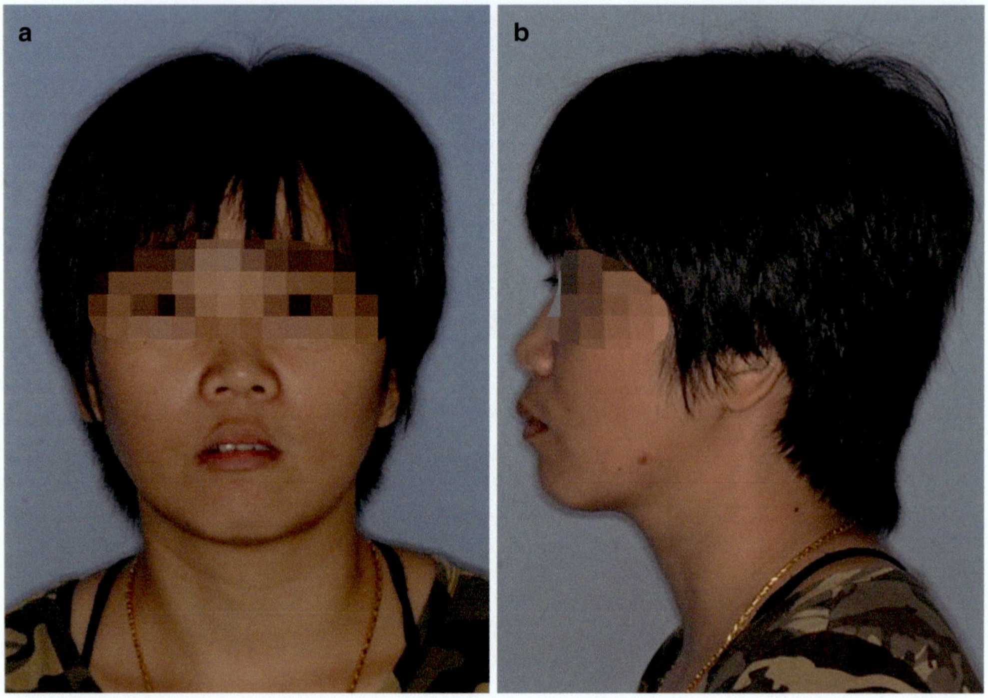

Fig. 4.105 Case I. Facial examination. There was mild asymmetry. The labial commissure was higher on the left than on the right. (**a**) Frontal view. (**b**) Lateral view

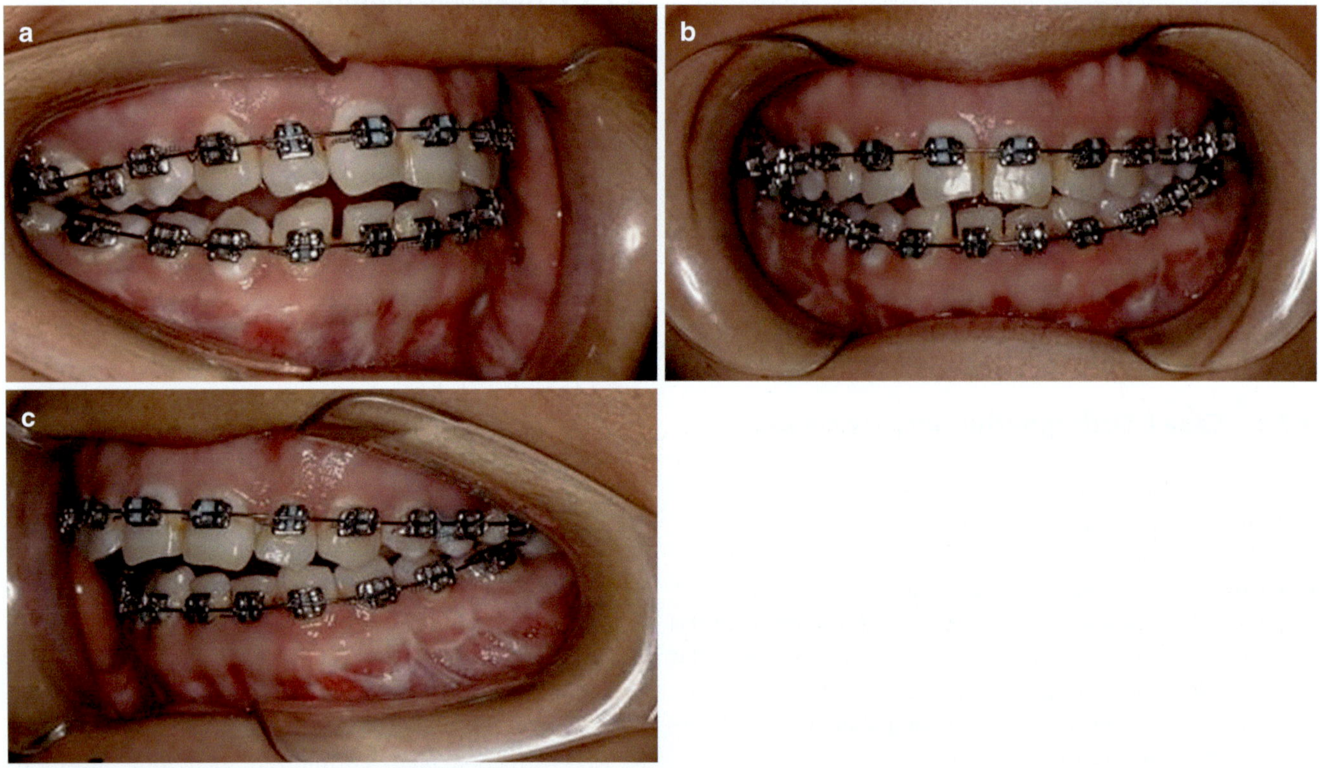

Fig. 4.106 Case I. Intraoral examination. There was an anterior open bite. The upper dental midline was 2 mm to the right. The lower dental midline was 1 mm to the left. The molars were in a Class III relationship. (**a**) Right occlusion. (**b**) Frontal occlusion. (**c**) Left occlusion

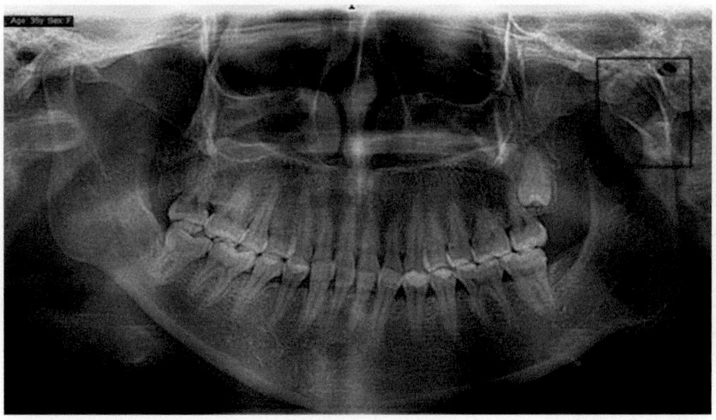

Fig. 4.107 Case I. Panoramic film prior to surgery at the other hospital. A tumor of the left condyle (red rectangle) and jaw deformity are noted. The pathology was osteochondroma

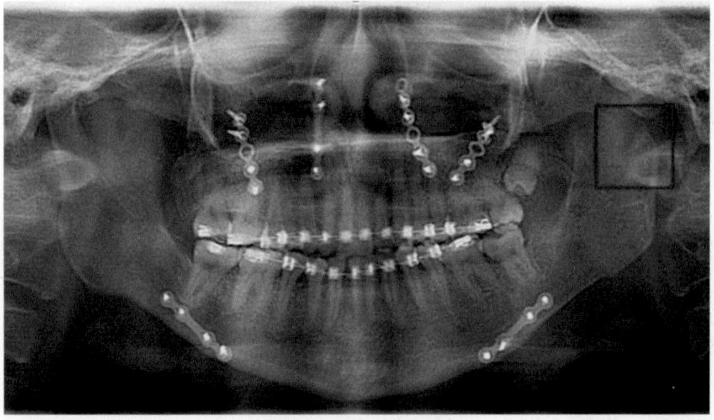

Fig. 4.108 Case I. Panoramic film after surgery at the other hospital. The tumor was removed and bimaxillary osteotomies were performed. The left condyle was short because it was not reconstructed (red rectangle)

4.7.4 Case I. Design and Processing of Total Joint Prostheses and Cutting Guides

Surgical simulation and prosthesis design (Figs. 4.111, 4.112 and 4.113)

- Prosthesis fabrication and fitting: the fabrication process is described in Sect. 2.5 in Chap. 2.

4.7.5 Case I. Surgical Procedure

Preoperative laboratory tests: the same as described in Sect. 3.2.5, Preoperative Laboratory Tests.

Preoperative preparation: the same as described in Sect. 3.2.5, Preoperative Preparation, and preparation of 200 mL of blood

4.7.5.1 Steps of Surgical Procedure

1. Surgical approach: preauriculotemporal incision, submandibular incision, and intraoral incision were used.
2. Prosthesis implant bed management: subcondylar osteotomy and articular eminence osteotomy to prepare the implant bed.
3. Orthognathic surgery: sagittal split osteotomy of the right mandibular ramus.
4. Intermaxillary ligation.
5. Implantation of the prosthesis.
6. The mandibular prosthesis neck is filled with postmandibular fat.

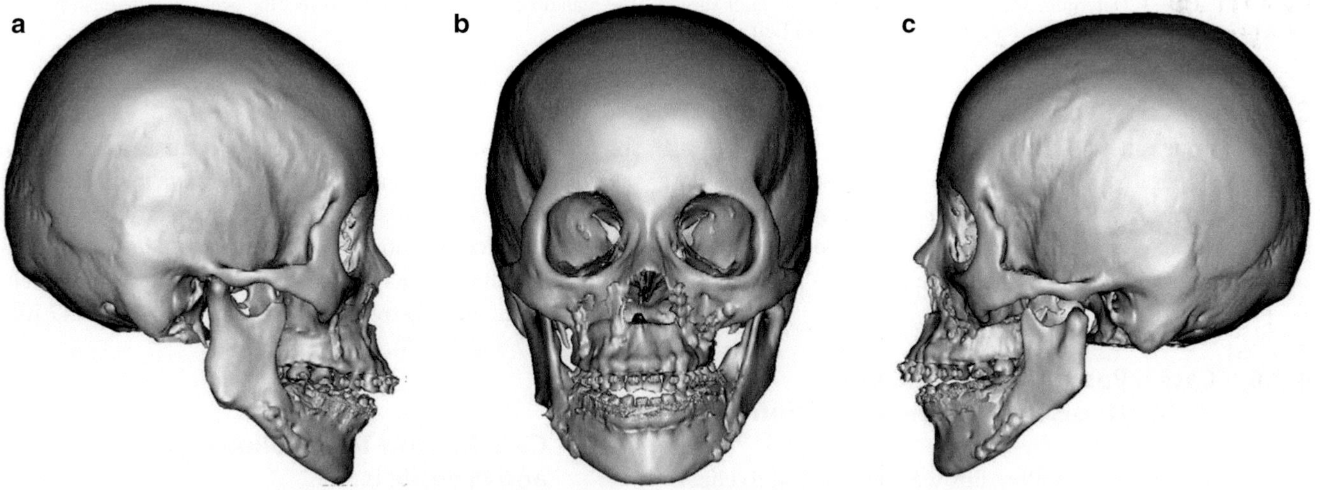

Fig. 4.109 Case I. 3D reconstruction of the maxillofacial CT after surgery at the other hospital. There is residual jaw deformity and malocclusion. The short residual left condyle has not been placed in the fossa. (**a**) Right view. (**b**) Frontal view. (**c**) Left view

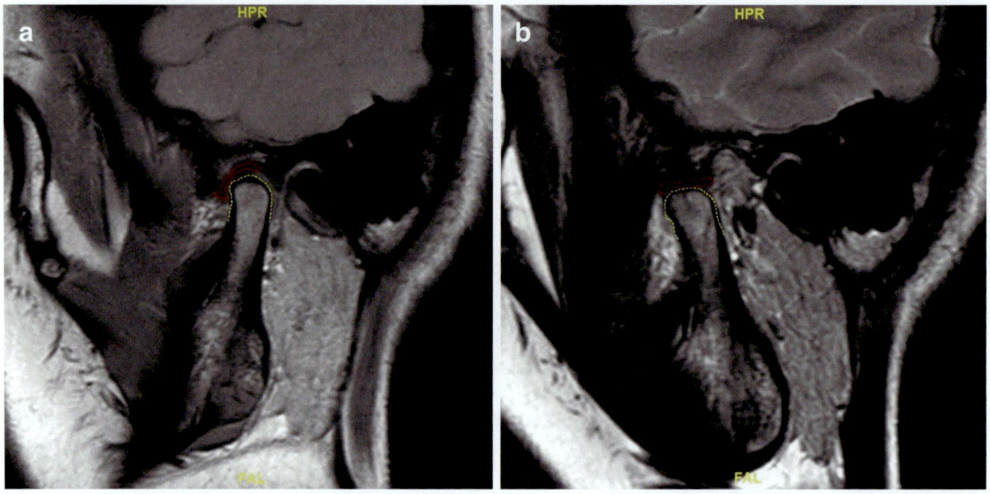

Fig. 4.110 Case I. Joint MRI. Right disc condyle in normal relationship. (**a**) Closed mouth position. (**b**) Open mouth position

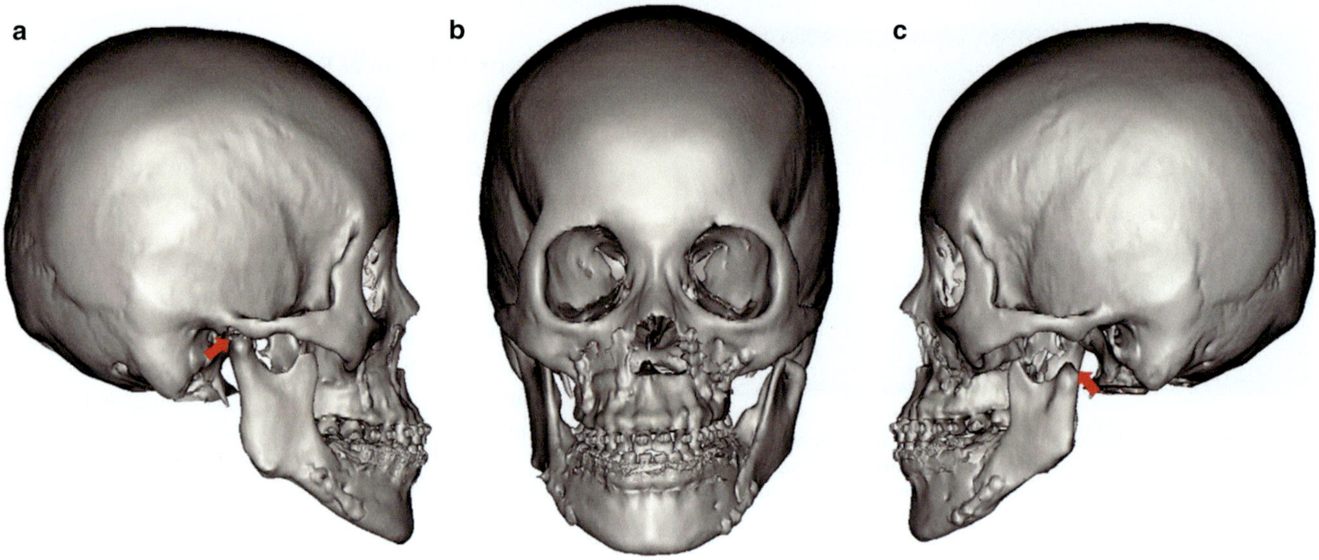

Fig. 4.111 Case I. Determine the position of the mandible after surgery. The mandible is repositioned to correct the occlusal relationship (indicated by red arrows). (**a**) Right view. (**b**) Frontal view. (**c**) Left view

- Joint prosthesis fitting.
- Postoperative orders and nursing care: see Sect. 3.2.5, Postoperative Orders and Nursing Care. In addition, intermaxillary elastic traction was performed and daily oral care was administered.

4.7.6 Case I. Postoperative Analysis of Prosthesis Implantation Precision

Regular postoperative follow-ups were performed to check for appearance (facial shape), function (mouth opening, mouth shape), and prosthesis evaluation (safety, accuracy).

Immediately after surgery: the intraoperative guide plate was accurately seated, and the prosthesis was installed smoothly (Figs. 4.114 and 4.115). The comparison between the preoperative design and the postoperative reconstruction showed that the prosthesis was accurately implanted (Fig. 4.116). Postoperative prosthesis installation error analysis showed that the maximum error of the core component was 1.31 mm, and the overall maximum error was 1.47 mm (Figs. 4.117 and 4.118).

4.7.7 Case A. Long-Term Follow-Up and Prognosis

4.7.7.1 1-Year Postoperative Follow-Up

There were no complaints of discomfort, the face was well shaped, and there was no redness, swelling, or other reactions in the operative area.

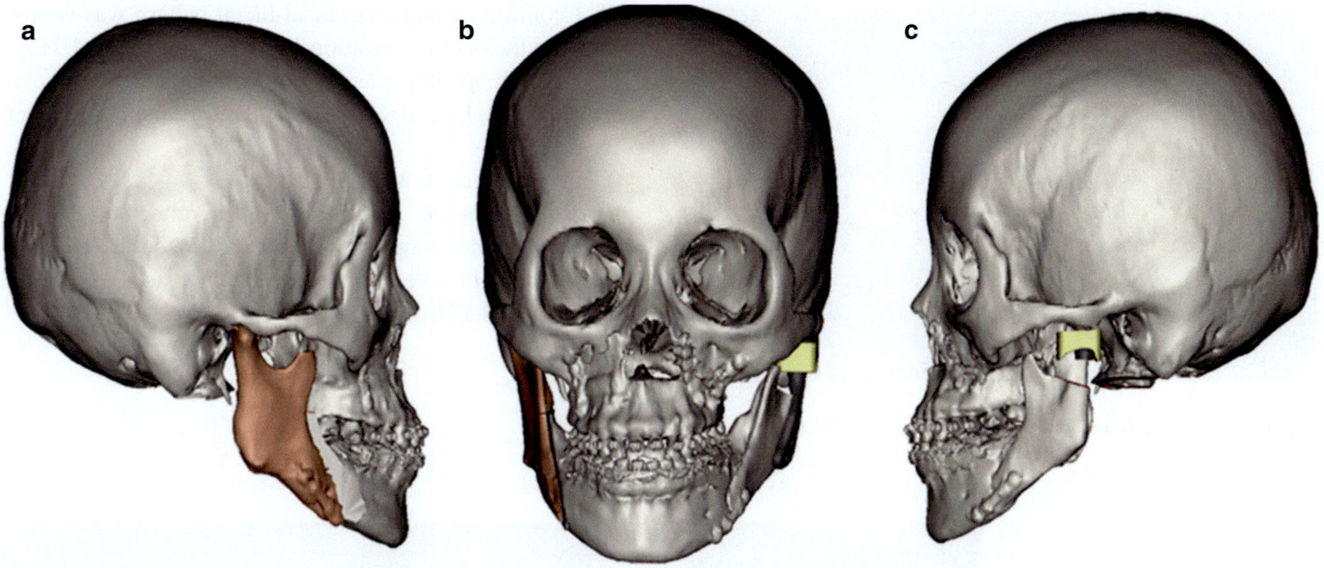

Fig. 4.112 Case I. Prosthesis and surgical design. Sagittal ramus osteotomy is performed on the right side, and the condyle is placed in the fossa. The core components of the TMJ prosthesis are positioned on the left side. (**a**) Right view. (**b**) Frontal view. (**c**) Left view

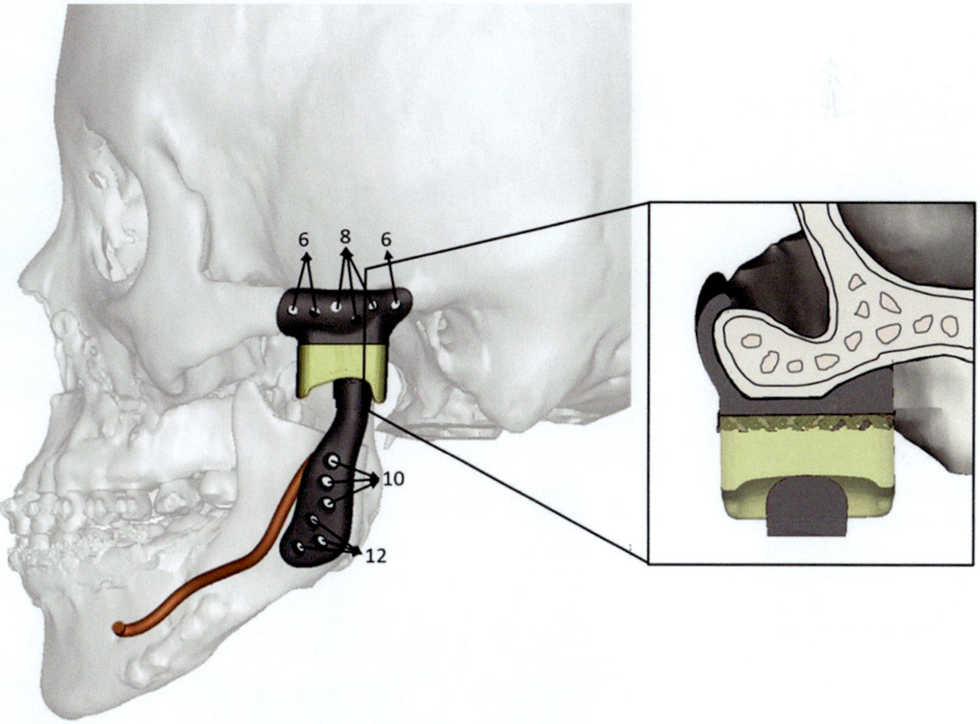

Fig. 4.113 Case I. Virtual design of the fixation components, and measurement of screw lengths. The fossa prosthesis has a fused metal-nonmetallic design to permit osseointegration. The thickness of the interface is 1.5 mm. Porosities in the surface of the titanium alloy are 900 μm

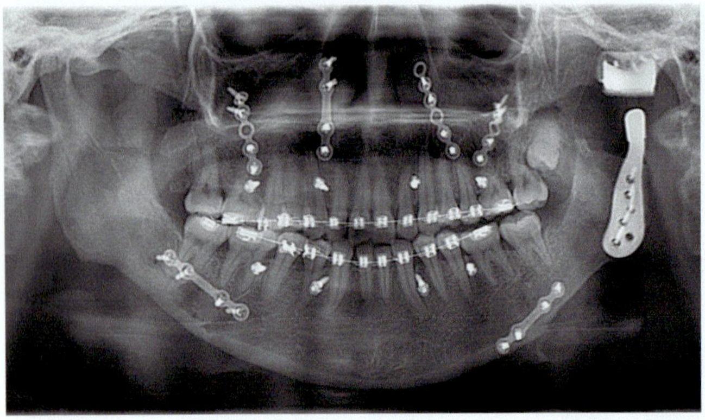

Fig. 4.114 Case I. Immediate postoperative panoramic film

The joint-mandibular-occlusal-facial pattern was coordinated, and the occlusal relationship was stable (Fig. 4.119).

The mouth opening was 37 mm, with 3 mm lateral movement to the right and 6 mm lateral movement to the left (Fig. 4.120).

Chewing function was normal.

Evaluation of the prosthesis: 1 year after surgery, the prosthesis had no complications such as infection, rejection, loosening, displacement, fracture, ectopic osteogenesis, and allergy (Figs. 4.121 and 4.122)

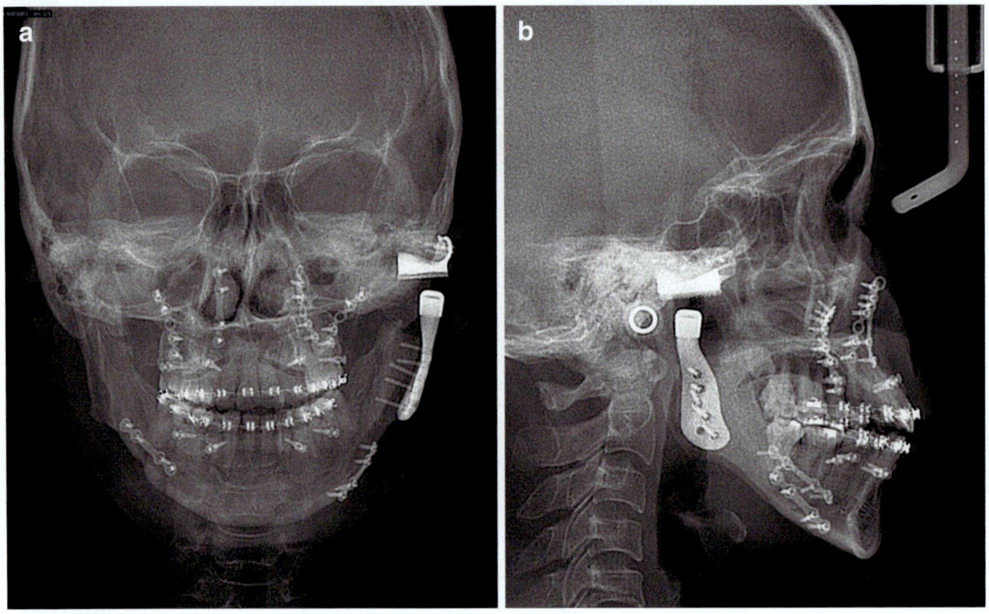

Fig. 4.115 Case I. Immediate postoperative cephalometric X-ray. (**a**) Frontal view. (**b**) Lateral view

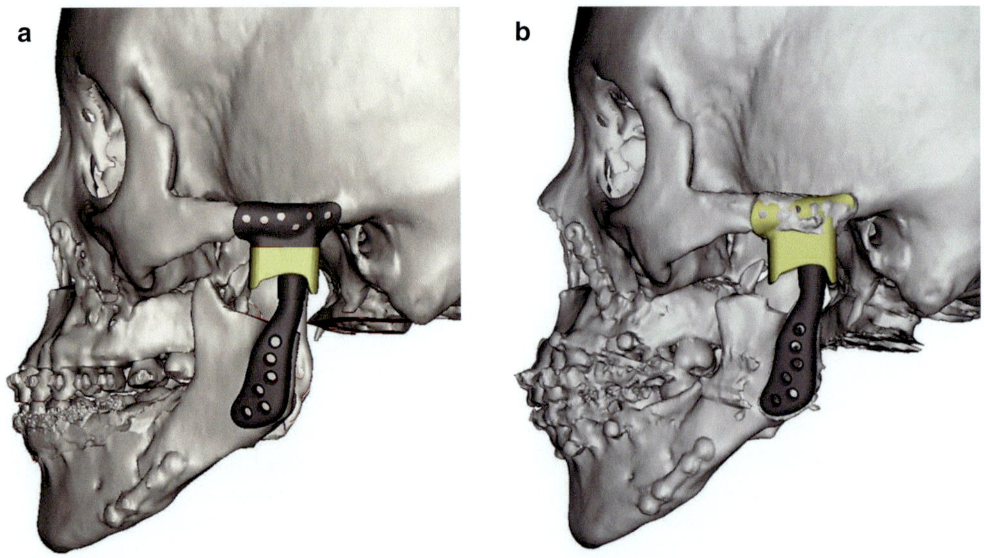

Fig. 4.116 Case I. Comparison of CT reconstruction showing precise prosthesis placement. (**a**) Preoperative design. (**b**) Immediate postoperative period

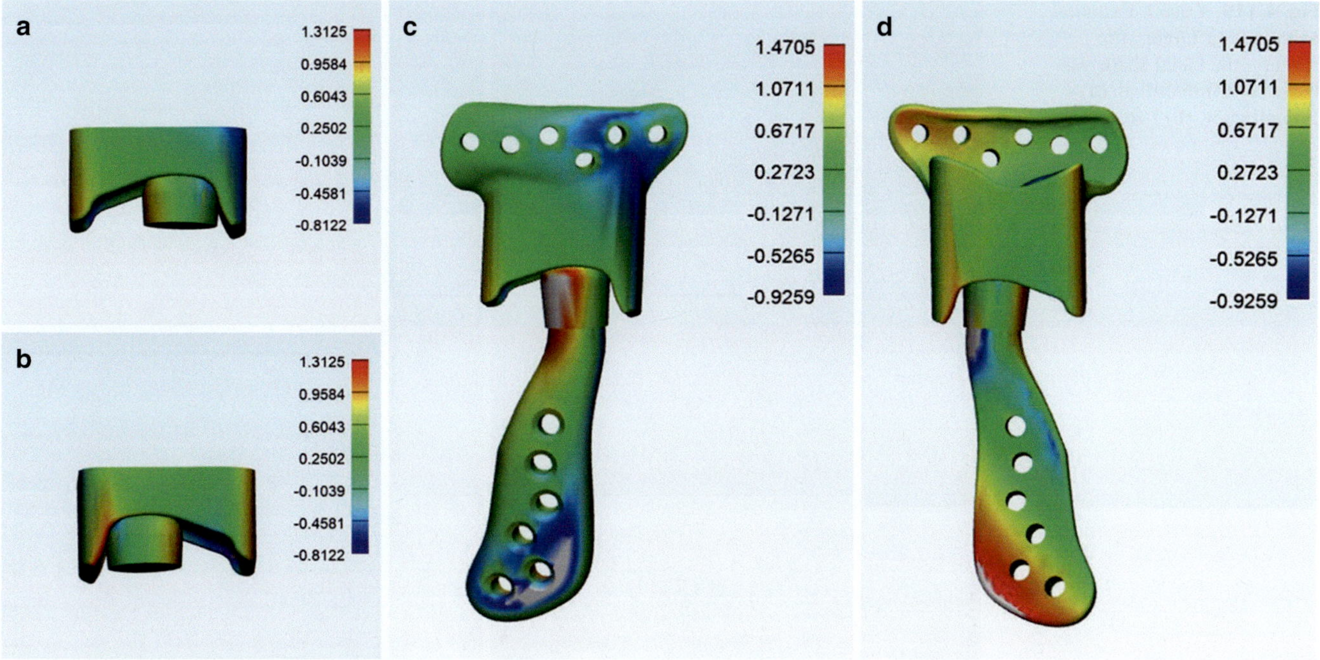

Fig. 4.117 Case I. Comparison of the postoperative prosthesis position with the preoperative design. The maximum error of the core component is 1.31 mm, and the maximum error of the whole is 1.47 mm; the error mainly has occurred in the condylar head component of the mandibular prosthesis. (**a**) Lateral side error of the core component. (**b**) Medial side error of the core component. (**c**) Overall lateral side error. (**d**) Overall medial side error

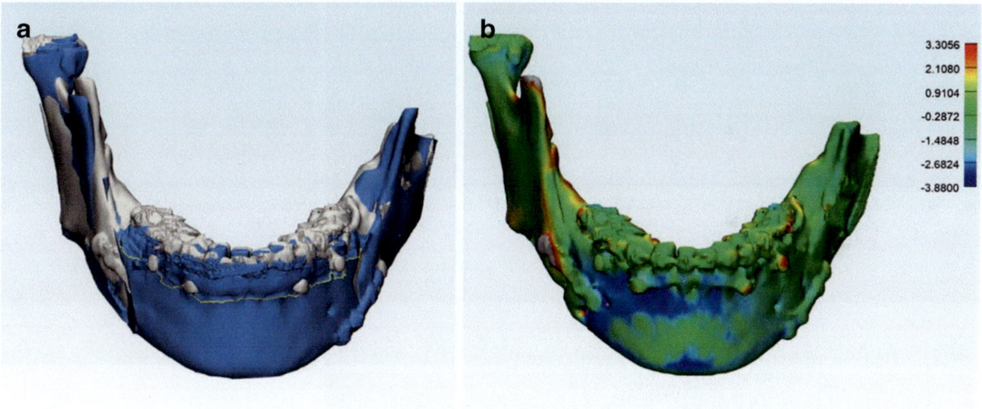

Fig. 4.118 Case I. Postoperative mandibular (white) position compared to design (blue). Errors were mainly present in the right mandibular ramus (offset forward and outward compared to design). (**a**) Mandibular match. (**b**) Mandibular error analysis

4.7.7.2 3-Year Postoperative Follow-Up

The degree of mouth opening was 38 mm, and the rest was the same as the one-year postoperative follow-up (Figs. 4.123 and 4.124).

4.7.8 Case I. Advantages and Disadvantages

Zhang ShanyongXie Qianyang, and Ma Zhigui

4.7.8.1 Advantages

Resolution of open bite and jaw deformity by joint reconstruction and sagittal split osteotomy of the contralateral mandibular ramus. It is shown that joint stability is essential for orthodontic-orthognathic treatment.

4.7.8.2 Disadvantages

In this case, the mandible still had a mild right deviation, and the maximum error of the prosthesis was close to 1.5 mm, which is a large error; the error should be controlled within 1 mm.

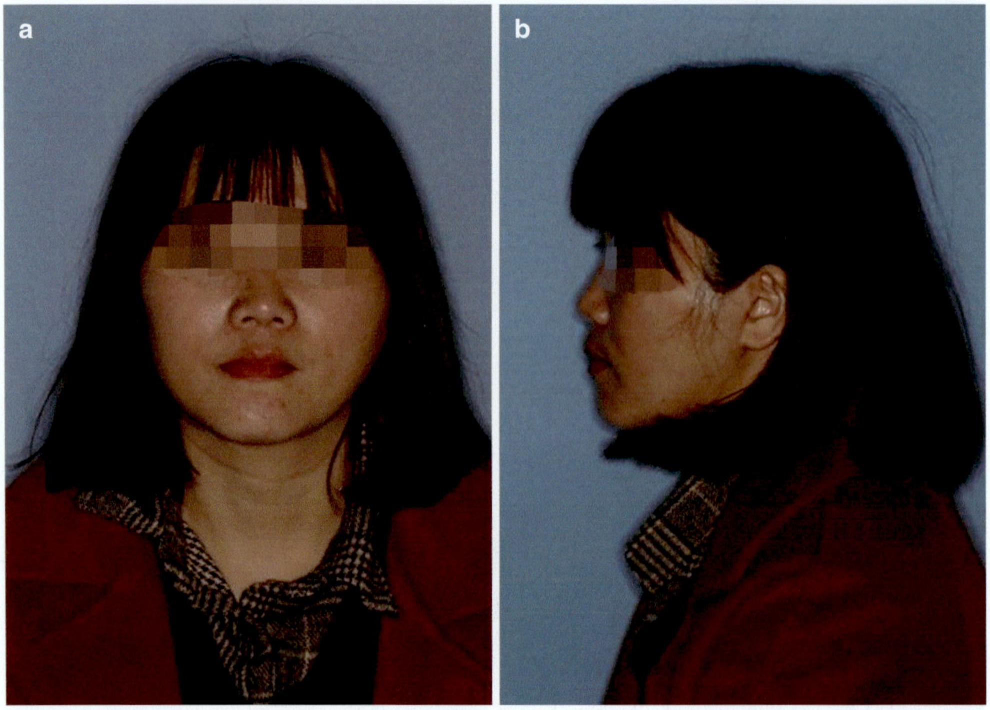

Fig. 4.119 Case I. Extraoral examination 1 year after surgery; the facial shape was basically symmetrical. (**a**) Frontal view. (**b**) Lateral view

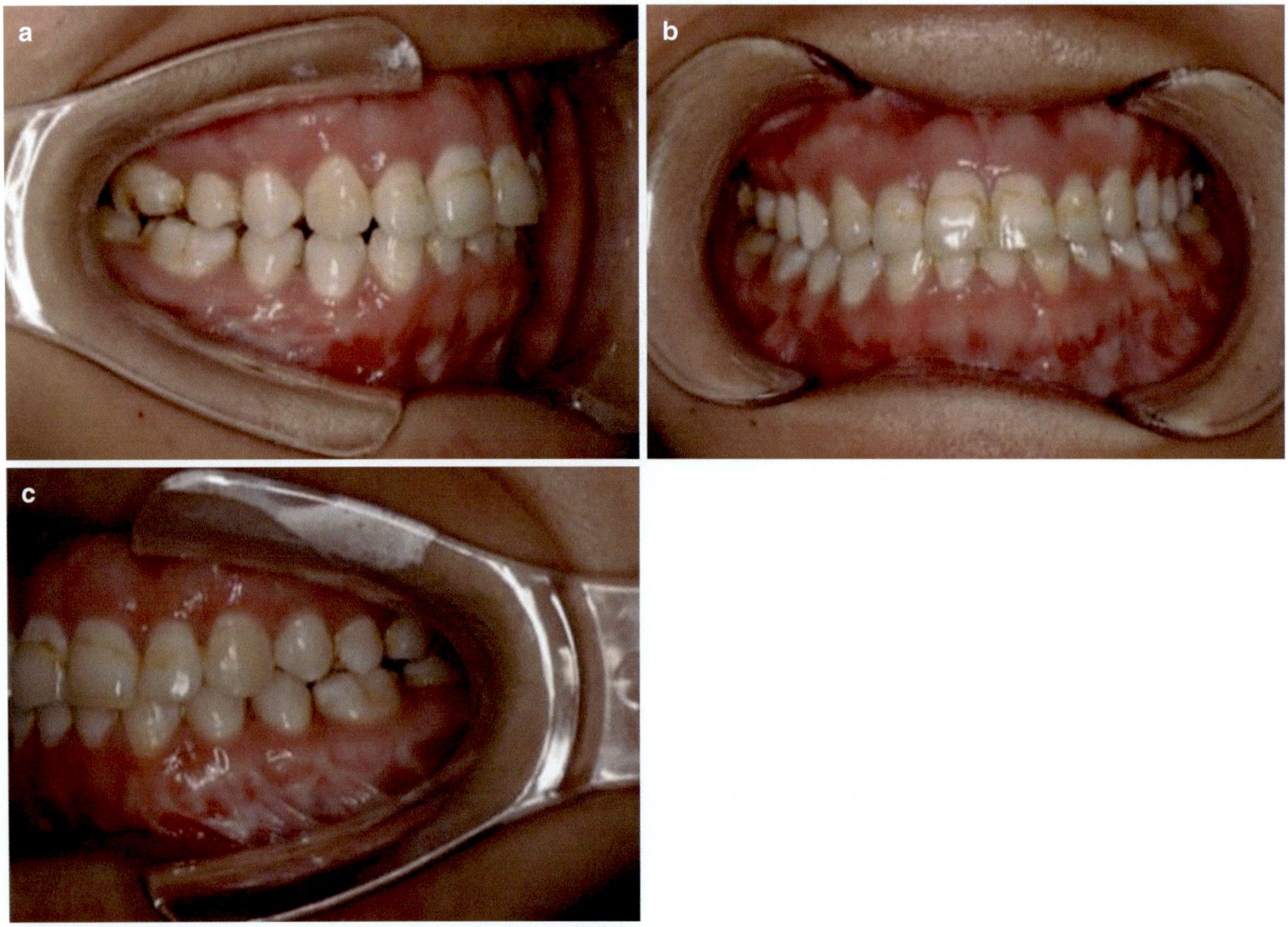

Fig. 4.120 Case I. Stable occlusal relationship on intraoral examination 1 year after surgery. (**a**) Right occlusion. (**b**) Frontal occlusion. (**c**) Left occlusion

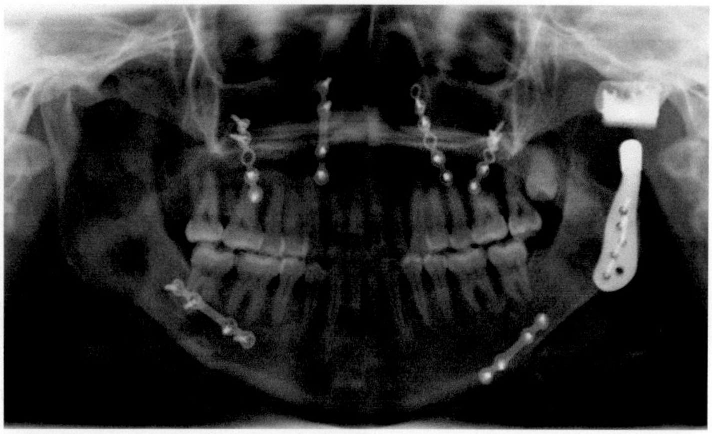

Fig. 4.121 Case I. One-year postoperative panoramic view with stabilized position of the joint prosthesis

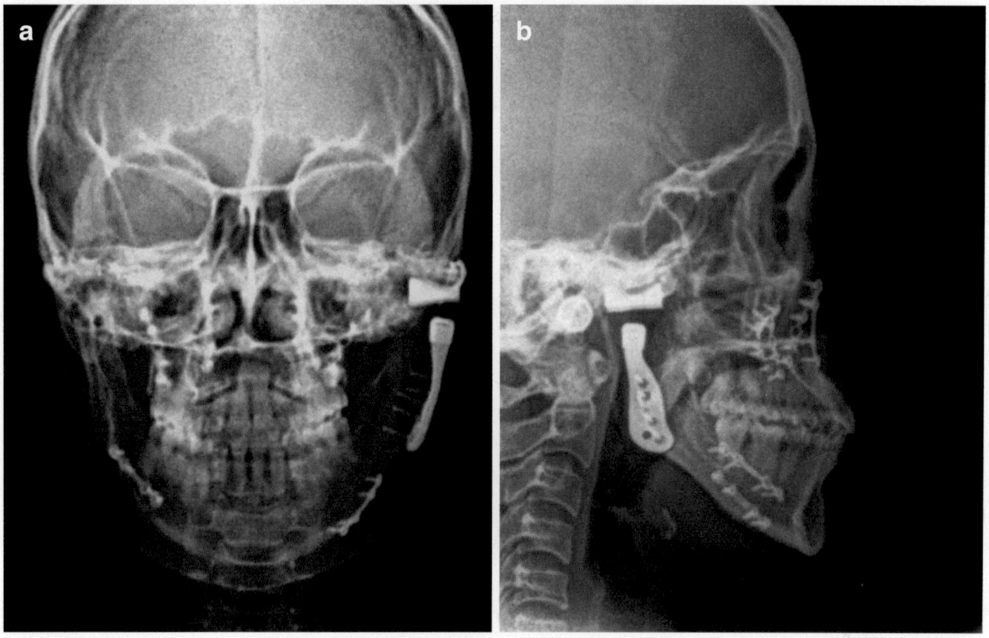

Fig. 4.122 Case I. Cephalometric X-ray at 1 year postoperatively. (**a**) Frontal view. (**b**) Lateral view

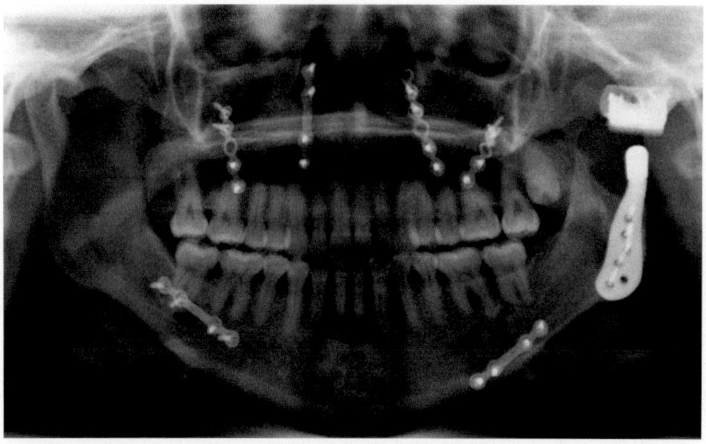

Fig. 4.123 Case I. Panoramic view 3 years after surgery. The position of the joint prosthesis was stable

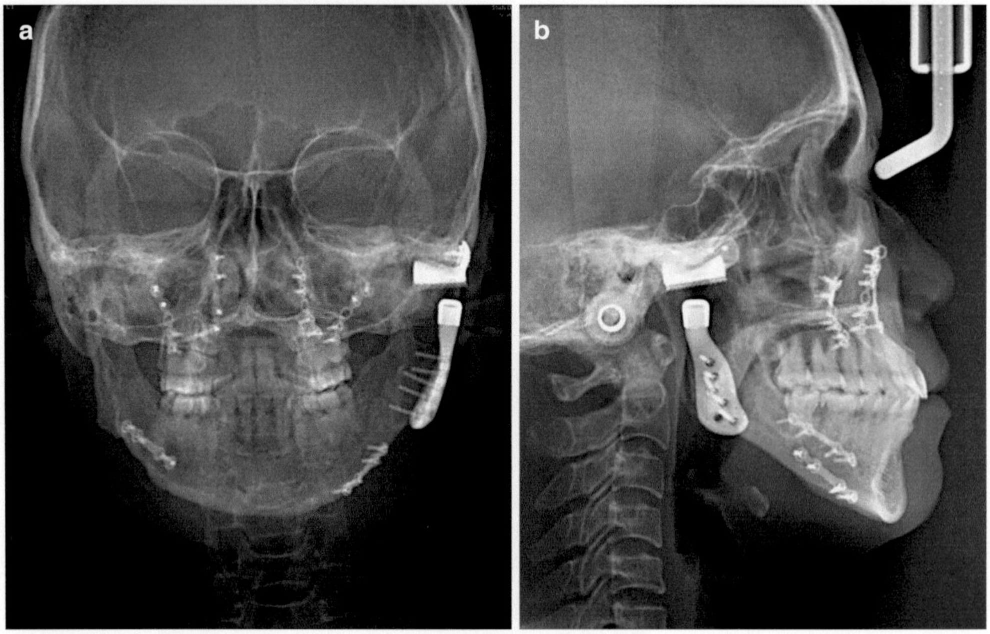

Fig. 4.124 Case I. Cephalometric X-rays at 3 years postoperatively. (**a**) Frontal view. (**b**) Lateral view

Joint Preservation Combined with Orthognathic Surgery for Temporomandibular Joint-Originated Dentofacial Deformities

5

Chi Yang, Qianyang Xie, and Xuzhuo Chen

This chapter addresses Class IIb of Yang's modified classification, i.e., Class II encompasses dental and maxillofacial deformities secondary to temporomandibular joint (TMJ) diseases, and within this, Class IIb includes only salvageable cases where the condyle is salvageable, in contrast to Class IIa, where the condyle is non-salvageable. Class IIb cases can be treated with a combination of joint preservation surgery and orthognathic orthodontics, but they do not require the use of a prosthesis joint replacement.

In this chapter, we will give:

- An overview of the definition of dentofacial deformity originating in joints
- The combined treatment mode of orthognathic surgery and surgery on salvageable joints
- Traditional fixation techniques of orthognathic surgery used in conjunction with surgery on salvageable joints
- Innovative fixation techniques with customized orthognathic surgical plates

Combined with the demonstration of these in clinical cases, we will focus on the key points of the design of customized orthognathic surgical plates and standardized surgical operations. The aim is to discuss how orthognathic surgery can maintain the stability of joint form and function through joint preservation surgery, while avoiding the occurrence of complications.

5.1 Overview

In the treatment of TMJ-Originated Dentofacial Deformities with salvageable Joint, the subject we are addressing is how to achieve joint preservation surgery and orthognathic surgery without the surgeries interfering with each other. In this section, we will introduce the basic concepts of the definition of dentofacial deformity with salvageable joint the treatment mode of combined joint preservation surgery and orthognathic surgery, and the traditional fixation techniques for orthognathic surgery and its problems, and we will propose innovative fixation techniques with customized plates to achieve precision in orthognathic surgery and maintain the stability of the TMJ joints. The process of joint preservation surgery and orthognathic surgery is also standardized accordingly.

5.1.1 Definition of TMJ-Originated Dentofacial Deformities with Salvageable Joint

If the morphology and quality of the articular disc and condyle indicate they are salvageable, the associated dental and maxillofacial deformities are called "TMJ-Originated Dentofacial Deformities with Salvageable Joint." Salvageable joints include:

Chi Y. (✉) · Qianyang X. · Xuzhuo C.
Shanghai Ninth People's Hospital, Shanghai Jiao Tong University School of Medicine, Shanghai, China

© People's Medical Publishing House, PR of China 2025

Chi Y. (ed.), *Atlas of Customized TMJ-Cranio-Jaw Prosthesis*, https://doi.org/10.1007/978-981-95-0611-8_5

1. An ankylosed joint with a condylar head and disc on the medial side of the joint
2. Some joint tumors, such as condylar osteochondroma with >50% preservation of the native condylar structure
3. Displacement of the disc consistent with the conditions necessary for reposition
4. Stable displacement of the disc with condylar resorption

5.1.2 Treatment Plan of Combined Orthognathic Surgery and Surgery That Preserves the Joint

Orthognathic surgeries that are commonly used together or at the same stage as preservation joint surgery include maxillary Le Fort I osteotomy, mandibular sagittal split osteotomy, and genioplasty.

The treatment modes of orthognathic surgery combined with simultaneous or staged preservative joint surgery are:

1. Simultaneous surgery: preserving the disc-condylar-muscle complex through surgical methods such as joint disc repositioning or lateral arthroplasty (ankylosis) or simple tumor removal (e.g., osteochondroma), along with orthognathic surgery at the same time.
2. Staged surgery: preservative joint surgery first and orthognathic surgery at a staged time. This is especially suitable for adolescent patients, such as those with adolescent joint disc displacement and condylar resorption with dentofacial deformity: first, carry out disc repositioning surgery. After they are adults, if there is still moderate to severe jaw deformity but the joint is stable, then carry out orthognathic surgery.
3. In adults, stabilization of joint disc displacement and controlled condylar resorption require orthognathic "unloading" techniques. The key is to keep the condylar position unchanged as much as possible during treatment and to use treatment methods that do not increase joint stress.

The basic conditions for stability of the joint and avoidance of condylar resorption in adults are:

1. The patient's growth and development have been completed.
2. There are no clinical symptoms.
3. The condylar bone cortex is continuous and intact.
4. There is no active degeneration of the joint.
5. There is disc-like change in the posterior region of the articular disc.
6. There has been no progressive change of the joints and dentition and jaws, as confirmed by two clinical and imaging follow-up visits at an interval of more than 6 months.

5.1.3 Traditional Fixation Techniques for Orthognathic Surgery Combined with Preservative Joint Surgery

Maxillary Lefort I osteotomy, sagittal split osteotomy of the mandibular ramus, and genioplasty are the most common orthognathic procedures used in conjunction with preserving joint surgery.

- Maxillary Le Fort I osteotomy fixation method

Multiple small titanium plates are standardly used for fixation: usually one at the outer edge of each pyriform foramen and one at the zygomatic alveolar ridge (Fig. 5.1). Pre-bending is required, which increases the operating time and decreases the mechanical strength of the titanium plates; at the same time, the titanium plates do not fit perfectly, resulting in a slight displacement of the bone block and a decrease in accuracy (Fig. 5.2).

3D-printed titanium plate fixation: the design and 3D-printing of customized titanium plates based on the preoperative analysis and osteotomy positioning avoid the need for an intraoperative pre-bending process. However, most of the designs are sloppy and oversized and not mechanically compatible with the human body, affecting bone healing (Fig. 5.3).

Although this procedure has no direct or indirect correlation with the condyle, joint surgery and double jaw surgery can still affect each other when performed concurrently, and thus the accuracy of their osteotomy and mobilization and the stability of their fixation are also important, i.e., concurrent surgery of the upper and lower jaws and the joints is also a matter of mutual impact.

- Fixation in sagittal split osteotomy of the mandible
- The three traditional fixation methods used are:

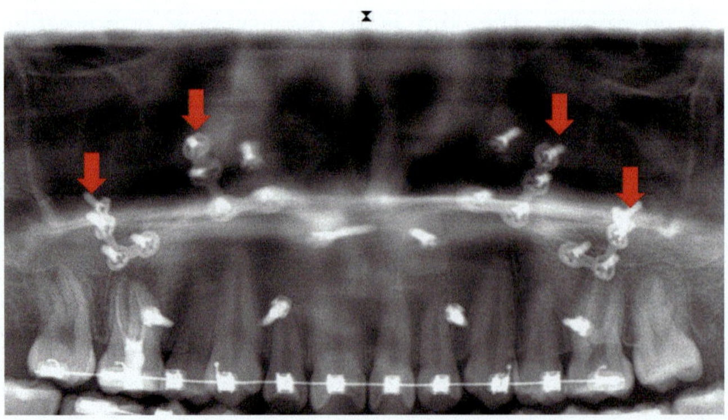

Fig. 5.1 Fixation of a preferred Le Fort I osteotomy of the maxilla; 4 small, standardized titanium plates are required, fixed along the bilateral nasofrontal and zygomatic buttress. Red arrows point to the pre-bent titanium plates

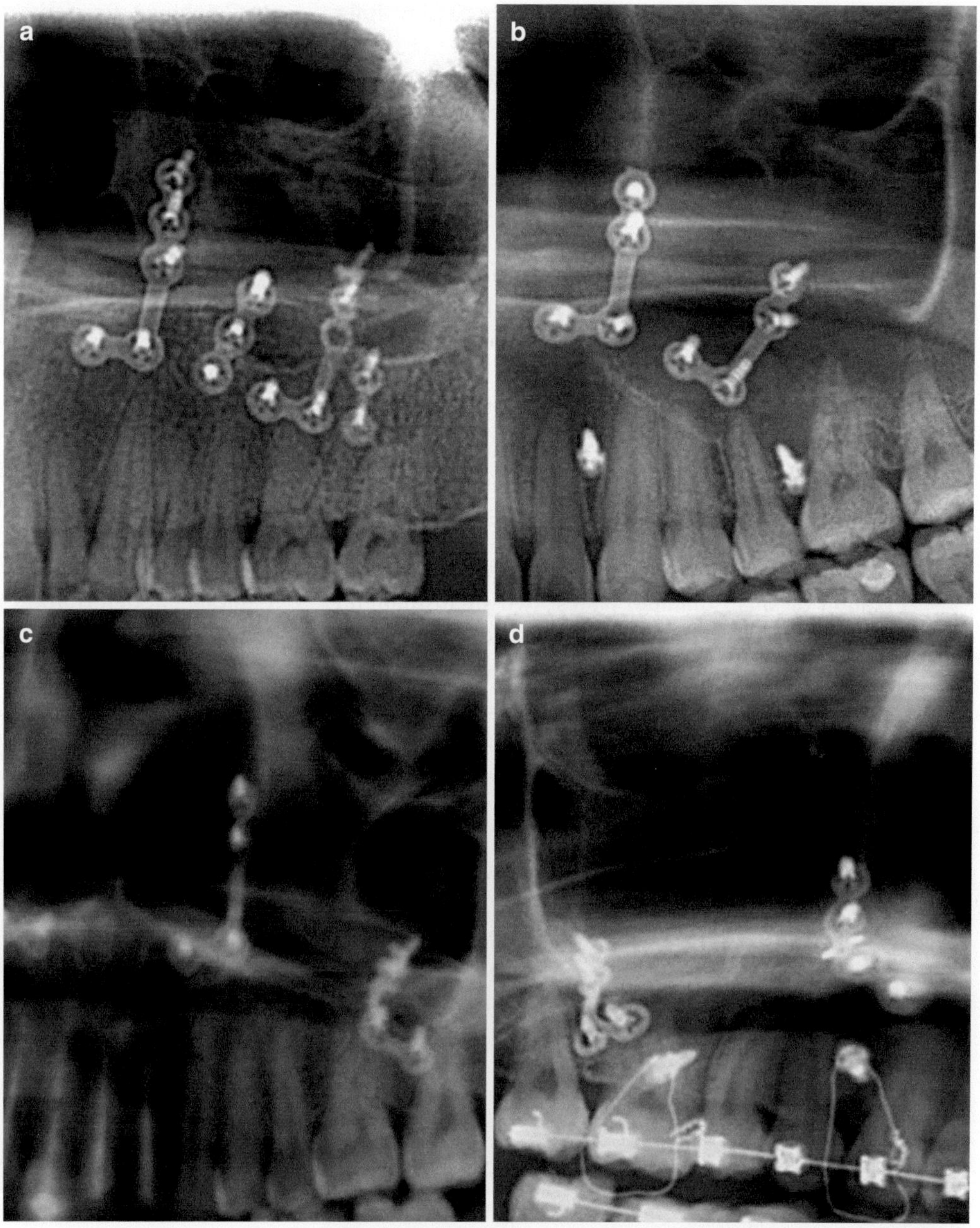

Fig. 5.2 Common problems in titanium plate fixation in maxillary Le Fort I osteotomy. (**a**) Too many fixed titanium plates. (**b**) Titanium plates in the posterior region are positioned too far forward. (**c**) Titanium plate bridges in the anterior region are too long. (**d**) Difficulty in fitting the titanium plates and excessive bending during the operation

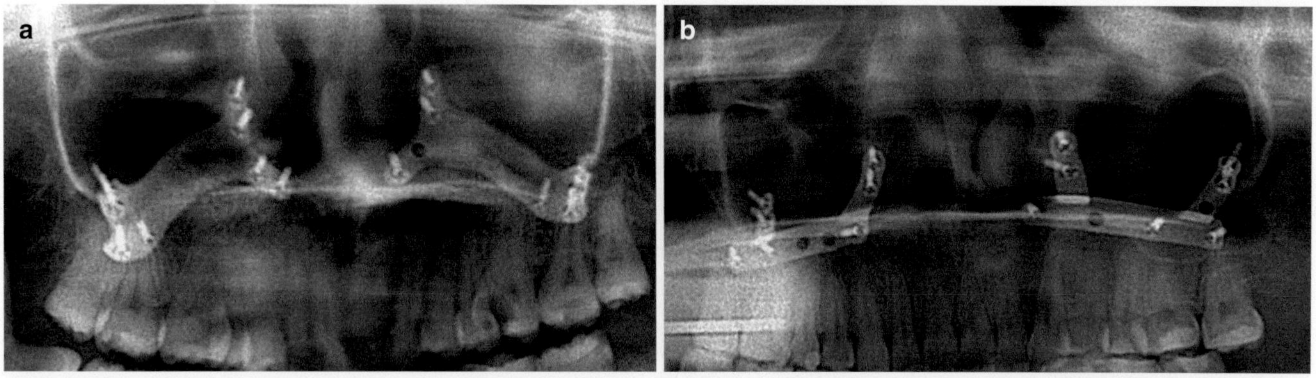

Fig. 5.3 3D printed titanium plates of different designs for maxillary Le Fort I osteotomy fixation. (**a**) Maxillary Le Fort I osteotomy fixation with wide plates. (**b**) Plate for Le Fort I osteotomy fixation with lower margin attachment

  - Small titanium plate fixation: typically, a four-hole titanium plate (Fig. 5.4a).
  - Long screw fixation: two to three long screws are used for double cortical bone fixation in the vertical bone surface behind the molar (Fig. 5.4b).
  - Hybrid fixation: a small titanium plate is fixed with one to two long screws (Fig. 5.4c).

All three fixation methods can induce positional changes of the condyle, resulting in mandibular ramus flaring, condylar displacement, and rotation, which may subsequently lead to condylar resorption. This complication is particularly prone to occur in cases of mandibular deviation deformity (Fig. 5.5) and mandibular retrognathia (Fig. 5.6).

- Titanium plate fixation in genioplasty
  - Standardized titanium plate fixation: standardized genioplasty fixation plates may be used (Fig. 5.7a).
  - Fixation of small titanium plates: two small titanium plates may be used for fixation on both sides (Fig. 5.7b).
  - Combined fixation: standardized titanium plate and small titanium plate co-fixation (Fig. 5.7c), titanium plate and long screw fixation, etc., may be used.

The three fixation methods mentioned above often lead to imprecise fixation or large displacement of the bone block after surgery due to the high strength of the chin muscles and the lack of intraoperative fit to the curvature, especially for two-layer genioplasty.

In addition, there are the following problems for patients with TMJ-originated dentofacial anomalies, due to the limited therapeutic effects of genioplasty:

1. Continuing joint instability in patients with anterior disc displacement and condylar resorption: joint instability will cause further mandibular retraction and/or anterior occlusion gaps after genioplasty.
2. Furthermore, genioplasty in patients with TMJ-originated dentofacial deformities presents several clinical challenges. Joint stability issues in patients with disc dis-

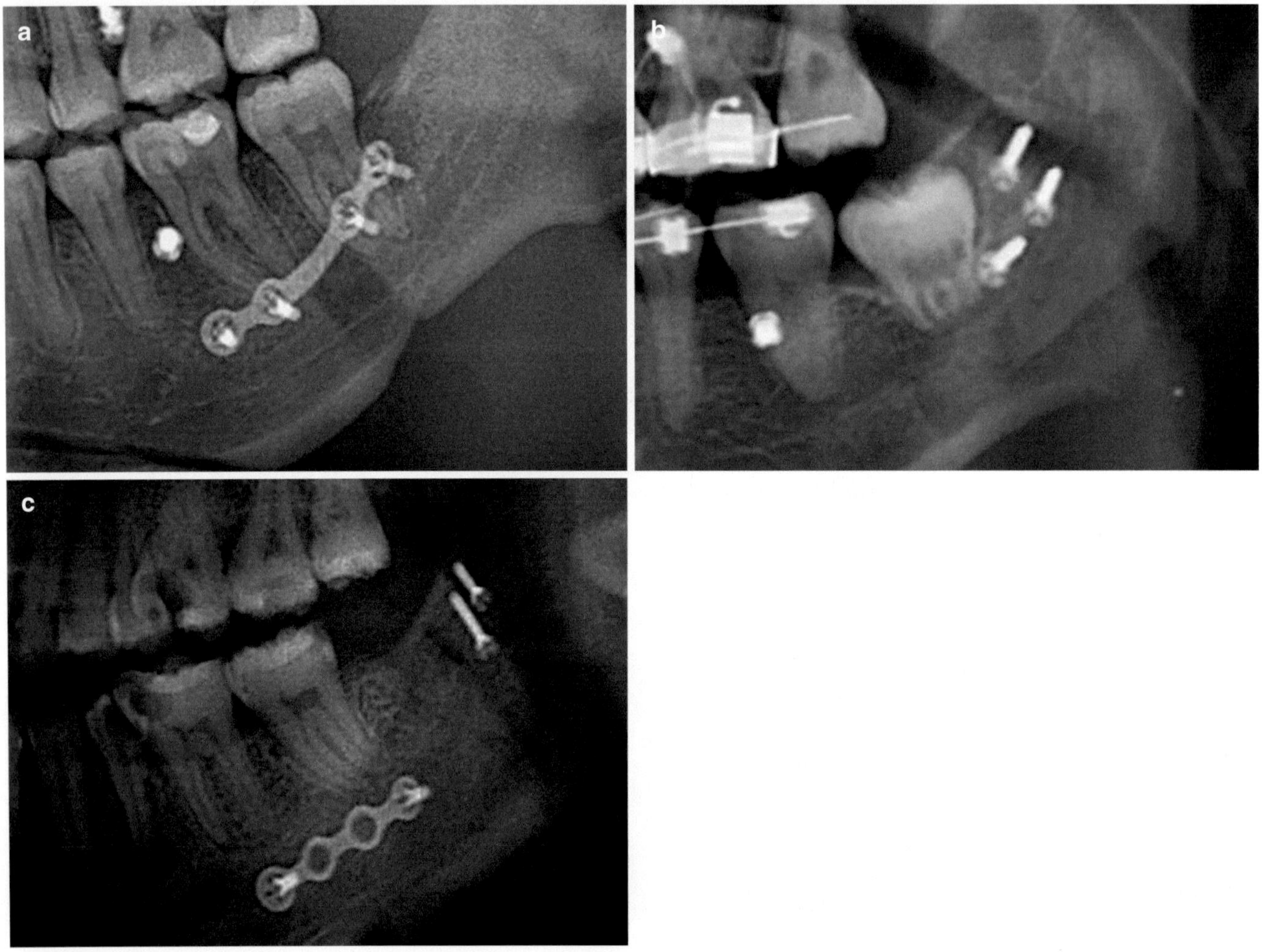

Fig. 5.4 Fixation of sagittal split osteotomy of the mandible. (**a**) Titanium plate fixation. (**b**) Long screw fixation. (**c**) Combined fixation

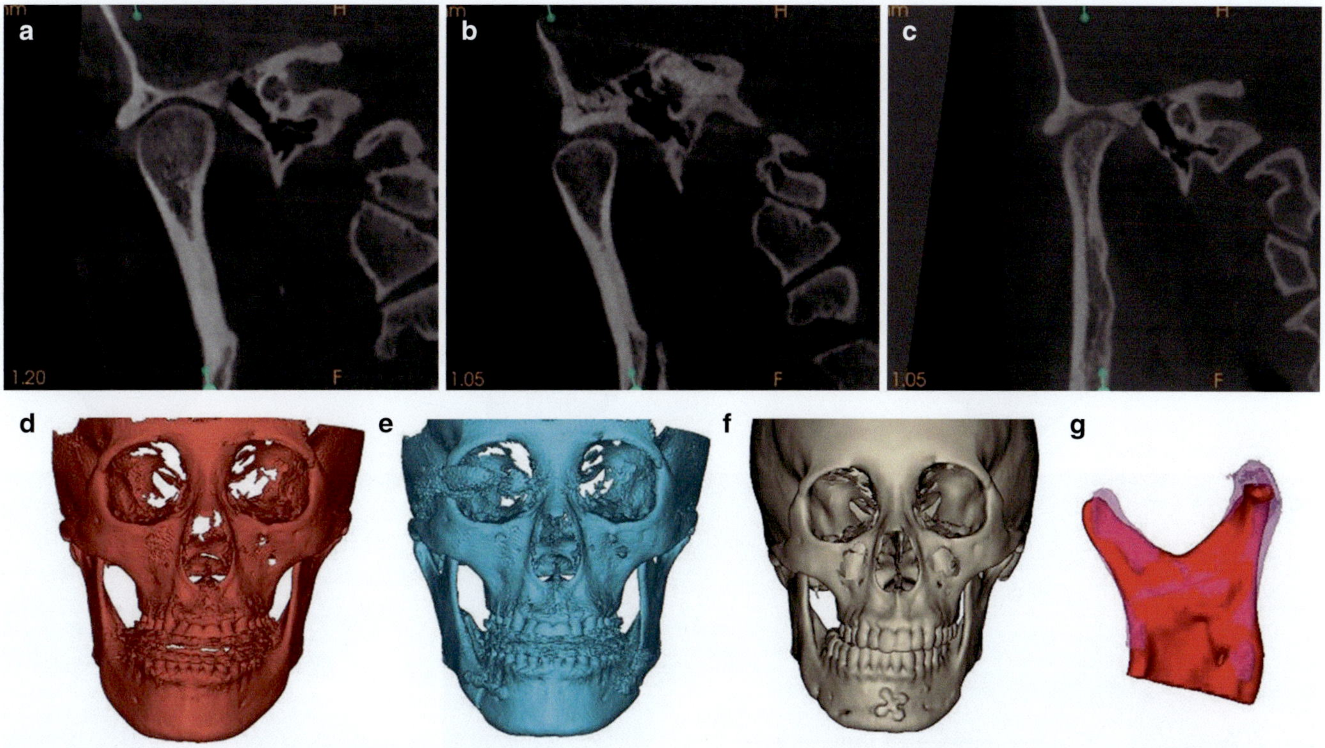

Fig. 5.5 Inadequate fixation following mandibular deformity surgery with mandibular sagittal splitting, resulting in condylar resorption and recurrence of mandibular deviation. The mandibular midline is seen to be corrected, while the right condyle is displaced outward. (**a**) Preoperative CT coronal view; (**b**) immediate postoperative CT coronal view, showing lateral dislocation of the condyle; (**c**) six months postoperatively, showing condylar resorption; (**d**) preoperative CT 3D reconstruction; (**e**) immediate postoperative CT 3D reconstruction; (**f**) six months postoperatively after further surgery, genioplasty, in CT 3D reconstruction mandibular deviation is seen to recur; (**g**) preoperative outline (purple, half transparent) of the volume of the right condyle compared with postoperative outline (red) shows a significant reduction of the condyle in the postoperative period

placement and condylar resorption: TMJ instability may lead to progressive mandibular retrusion and/or anterior open bite following genioplasty. Aesthetic and functional limitations of genioplasty: Excessive single-layer advancement may result in an overly pronounced labiomental fold, compromising lateral profile aesthetics. Silicone implants (commonly used in plastic surgery) fail to address concomitant upper airway stenosis. Conventional genioplasty yields suboptimal outcomes in cases of severe mandibular deficiency (Fig. 5.8).

5.1.4 Innovative Fixation Methods for Customized Bone Graft Fixation Plates in Orthognathic Surgery

The difficulties faced by orthognathic surgery combined with joint preservation surgery include:

1. Sagittal split osteotomy of mandibular ramus, how to ensure that the condyle does not rotate or move, especially since this problem is more pernicious when orthognathic deformity is treated with simultaneous orthognathic surgery and articular disc reposition.
2. How to ensure that the genioplasty can achieve satisfactory aesthetic results along with stability of the joints, producing centering of chin midpoint, precise anterior advancement, beautiful lateral appearance of the lower third of the face, stable fixation, etc.
3. Le Fort I osteotomy, how to improve precision of the osteotomy and bone block repositioning, as well as precision of the fixation site. At the same time, we want to improve stress transmission and eliminate the need for intermaxillary ligation.

Improved and innovative fixation techniques include: the stress-conducting "H" and "Y" customized plate for the maxilla, the mandibular condylar stabilized sagittal split fixation plate, and the customized genioplasty fixation plate.

- Stress-conducting H and Y shape-type customized maxillary plates

For fixation of Le Fort I osteotomies of the maxilla. Stresses in the maxilla are transmitted along the three buttresses: the nasomaxillary, zygomaticomaxillary, and pterygomaxillary buttresses, with the lateral margin of the pyriform foramen and the zygomatic alveolar ridge being the

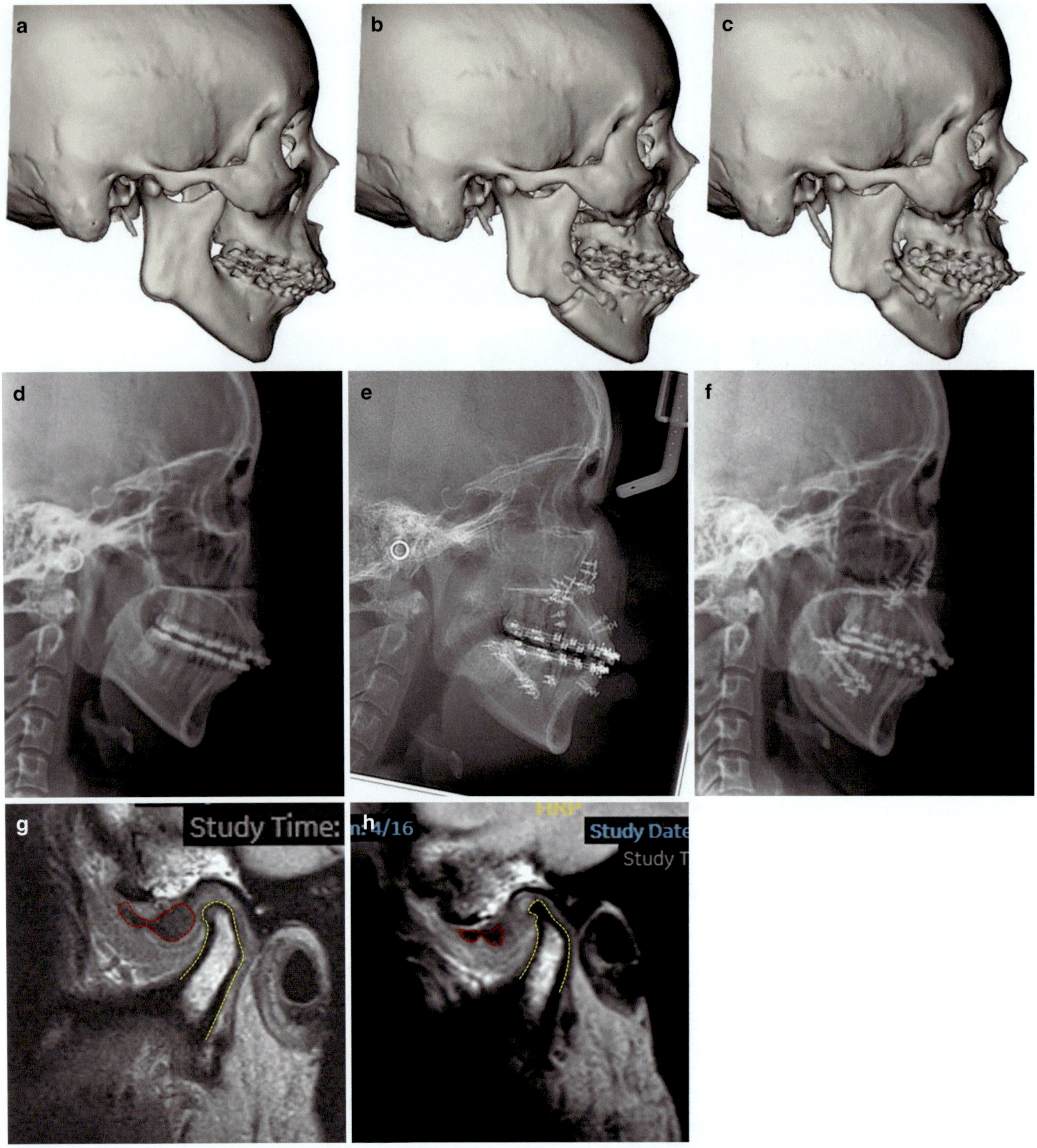

Fig. 5.6 Recurrence of condylar resorption due to improper fixation of mandibular sagittal split. (**a–c**) CT reconstruction of skull: preoperative, immediate postoperative, and 1-year postoperative of orthognathic surgical reconstruction. (**d–f**) lateral radiographs: preoperative, immediate postoperative, and 1-year postoperative. (**g** and **h**) MRI of TMJ joint: preoperative, 1 year

optimal areas for placing the plate. Depending on the individual anatomical shape and direction of stress transmission, the H and Y shape series of customized bone grafting plates can better carry the occlusal force, reduce the displacement of the maxillary mass after surgery, and improve the stability of orthognathic surgery (Fig. 5.9).

- Individualized mandibular plates for condylar stabilization

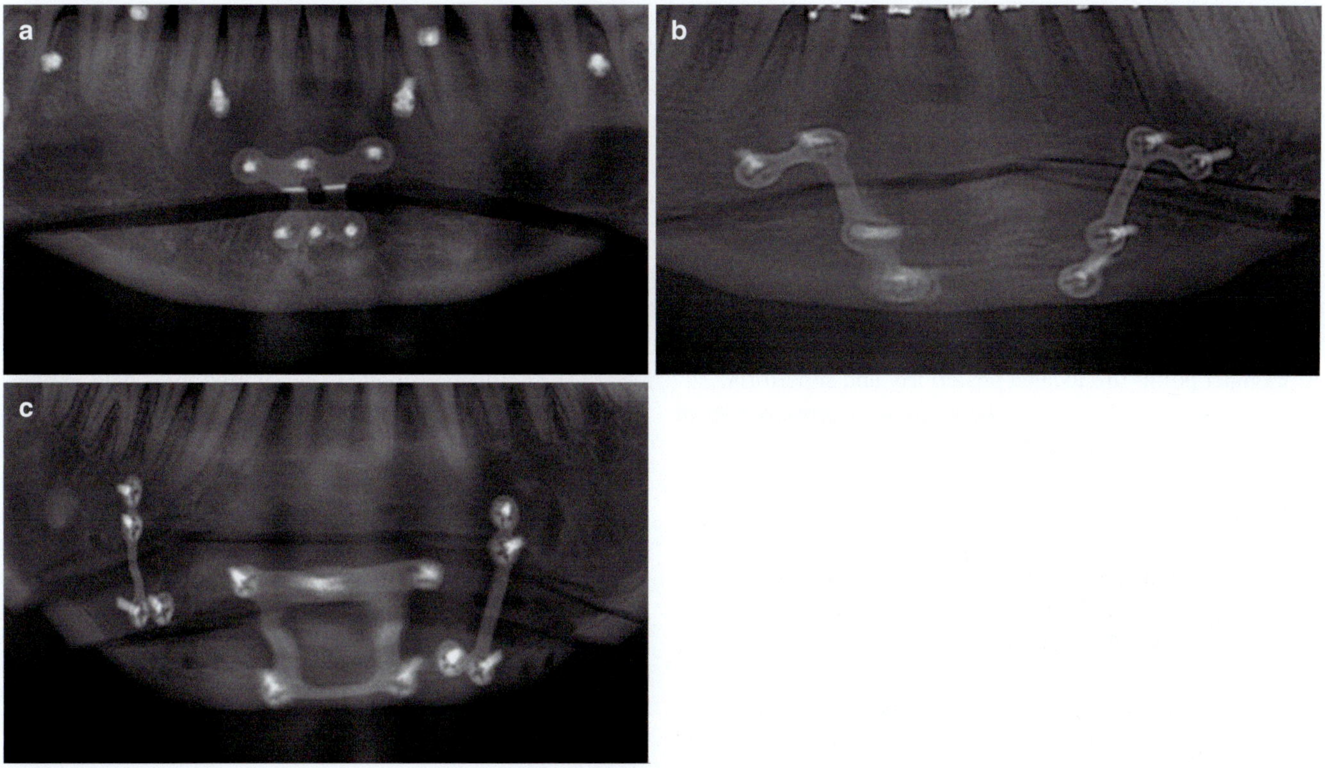

Fig. 5.7 Methods of fixation in genioplasty. (**a**) Standardized titanium plate. (**b**) Small titanium plate fixation. (**c**) Combined fixation

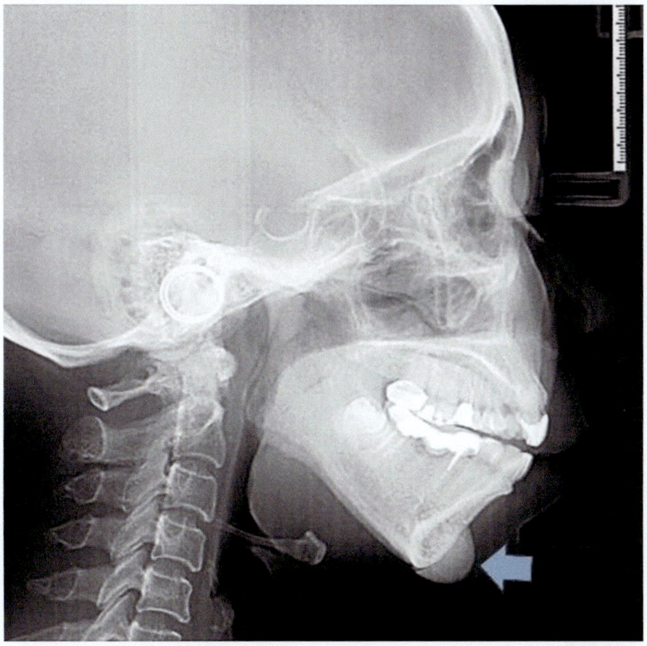

Fig. 5.8 Deficiencies of chin prostheses. Joint instability can cause the mandible to undergo further retraction and/or open a gap between upper and lower anterior teeth; silicone prostheses (arrow) do not solve the problem of a narrow upper airway and poor occlusion

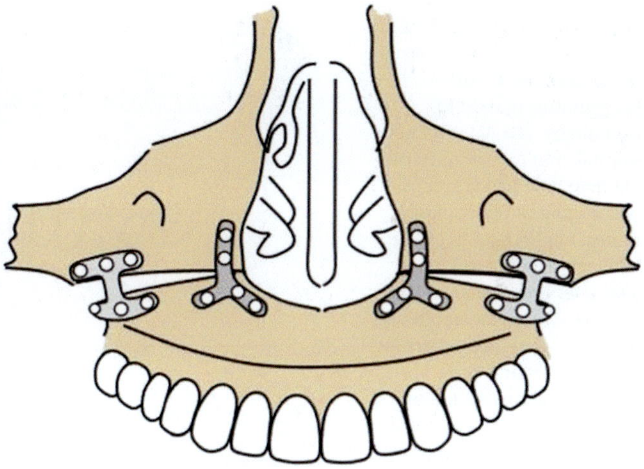

Fig. 5.9 H and Y shape series of customized plates

Patient-specific condylar positioning plates for fixation in sagittal split ramus osteotomy.

In patients with mandibular deviation, bilateral sagittal split ramus osteotomy (BSSRO) can correct mandibular position. However, during this correction process, the angulation and contact points between the proximal and distal segments differ significantly between the two sides. Uncontrolled correction may lead to condylar torsion and medial/lateral displacement issues.

Typically, on the deviated side:

- Contact points are located posteriorly and superiorly
- A wedge-shaped gap exists between the anterior border of the lateral plate and medial plate.

On the contralateral side:

- Contact points are positioned anteriorly and inferiorly.
- The gap between lateral and medial plates progressively increases toward the distal aspect.

Therefore, during surgical planning, precise measurement of these inter-segmental gaps is crucial. Custom-designed osteosynthesis plates should be fabricated to control ramus and condylar positioning (Fig. 5.10).

- Genioplasty customized plates
  - Single-layer genioplasty osteotomy: the use of a customized bone graft fixation plate to perform a conventional genioplasty, combined with a cutting guide, greatly reduces the difficulty and trauma of the procedure and improves the accuracy of the bone block positioning.
  - Single-layer genioplasty osteotomy + sandwich bone grafting: in the case of insufficient vertical height of the chin, the chin bone block can be placed forward vertically and autogenous bone implanted in the gap. The autogenous bone material mixture is held in place using the support of a customized fixation plate to achieve vertical lengthening of the chin (Fig. 5.11).
  - Double-layer genioplasty osteotomy: in patients with severe underdevelopment of the chin, too much genioplasty anterior displacement may lead to complications such as bone disconnection, and the postoperative contour of the mandibular body may appear to be obviously uneven, which affects the surgical result. In this case, double osteotomies should be performed, and the middle osteotomy line should be extended to the distal center in front of the anterior angular notch, to make the lower contour of the jaw look natural and beautiful after surgery (Fig. 5.12).

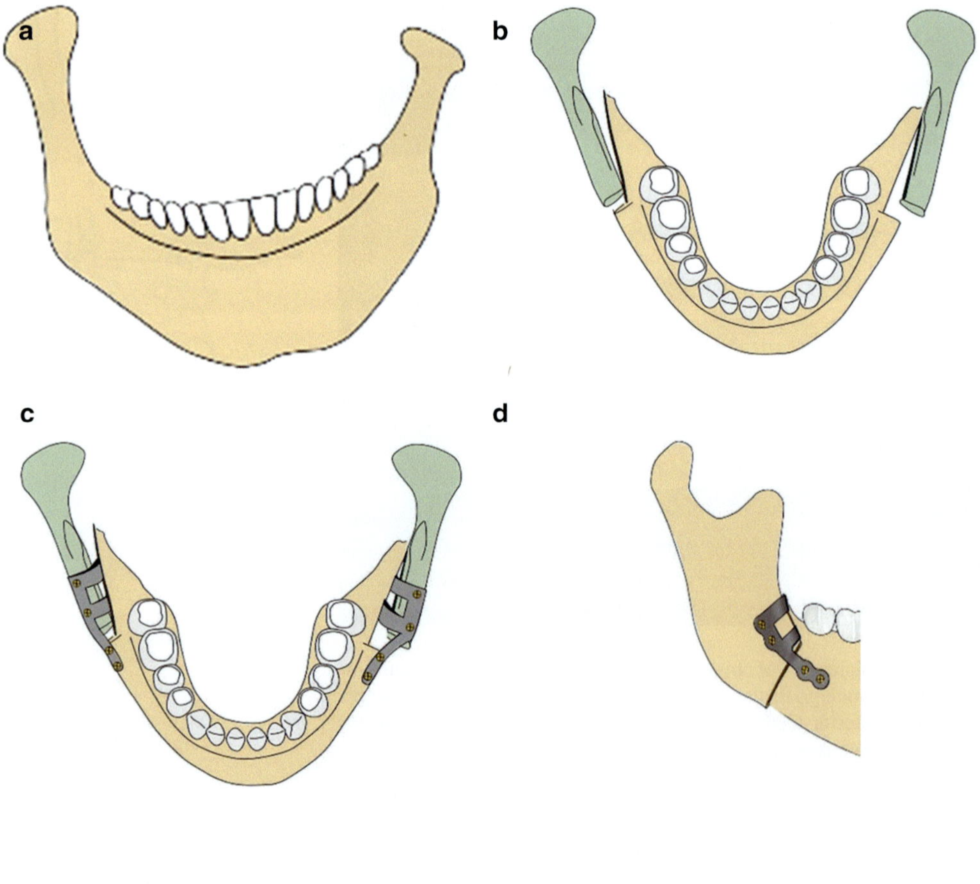

Fig. 5.10 Sagittal split of the mandible, bilateral, to correct facial asymmetry. (**a**) Preoperative mandible asymmetry. (**b**) After bilateral sagittal split osteotomies of the mandible and corrective positioning of the mandible ramus, angles, and gaps between the bilateral inner and outer jaw segments are seen. (**c**) Condylar stabilizing plates are designed according to the angles and gaps between the inner and outer jaw segments. (**d**) Lateral view of right condylar process

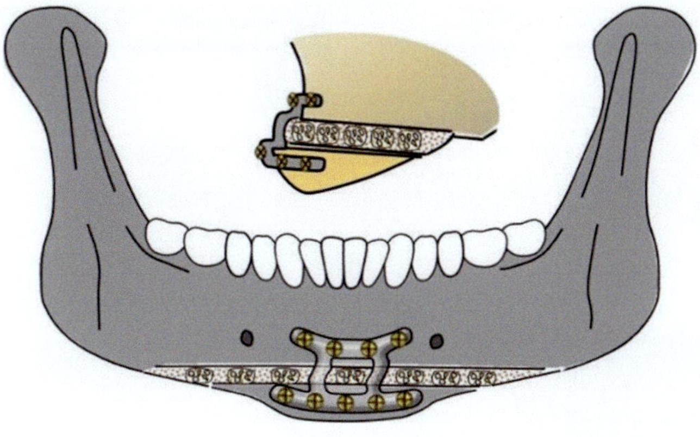

Fig. 5.11 Customized fixation plate for single-layer genioplasty osteotomy + sandwich bone graft

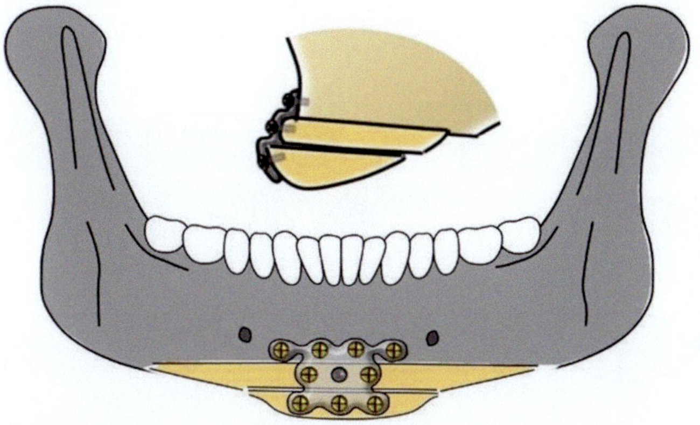

Fig. 5.12 Double-layer genioplasty osteotomy customized plate

– Double-layer genioplasty combined with sandwich bone grafting: patients with severe underdevelopment of the chin both horizontally and vertically may require a combination of both above procedures to achieve substantial anterior displacement and vertical increase at the same time (Fig. 5.13).

5.1.5 Indications and Contraindications

Indications: in principle, these customized plates can be designed for patients who are candidates for orthognathic surgery, including, but not limited to, the indications expressed in Chap. 4.

Contraindications: see contraindications to total TMJ prosthesis in Chap. 3.

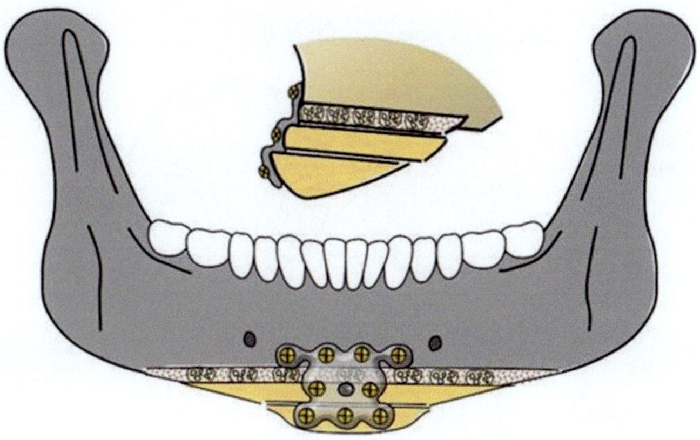

Fig. 5.13 Double-layer genioplasty combined with sandwich bone grafting

5.1.6 The General Digital Design Process for Customized Orthognathic Surgical Bone Graft Fixation Plates

Orthognathic surgical precision and stabilization of condylar morphology are essential for long-term stability of the results of simultaneous/staged orthognathic surgery in patients with condylar resorption and articular ankylosis. Surgical options typically include Le Fort I osteotomy of the maxilla, bilateral sagittal split ramus osteotomy (BSSRO), and genioplasty. This chapter focuses on a modified fixation technique for orthognathic surgery. The general process consists of the design of the orthognathic osteotomy plan, the design and manufacture of the guides and plates, and the surgical procedure (Fig. 5.14).

- Orthognathic osteotomy plan design

CT data are first used to model a reconstruction of the patient's skull, measurement and analysis are done to evaluate the severity of the deformity, and then the osteotomy lines and the surgical plan are designed.

- Design and manufacture of guides and plates

3D-printed cutting guides are designed according to the osteotomy plan, customized plates are designed according to the bone block repositioning plan, and these are positioned precisely through shared screw holes.

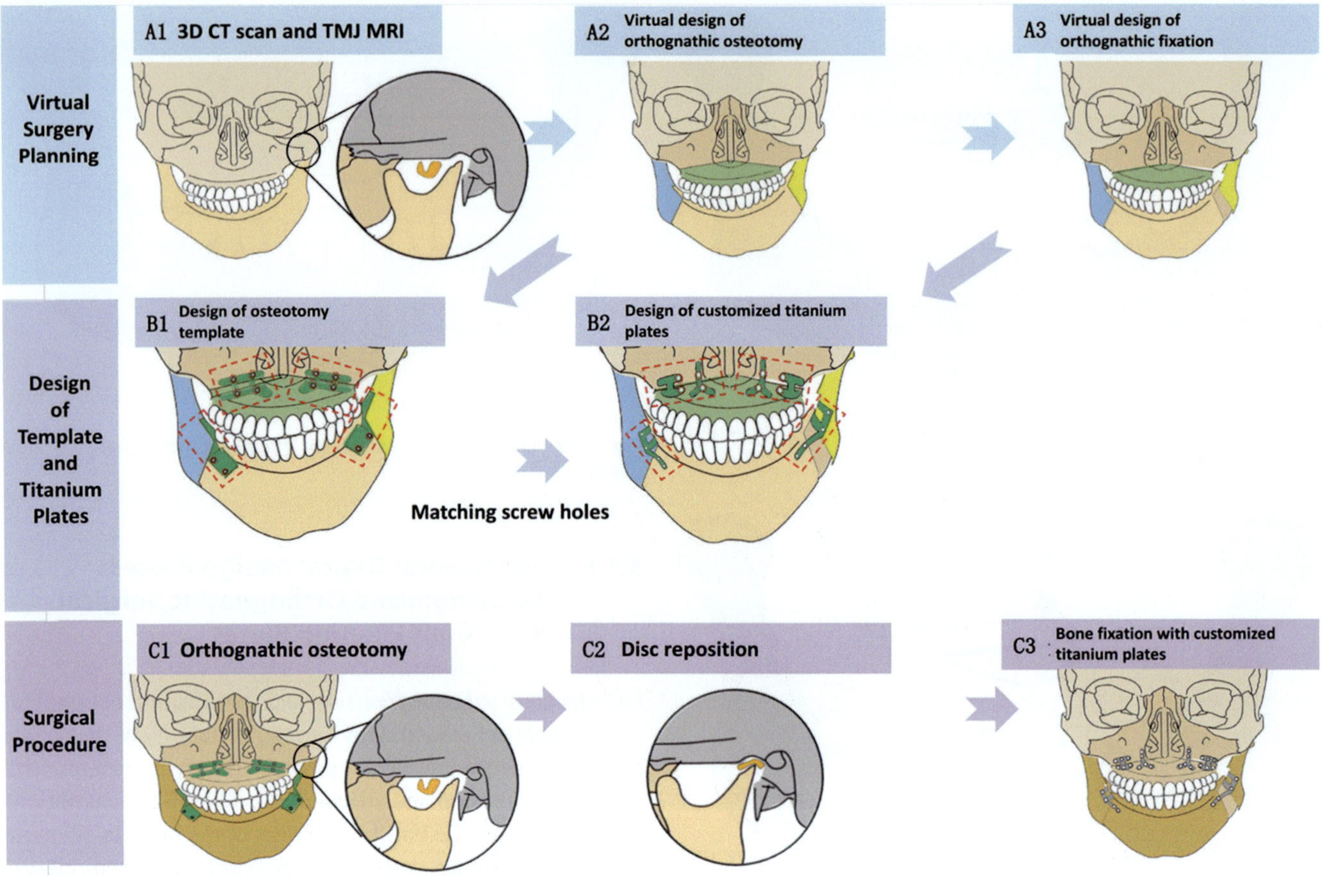

Fig. 5.14 General digital design process for customized bone fixation plates for orthognathic surgery. Simulation of osteotomy surgery: (**a1**) First, model the patient's cranium using CT data, and do measurement and analysis to evaluate the severity of deformity. (**a2**). Design the osteotomy lines. (**a3**) Design the surgical repositioning scheme. (**b1**) Design and manufacture 3D-printed osteotomy positioning guides according to the osteotomy plan. (**b2**) Design and manufacture customized fixation plates according to the bone repositioning plan, noting that they need to be positioned through the screw holes shared with the cutting guides. (**c1**) Surgical procedure: first, perform maxillary surgery. (**c2**) Then reposition the articular disc in the correct position. (**c3**) Last, perform mandibular surgery and utilize the customized bone fixation plates to stabilize the mandible

- Surgical procedure

In the case of articular disc displacement and condylar resorption with dentofacial deformity, the surgical plan is to reposition the articular disc with simultaneous orthognathic surgery. The standard surgical sequence is: (1) maxillary osteotomy, (2) articular disc repositioning, and (3) mandibular osteotomy.

5.2 TMJ Preservation with Orthognathic Surgery: Clinical Application of Customized Orthognathic Fixation Plates

Ensuring satisfactory results and avoiding TMJ complications in orthognathic surgery, while attaining the goal of preserving the condyle and its articular motion, requires precision in the performance of osteotomies and bone block repositioning.

The author's team used digital design and customized orthognathic fixation plates to try to solve the above issues of precision in osteotomy and bone block repositioning, and after a minimum 24-month follow-up period, the results have met the goals. In this section, two clinical cases are shown to illustrate the design and application of the customized bone grafting plates.

5.2.1 Case J. Design and Application of Customized Orthognathic Fixation Plates for Simultaneous TMJ Disc Repositioning

- Patient information: female, 26 years old.
- Complaint: facial deviation with poor occlusal relationship for more than 15 years.
- History: the patient had incidentally noticed facial deviation since primary school, and it gradually worsened with age.

- Previous history: the patient reported being in good health and denied a history of systemic disease or drug and food allergies.
- Clinical examination: facial asymmetry with chin deviation to the left. Oral commissures: left side elevated compared to the right. Mouth opening pattern: centered. Dentition: permanent dentition with lower dental midline deviation to the left. Occlusion: right first molar, Angle's Class III relationship. Left first molar: Angle's Class I relationship (Figs. 5.15 and 5.16).
- Diagnostic imaging: CT of the maxillofacial region showed mandibular asymmetry (unilateral mandibular deviation deformity); MRI of the joints showed anterior disc displacement without reduction of the left TMJ (Figs. 5.17, 5.18, and 5.19).
- Diagnosis: left TMJ anterior disc displacement without reduction; mandibular deviation deformity.

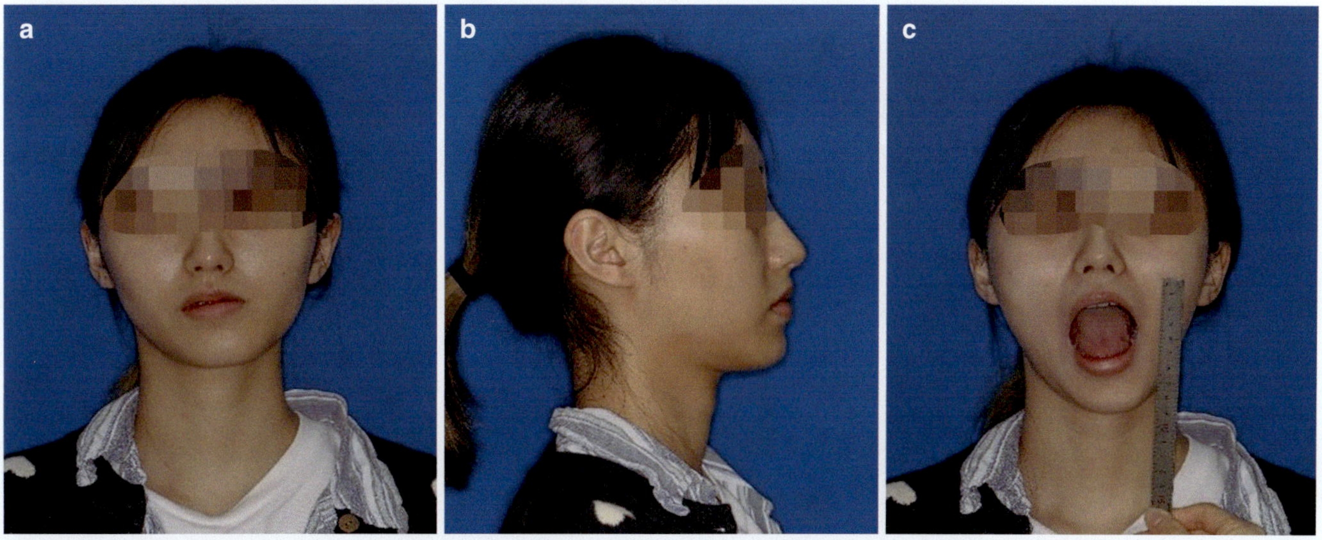

Fig. 5.15 Case J. Facial examination. (**a**) Lateral view. (**b**) Frontal view with left deviation of the chin. (**c**) Mouth opening of 37 mm

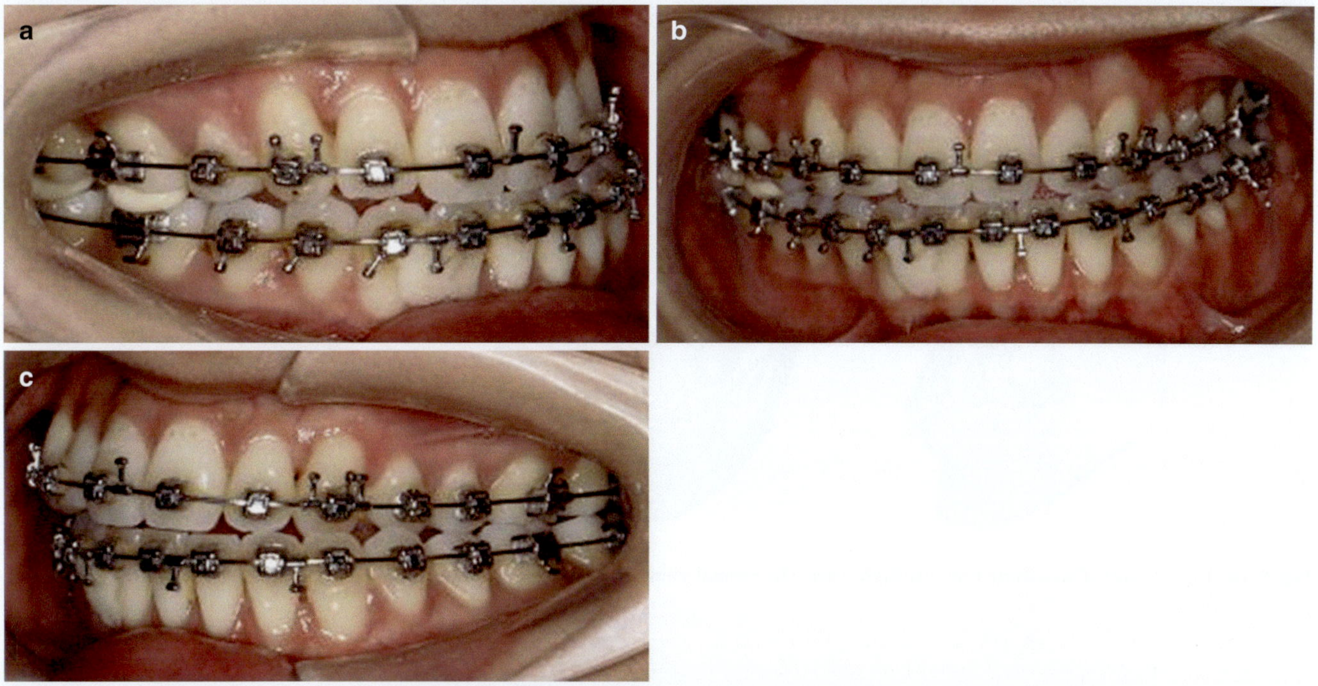

Fig. 5.16 Case J. Intraoral examination. The lower dental midline was deviated to the left, with Angle's Class III molar on the right and Angle's Class I molar and a crossbite on the left. (**a**) Right occlusion. (**b**) Frontal occlusion. (**c**) Left occlusion

Fig. 5.17 Case J. Diagnostic imaging. Radiological examinations demonstrate the mandibular asymmetry and the occlusal cant. (**a**) Panoramic film. (**b** and **c**) Cephalometric radiographs

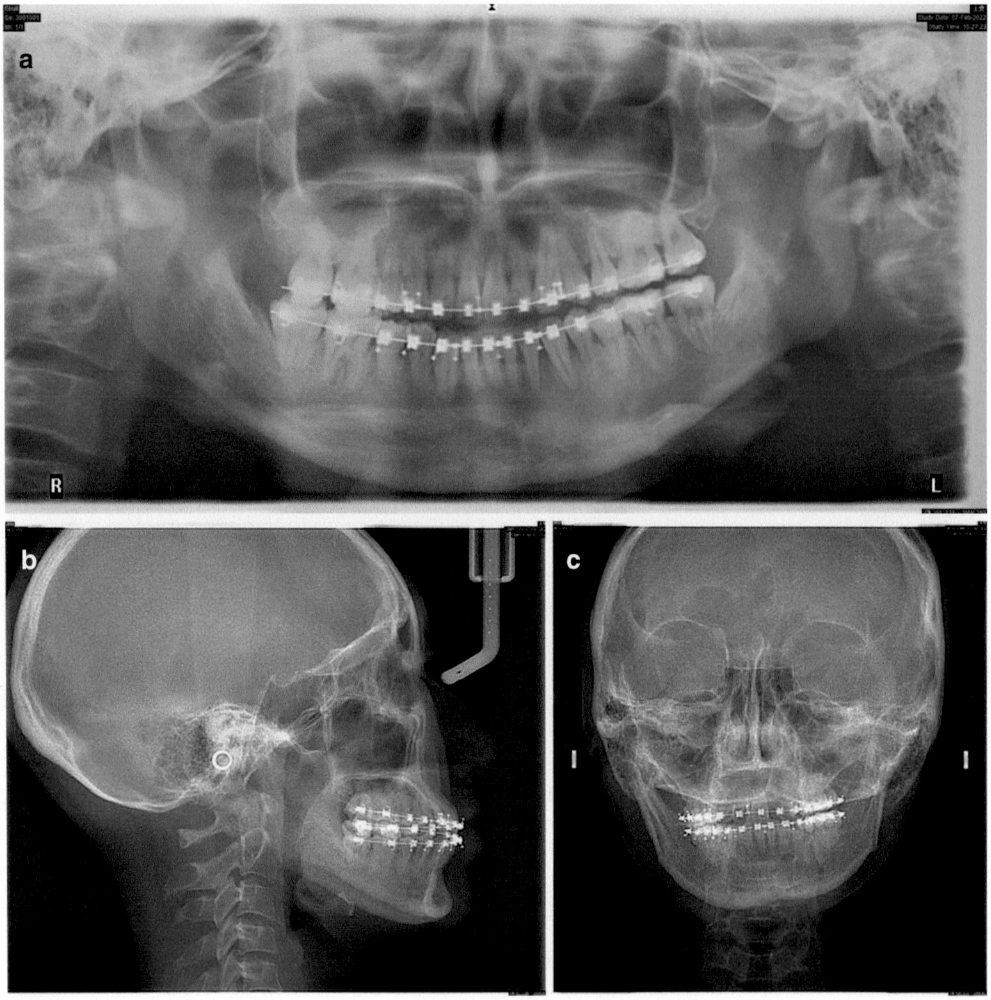

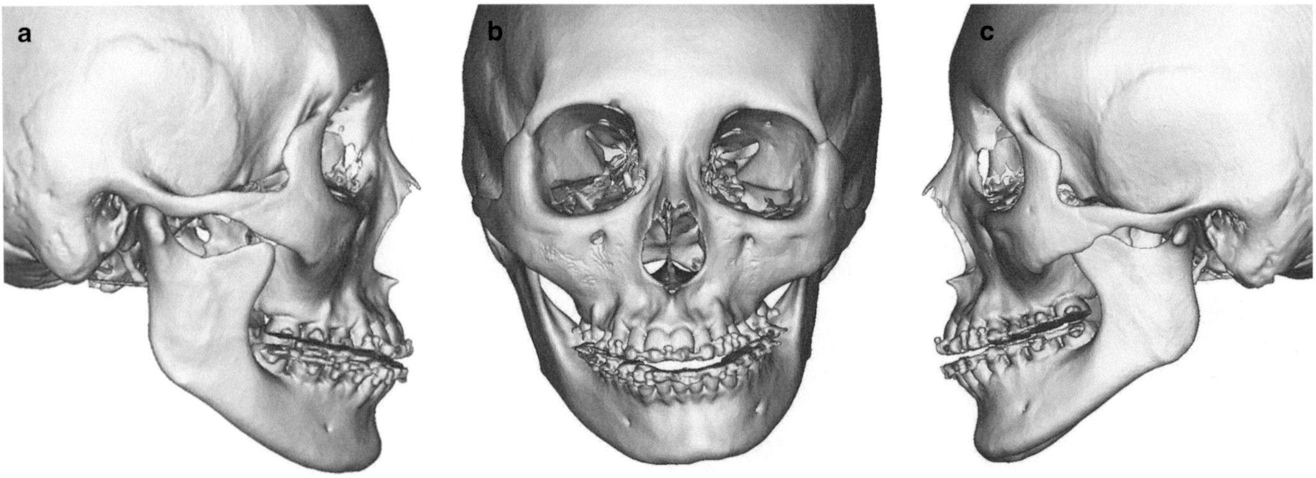

Fig. 5.18 Case J. 3D CT reconstruction. (**a**) Right view. (**b**) Frontal view. (**c**) Left view

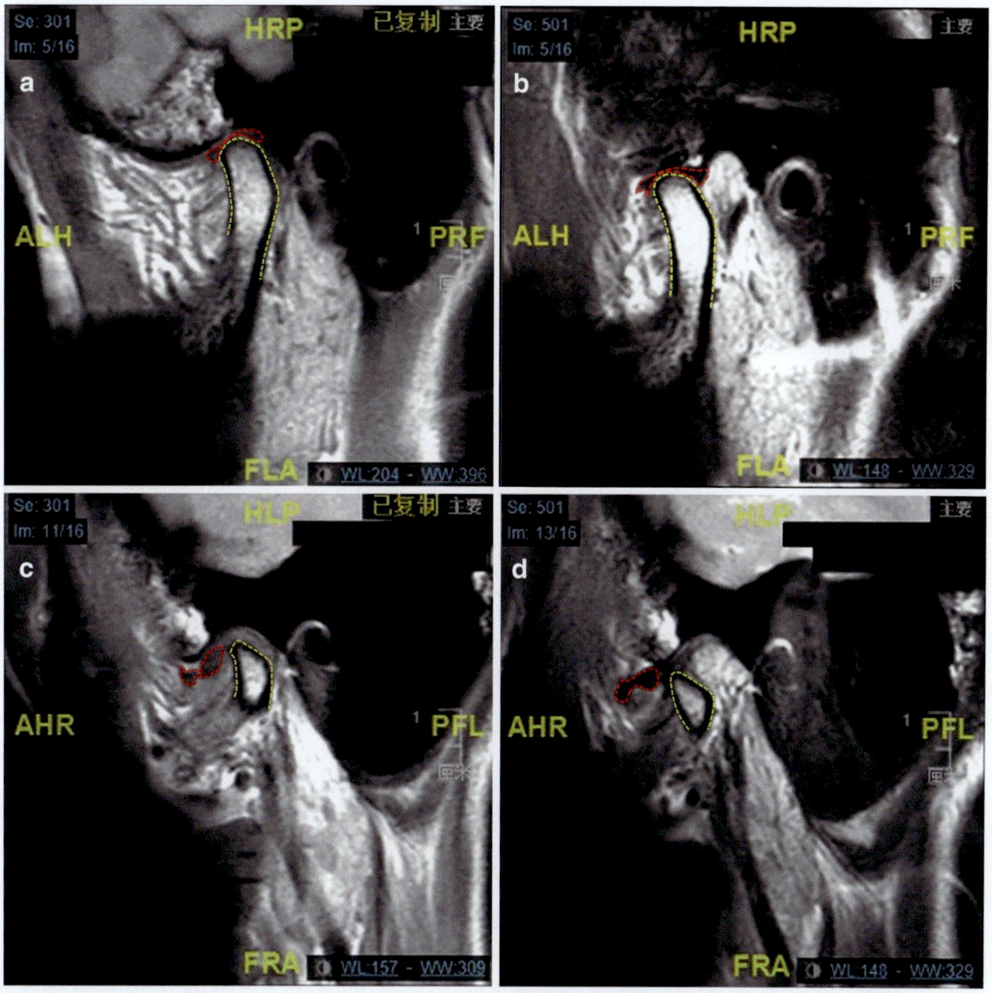

Fig. 5.19 Case J. MRI showed that the right side is normal. The left side shows anterior disc displacement, without reduction. (**a**) Right closed mouth position. (**b**) Right open mouth position. (**c**) Left closed mouth position. (**d**) Left open mouth position (yellow dotted lines indicate condylar head, red dotted lines indicate articular disc)

5.2.2 Case J. Diagnostic Imaging

5.2.3 Case J. Treatment Plan

- Overall treatment plan: left articular disc repositioning and simultaneous orthognathic surgery. Specifically:
  1. Preoperative immobilization and orthodontic decompensation
  2. Left articular disc repositioning and suture fixation, simultaneous bimaxillary orthognathic surgery
  3. Postoperative orthodontics
- The order of the surgical procedure is as follows:
  1. Le Fort I osteotomy of the maxilla
  2. Left articular disc repositioning and suture fixation
  3. BSSRO

5.2.4 Case J. Design and Processing of H-Y-Shaped Plates and Condylar Stabilizing Plates and Guides

- H-Y-shaped fixation plate design

Design the shape of the fixation plate for stress conduction with reference to the stress conduction lines of bony buttress of the maxilla (Figs. 5.20 and 5.21).

- Condylar stabilizing fixation plates design: rotation of the mandible

This case is one of a mandibular deviation deformity, and when designing a bilateral sagittal split osteotomy of the mandibular ramus to correct the mandibular position, a large gap between the inner and outer plates on both sides will be found to occur due to the large rotation required at the inner segment of the jaw (Fig. 5.22).

- Condylar stabilizing fixation plate design: the medial wing of the fixation plate is angled inward from the external oblique line and embedded in the bone segment space to stabilize the condyle (Fig. 5.23).
- Design and machining of digital guides: design of cutting guides (pink) according to the maxillary Le Fort I osteotomy line, and design of positioning plates (gray) to be used intraoperatively to reset the maxillary block to the desired position (Fig. 5.24).

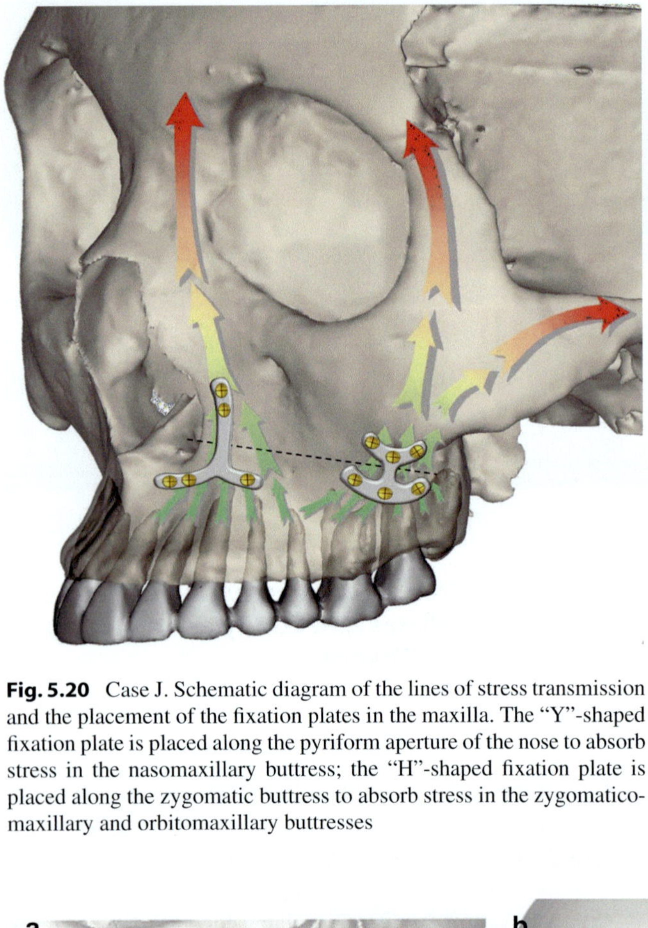

Fig. 5.20 Case J. Schematic diagram of the lines of stress transmission and the placement of the fixation plates in the maxilla. The "Y"-shaped fixation plate is placed along the pyriform aperture of the nose to absorb stress in the nasomaxillary buttress; the "H"-shaped fixation plate is placed along the zygomatic buttress to absorb stress in the zygomatico-maxillary and orbitomaxillary buttresses

5.2.5 Case J. Surgical Procedure

Preoperative laboratory tests: the same as described in Sect. 3.2.5, Preoperative Laboratory Tests.

Preoperative preparation: the same as described in Sect. 3.2.5, Preoperative Preparation and preparation of 400 mL of blood.

- Surgical sequence:
  Le Fort I osteotomy of the maxilla, followed by left arthroscopic disc repositioning and suture fixation, and finally BSSRO
  1. Le Fort I osteotomy and repositioning of the maxilla are shown in Figs. 5.25 and 5.26.
  2. Left arthroscopic disc repositioning and suture fixation (Fig. 5.27).
  3. BSSRO (Fig. 5.28).
  4. Postoperative medical advice and care: daily oral care and intermaxillary elastic traction if necessary.

5.2.6 Case J. Postoperative Analysis of Prosthesis Implantation Precision

Regular postoperative follow-ups were performed for appearance (facial shape), function (degree of mouth opening, mouth opening shape), and plate evaluation (safety, accuracy).

Immediately after surgery: the intraoperative guides were accurately positioned, and the fixation plates were installed smoothly (Fig. 5.29). The positions of the bilateral condyles were stable, and the position of the left condyle was slightly lower than the preoperative position due to the increase in the upper posterior articular space after the articular disc was reset and the condyle was shifted forward and downward (Fig. 5.30), as was planned for rectification of facial symmetry.

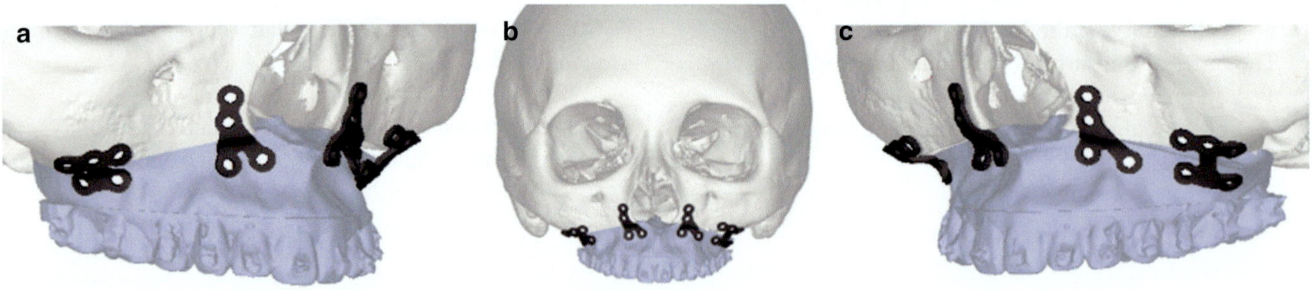

Fig. 5.21 Case J. H-Y-shaped fixation plate design, designed after determination of the maxillary position to be obtained through orthognathic surgery. (**a**) Right side. (**b**) Front. (**c**) Left side

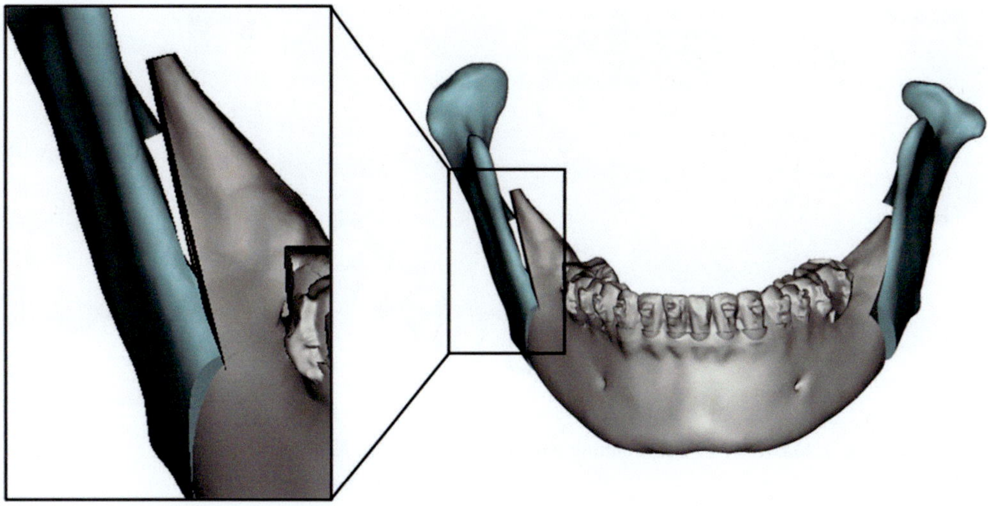

Fig. 5.22 Case J. Sagittal split osteotomy design of the right mandibular ramus showing inner and outer gaps in segments of mandibular bone in enlarged view in box on left. The sagittal split osteotomy will allow the right mandibular ramus to be slightly shortened and rotated, and the left to be slightly lengthened

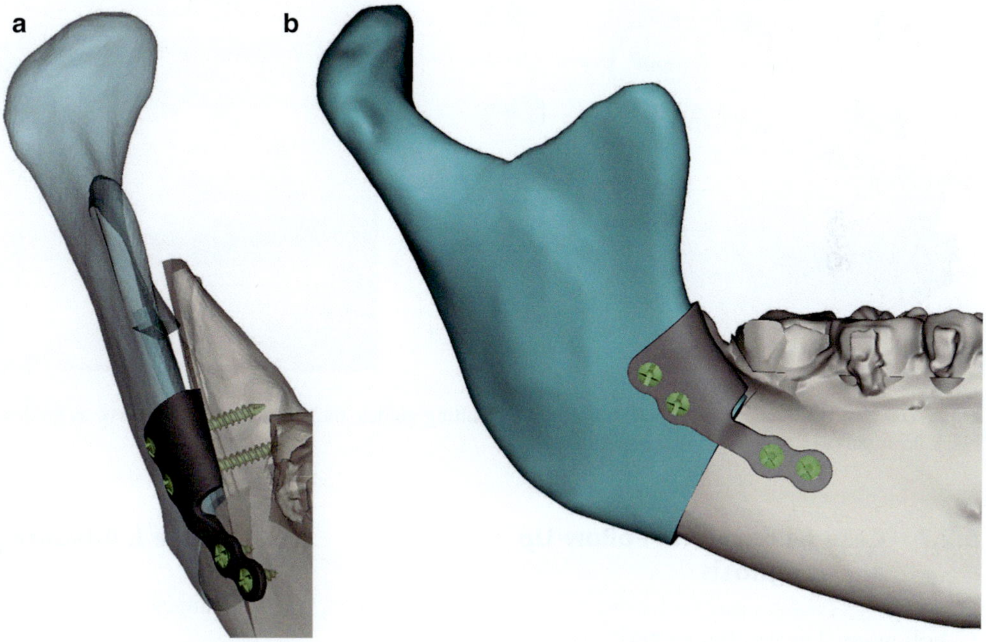

Fig. 5.23 Case J. Mandibular splice fixation plate design, with medial wing angled inward from the external oblique line, stabilizes the condyle. (**a**) Frontal view. (**b**) Lateral view

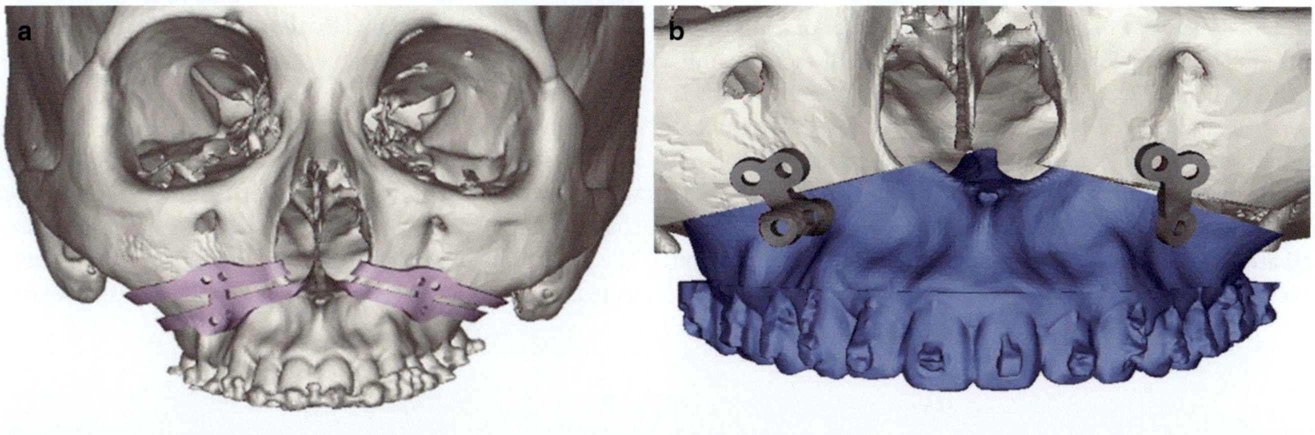

Fig. 5.24 Case J. Design of cutting guides and positioning plates. The screw holes of the former guide set the position of the latter. (**a**) Cutting guide plate design (pink). (**b**) Positioning plate design (gray) to be used intraoperatively to reset the maxillary block to the desired position

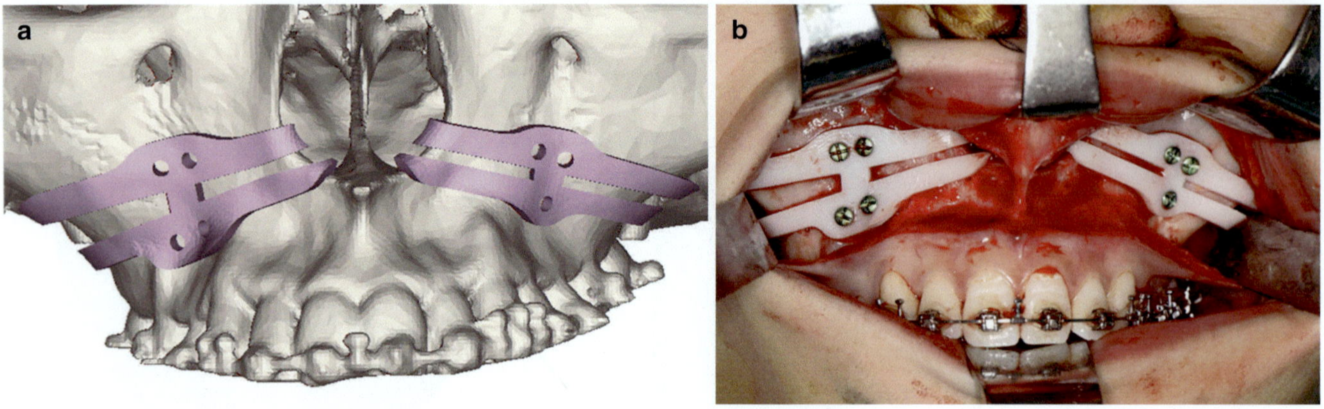

Fig. 5.25 Case J. Maxillary Le Fort I cutting guides. (**a**) Design. (**b**) Actual

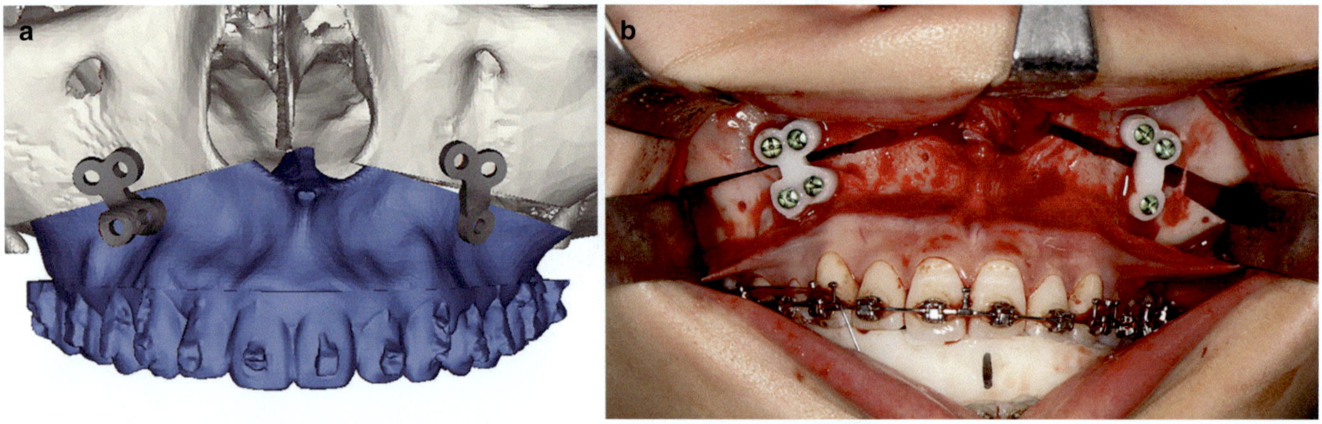

Fig. 5.26 Case J. In matching the screw holes of the cutting guides, the positioning plates serve as guides to determine the corrected maxillary block position. (**a**) Design. (**b**) Actual

5.2.7 Case J. Long-Term Follow-Up and Prognosis

- Follow-up 2 years after surgery

The face is symmetrical and free of deviation (Fig. 5.31).

Good recovery of joint function, no pain or discomfort in the joint area, stable joint-mandibular-occlusal-facial coordination, and stable occlusal relationship (Fig. 5.32).

Evaluation of the bone graft fixation plates: no complications such as rejection, loosening, fracture, heterotopic osteogenesis, or material allergy were observed (Fig. 5.33).

The left articular disc was properly reset and stabilized in position with normal disc-condylar relationship and good condylar mobility (Fig. 5.34).

5.2.8 Case J. Advantages and Disadvantages

- Advantages

The design of the H-Y-shaped plates in accordance with the biological stress lines in fixation of the maxilla in Le Fort I surgery theoretically makes the fixation more scientific, more precise, more stable, and easier for surgical performance.

Condylar resorption after orthognathic surgery is an important factor in the recurrence of mandibular deviation, which occurs mostly due to improper fixation, resulting in a change in condylar position and increased surface pressure. The probability of condylar resorption after surgery is greatly increased, especially in the presence of disc displacement

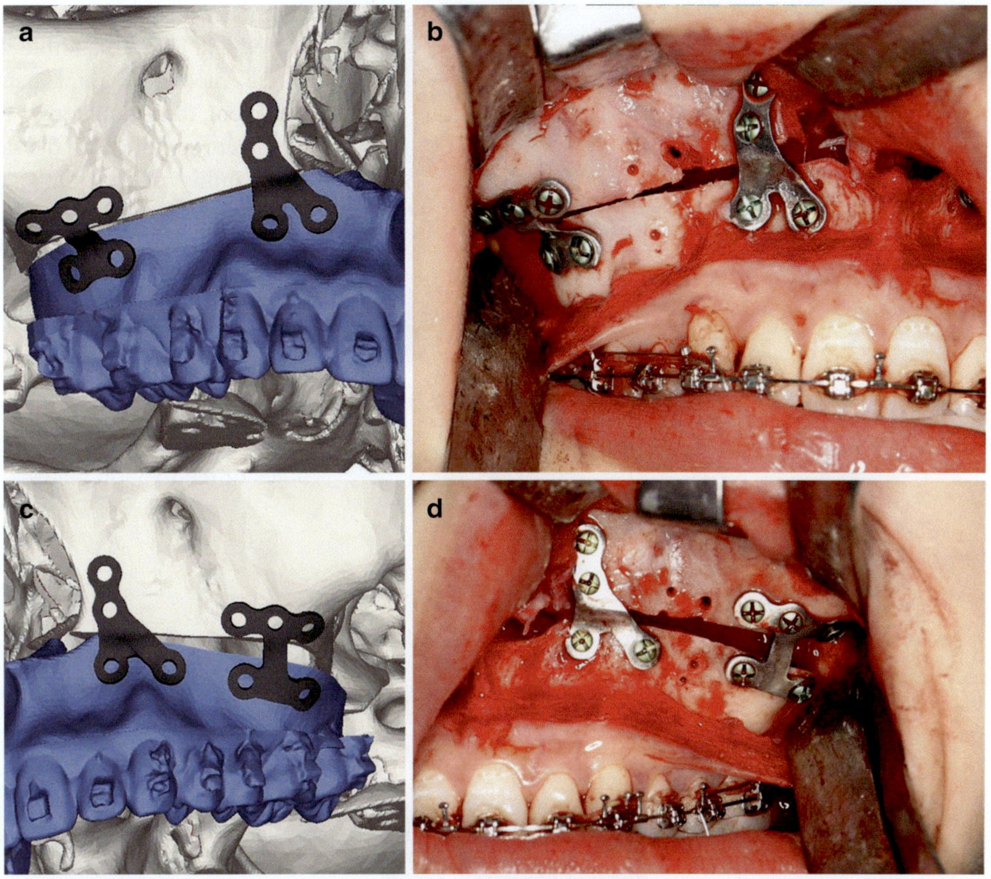

Fig. 5.27 Case J. H-Y-shaped fixation plate implantation; note that they are 3D and have the effect of moving the bone block slightly posteriorly as well, which will help in occlusion with the lower teeth. (**a**, **c**) Design. (**b**, **d**) Actual. After the permanent fixation with the titanium plates, the plastic positioning plates were removed

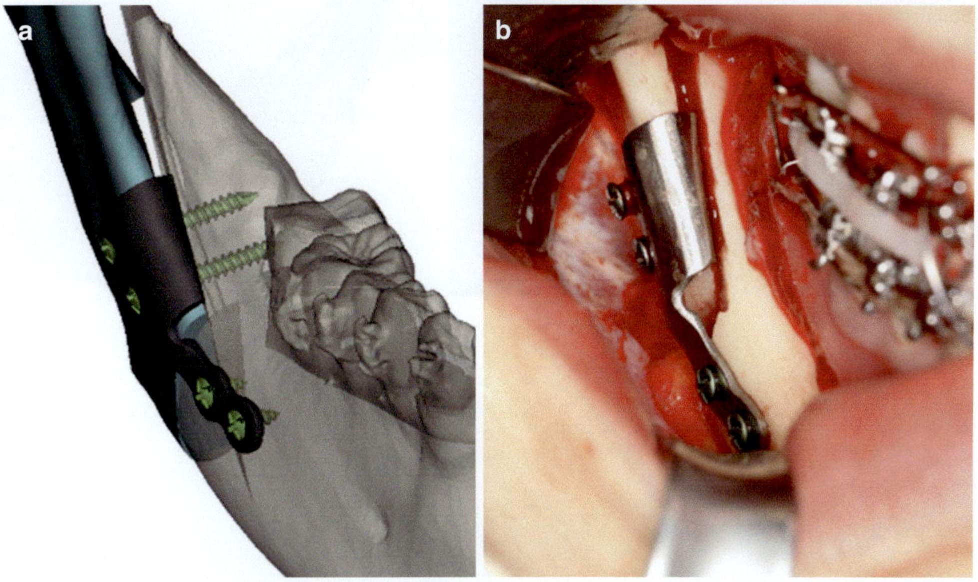

Fig. 5.28 Case J. Stabilizing condylar fixation plate implantation after sagittal split osteotomy of the right mandibular ramus, for slight rotation and shortening. (**a**) Design. (**b**) Actual

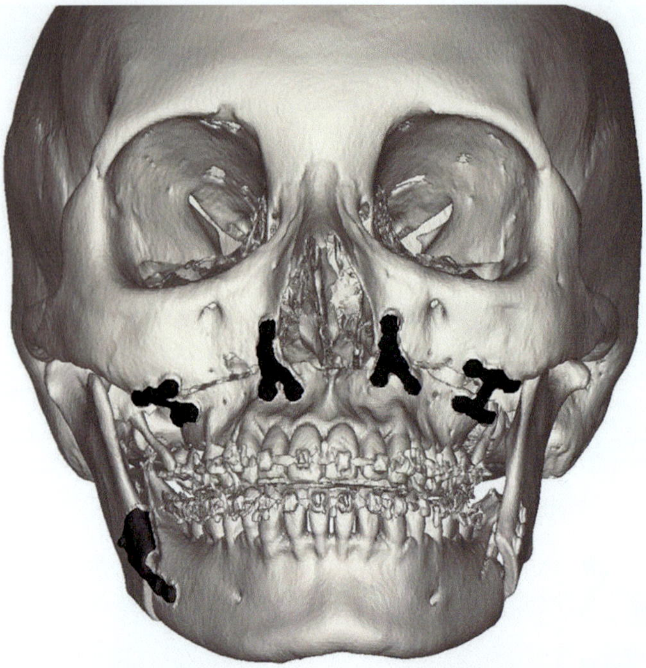

Fig. 5.29 Case J. Postoperative CT showing the fixation plates in good position

(Fig. 5.6). In this case, the left articular disc had been displaced and led to mandible deformity. But through the innovative model of joint-mandibular-occlusion combination treatment, the articular disc reposition, and orthognathic surgery were completed at the same time. This served to improve the stability of the joints; customized bone graft fixation plates were used to maintain the gap between the bone segments, thus stabilizing the condylar eminence.

- Disadvantages

The cutting guides as designed were too large for easy maneuvering, and it would have been more manageable if the screw holes of the cutting guide plate matched the screw holes of the fixation plates.

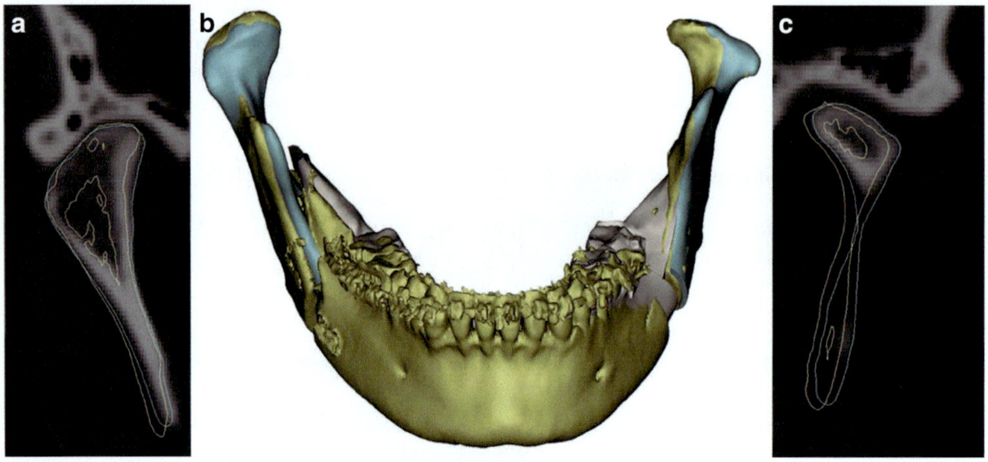

Fig. 5.30 Case J. Postoperative CT comparison (preoperative design, blue contour lines; actual postoperative, yellow contour lines). (**a**) Stabilization of the right condylar position. (**b**) 3D reconstruction of the whole mandible. (**c**) Left condylar position

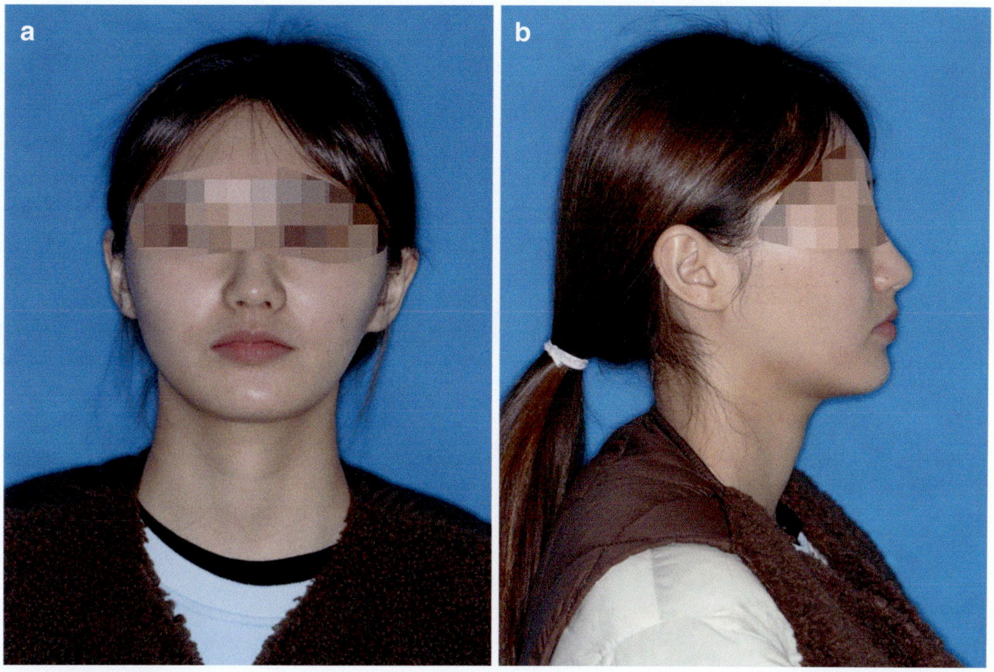

Fig. 5.31 Case J. Follow-up 2 years after surgery with good facial features. (**a**) Frontal view, (**b**) lateral view

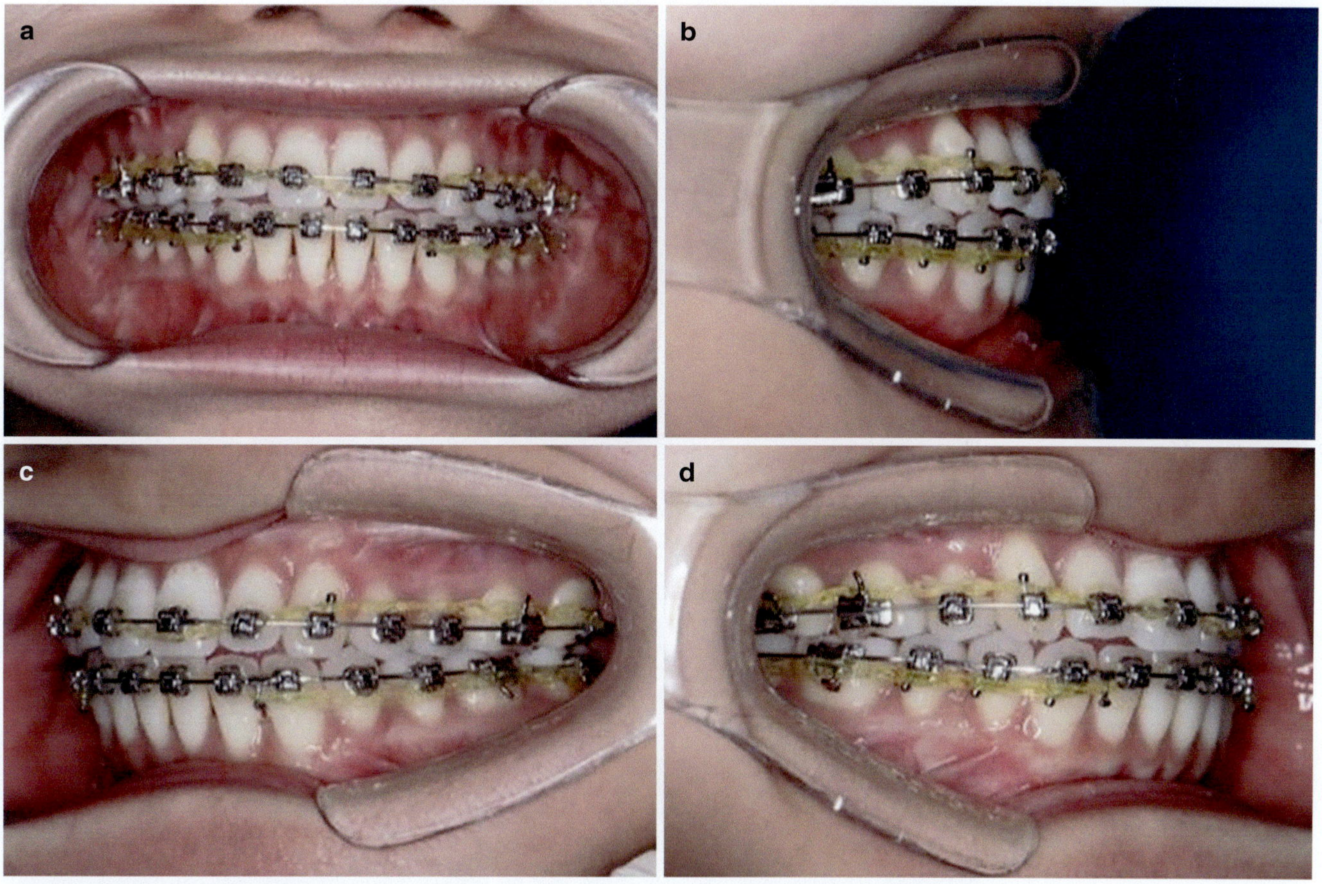

Fig. 5.32 Case J. Intraoral examination 2 years after surgery with stable occlusal relationship. (**a**) Frontal occlusion. (**b**) 90° lateral occlusion. (**c**) Left occlusion. (**d**) Right occlusion

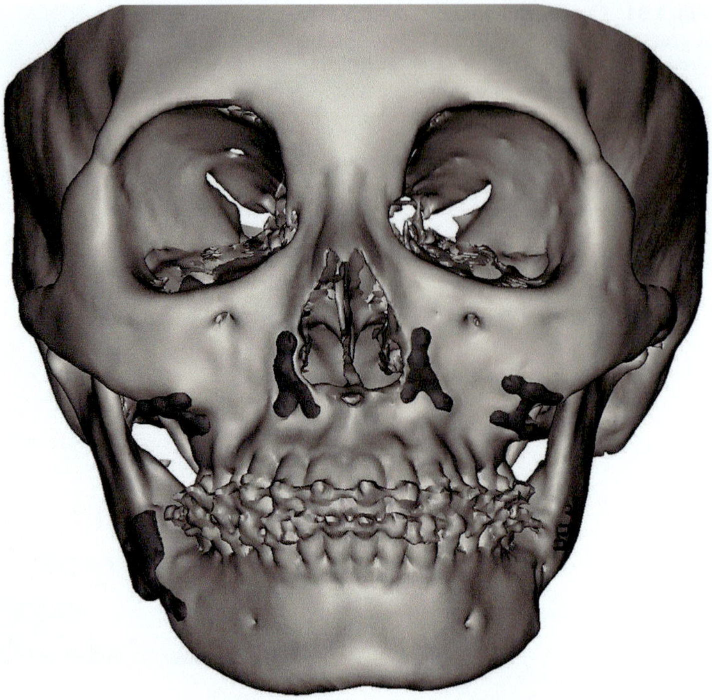

Fig. 5.33 Case J. CT at 2 years postoperatively showing good bone healing and stable positions of the plates

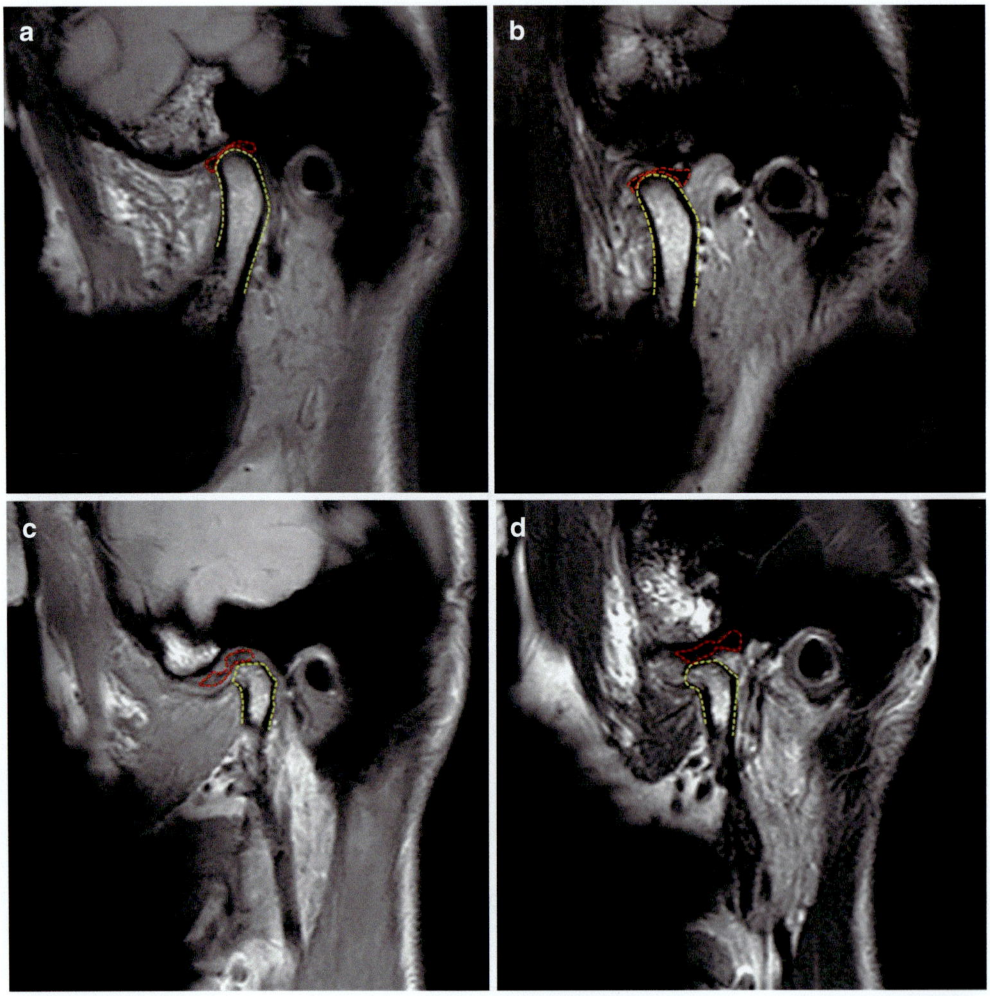

Fig. 5.34 Case J. MRI shows the left side joint after repositioning, with normal disc-condylar relationship and stabilized condylar eminence without resorption, and even some new bone formation. (Red dotted line highlights the articular disc, yellow the condylar head.) (**a**) Right closed mouth position. (**b**) Right open mouth position. (**c**) Left closed mouth position. (**d**) Left open mouth position

5.3 Case K. TMJ Preservation with Orthognathic Surgery: Design and Application of Customized Plates for Staged Genioplasty with Articular Disc Repositioning

Qianyang Xie and Xuzhuo Chen

5.3.1 Case K. Customized Plates for Staged Genioplasty and Articular Disc Repositioning

- Patient information: female, 18 years old.
- Complaint: mandibular retrognathia and open bite of anterior teeth for 8 years.
- History: the patient presented with progressive mandibular retrognathia and open bite in anterior occlusion 8 years ago. She was diagnosed with bilateral anterior disc displacement without reduction 3 years ago and underwent bilateral arthroscopic articular disc repositioning and fixation.
- Previous history: the patient reported being in good health and denied a history of systemic disease, or drug and food allergies.
- Clinical examination: mandibular retraction, mouth opening of 38 mm, centered mouth opening, permanent teeth in the mouth, stable occlusal relationship (Fig. 5.35).
- Diagnostic imaging examination: joint MRI showed that after bilateral arthroscopic surgery, the relationship between the discs and condyles was good (Fig. 5.36); maxillofacial CT showed that the condylar bones were stable (Fig. 5.37).
- Diagnosis: bony Class II malocclusion.

5.3.2 Case K. Treatment Plan

Overall treatment plan: 3 years after bilateral articular disc repositioning, the condyles were evaluated as to whether they were stabilized (Fig. 5.36). The following orthodontic and orthopedic options for the problem of mandibular retraction were offered:

Option 1: fixed orthodontic decompensation, bilateral sagittal split ramus osteotomy (BSSRO), possible adjunctive maxillary Le Fort I osteotomy.

Option 2: compensatory fixed orthodontic treatment, genioplasty to improve mandibular retrusion.

The patient and family opted for Option 2 after being thoroughly informed of its therapeutic limitations during preoperative counseling.

5.3.3 Case K. Design and Processing

- Surgical osteotomy design: digital simulation of surgical and genioplasty fixation plate design (Figs. 5.38 and 5.39).
- Design of the cutting guide (Fig. 5.40).

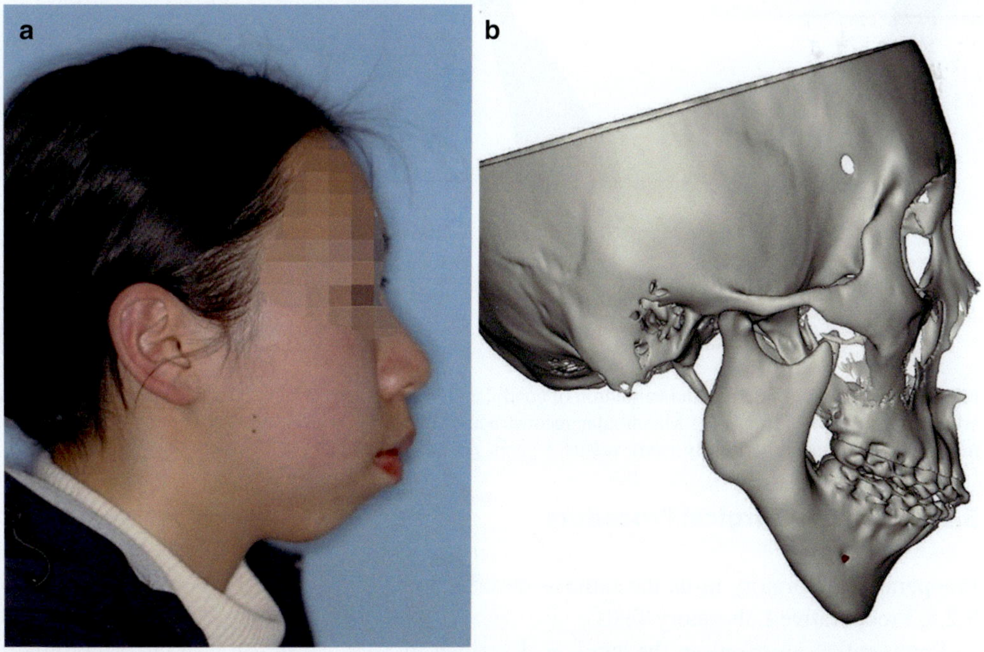

Fig. 5.35 Case K. Facial examination. Mandibular retrognathia, bony Class II deformity with high mandibular and occlusal plane angles. (**a**) Lateral view. (**b**) Preoperative CT reconstruction

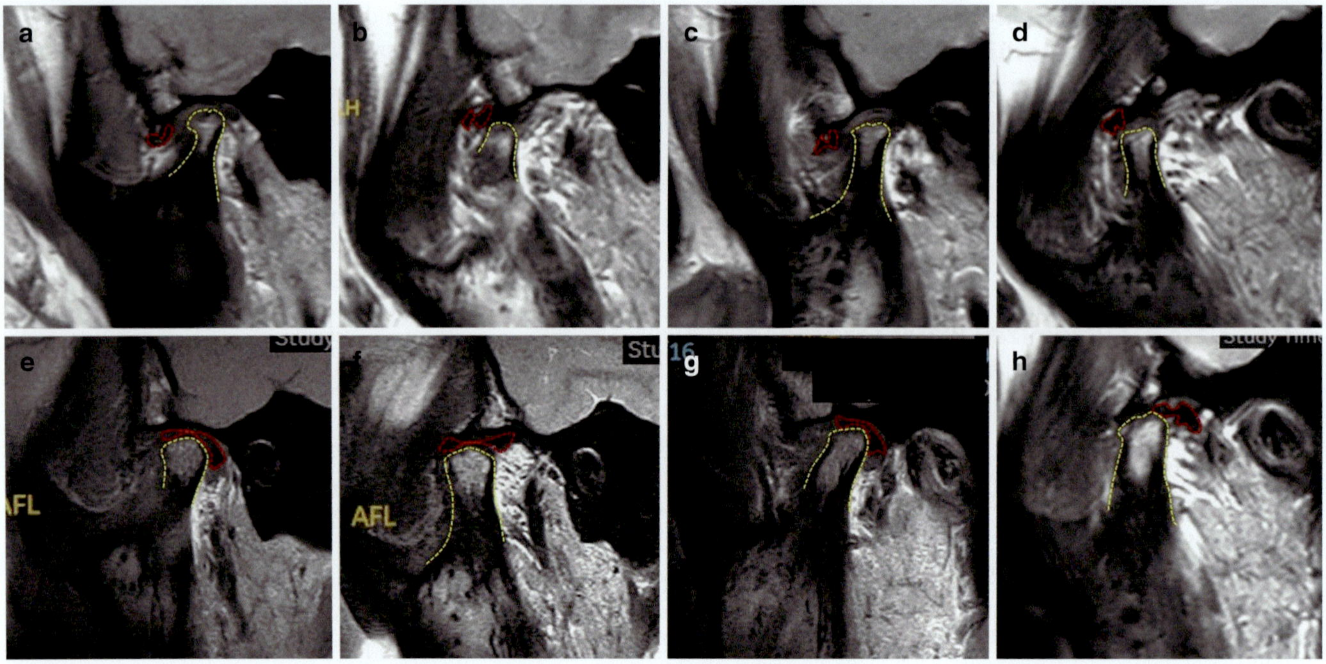

Fig. 5.36 Case K. Preoperative and 2-year postoperative MRIs. Preoperative MRIs showed anterior disc displacement without reduction on both sides. Postoperative MRIs showed normal disc-condylar relationships and thickening of the condylar heads after surgical repositioning; the disc-condylar relationship was stabilized (or even overcorrected). (Yellow dotted lines indicate condylar head; red dotted lines indicate articular disc.). Preoperative (**a**–**d**): (**a**) right close mouth position; (**b**) right open mouth position; (**c**) left close mouth position; (**d**) left open mouth position. Postoperative (**e**–**h**): (**e**) right close mouth position; (**f**) right open mouth position; (**g**) left close mouth position; (**h**) left open mouth position

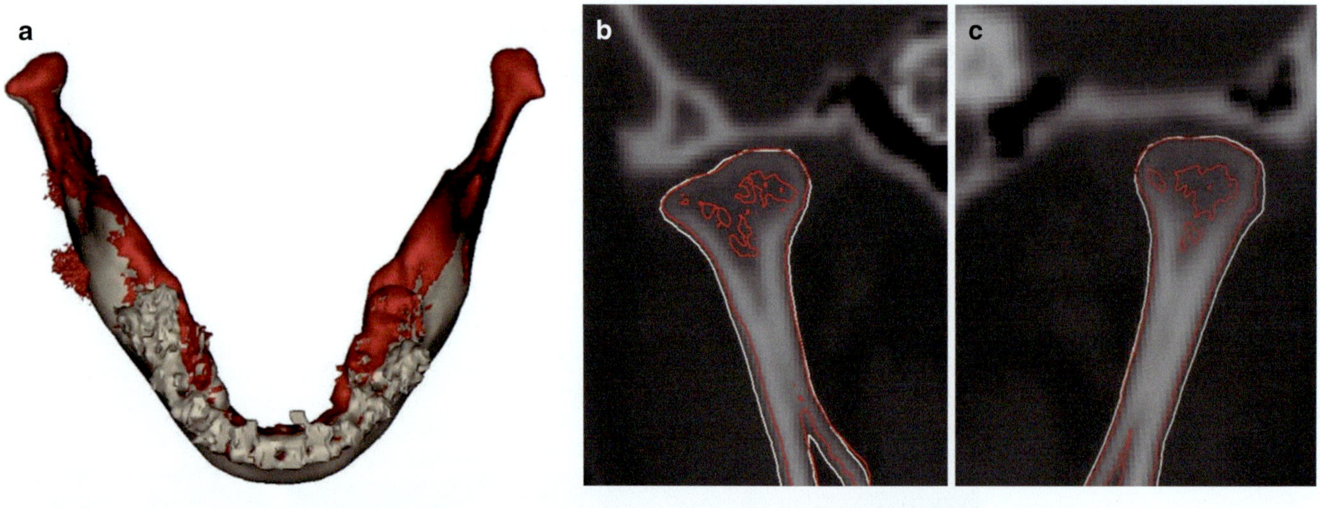

Fig. 5.37 Case K. Follow-up and validation of condylar stability after articular disc repositioning. (**a**) Mandibular reconstruction and alignment at 2 years postoperatively (red) versus 3 years postoperatively (white). (**b**) Good overlap of right coronal contours. (**c**) Good overlap of left coronal contours

5.3.4 Case K. Surgical Procedure

Preoperative laboratory tests: the same as described in Sect. 3.2.5, Preoperative Laboratory Tests.

Preoperative preparation: the same as described in Sect. 3.2.5, Preoperative Preparation.

Surgical sequence and approach: genioplasty with conventional incision exposure, fixation of the cutting guide, guide plate-assisted completion of the osteotomy, and stabilization with the genioplasty fixation plate after anterior extension of the osteotomy block.

Postoperative medical advice and care: daily oral care.

5.3.5 Case K. Postoperative Analysis of Prothesis Implantation Precision

Regular postoperative follow-ups were performed for appearance (facial shape), function (degree of mouth opening, mouth opening shape), and plate evaluation (safety, accuracy).

Immediately postoperatively: accurate positioning of the intraoperative guides, smooth installation of the plates, stabilization of the bilateral condylar position, significant improvement of the lateral shape, and harmonization of the lower third of the facial form (Fig. 5.41). Postoperative CT showed no loosening, dislocation, displacement, or fracture of the plate (Fig. 5.42).

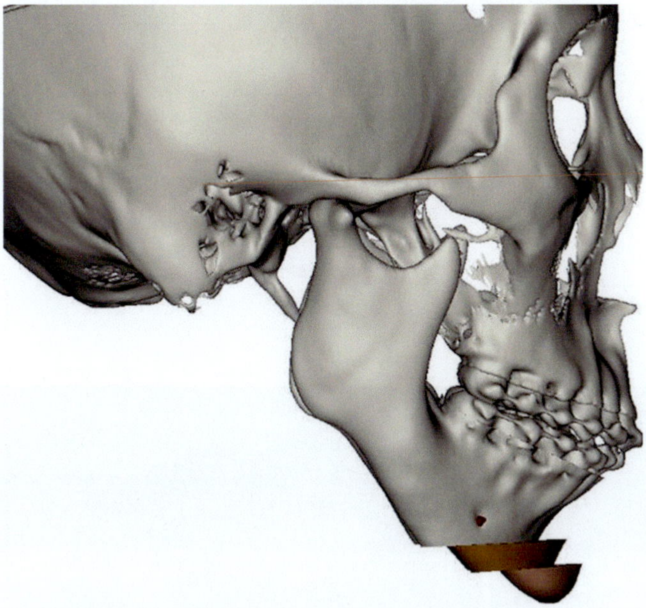

Fig. 5.38 Case K. Design of a double-layer genioplasty osteotomy. The osteotomy line is parallel to the orbital auricular plane, and the chin is moved forward without affecting the rest of the lower third of the face

5.3.6 Case K. Long-Term Follow-Up and Prognosis

- Follow-up 6 months after surgery

There were no complaints of discomfort, the face was well shaped, and there was no redness, swelling, or other reactions in the operative area.

The joint-mandibular-occlusal-facial shape was harmonized, and at the end of orthodontic treatment, the occlusion was significantly improved from the preoperative period (Fig. 5.43).

Mouth opening 36 mm, lateral movement 5 mm to the right and 6 mm to the left.

Evaluation of the bone graft fixation plate: there were no complications such as rejection, loosening, breakage, ectopic osteogenesis, and material allergy. The position of the chin was significantly improved after surgery compared with the preoperative period, and the surgical result was stable (Figs. 5.44 and 5.45).

- 2-year postoperative follow-up

The degree of mouth opening was 37 mm, and the rest was the same as the 1-year postoperative follow-up.

5.3.7 Case K. Advantages and Disadvantages

- Advantages

Less invasive, the procedure is quick and precise and drastically improves the shape of the chin.

- Disadvantages

None currently.

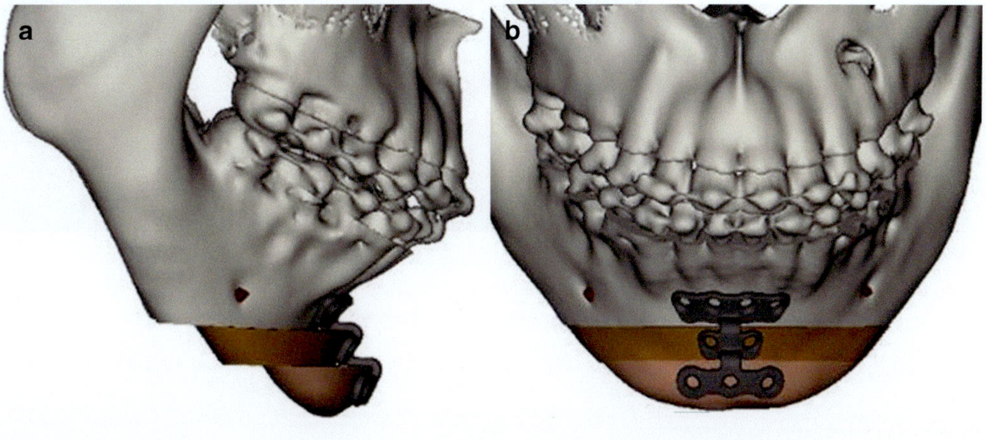

Fig. 5.39 Case K. Virtual design of the fixation plate for a double-layer chin advancement. The line of advancement parallels Frankfort horizontal, so it does not alter the height of the lower 1/3 of the face. (**a**) Lateral view. (**b**) Frontal view

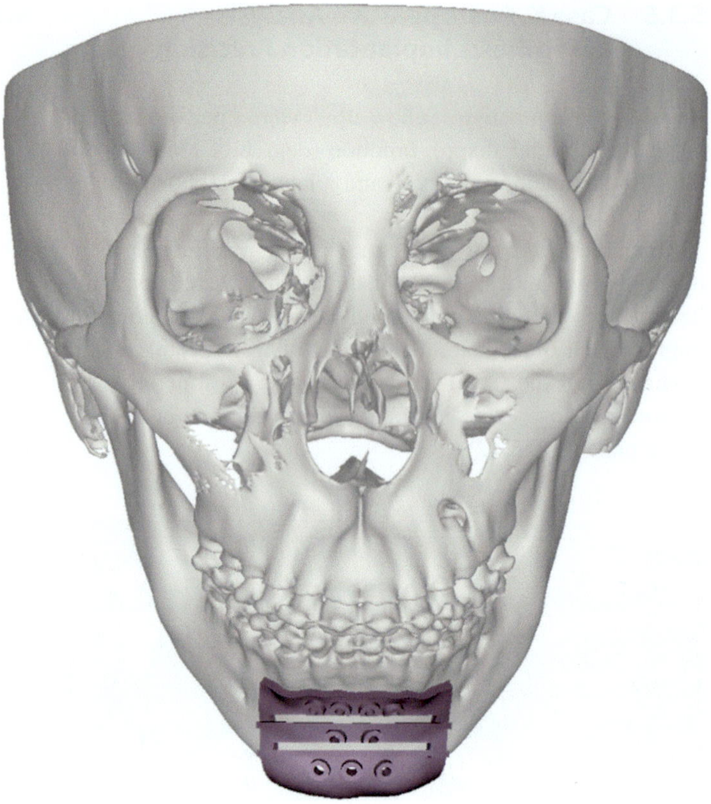

Fig. 5.40 Case K. Double osteotomy cutting guide design, with the guide screw holes planned to match those of the genioplasty fixation plate

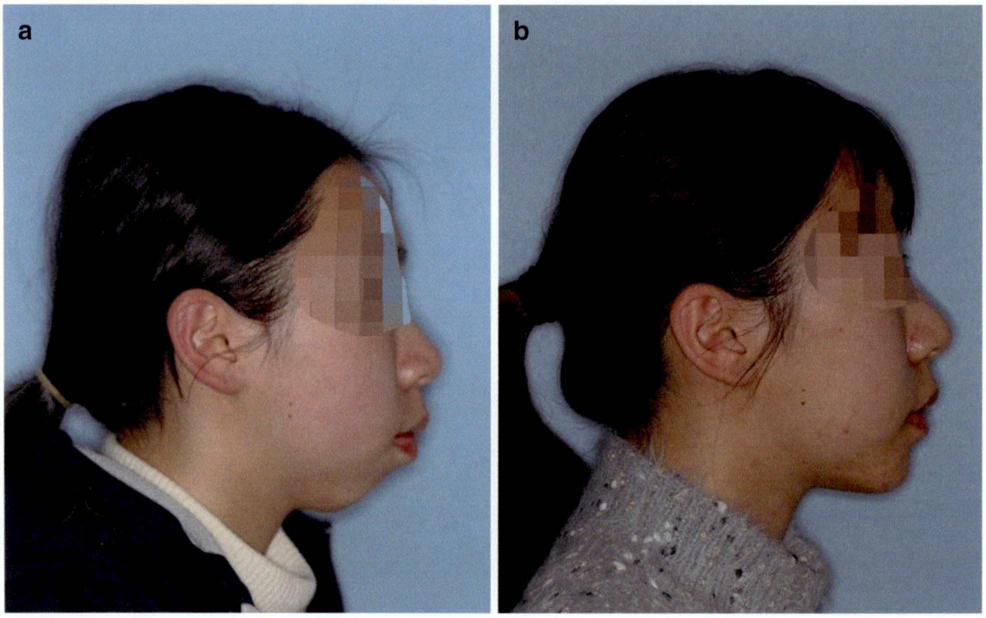

Fig. 5.41 Case K. Comparison of preoperative and postoperative lateral views. Significant improvement in the lateral profile and harmonization of the lower third of the face after surgery. (**a**) Preoperative lateral view. (**b**) Postoperative lateral view

Fig. 5.42 Case K. Immediate postoperative CT reconstruction. There was no loosening, dislocation, displacement, or fracture of the plate

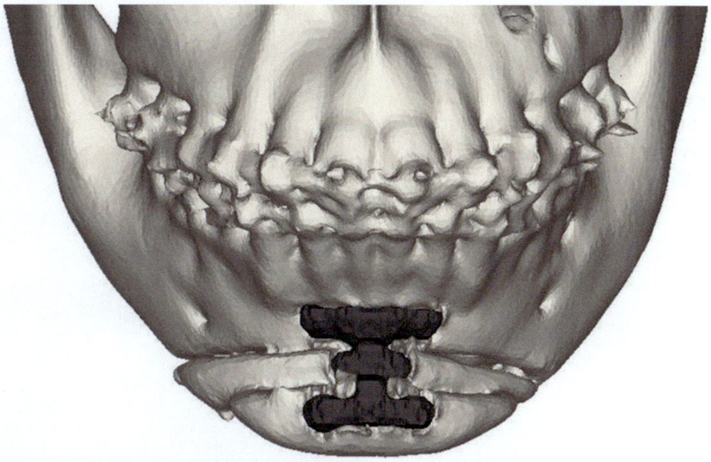

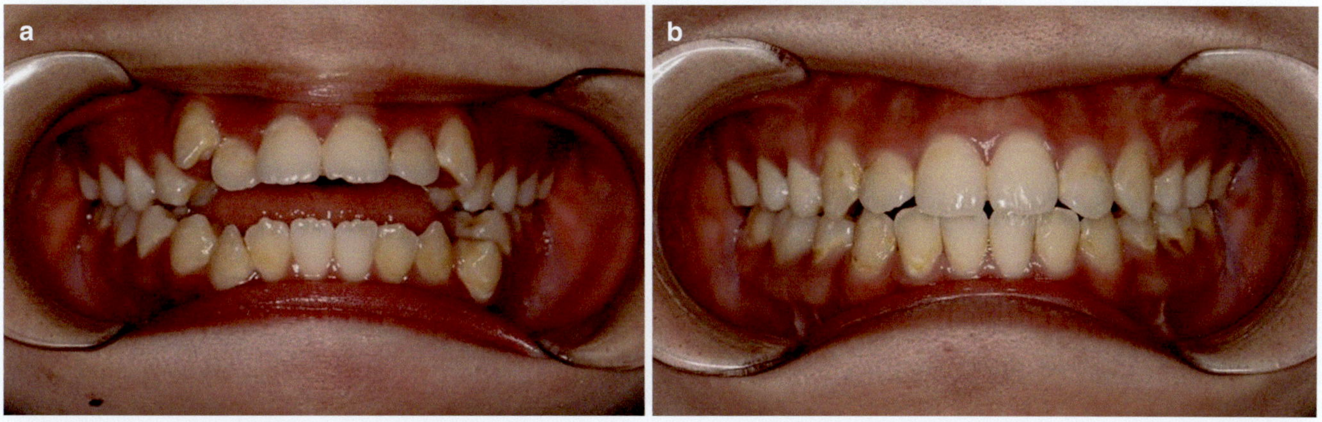

Fig. 5.43 Case K. Comparison of occlusion before and after orthodontic treatment, showing significant improvement in occlusion. (**a**) Preoperative occlusion. (**b**) Occlusion after completion of orthodontic treatment (6 months postoperatively)

Fig. 5.44 Case K. Six-month postoperative panoramic view. There was no loosening, displacement, dislocation, or fracture of the genioplasty fixation plate

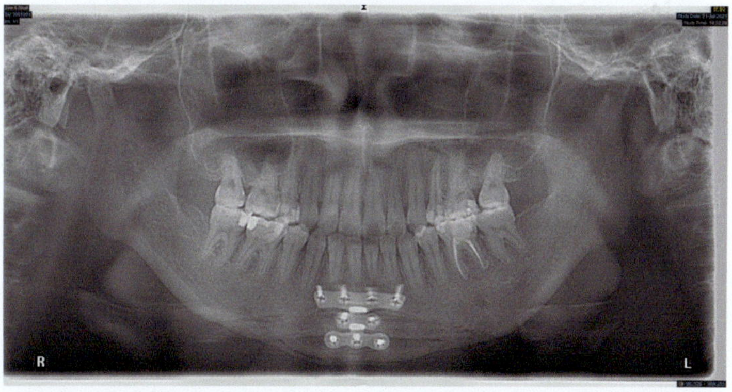

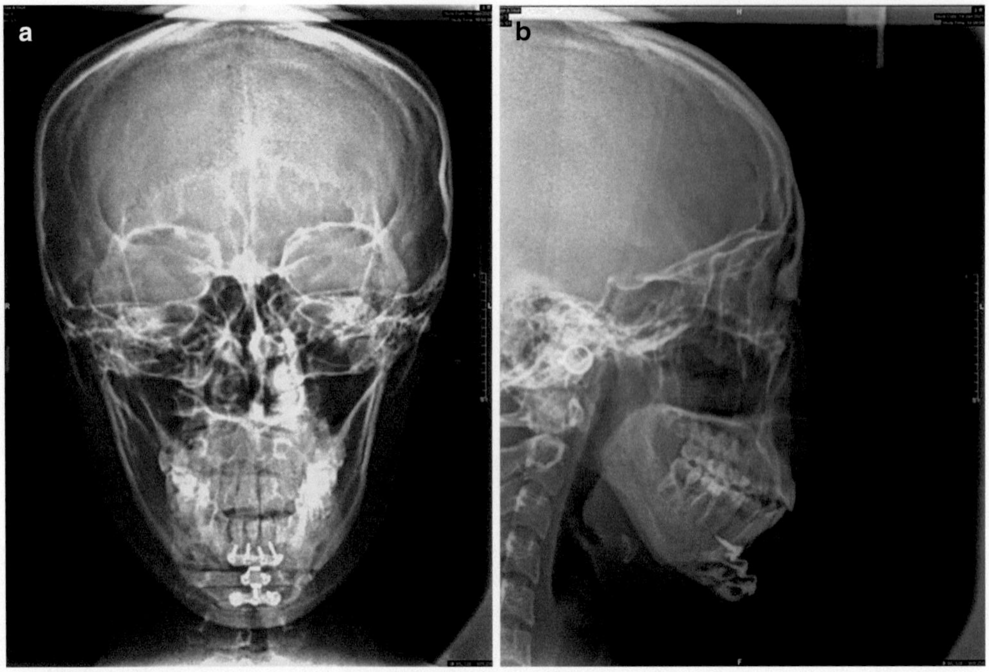

Fig. 5.45 Case K. Six-month postoperative cephalometric film. The position of the genioplasty fixation plate is stable, and the bone is healing well. (**a**) Frontal view. (**b**) Lateral view

6 Prosthetic Reconstruction of Combined Temporomandibular TMJ-Skull Base Diseases

Minjie Chen, Jisi Zheng, Hao Wu, Zhaoyan Wang, and Chi Yang

This chapter addresses Class IIIa of Yang's new classification, which deals with combined temporomandibular joint (TMJ) and skull base diseases affecting the skull base and the joints and involving the ear canals and infratemporal fossa. This Class IIIa covers cases in which the condyle cannot be preserved, and it falls under the larger category of complexes involving the upward connections of the articular joint.

The TMJ is located centrally in the lateral view of the skull, above the skull base (the articular fossa is at the subtemporal portion of the skull base, with its surface sitting approximately 1 mm from the nearest surface of the brain), behind the ear canal (the anterior wall of the ear canal is the posterior wall of the articular fossa), and within the inferior side of the temporal fossa (separated only by the thin articular capsule). This positioning gives us some sense of the delicacy of surgery in this area.

When a tumor in this region has affected two or more anatomical regions, tumor removal will result in a combined joint and skull base defect, the repair and reconstruction of which is a formidable challenge for oral and maxillofacial surgery, otorhinolaryngology, and neurosurgery. The main challenges are:

- Precise osteotomy of the tumor in resection to avoid recurrence and facilitate reconstruction
- Precise reconstruction of bone defects to restore joint function, mastication function, and craniomaxillofacial morphology
- Avoiding the need to harvest autogenous bone, to reduce trauma for the patient and surgical difficulty and risk.

Only the customized prosthesis can meet the above requirements, given the large scope of rehabilitation and reconstruction. There are few systematic reports of similar reconstruction methods at home and abroad that achieve satisfactory therapeutic results.

Based on the successful experience of applying total joint prostheses designed personally for the individual, the author's team extended the coverage of the prosthesis according to the needs for repair and reconstruction, and constructed a customized TMJ-skull base prosthesis system that can encompass the base of the skull, the lateral cranium, and the zygomatic arch. This prosthesis system has been gradually optimized and perfected and has been clinically applied and followed up for the longest time. It has shown satisfactory efficacy, and it will be described in detail in explaining the design and application of the system.

6.1 Overview

This section proposes a definition and a new classification of joint-craniofacial diseases, and after reviewing traditional prosthetic reconstruction methods and the recurrent problems with them, it proposes an innovative reconstruction method utilizing customized temporomandibular joint (TMJ)-craniofacial joint prostheses and their digital design process. The aim is to provide new concepts and techniques for specialists in oral and maxillofacial surgery, otorhinolaryngology, and neurosurgery to deal with this kind of complex and difficult disease.

6.1.1 Definition of Combined TMJ-Skull Base Lesions

This definition applies to cases where the joints and the skull base are jointly involved in the lesion. It is caused by tumors, tumorlike lesions, and congenital diseases in the joints and skull base area and may involve the ear canal or the infratemporal fossa and may also invade important peripheral nerves (facial nerve and mandibular branch of the trigeminal nerve) and blood vessels (internal carotid artery, internal jugular

Minjie C. · Jisi Z. · Hao W. · Zhaoyan W. · Chi Y. (✉)
Shanghai Ninth People's Hospital, Shanghai Jiao Tong University School of Medicine, Shanghai, China

© People's Medical Publishing House, PR of China 2025

Chi Y. (ed.), *Atlas of Customized TMJ-Cranio-Jaw Prosthesis*, https://doi.org/10.1007/978-981-95-0611-8_6

vein, and internal maxillary artery and vein). Clinical manifestations are usually characterized by limitation of mouth opening and swelling and pain in the preauricular and temporal regions, sometimes accompanied by hearing loss or numbness of the lower lip. The treatment of choice is surgical resection, often requiring collaboration between TMJ surgeon, Ear, Nose and Throat (ENT) surgeon, and neurosurgeon, and opinions vary as to whether and how TMJ-skull base reconstruction is required.

6.1.2 Classification of Combined TMJ-Skull Base Lesions

The classification of joint-craniofacial joint diseases has not been clearly reported in the past, nor is there a consensus. The author has proposed two classifications: (1) classification according to the origin of the disease and (2) classification according to the scope of the disease, and the contents of this chapter and Chap. 7 are mainly planned according to this classification. This classification according to scope is related to the design of prostheses.

6.1.2.1 Classification According to the Origin of the Lesion

Previously, the lesions were divided into categories according to their origin: Category I is a primary temporal bone lesion that invades the articular fossa and even involves the entire joint and surrounding tissues, and the most common type of this lesion is a giant cell lesion of the temporal bone. This category can be further divided into two subcategories: Category Ia involves only the articular fossa and supra-articular cavity, with a normal disc and condyle (Fig. 6.1), and Category Ib involves the entire joint and surrounding tissues (Fig. 6.2).

Class II is a primary lesion of the joint that invades the skull base, causing perforation of the skull base and protrusion into the skull, such as osteochondroma of the condyle, synovial chondromatosis, or diffuse giant cell tumor of the tendon sheath (Fig. 6.3).

6.1.2.2 Classification According to the Extent of the Lesion

The author has proposed a new classification based on the extent of the lesion, as follows:

- Class I (condyle preserved) is the involvement of the skull base and joint fossa, but not protruding into the infratemporal fossa, and the condyles and disc are not involved or only have synovial involvement, suggesting that the condyles and disc may be preserved.
- Class II (condyle temporarily moved aside but preserved) is the involvement of the skull base and joint fossa and protruding into the infratemporal fossa, but the condyles and disc are not involved or only have synovial involvement, suggesting that the condyles and disc may be preserved, but the condyles must be temporarily cut in order to remove the tumor of the infratemporal fossa.
- Class III (condyle not preserved) is the involvement of the skull base, articular fossa, condyle, and articular disc, but not exceeding the mandibular foramen.
- Class IV (condyle not preserved, jaw much diseased) is the involvement of the skull base, articular fossa, condyle, and articular disc and exceeding the mandibular foramen (Fig. 6.4).

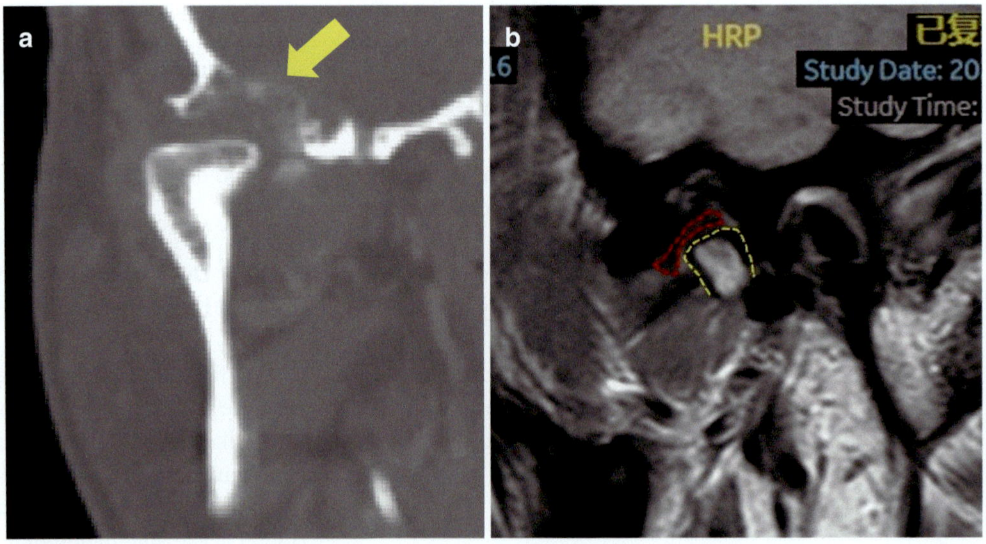

Fig. 6.1 Primary temporal bone giant cell lesion involving the skull base and articular fossa (subcategory Ia). The yellow arrow points to bone destruction in the articular fossa and upper-articular cavity, and the red dotted line shows the articular disc with good positional morphology. (**a**) Maxillofacial CT; (**b**) MRI of the joints, with the articular disc shown by the red dotted line and the condyle outlined with the yellow dotted line

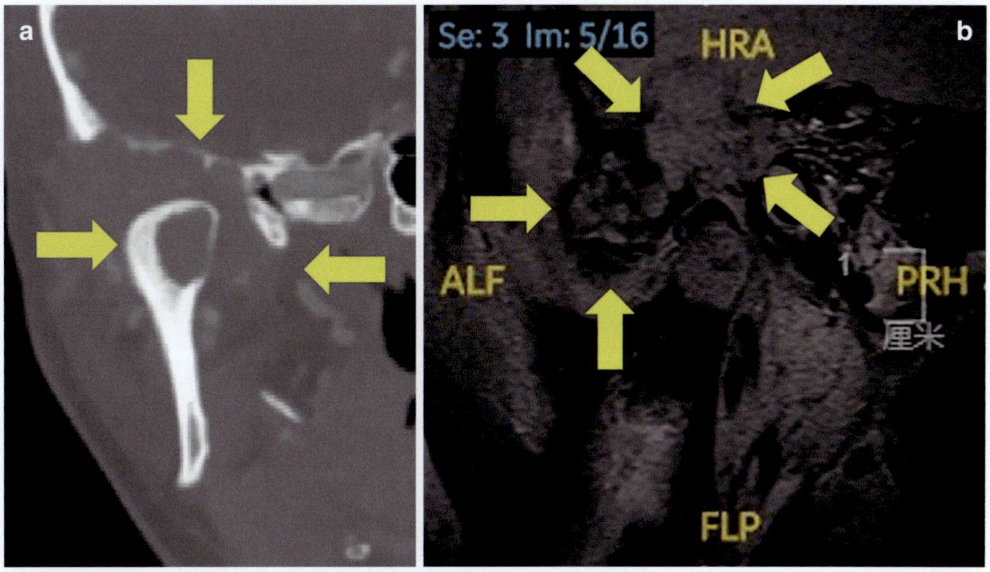

Fig. 6.2 Primary giant cell lesion of the temporal bone involving the skull base, total joint, and surrounding tissues (Class Ib). Yellow arrows indicate destruction of the skull base, total joints, and surrounding tissues. (**a**) Maxillofacial CT. (**b**) Joint MRI

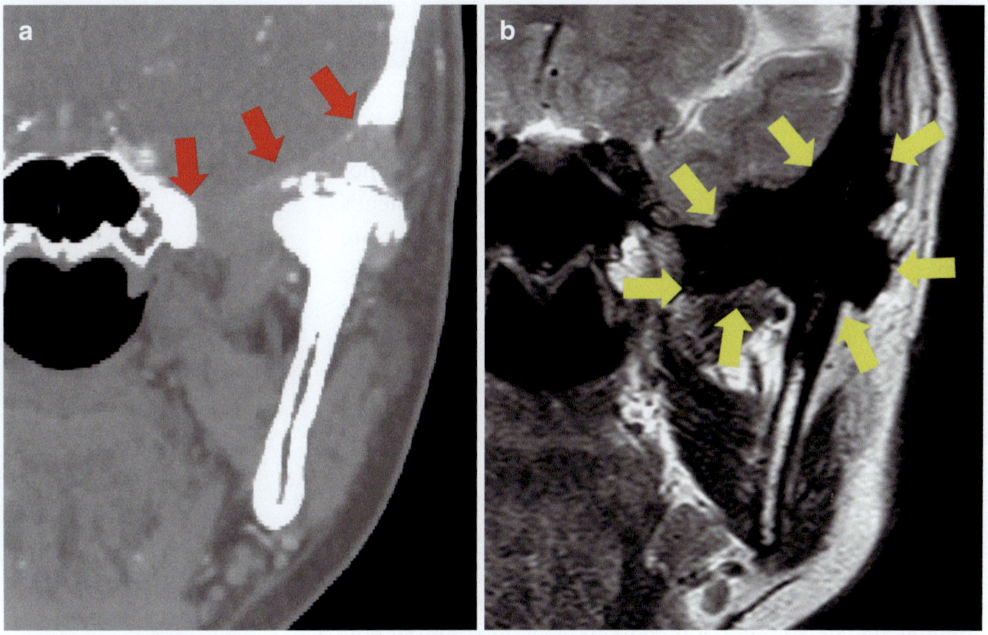

Fig. 6.3 Synovial chondrosarcoma causing perforation of the skull base (Class II). Yellow arrows show articular primary synovial chondrosarcoma encroaching into the skull base causing bone destruction of the skull base and protruding into the skull. (**a**) Maxillofacial CT (red arrows show the extent of the perforation of the skull base). (**b**) Maxillofacial MRI (yellow arrows show the lesion at the skull base)

6.1.3 Traditional Prosthetic Reconstruction of Combined TMJ-Skull Base Lesions

Traditional repair and reconstruction of TMJ-skull base lesions include reconstruction utilizing soft tissue flap filling, skull base titanium mesh, and autologous bone. However, these repair and reconstruction methods have many shortcomings and drawbacks that need to be improved.

6.1.3.1 Previous Methods of Resection of Combined TMJ-Skull Base Lesions

The conventional surgical approach for TMJ-skull base diseases primarily utilizes postauricular and hemicoronal incisions, requiring drilling of the superior external auditory canal and resection of lateral temporal bone and glenoid fossa to expose tumors. For benign or borderline tumors, intracapsular enucleation is typically performed in a top-

Fig. 6.4 Classification of TMJ-skull base lesions. (Green illustrates the tumor.) (**a**) Class I, condyle can be preserved. (**b**) Class II, the condyle should be temporarily cut in order to remove the tumor. (**c**) Class III, the condyle cannot be preserved, but the lesion does not exceed the mandibular foramen. (**d**) Class IV, the condyle cannot be preserved, and the lesion exceeds the mandibular foramen

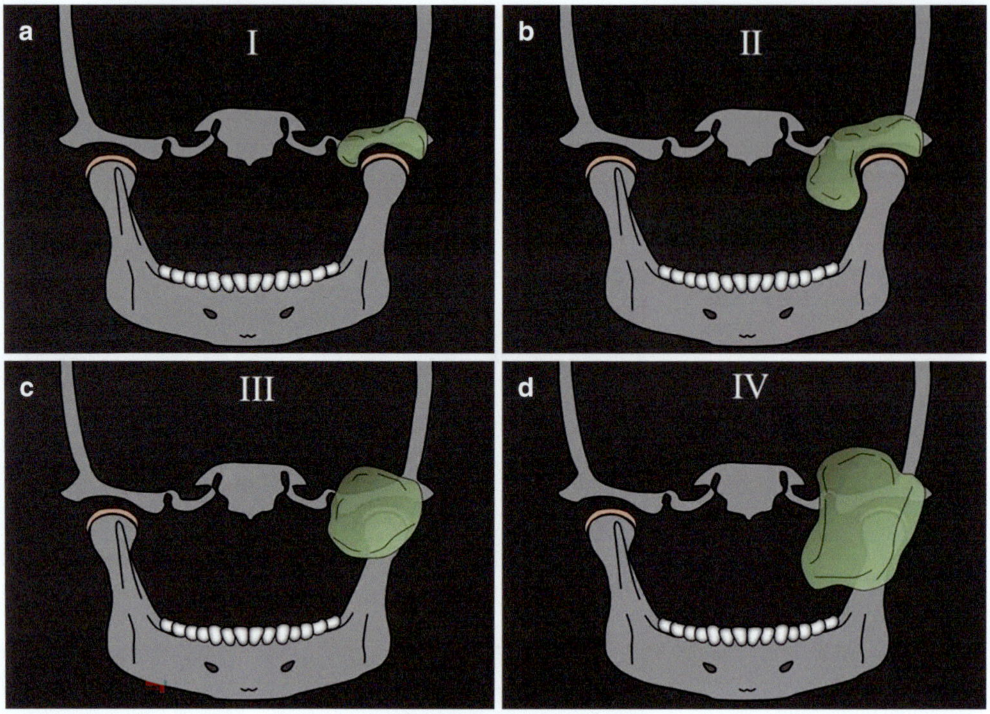

down manner, with condylectomy executed when the tumor encases the condylar neck. However, the author contends that this approach often leads to insufficient tumor exposure (Fig. 6.5), making en bloc resection challenging and resulting in unnecessary condylar sacrifice. Complete tumor exposure and intact removal are essential for minimizing recurrence rates.

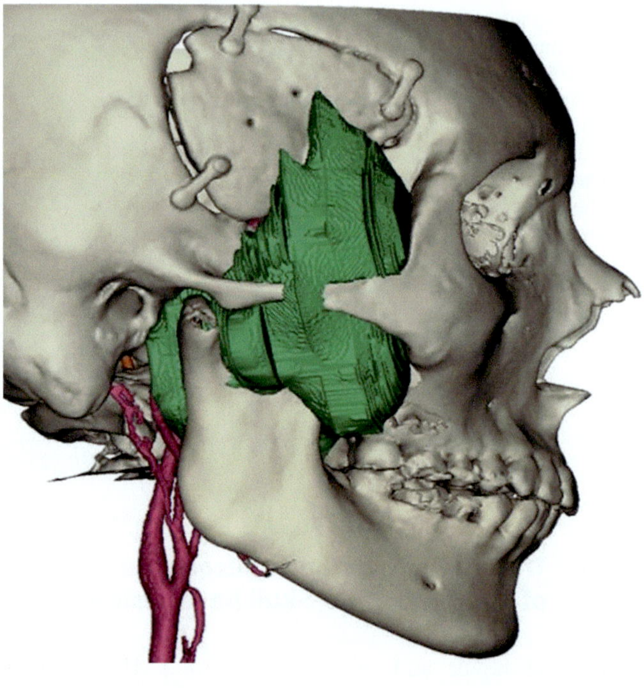

Fig. 6.5 In this case, inadequate exposure of the tumor during surgery on a combined TMJ-skull base lesion resulted in incomplete removal of the extracranial portion of the tumor, and this led to postoperative recurrence

6.1.3.2 Previous Restorations for TMJ-Skull Base Combination Lesions

The current prevalent approach across oral-maxillofacial surgery, otolaryngology, and neurosurgical specialties involves using temporalis muscle flaps for cavity obliteration without bony reconstruction (Fig. 6.6). While this method remains widely adopted, it inevitably leads to temporal hollowing and partial loss of joint function, which constitute the primary quality-of-life concerns for patients postoperatively.

The reconstruction of skull base defects with titanium mesh supplemented by fat grafts to separate the dura mater can partially restore facial contour but demonstrates limited load-bearing capacity for masticatory forces, consequently compromising the patient's masticatory efficiency (Fig. 6.7).

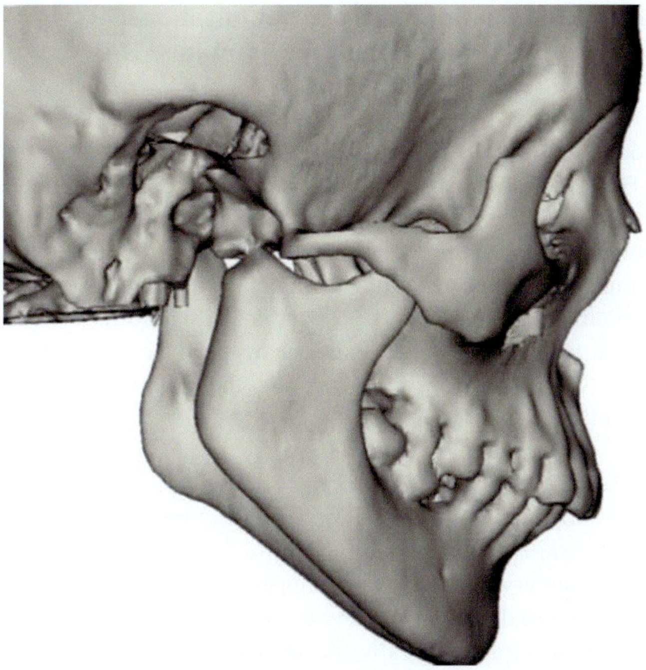

Fig. 6.6 In this case, defective bone tissue was not reconstructed after resection of a combined TMJ-skull base lesion

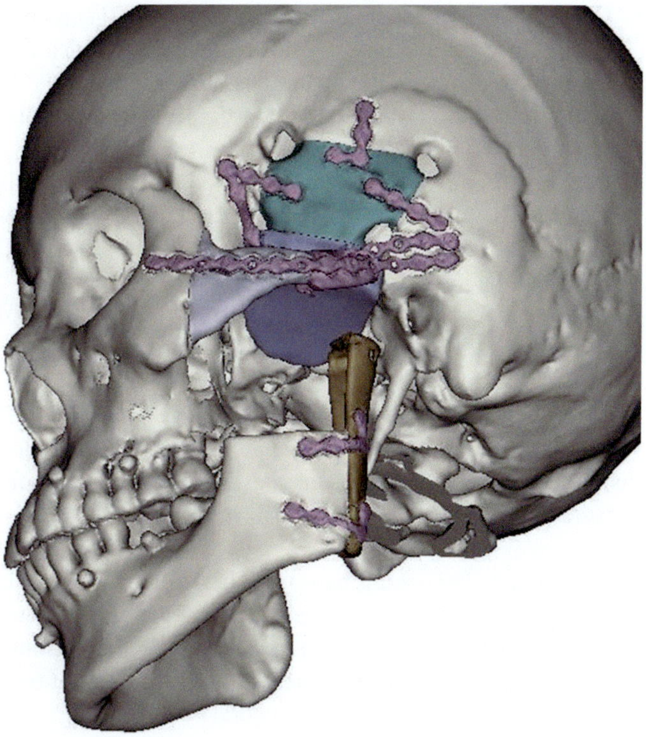

Fig. 6.8 Autologous iliac bone (purple) repair of the skull base after resection of a combined TMJ-skull base lesion and hemi-sternoclavicular joint repair of the condyle. The zygomatic arch (light purple) and temporal bone (blue) were temporarily resected and moved aside to remove the tumor and then reattached

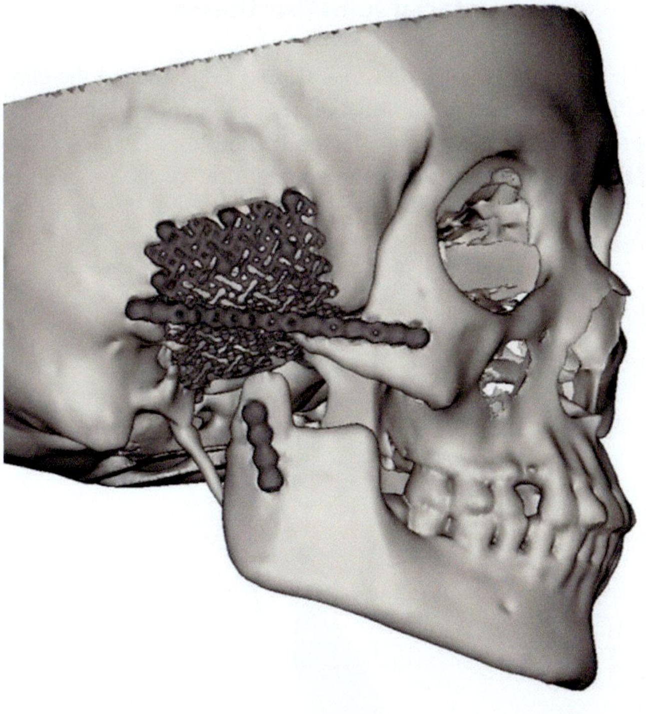

Fig. 6.7 Titanium mesh (dark gray) repair of the skull after resection of a combined TMJ-skull base lesion. The condyle was not reconstructed

The author has employed autologous bone grafts for skull base reconstruction using split-thickness iliac crest or temporal bone grafts, combined with either free rib cartilage grafts or pedicled hemi-sternoclavicular joint transfers for condylar reconstruction (Fig. 6.8). This approach has demonstrated satisfactory therapeutic outcomes, effectively restoring both facial contour and joint function. However, donor site morbidity and the technical complexity of the reconstructive procedure remain significant clinical challenges.

6.1.4 Innovative Prosthetic Reconstruction with Customized Combined TMJ-Skull Base Prosthesis

For Class III and IV lesions in the new classification, we constructed personalized TMJ-skull base prosthesis design plans and surgical plans. We adopted digital design, 3D printing, and the 5-axis machining process to customize the TMJ-skull base prostheses, aiming to accurately resect the lesions and repair the joint and the base of the skull at the same time, while making the complex reconstruction simple, accurate, stable, and efficient.

The reconstruction options for each type of case and the chapters of this book where they are addressed are summarized as follows:

- Class I (condyle can be preserved) and Class II (condyle temporarily cut and moved aside to clear the tumor): it is appropriate to use the skull base-fossa prosthesis to achieve the preservation of the articular disc, condylar process, and lateral pterygoid muscle; see Chap. 7.
- Class III (condyle cannot be preserved, but the lesion is small): it is appropriate to use the TMJ-skull base prosthesis to realize the combined reconstruction of the skull base and the joints; see cases in the following sections.

6.1.4.1 Types of Design of TMJ-Skull Base Prostheses

Two types of TMJ-skull base prostheses have been designed (but in future applications not limited to two), and these are distinguished by differences in the skull base component prosthesis design and its means of fixation.

- Edge-fixed TMJ-skull base prosthesis: this prosthesis relies on the peripheral bone tissue of the lateral skull base remaining after defect removal to hold the titanium skull base prosthesis component in place, with additional titanium plate fixation of the temporal bone flap (Fig. 6.9).
- Temporal bone flap-fixing TMJ-skull base prosthesis: this prosthesis is designed to serve to simultaneously attach the temporal bone flap and the prosthesis. The design is based on the biological stress lines, and it is effective in absorbing occlusal forces. It eliminates the need for additional titanium plates to reattach the temporal bone flap at the surgical opening (Fig. 6.10).

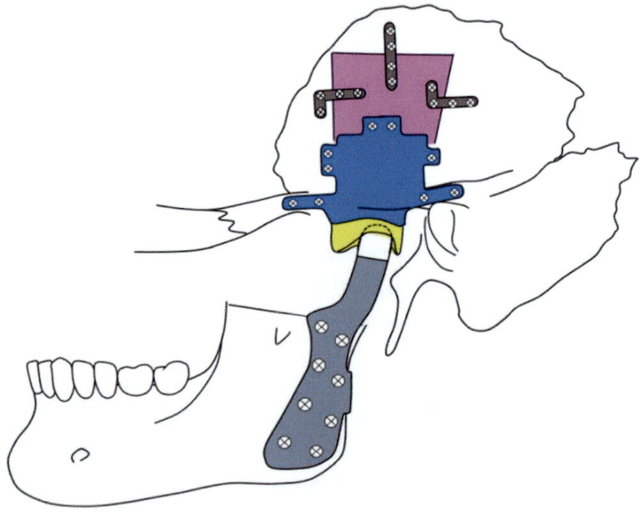

Fig. 6.9 Edge-fixed TMJ-skull base prosthesis. Blue shows the titanium skull base component, yellow shows the articular fossa component of ultrahigh-molecular-weight polyethylene, gray shows the mandibular extension component, white between yellow and gray shows the condylar head of the prosthesis, bright pink shows the temporal bone flap opening with bone replaced in original position after tumor removal, and dark gray shows the titanium fixation plates used for reattachment of the temporal bone flap

6.1.4.2 Indications and Contraindications for Application of the Combined TMJ-Skull Base Prostheses

6.1.4.2.1 Indications

This application is indicated for combined joint-craniofacial lesions in adults, mainly in cases of benign or borderline tumor and tumorlike lesions, in cases where malignant tumors are expected to be completely resected, quiescent inflammatory lesions, post-surgically acquired joint-craniofacial union defects, and osteolysis in the stable phase, and where both the condyle and the articular disc are involved.

6.1.4.2.2 Contraindications

This application should be used with caution, mainly in the acute stage of inflammatory lesions, in cases with incomplete surgery for malignant tumors, in adolescents during growth and development, and if soft tissue is insufficient to cover the implant area after defect removal.

6.1.5 General Digital Design Process for Customized Combined TMJ-Craniofacial Joint Prostheses

This chapter focuses on Class III and IV lesions in the classification of joint-craniofacial lesions (condyle cannot be preserved, lesion extends to the mandible), of which Class III is more common. So, the general flow of the procedures

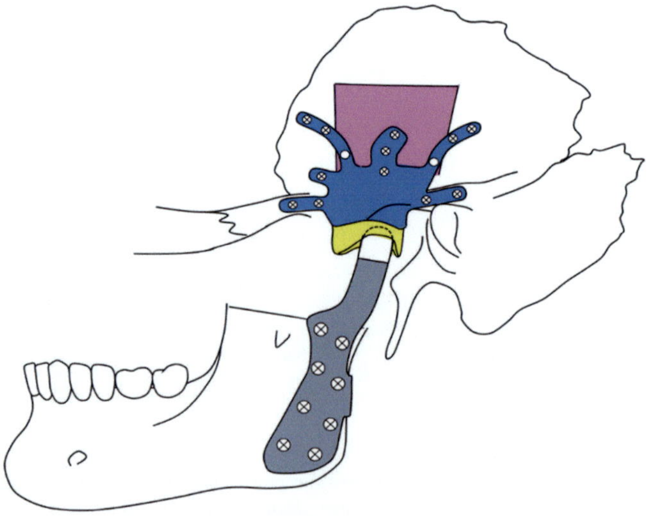

Fig. 6.10 Temporal bone flap-fixing TMJ-skull base prosthesis. As in Fig. 6.9, blue shows the titanium skull base component, yellow shows the articular socket component made of UHMWPE, gray shows the mandibular extension, white between yellow and gray shows the condylar head, and bright pink shows the temporal bone as repositioned after intraoperative opening

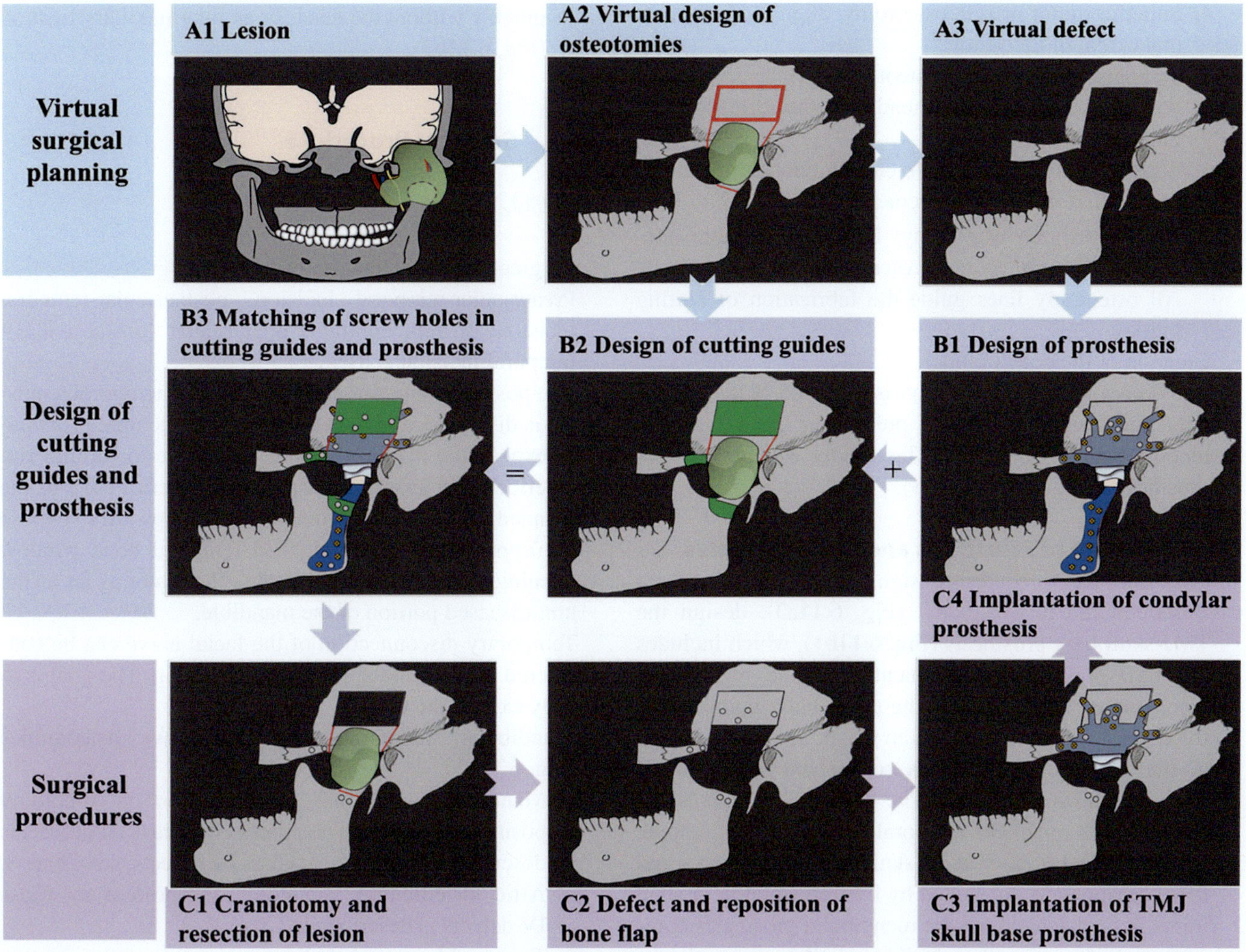

Fig. 6.11 The general flow of surgical design and procedures for digitally designed TMJ-skull base prostheses. (**a1**) From 3D reconstruction based on CT data, define the scope of the lesion (transparent light green), and mark the course of the mandibular nerve (yellow), the internal carotid artery (red), and the internal jugular vein (blue—between the red and yellow). (**a2**) Design the osteotomy lines (red lines), while protecting the ear canal. (**a3**) Obtain the defect space model of the skull after osteotomies. (**b1**) Design the shape of the prosthesis (blue and gray) based on the defect model. (**b2**) Design the cutting guides (green) according to the osteotomy lines. (**b3**) Transfer the position of the prosthesis screw holes to the cutting guides. (**c1**) Surgically perform the osteotomies according to the fixed placement of the cutting guides. (**c2**) Reimplant the temporal bone flap after resection of the lesion. (**c3**) Install the upper components of the TMJ-skull base prosthesis. (**c4**) Install the mandibular component of the prosthesis

is exemplified (Fig. 6.11) by the process for Class III and IV lesions, encompassing three aspects, i.e., simulated surgery for osteotomies for the lesion removal and reconstruction, prosthesis and cutting guides design (here in Sect. 6.1.5), and surgical procedure (Sect. 6.1.6).

6.1.5.1 Simulated Surgery for Osteotomies for Lesion Removal and Reconstruction

- Plan the scope of lesion: CT datasets in DICOM format are processed through surgical planning software to delineate pathological boundaries. Critical anatomical structures (e.g., foramen ovale, auditory canal) require explicit tagging of the mandibular nerve, facial nerve, internal carotid/jugular vessels, and auricular components (Fig. 6.11a1).
- Design of osteotomy lines:
  1. Anterior tumor margin osteotomy: ensures safe lesion resection.
  2. Mandibular osteotomy: facilitates pathological tissue removal. For Class IV disease, a dedicated osteotomy line is designed to mobilize the inferior alveolar neurovascular bundle.
  3. Posterior tumor margin osteotomy: maximizes auricular structure preservation while achieving complete resection.

4. Superior tumor margin osteotomy: aligns with the cranial extent of the lesion.
5. Temporal bone window osteotomy:
   Anterior/posterior lines extend from the corresponding tumor margins.
   Superior line adapts to intracranial tumor dimensions and brain retraction requirements (Fig. 6.11a2).
6. Zygomatic arch osteotomy: balances exposure adequacy with architectural preservation.
   All osteotomy lines guide the fabrication of cutting guides.

- Creation of the defect model
  The defect left after the lesion is removed at the osteotomy lines, with the goal of preserving the nerves and blood vessels, is modeled. This model will be used for prosthesis design (Fig. 6.11a3).

6.1.5.2 Design of Prosthesis and Cutting Guides

- TMJ-skull base prosthesis design:
  Based on the defect model (Fig. 6.11a3), design the TMJ-skull base prosthesis (Fig. 6.11b1), which includes the TMJ-skull base components and the mandibular components. The design of the mandibular components for Class III defects is shown in Chap. 3, and the design of the mandibular prosthesis component for Class IV defects is shown in Chap. 8. The TMJ-skull base prosthesis is used to repair the temporal bone, zygomatic bone, and fossa, and it consists of skull base components and fossa components connected by friction welding or snap joints. It is matched with the mandibular prosthesis components to form together the TMJ-skull base prosthesis. The final design of the prosthesis screw holes (screw holes shared with the cutting guides) allows the skull base and articular socket components of the prosthesis to be stabilized in position flush with the temporal bone and zygomatic bone, plus the mandibular prosthesis component smoothly aligned with the residual mandible.
- Osteotomy positioning guides' design:
  Following the osteotomy lines (Fig. 6.11a2), design the osteotomy positioning guides.
  1. Mandibular cutting guide design: for Class III defects, see Chap. 3, and for Class IV defects, see Chap. 8.
  2. Skull base-articular fossa cutting guides: these encompass the temporal bone window opening, anterior and posterior skull base osteotomies, and zygomatic arch osteotomies, as described in Case L (Fig. 6.11b2).
  3. Match the cutting guide screw holes to the prosthesis screw holes: overlay Fig. 6.11b1 and B2 on the image to determine the screw holes of the cutting guides according to the position of the prosthesis screw holes. The positioning is such that not only is the osteotomy precise, but the prosthesis can be fitted more easily and quickly without the need for an intermaxillary ligation (Fig. 6.11b3).

6.1.6 Surgical Procedure

Yang Chi, Zheng Jisi, and Chen Minjie

- Surgical approach and tumor exposure:
  Preauricular-temporal incision, postauricular-temporal incision, or submandibular-preauricular (postauricular)-temporal incision is used.
  The posterior-superior attachment of the temporalis muscle is dissected, and then the outer flesh is turned forward to expose the zygomatic bone and posterior orbital rim anteriorly, backward to the farthest posterior edge of the planned implantation of the prosthesis, upward to expose the upper edge of the planned temporal bone window opening, and downward to expose the tumor as far as the non-diseased portion of the mandible.
  Temporary disconnection of the facial nerve can be considered appropriate if the tumor is too big. The goal is to fully expose the tumor.
- Mandibular, temporal, and skull base osteotomies (Fig. 6.11c1):
  1. Mandibular osteotomy after fixation of osteotomy positioning guides. The process for Class III defects is described in Chap. 3; for Class IV defects, see Chap. 8. Articular eminence osteotomy: the process for Class IV defects is described in Chap. 8.
  2. Temporal bone and skull base osteotomy after fixation of the osteotomy positioning guide plates. Use a piezosurgery to perform temporal bone window opening, skull base osteotomy, and zygomatic arch truncation, respectively, as described in Case L.
- Prosthesis installation:
  1. Place the temporal bone flap back into the cranium window opening (Fig. 6.11c2).
  2. Implant the upper components of the TMJ-skull base prosthesis according to the position of the screw holes left by the cutting guides and check the degree of affinity between the prosthesis and the bone surface to set the precise position of the prosthesis. Complete the fixation with the screws.
  3. Install the mandibular component of the prosthesis, while ensuring that the occlusal relationship is matching and stable. See Chap. 3 (Fig. 6.11c3).
- Soft tissue management: intraoperative dural rupture can be repaired by suturing, fascia, or patch grafting. The space between the brain tissue and the skull base-articular fossa prosthesis is filled with free fat grafts, while dead spaces around the mandibular prosthesis are

packed with buccal fat pads or free fat grafts. If combined with otolaryngology procedures such as radical mastoidectomy, radical middle ear surgery, or eustachian tube closure, the resulting cavities can also be filled with free fat grafts.

6.2 Prosthetic Reconstruction Techniques for Customized TMJ-Skull Base Combined Prosthesis

Following the definition and classification of TMJ-skull base lesions, this section focuses on two clinical cases that exemplify the excellent results of customized joint prostheses in clinical practice. These cases illustrate Class III in the classification of the scope of the lesion, i.e., the condyle cannot be preserved, but the lesion does not extend beyond the mandibular foramen.

- Case L: This case demonstrates application of a combined TMJ-skull base prosthesis to repair a TMJ-skull base defect after resection of a giant osteochondroma. After much experience with total joint prostheses, the author's team took the lead in designing the combined TMJ-skull base prosthesis, which consists of a skull base-joint fossa prosthesis and a mandibular prosthesis together. This is the edge-fixed prosthesis shown in Fig. 6.9, with square edges and many small titanium plates for fixation of the temporal bone flap window. The innovation is that the 3D-printed titanium alloy skull base component and the ultrahigh-molecular-weight polyethylene joint fossa component constitute a stable connection, even with the movement of the joint, and together, they can realize the restoration of the skull base and the joint structure and function, while avoiding the use of autologous bone graft.
- Case M: Following Case L, the author's team further improved the fixation design of the combined TMJ-skull base prosthesis, obviating the need for several small plates. Moreover, the design considered the characteristics of craniomaxillofacial bone and joint stress distribution and integrated fixation of the temporal bone flap window into the design. The TMJ-skull base prosthesis, also applying metal-nonmetal friction welding technology to connect the components, can reconstruct cases of TMJ-skull base giant cell lesions This is the prothesis shown in Fig. 6.10. The prosthesis design not only meets the requirements of mechanical force conduction properties and long-term stability but also achieves the integrated fixation of the temporal bone flap, which has both morphological and functional advantages.

6.2.1 Case L: Design and Application of an Edge-Fixed Combined TMJ-Skull Base Prosthesis

- Patient information: female, 53 years old.
- Complaint: right preauricular pressure and pain, limited mouth opening with hearing loss for more than 10 years.
- History: the patient presented to our department with right-sided preauricular pressure and pain, limited mouth opening, and hearing loss for the past 10 years, after she was diagnosed with right TMJ tumor at an outside hospital.
- Past history: she was physically fit and denied history of otitis media, systemic diseases, or drug and food allergies.
- Clinical examination: facial deviation to the left, no significant swelling. Mild tenderness in the right TMJ region. Maximal mouth opening: 3 mm, with deviation to the left. Stable occlusal relationship intraorally, but poor periodontal condition of the entire dentition (Fig. 6.12). Preauricular pain VAS score: 4.
- Imaging examination: panoramic radiograph, shows extensive bony fusion involving the right TMJ, skull base, and mandibular ramus (Fig. 6.13). CT scan: reveals a tumor (60 × 71 × 45 mm) involving the TMJ, skull base, infratemporal fossa, pterygomandibular space, and parapharyngeal space. Skull base perforation (20 × 28 mm) (Fig. 6.14). Tumor erodes the middle ear and anterior wall of the external auditory canal, but the cochlear structure remains intact (Fig. 6.15). Tumor in contact with the facial nerve, mandibular nerve (Fig. 6.16), as well as the internal carotid artery (red arrow), internal jugular vein (blue arrow), and maxillary artery (yellow arrow) (Fig. 6.17). PET-CT: suggests a right TMJ osteogenic tumor, likely benign or low-grade malignant. Audiometry test exhibited moderate conductive deafness on the right side.
- Diagnosis: osteochondroma of the right TMJ-skull base.

6.2.2 Case L. Diagnostic Imaging

6.2.3 Case L. Treatment Plan

- Overall treatment plan: resection of the right TMJ-skull base osteochondroma, the diseased condyle, and the involved skull base, and repair and reconstruction with a customized combined TMJ-skull base prosthesis (edge-fixed type)
- Surgical resection design
  Resection scope design: resection of the tumor in pieces, resection of the diseased condyle (condylar head to man-

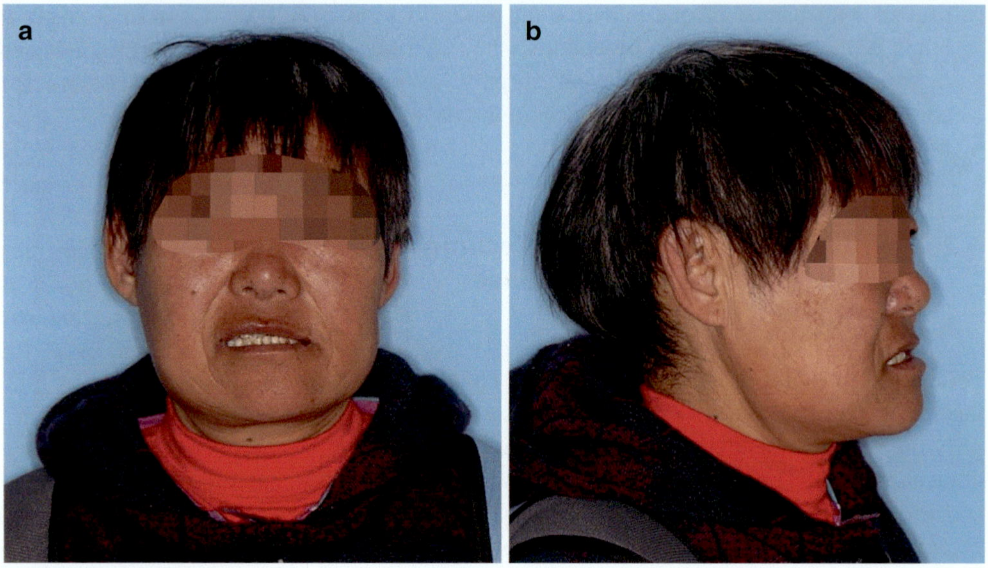

Fig. 6.12 Case L. Extraoral examination. There is mild overall asymmetry. The right mandible is longer than the left, with deviation of the chin to the left. (**a**) Frontal view. (**b**) Lateral view

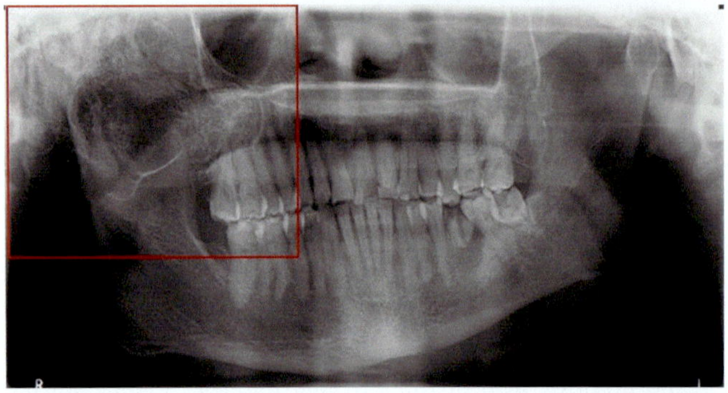

Fig. 6.13 Case L. Panoramic X-ray film. A large bony lesion involves the right TMJ, skull base, and mandibular ramus

dibular foramen), and resection of the skull base (posterior border to the anterior wall of the external auditory canal, anterior border to the anterior margin of the tumor, and internal border to the foramen ovale); this case is a Class III defect.

- Digital simulation surgery
  - Temporary osteotomy of the zygomatic arch: the anterior and posterior osteotomy lines of the zygomatic arch are determined, and the zygomatic arch is truncated, preserving the masseter muscle attachment while pushing the zygomatic arch forward and down during the surgery (Fig. 6.18).
  - Condylar osteotomy: a segmented osteotomy and resection of the condylar-mandibular ramus is performed (Fig. 6.19).
  - Segmental resection of the tumor: the lower portion of the tumor is segmented and resected (Fig. 6.20).
  - Temporal bone craniotomy: design the temporal bone flap window opening location (Fig. 6.21).
  - Resection of the skull base and the upper part of the tumor: partial excision of the skull base and the upper part of the tumor, while protecting the petrous part of the temporal bone and the internal carotid artery and internal jugular artery (Fig. 6.22).
  - Excision of the tumor around the styloid process: great care is required because of the proximity to important blood vessels and facial nerves (Fig. 6.23).
  - Post-excision defect model: the internal carotid artery and facial and mandibular nerves are preserved after the tumor, TMJ, and skull base are resected (Fig. 6.24).

6.2.4 Case L. Design and Processing of the Edge-Fixed TMJ-Skull Base Prosthesis and the Osteotomy Positioning Guides

- Edge-fixed combined TMJ-skull base prosthesis design
  The core components are introduced as described in Sect. 2.4.1 in Chap. 2 (Fig. 6.25).
- Skull base extension design: when designing the skull base extension, there should be a gap left between the oval foramen and the medial side of the prosthesis. The anterior wall of the ear canal and the posterior side of the prosthesis, and the skull base component and the articulating fossa component are connected by a snap joint and screws (Fig. 6.26), and then the mandibular extension component is designed (Fig. 6.27), which will complete the final design of the joint prosthesis (Fig. 6.28).
  Osteotomy and screw hole depth measurements: measure the thickness of the temporal bone at the craniotomy locations, the depth of the skull base osteotomy, and the depth

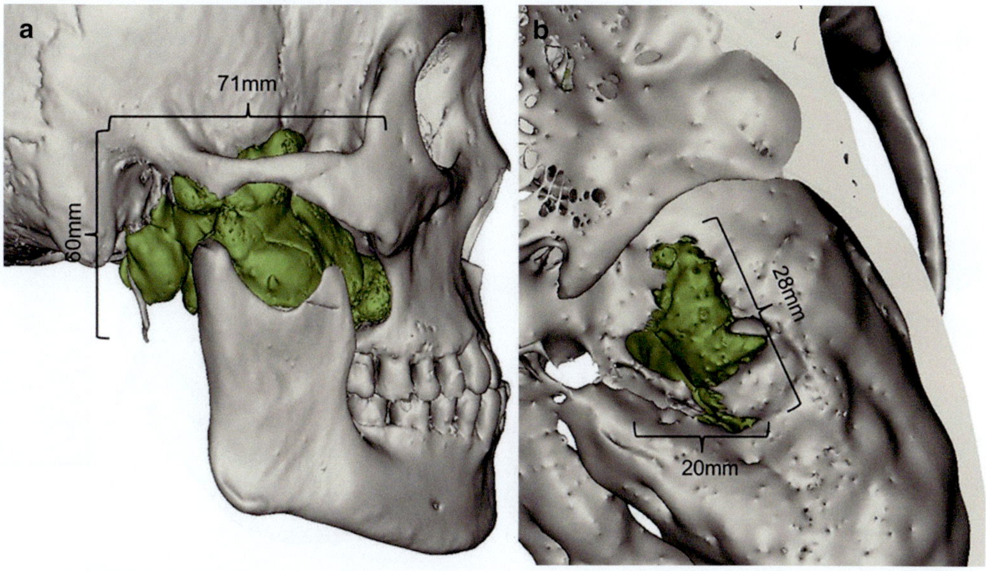

Fig. 6.14 Case L. 3D reconstruction of the maxillofacial CT. A 60 × 71× 45 mm mass (in green false color) involved the TMJ, skull base, infratemporal fossa, pterygomandibular space, and parapharyngeal space. There was a skull base perforation of 20 × 28 mm. (**a**) Right lateral view. (**b**) Cerebrofacial view

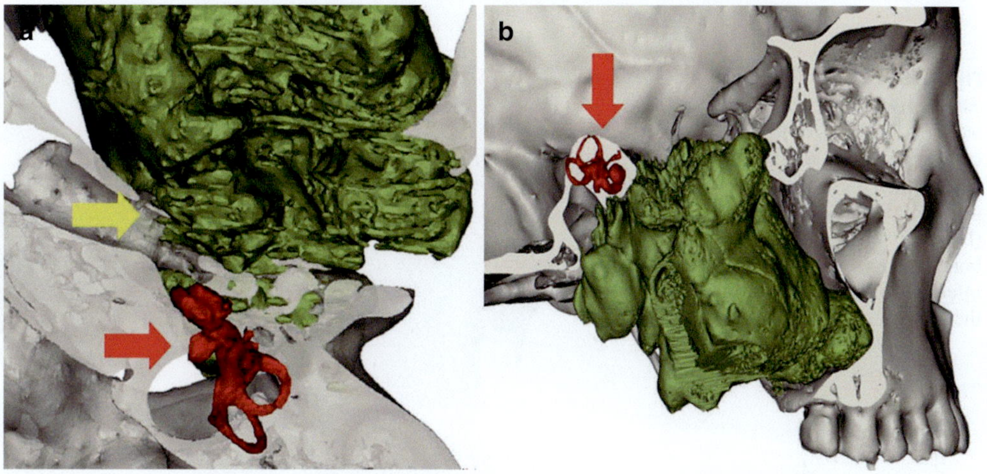

Fig. 6.15 Case L. Relationship of the mass to the ear. The mass has destroyed the ossicles of the middle ear and the anterior wall of the external auditory canal (yellow arrow). The cochlea was normal (red arrow). (**a**) Axial position. (**b**) Sagittal position

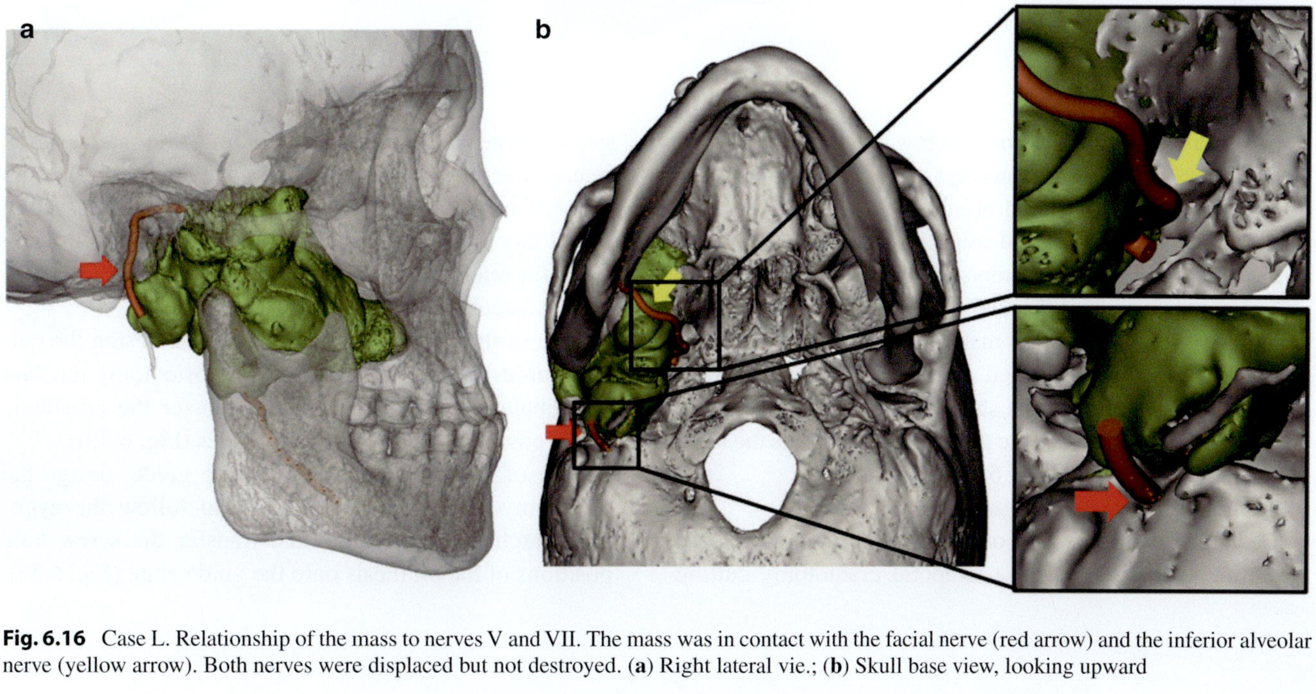

Fig. 6.16 Case L. Relationship of the mass to nerves V and VII. The mass was in contact with the facial nerve (red arrow) and the inferior alveolar nerve (yellow arrow). Both nerves were displaced but not destroyed. (**a**) Right lateral vie.; (**b**) Skull base view, looking upward

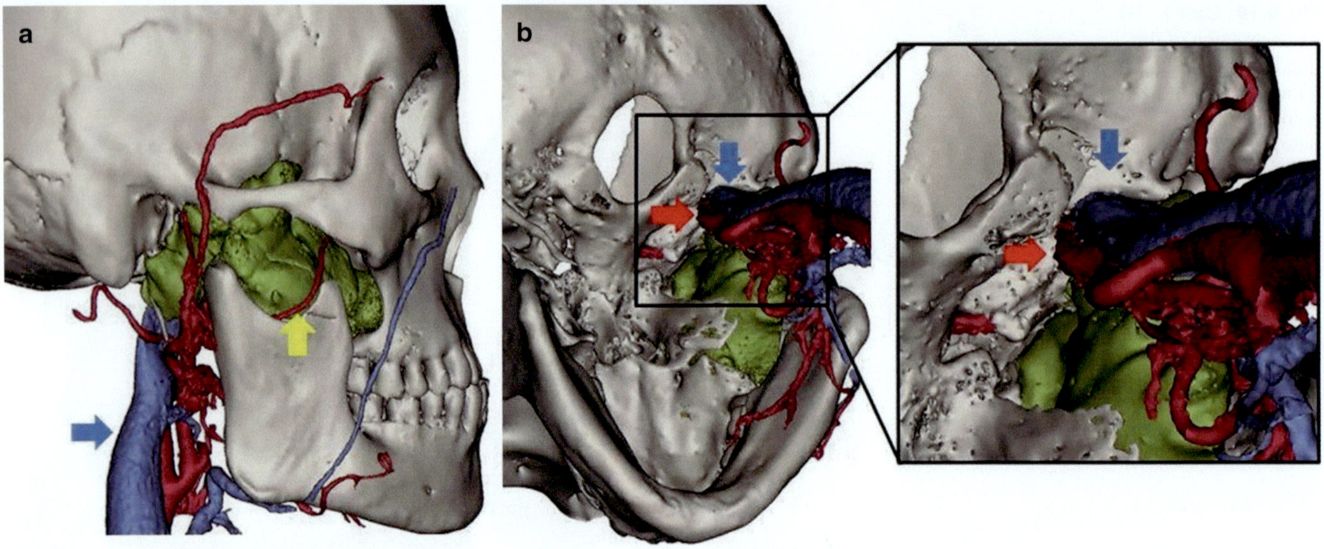

Fig. 6.17 Case L. Relationship of the mass to adjacent blood vessels. The mass is in contact with the internal carotid artery (red arrows), internal jugular vein (blue arrows), and internal maxillary artery (yellow arrow). (**a**) Right lateral view (**b**) Skull base view

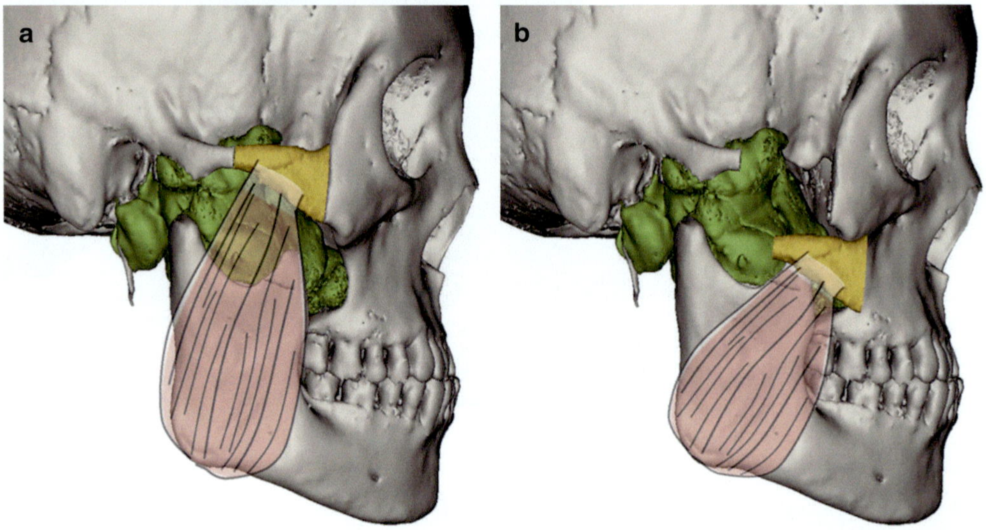

Fig. 6.18 Case L. Temporary osteotomy of the zygomatic arch. (**a**) The osteotomy lines on the zygomatic arch were determined, preserving the origin of the masseter muscle. (**b**) After the osteotomies, the bone is moved anteriorly and inferiorly to allow access to the tumor

of all screw holes to determine screw lengths to be used in intraoperative implantation (Figs. 6.29, 6.30 and 6.31).

- Prosthesis fabrication and fitting: the titanium skull base component was fabricated using a metal 3D printer, and the UHMWPE fossa component was fabricated using 5-axis finishing, and the two were connected using snap joint and screws. Specific material selection and machining methods are described in detail in Chap. 2. After machining, the prosthesis should be test fitted on a resin head mold to observe if the prosthesis closely fits the bone surface and is stable (Fig. 6.32).
- Design of digital cutting guides

  Design of the temporal bone craniotomy and skull base cutting guides: design the temporal craniotomy cutting guides along the temporal osteotomy line and position retention screw holes for intraoperative osteotomy. Design the skull base cutting guide with reference to the resection osteotomy lines for the tumor, and position fixation screw holes for retention of the guide plates during the intraoperative osteotomy (Fig. 6.33).

  Design of the mandibular cutting guides: design the cutting guides to follow the mandibular osteotomy line and mandibular inferior border; then transfer the prosthetic screw positions onto the cutting guides (Fig. 6.33).

  Design of the zygomatic arch cutting guide: design the osteotomy positioning guide plate to follow the zygomatic arch osteotomy line and transfer the screw hole positions of the prothesis onto the guide plate (Fig. 6.33).

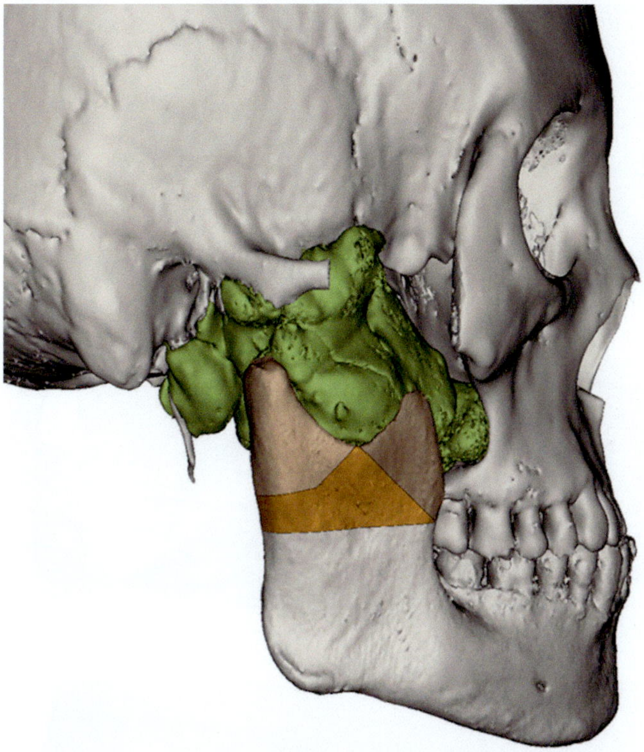

Fig. 6.19 Case L. Segmented osteotomy and resection of the condylar-mandibular ramus. The green shows the tumor, and the brown, orange, and tan colors show the condyle and mandibular ramus that is to be removed in sections

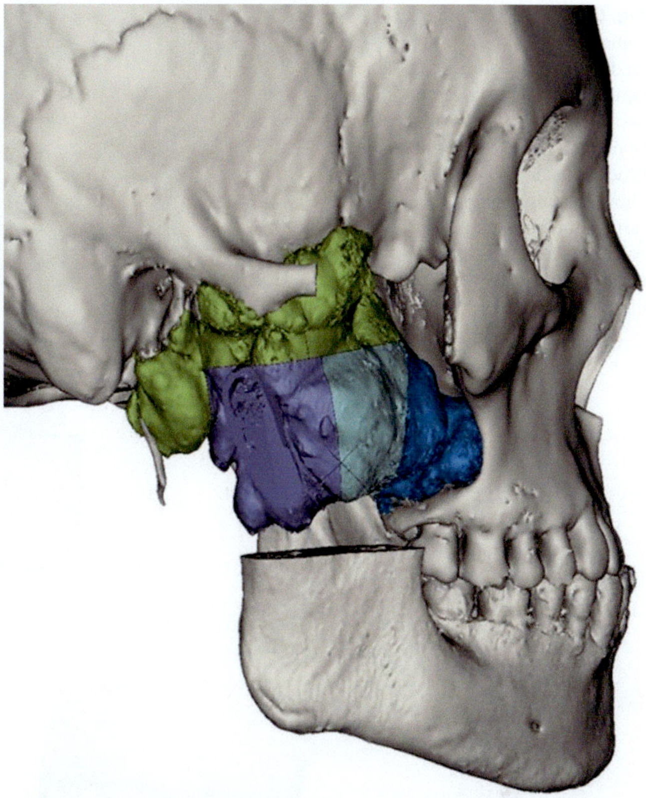

Fig. 6.20 Case L. Planned segmented resection of the lower part of the tumor in blocks (purple, light blue, dark blue)

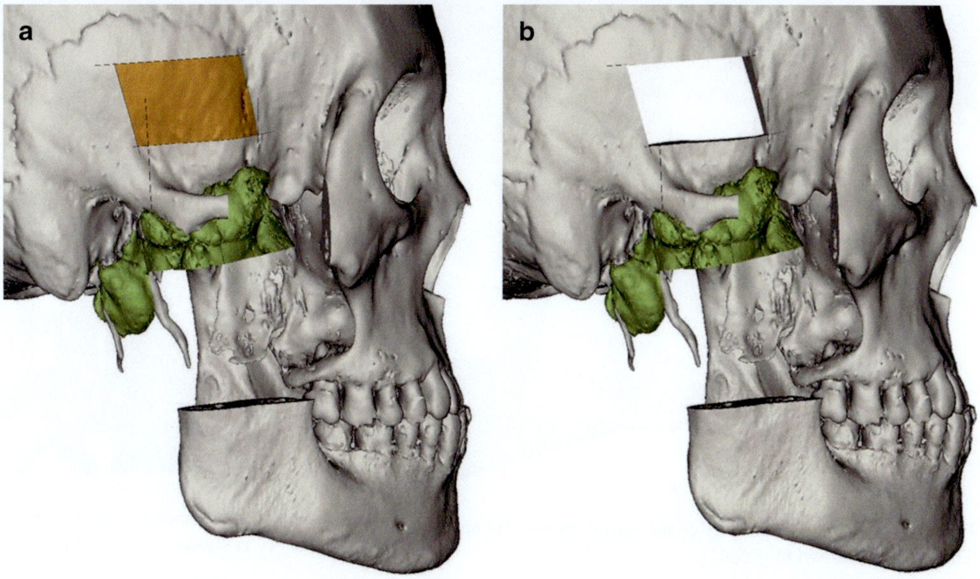

Fig. 6.21 Case L. Temporal bone craniotomy. Green color shows the tumor, and orange color shows the temporal bone window opening. (**a**) Temporal bone craniotomy design. (**b**) After temporal bone craniotomy

Fig. 6.22 Case L. Anterior (blue arrow) and posterior (red arrow) osteotomies of the skull base. The orange color shows the truncated skull base bone, and the green, light blue, and dark blue colors show the upper part of the tumor that was segmented to be removed in pieces. (**a**) Right lateral view. (**b**) Cerebrofacial view

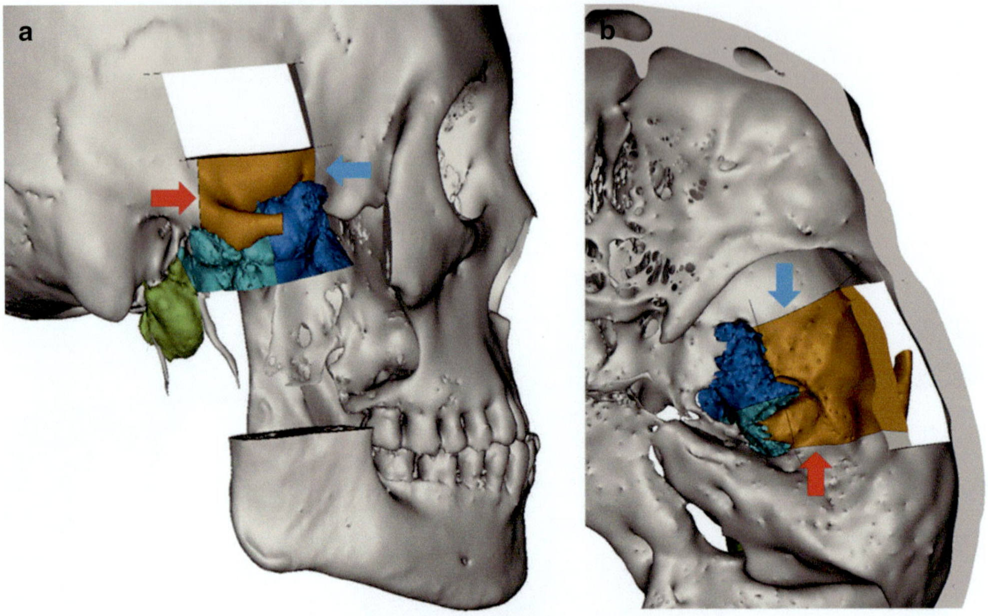

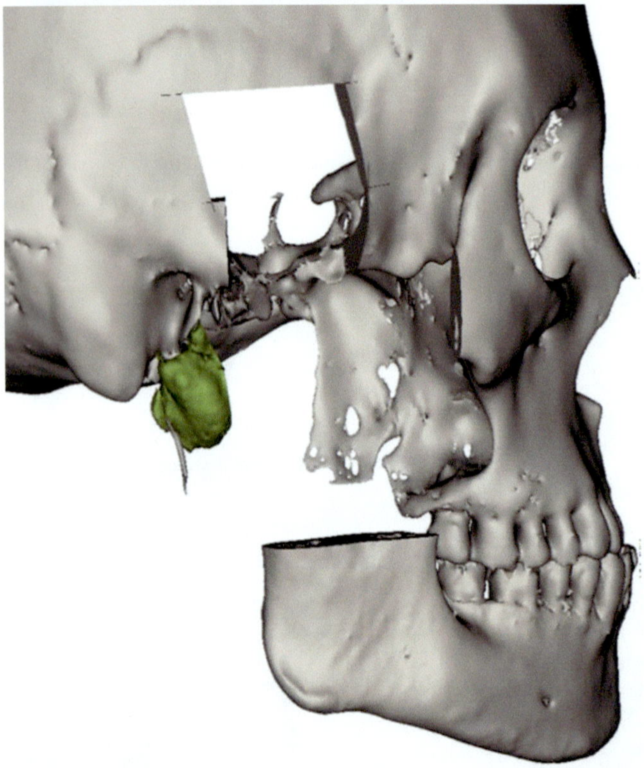

Fig. 6.23 Case L. Osteotomy of the tumor around the styloid process. The tumor is shown in green

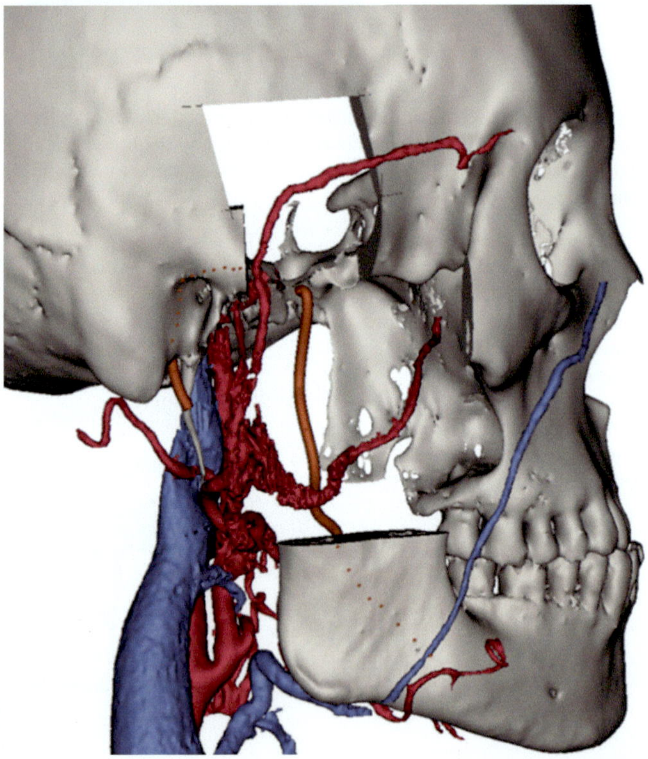

Fig. 6.24 Case L. Defect model after resection. The maxillofacial artery is shown in red and the maxillofacial vein in blue

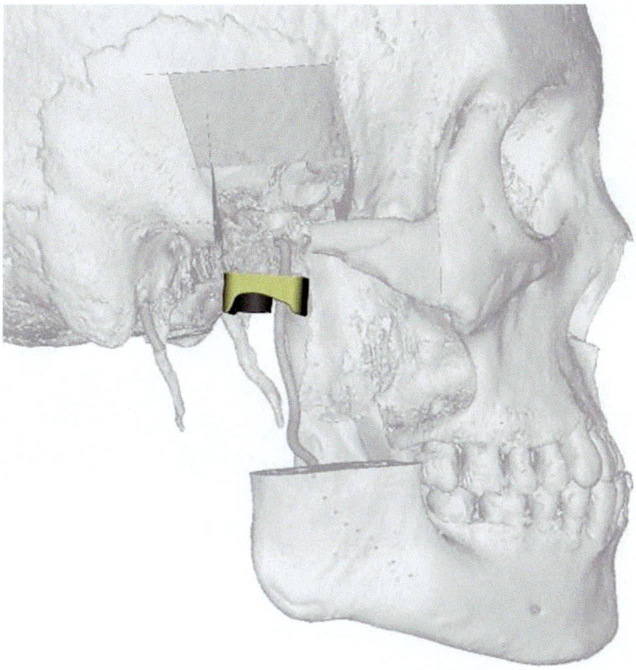

Fig. 6.25 Case L. Position determination for the joint fossa core component (yellow) and condyle head core component (dark gray)

6.2.5 Case L. Surgical Procedure

Preoperative laboratory tests: the same as described in Sect. 3.2.5, Preoperative Laboratory Tests.

Preoperative preparation: prepare the skin of the patient's affected side in the temporal, periapical, and submandibular areas. Prepare at least 600 mL of blood and special neurosurgical instruments such as an ice bucket, mannitol, cerebral pressure plate and cerebral sponges, and a microscope and facial nerve detector if the surgery is combined with the ENT department. For the rest of the preparation, please refer to Sect. 3.2.5, Preoperative Preparation.

6.2.5.1 Steps of the Surgical Procedure

Surgical approach: a modified preauricular-temporal incision combined with a parotidectomy incision was used to temporarily sever the facial nerve and expose the temporal bone squamous area, the joint, the mandibular ramus, and the mandibular angle (Figs. 6.34, 6.35 and 6.36).

- Temporary removal of the zygomatic arch and installation of the cutting guides: after the zygomatic arch is temporarily cut off and placed to the side with its muscle attachments, the condylar osteotomy and the removal of the lower portion of the tumor in segments are carried out (Fig. 6.37), and then cutting guide is installed (Fig. 6.38).
- Temporal bone craniotomy: temporal bone incision following the guide plate using piezoelectric saw (Fig. 6.39).
- Skull base osteotomy: use an oscillating saw to perform a skull base osteotomy following the cutting guide (Fig. 6.40).
- Resection of the lesion: complete removal of the tumor, joint, and diseased bone at the base of the skull, in segments (Figs. 6.41 and 6.42).
- Repositioning and fixation of the temporal bone flap window: the temporarily removed temporal bone flap was repositioned and fixed with titanium plates and screws (Fig. 6.43).
- TMJ-skull base prosthesis implantation and fixation: after the temporal bone flap and zygomatic arch have been repositioned, the TMJ-skull base prosthesis is implanted and secured with titanium screws (Fig. 6.44).
- Mandibular prosthesis implantation and fixation: after implantation of the TMJ-skull base prosthesis, the mandibular prosthesis component is fitted in place and fixed with titanium screws (Fig. 6.45).

Buccal fat pad used to fill the dead space: buccal fat pad is harvested to fill the dead space, and facial nerve was reanastomosed to recover the nerve function (Fig. 6.46).

6.2.6 Case L. Postoperative Analysis of Prosthesis Implantation Precision

Regular postoperative follow-ups were performed for appearance (facial shape), function (mouth opening, mouth shape), and prosthesis evaluation (safety, accuracy).

Immediately after surgery: the intraoperative cutting guides were accurately seated, and the prosthesis was installed smoothly (Fig. 6.47), and the comparison between the preoperative design and the postoperative reconstruction showed that the prosthesis position was accurate (Fig. 6.48). Postoperative prosthesis installation error analysis showed that the error of the core component was 1.01 mm and the overall error of the combined prosthesis was 1.47 mm (Figs. 6.49 and 6.50).

6.2.7 Case L. Long-Term Follow-Up and Prognosis

6.2.7.1 Five-Year Postoperative Follow-Up

No recurrence of pre-existing diseases, good facial shape without abnormalities, no redness, swelling, or other reactions in the operated area.

The preauricular pain improved, the VAS score improved to 1, and the joint-mandibular-occlusal-facial pattern was harmonized with a stable occlusal relationship (Fig. 6.51).

The mouth opening improved to 24 mm, with 7 mm of lateral movement to the affected side and 2 mm of lateral

Fig. 6.26 Case L. Skull base extension component (blue). The red arrow points to the oval foramen at the medial side of the designed prosthesis position, and the blue arrow points to the anterior wall of the ear canal at the posterior side of the designed prosthesis position, where a small gap has been left. (**a**) Right lateral facial view. (**b**) Skull base view

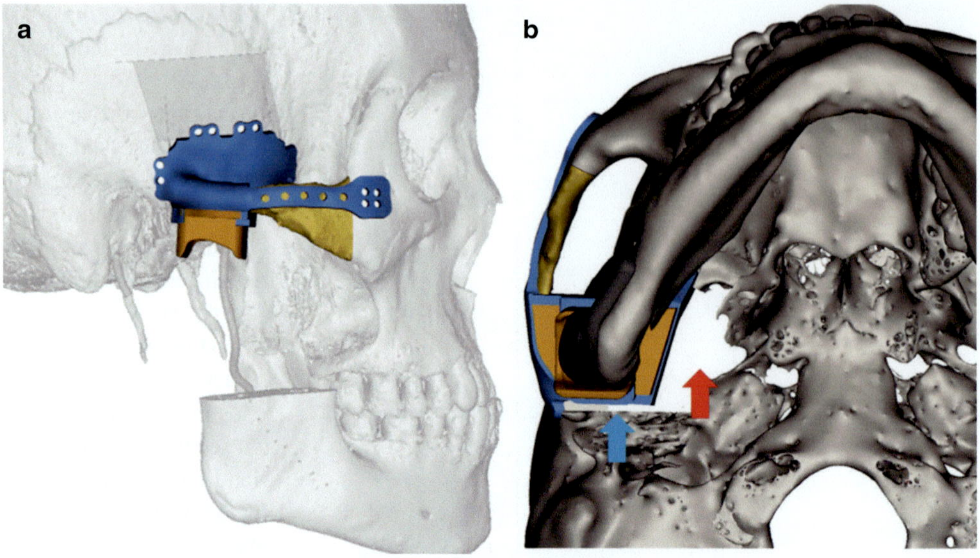

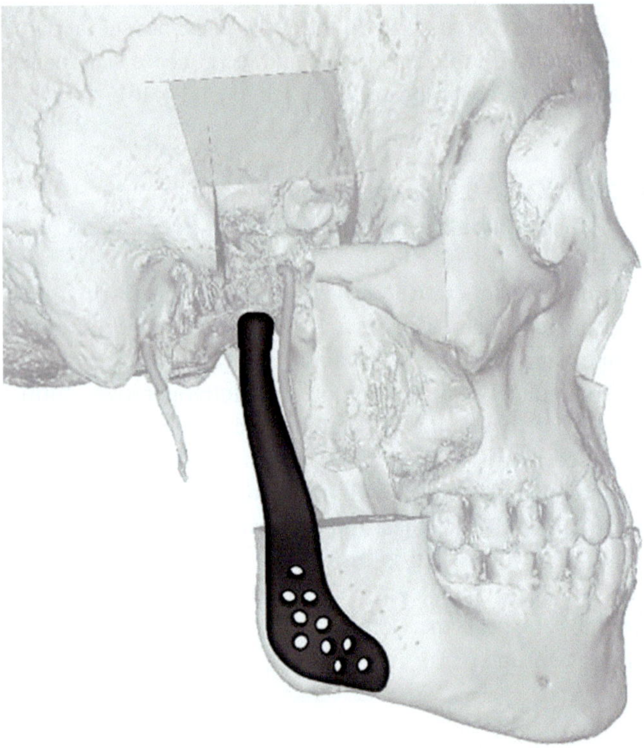

Fig. 6.27 Case L. Mandibular extension component (dark gray) design

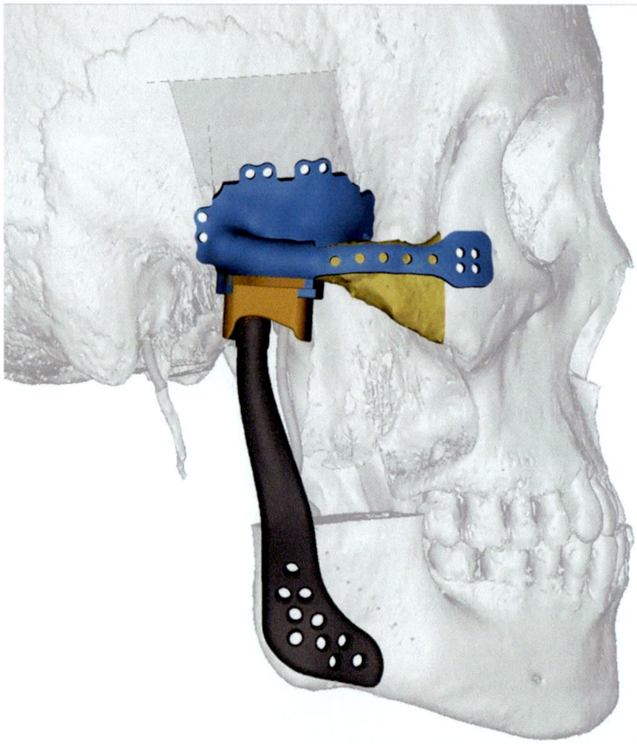

Fig. 6.28 Case L. Combined TMJ-skull base prosthesis design. Blue shows the skull base extension component, orange shows the articular fossa component, dark gray shows the mandibular extension component, and yellow shows the zygomatic arch as replaced in its original position after removal of the tumor

movement to the healthy side, and mouth opening with a deviation of 5 mm toward the affected side.

Prosthesis evaluation: no complications such as prosthesis infection, rejection, loosening, fracture, displacement, ectopic osteogenesis, or allergy (Fig. 6.52).

Others: mild deviation of the angle of the mouth on the affected side, no numbness in the maxillofacial region, significant recovery of facial nerve function compared to the immediate postoperative period, and hearing function similar to that of the preoperative period.

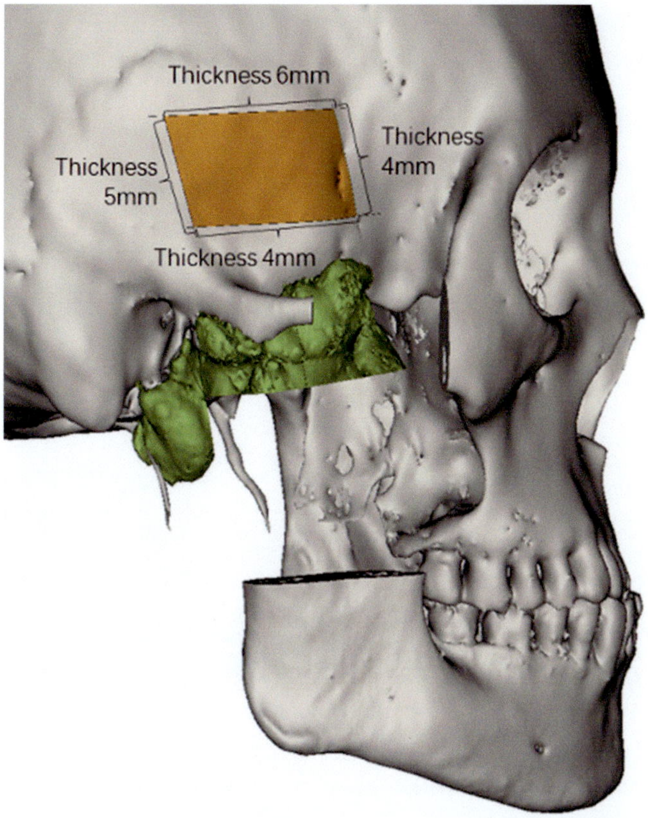

Fig. 6.29 Case L. Temporal bone window bone (orange) thickness measurements (in mm)

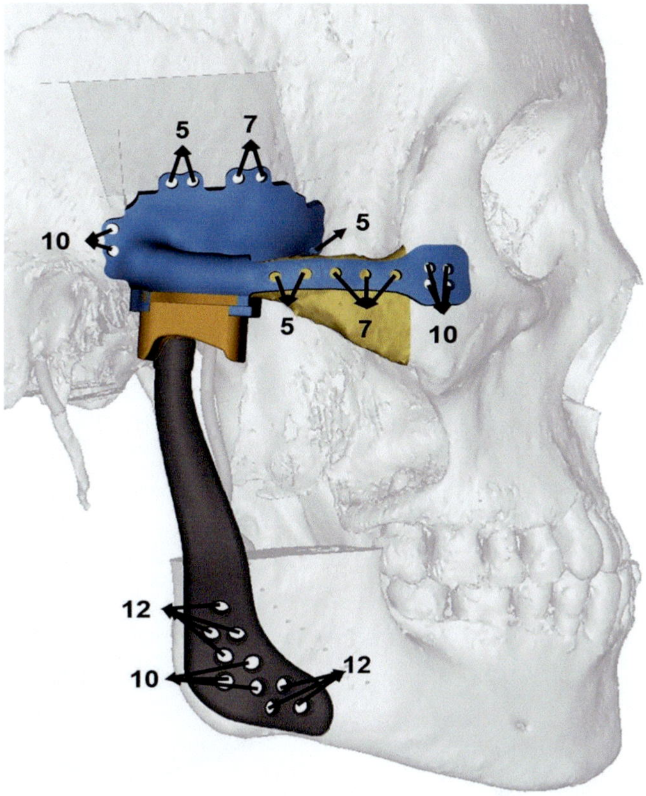

Fig. 6.31 Case L. Screw hole depth measurement (in mm) for prosthesis attachment. Blue shows skull base extension component, orange shows fossa component, dark gray shows mandibular extension component, and yellow shows zygomatic arch

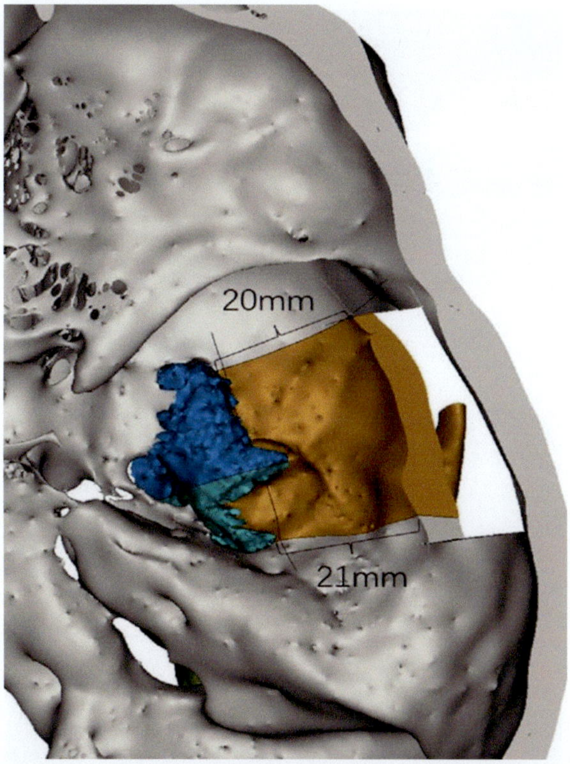

Fig. 6.30 Case L. Skull base osteotomy (orange) depth measurement (in mm)

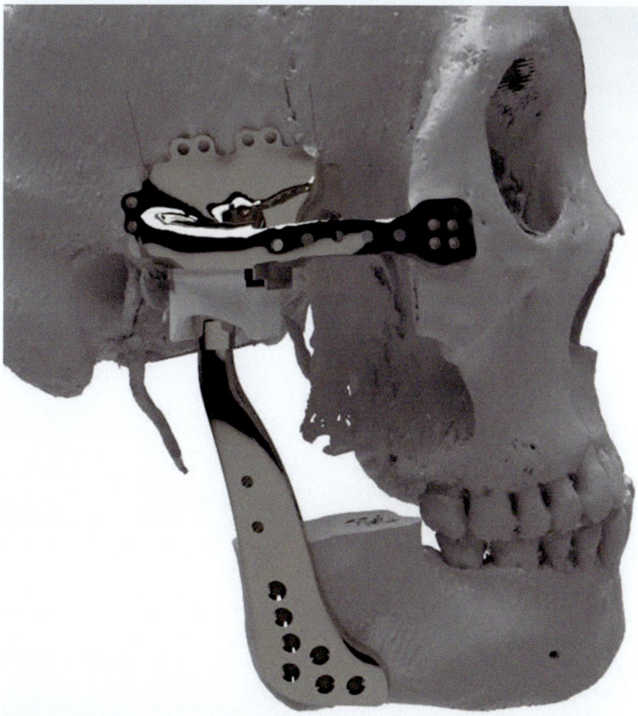

Fig. 6.32 Case L. Prosthesis fabrication and fitting on a resin model

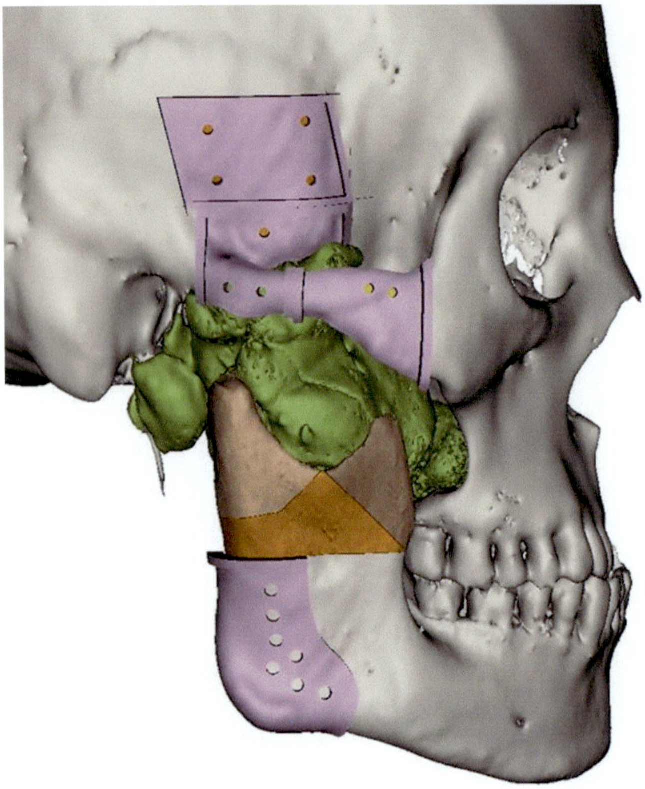

Fig. 6.33 Case L. Design of zygomatic arch osteotomy, temporal bone craniotomy, mandibular osteotomy, and skull base cutting guides (pink)

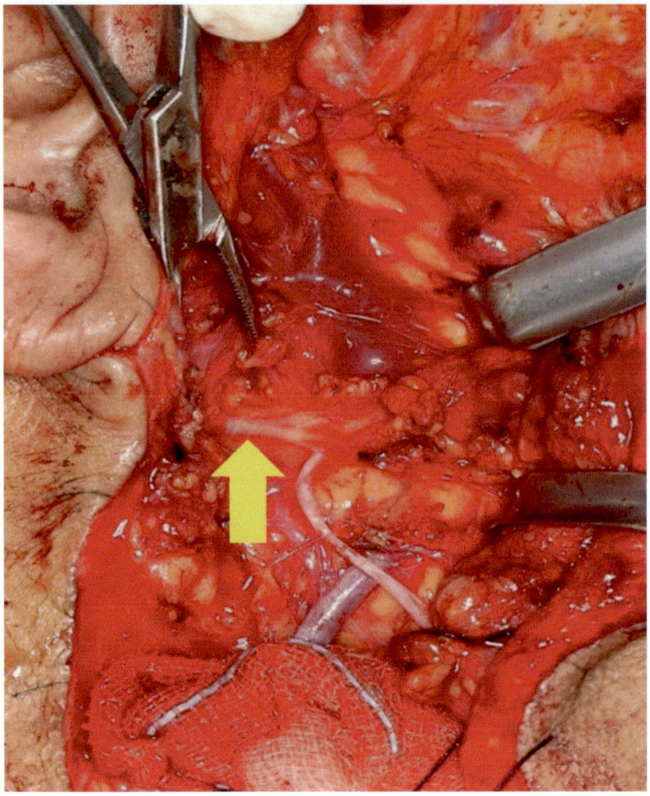

Fig. 6.35 Case L. Exposure of the facial nerve for temporary transection of the main trunk. The yellow arrow points to the main trunk of the facial nerve

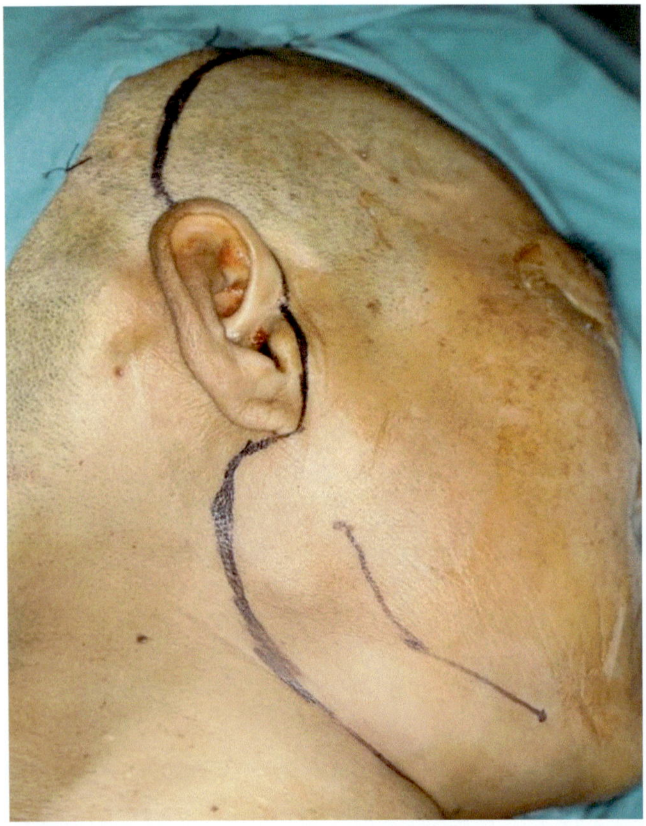

Fig. 6.34 Case L. Modified preauricular-temporal incision is combined with a parotidectomy incision for wide exposure of the surgical site

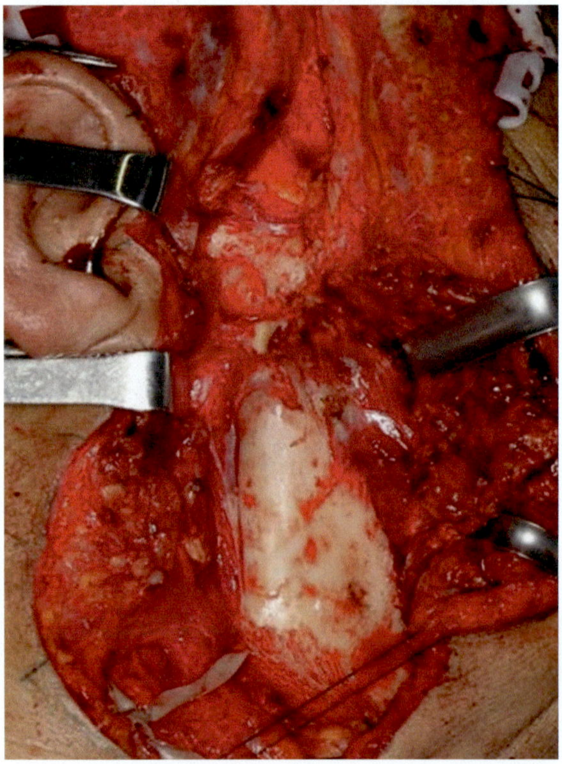

Fig. 6.36 Case L. Exposure of the TMJ, mandibular ramus, and mandibular angle

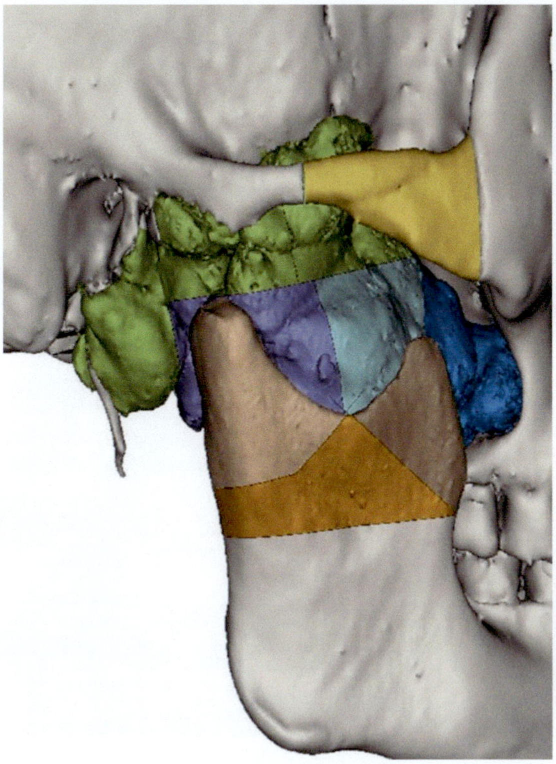

Fig. 6.37 Case L. Temporary osteotomy of the zygomatic arch, osteotomies of the condyle, coronoid process, and upper ramus, and piecemeal resection of the lower part of the mass

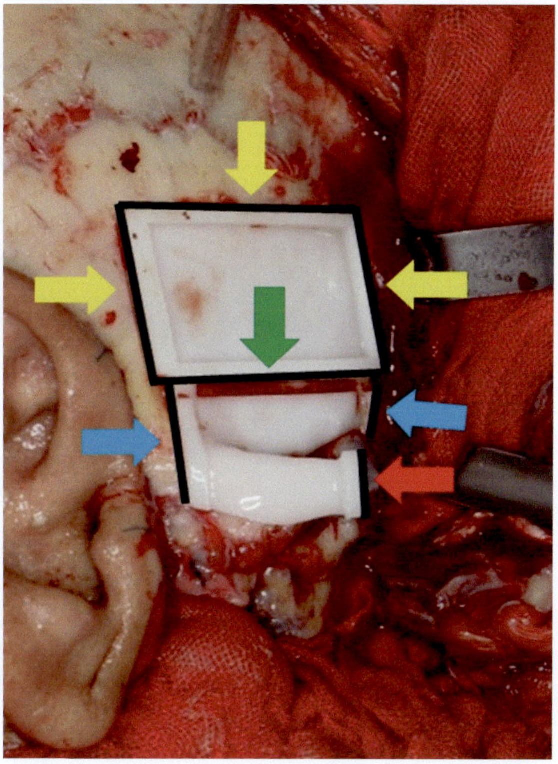

Fig. 6.38 Case L. Composite cutting guide for the temporal craniotomy (yellow arrows), skull base resection (blue arrows), and zygomatic arch osteotomy (red arrow)

Fig. 6.39 Case L. Temporal bone craniotomy. (**a**) Piezoelectric assisted osteotomy. (**b**) Temporal bone window opening. The temporal bone block will be replaced after the intracranial part of the tumor is excised

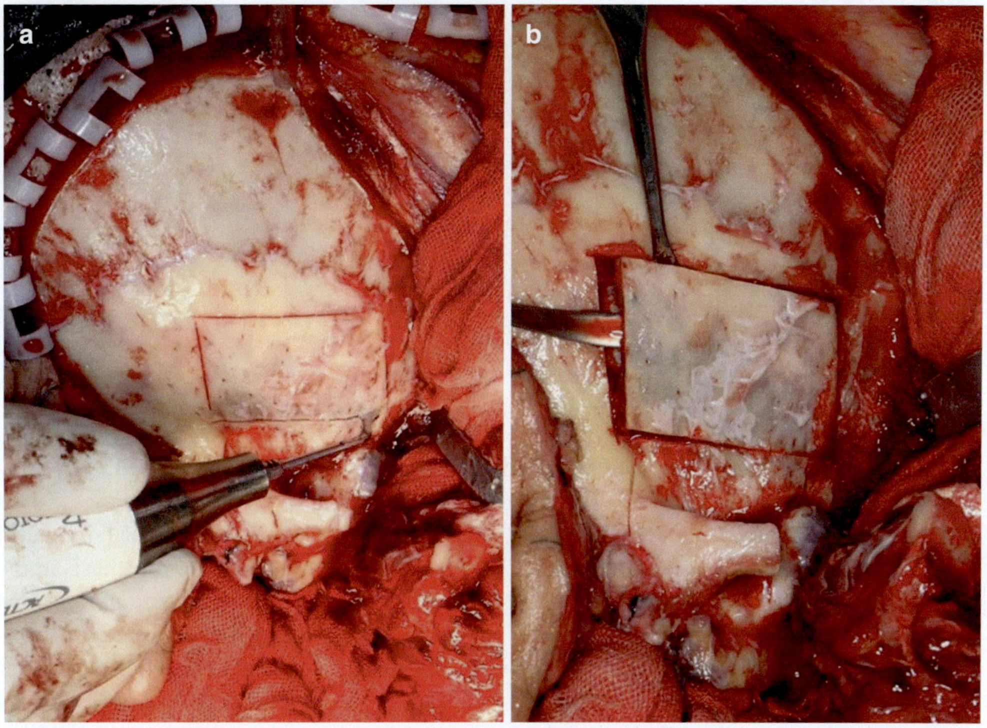

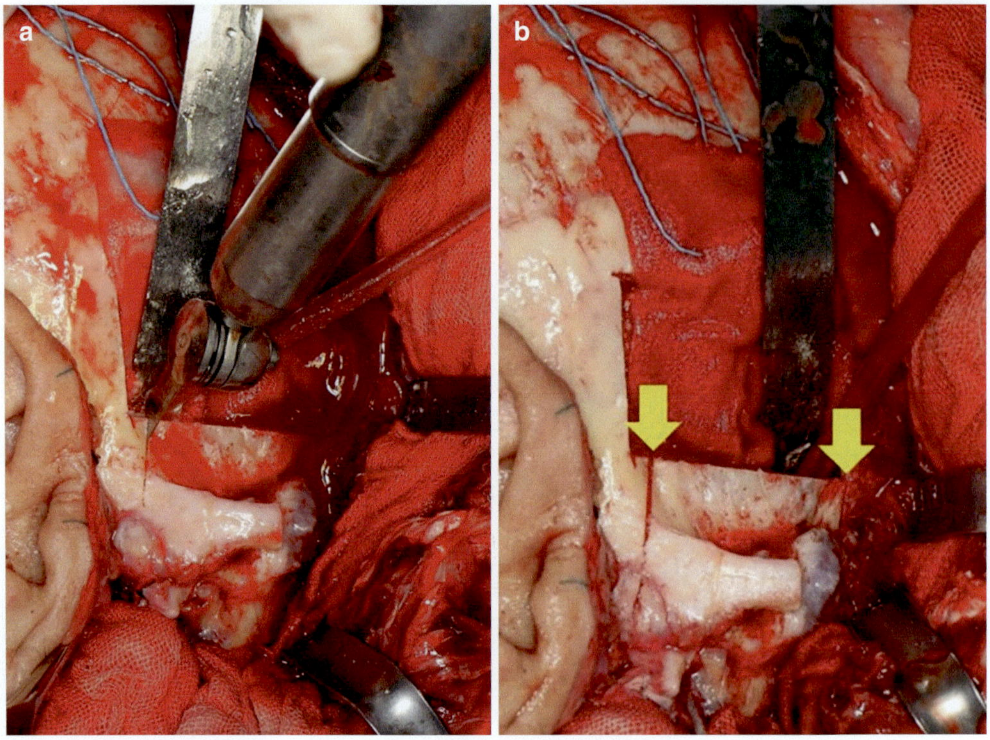

Fig. 6.40 Case L. Skull base osteotomy (yellow arrows). (**a**) Oscillating saw osteotomy. (**b**) Anterior and posterior osteotomy lines of the skull base

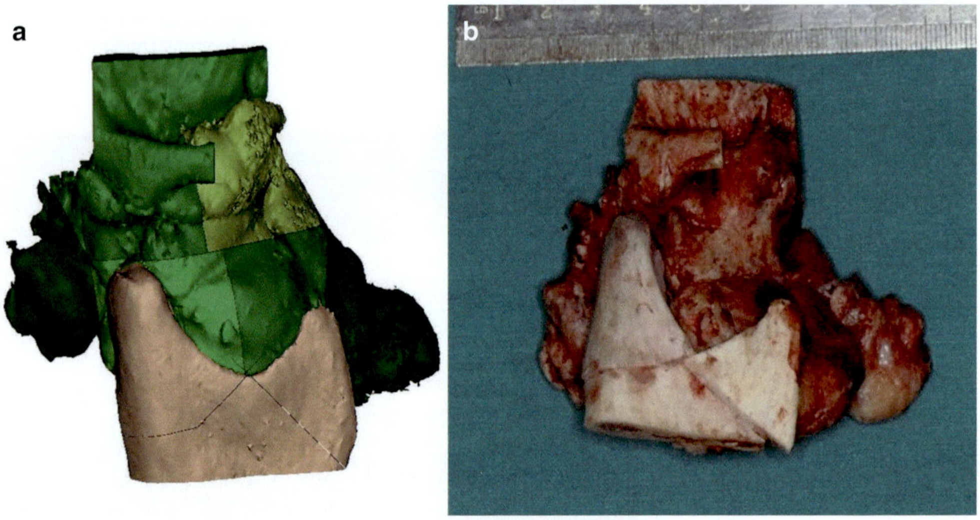

Fig. 6.41 Case L. Comparison of the preoperative design and the intraoperative tumor. (**a**) Design. (**b**) Actual

6.2.8 Case L. Advantages and Disadvantages

6.2.8.1 Advantages

Successful repair of an extensive TMJ-skull base lesion was achieved without harvesting autologous tissue, using only the prosthesis.

After 5 years of follow-up, the prosthesis was stable, safe, and accurately aligned.

The 3D-printed complex TMJ-skull base prosthesis was effective for combined joint and skull base restoration in form and function.

6.2.8.2 Disadvantages

The TMJ-skull base prosthesis fixation was designed to cover the normal bone perimeter of the bone defect, but it was prone to prosthesis immobilization due to multiple intraoperative resections, and the prosthesis was not planned with stress line distribution.

The connection of the nonmetallic articular socket to the metal skull base prosthesis was not strong enough and has micro movements.

Additional titanium plate fixation was required to close and stabilize the temporal bone window opening.

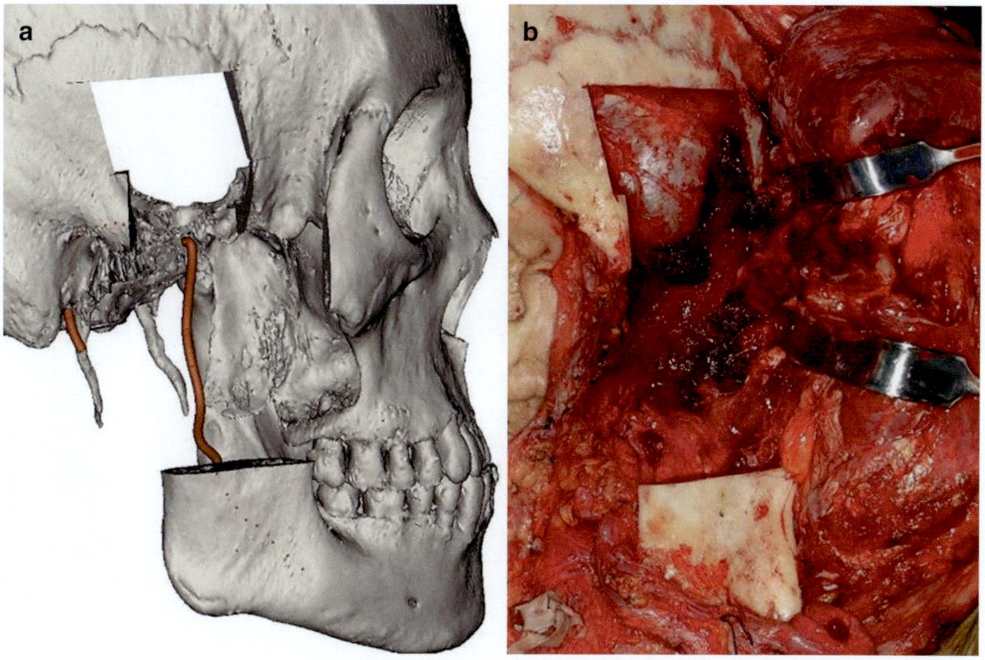

Fig. 6.42 Case L. Combined TMJ-skull base defect space left after complete removal of tumor. (**a**) Design. (**b**) Actual

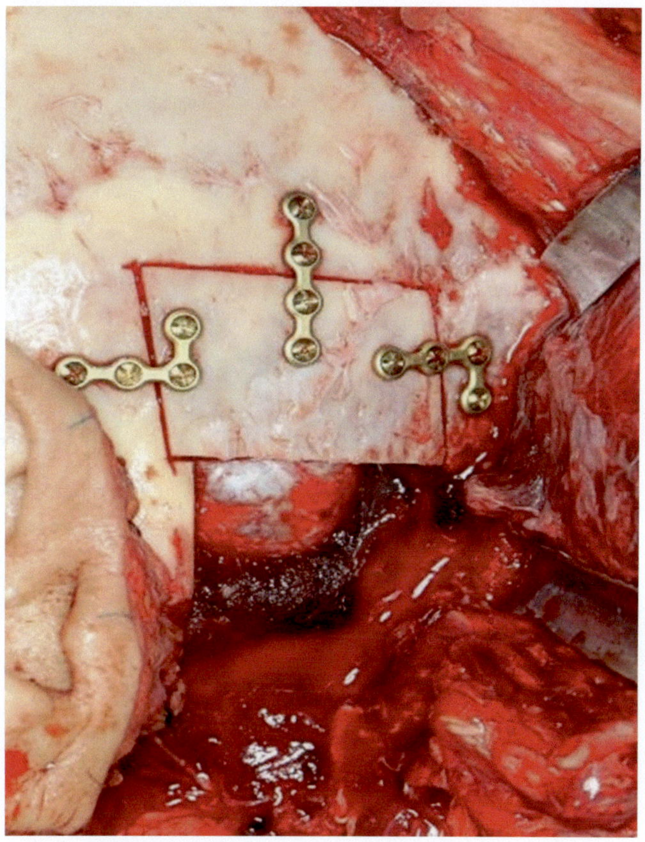

Fig. 6.43 Case L. Bone flap repositioning and titanium plate fixation to close temporal bone window

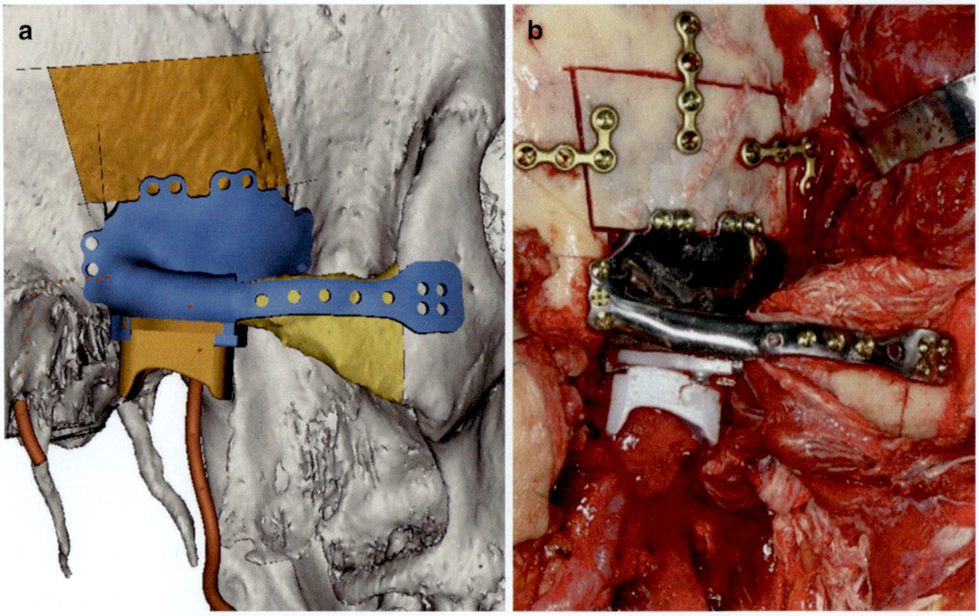

Fig. 6.44 Case L. TMJ-skull base prosthesis implantation and fixation, together with zygomatic arch repositioning and fixation. (**a**) Design. (**b**) Actual

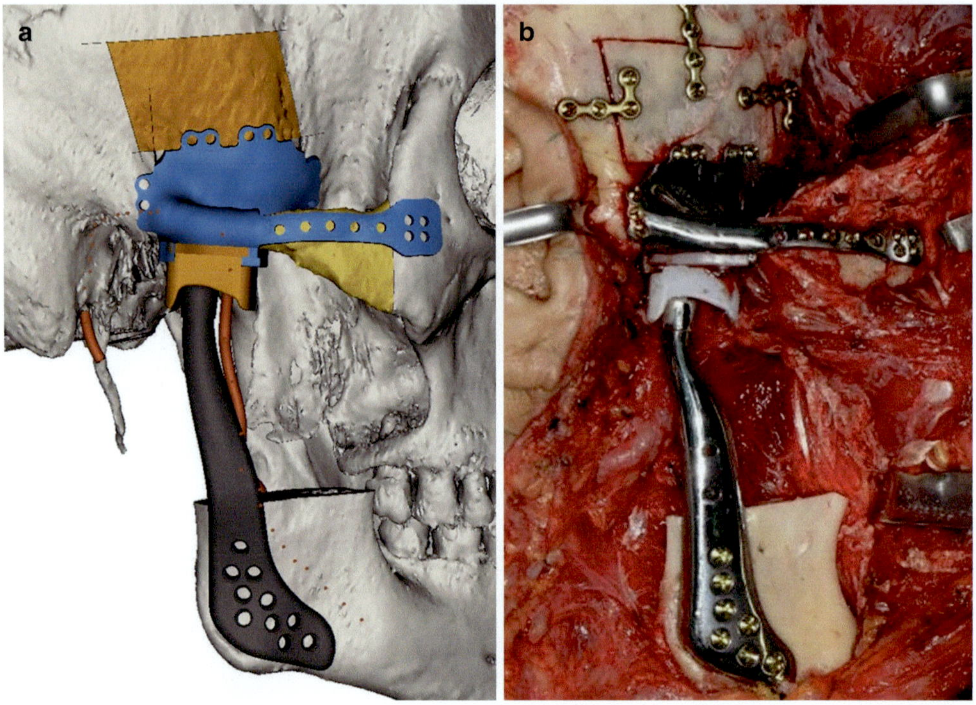

Fig. 6.45 Case L. Mandibular prosthesis implantation and fixation. (**a**) Design. (**b**) Actual

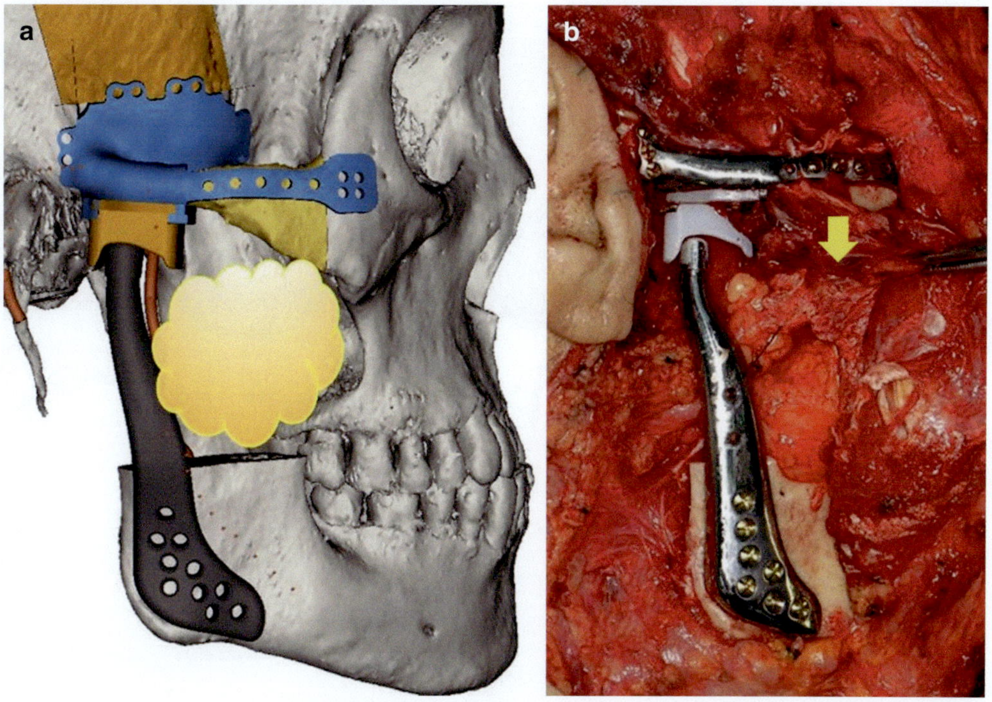

Fig. 6.46 Case L. Buccal fat pad filling dead space left after removal of the diseased tissue (yellow arrow). Facial nerve reanastomosed. (**a**) Design. (**b**) Actual

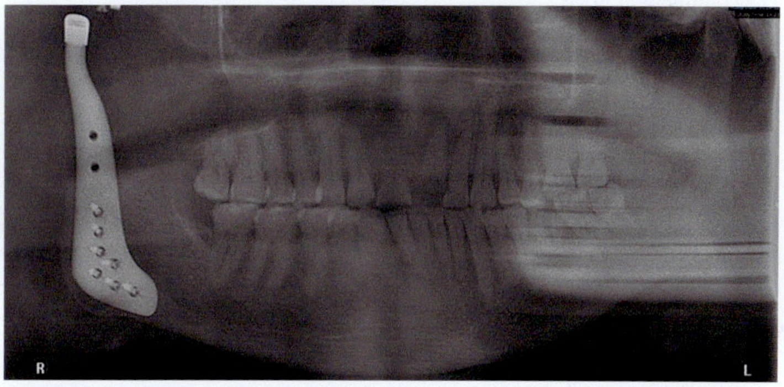

Fig. 6.47 Case L. Immediate postoperative panoramic film

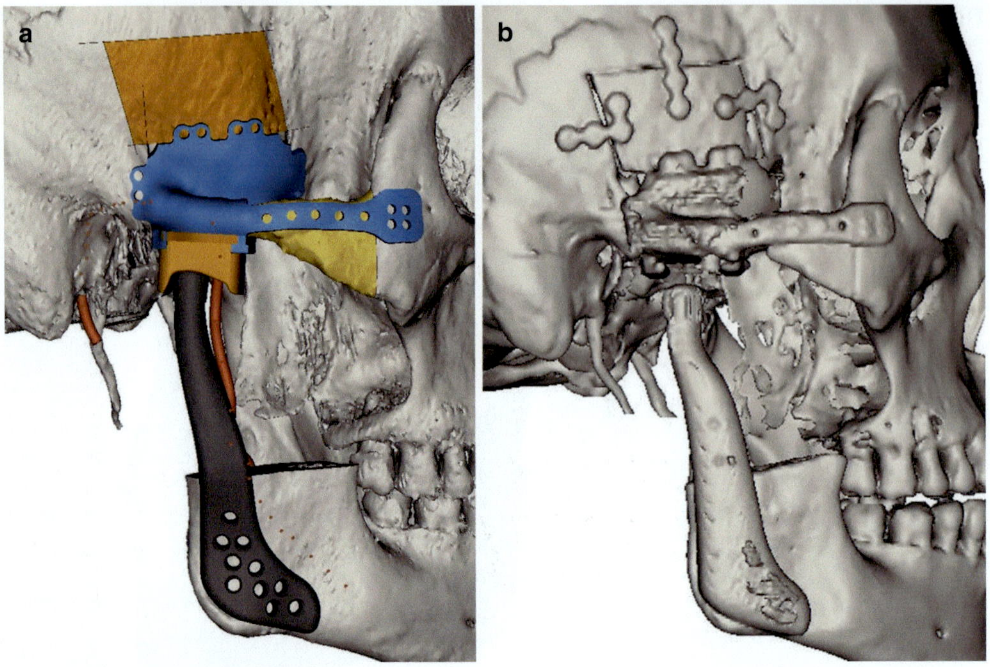

Fig. 6.48 Case L. Preoperative design versus immediate postoperative CT comparison showing precise prosthesis seating. (**a**) Preoperative design. (**b**) Immediate postoperative

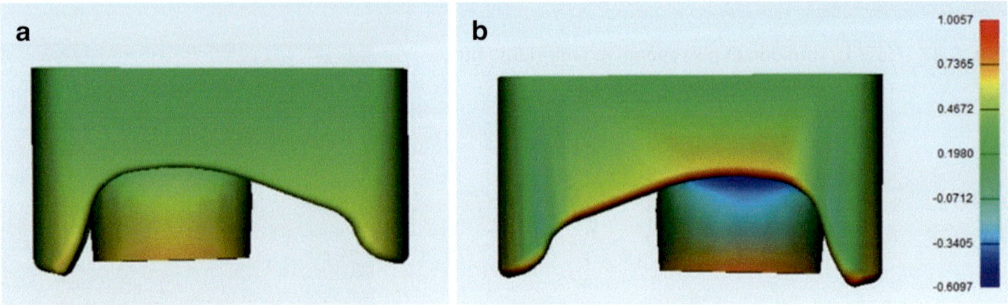

Fig. 6.49 Case L. Prosthetic core component error 1.01 mm. (**a**) Lateral error. (**b**) Medial error

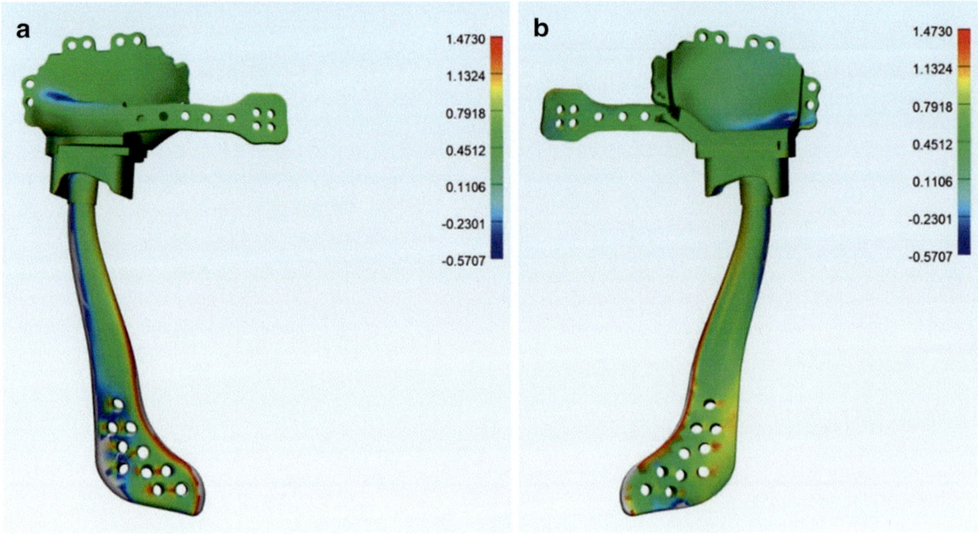

Fig. 6.50 Case L. Overall error of the TMJ-skull base combined prosthesis 1.47 mm. (**a**) Lateral error. (**b**) medial error

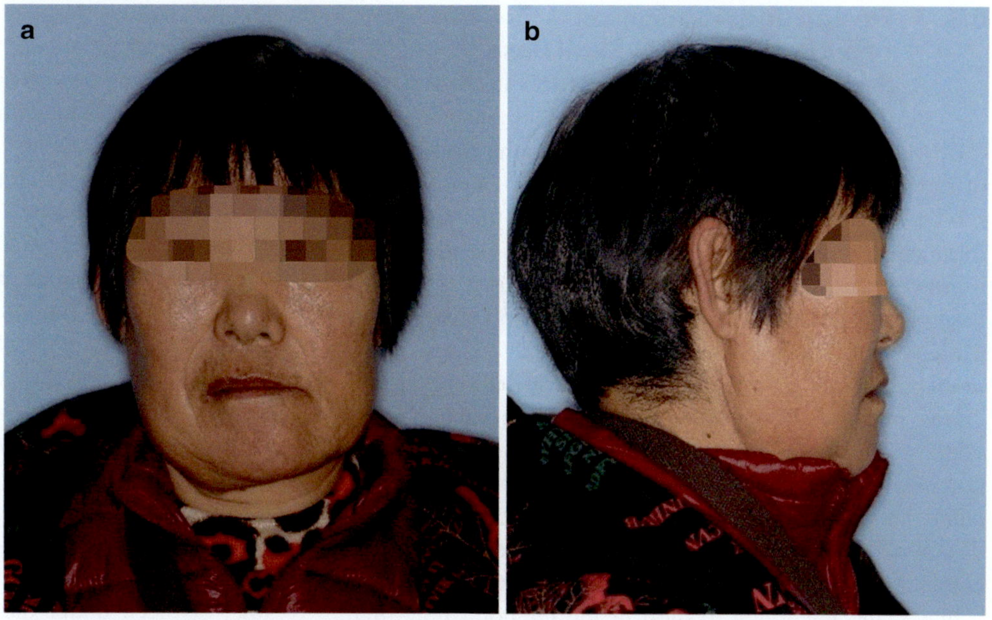

Fig. 6.51 Case L. Follow-up 5 years after surgery. (**a**) Frontal view. (**b**) Lateral view

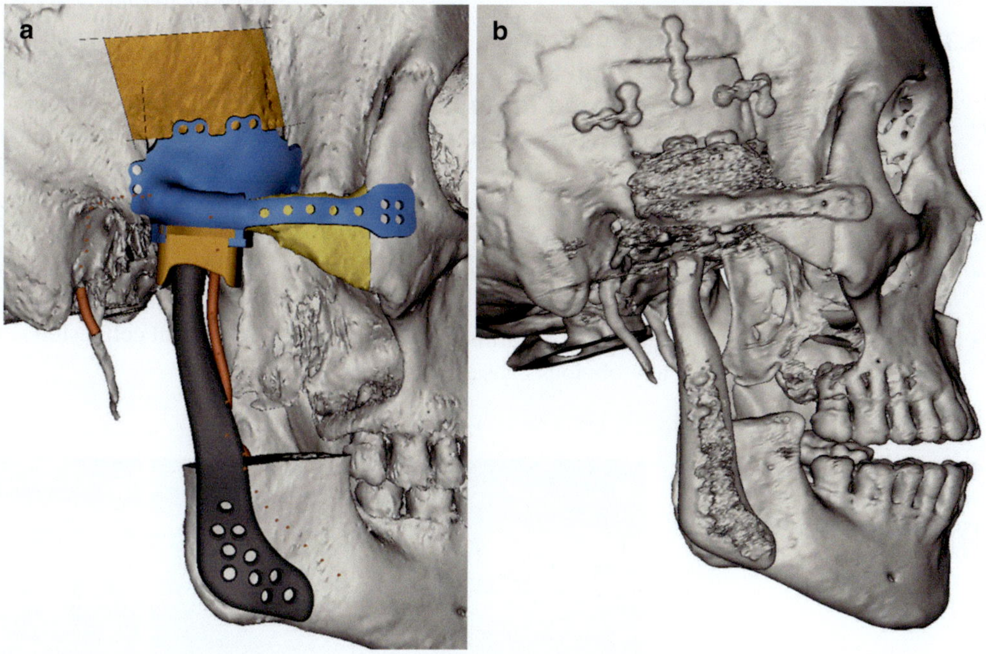

Fig. 6.52 Case L. Comparison between preoperative design and 5-year postoperative CT showing precise prosthesis seating. (**a**) Preoperative design. (**b**) 5-year postoperative

6.3 Design and Application of a Combined TMJ-Skull Base Prosthesis with Integrated Fixation

Case M: This case also illustrates Class III in the classification of the scope of the lesion, i.e., the condyle cannot be preserved, but the lesion does not extend beyond the mandibular foramen. Following Case L, the author's team further improved the fixation design of the combined TMJ-skull base prosthesis, obviating the need for several small plates. Moreover, the design considered the characteristics of craniomaxillofacial bone and joint stress distribution and integrated into the design fixation of the temporal bone flap window. The TMJ-skull base prosthesis also applies metal-nonmetal friction welding technology to connect the components. This is the prosthesis shown in Fig. 6.10. The prosthesis design not only meets the requirements of mechanical force conduction properties and long-term stability but also achieves the integrated fixation of the temporal bone flap, which has both morphological and functional advantages.

6.3.1 Case M. Design and Application of a Combined TMJ-Skull Base Prosthesis with Integrated Temporal Bone Flap Fixation and Stress Force Conduction

- Patient information: female, 26 years old.
- Complaint: pain in the left preauricular region with limited mouth opening for more than 2 years.
- History: the patient presented to our department with left preauricular pain without any obvious cause, which was not taken seriously, and then later she presented with limited mouth opening.
- Past history: she was physically fit, denied history of systemic diseases, and denied history of drug and food allergy.
- Clinical examination: chin point slightly deviated to the right, left preauricular mass, hard, indistinct, about 30 mm × 20 mm (Fig. 6.53). Mouth opening was limited, with a degree of 16 mm, and the mouth opening was deviated leftward. The intraoral occlusion was stable, with no dental or periodontal problems (Fig. 6.54). Preauricular pain VAS score was 5 of 10.
- Imaging: MRI of the joint showed the left TMJ mass, possible diagnosis of synovial chondromatosis or pigmentated villous nodular synovitis (PVNS) (Fig. 6.55). Advanced CT of the maxillofacial region showed that the bone of the left joint surface (condyle and temporal bone) was thickened, and multiple cystic bone destruction was seen under the joint surface, and soft tissue lesions were seen in the periphery of the joint, with a size of about 3.3 mm × 2.2 mm, CT-:137 HU, the joint space of the left TMJ was slightly narrowed, and there were no obvious abnormal and significant lymph node shadows in the neck bilaterally (Fig. 6.56). The tumor did not disrupt the ear canal or involve the internal carotid arteries (Fig. 6.56).
- Diagnosis: giant cellular lesion of the left joint and skull base.
- Postoperative pathology: microscopic description, giant cell lesion, mononuclear cell tumorlike hyperplasia, and osteoid matrix formation. The left TMJ was consistent with a giant cell lesion (Fig. 6.57).

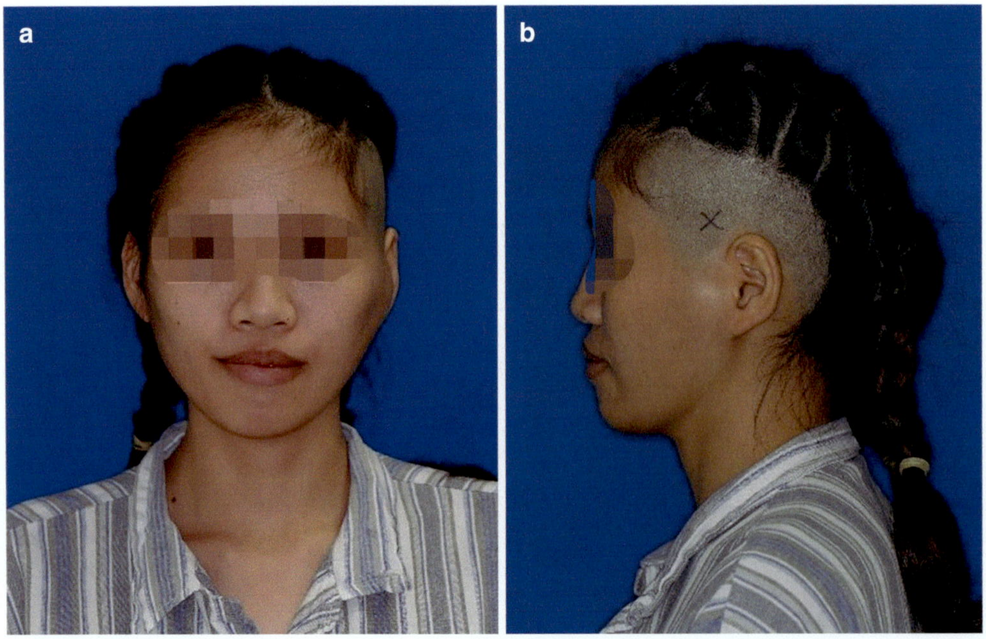

Fig. 6.53 Case M. Extraoral examination. Swollen left preauricular region. (**a**) Frontal view. (**b**) Lateral view

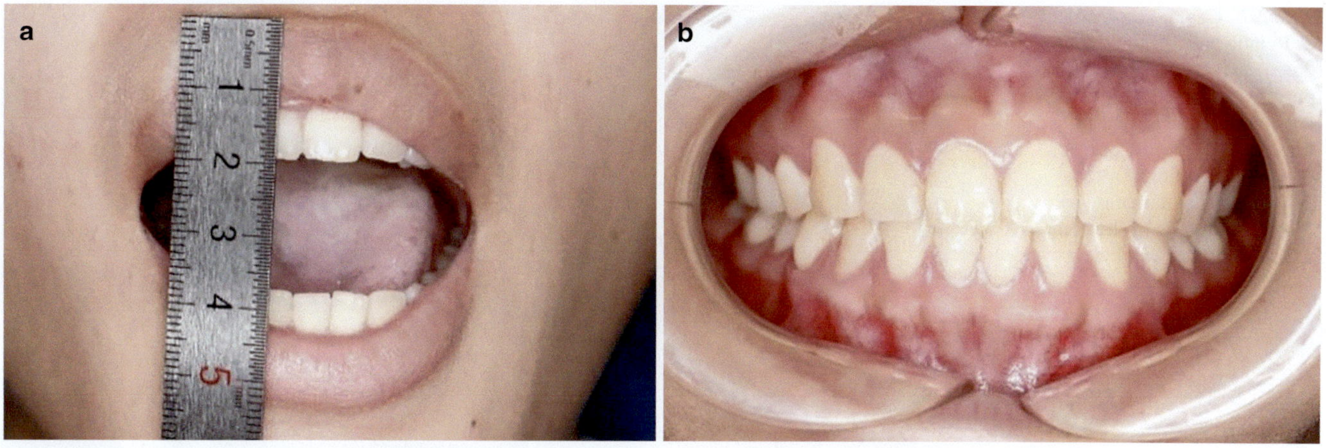

Fig. 6.54 Case M. Intraoral examination shows a 16 mm mouth opening with a left-sided mouth opening pattern and a stable intraoral occlusal relationship. (**a**) Mouth opening. (**b**) Occlusal relationship

Fig. 6.55 Case M. MRI of joints showed left TMJ-skull base occupied by lesion. (**a**) Lateral. (**b**) Medial

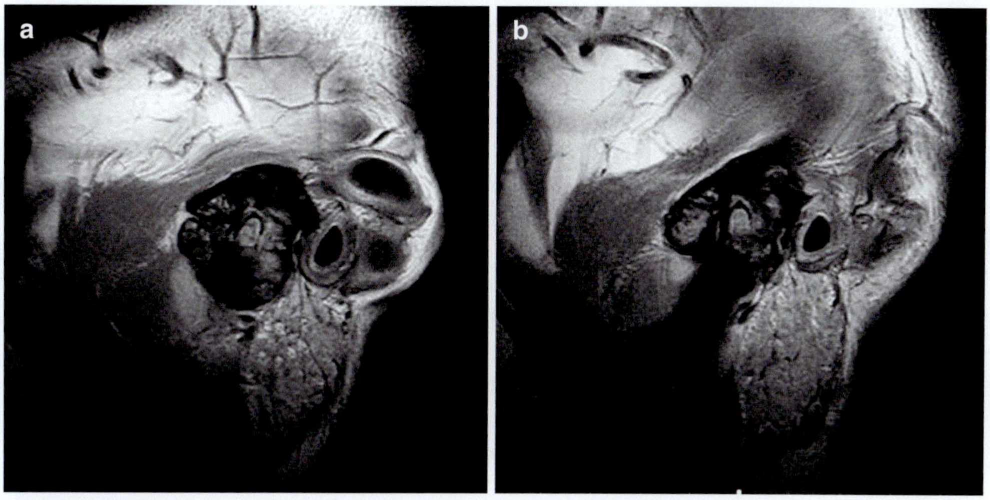

Fig. 6.56 Case M. Three-dimensional reconstruction of maxillofacial CT showing the extent of the tumor (green) in mm. (**a**) Lateral view. (**b**) Cerebrofacial view

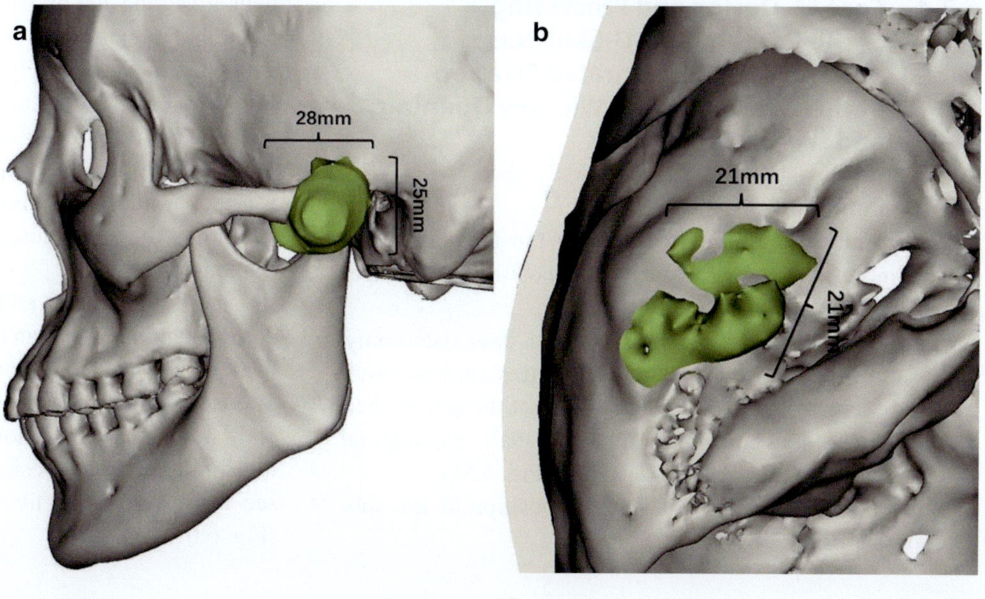

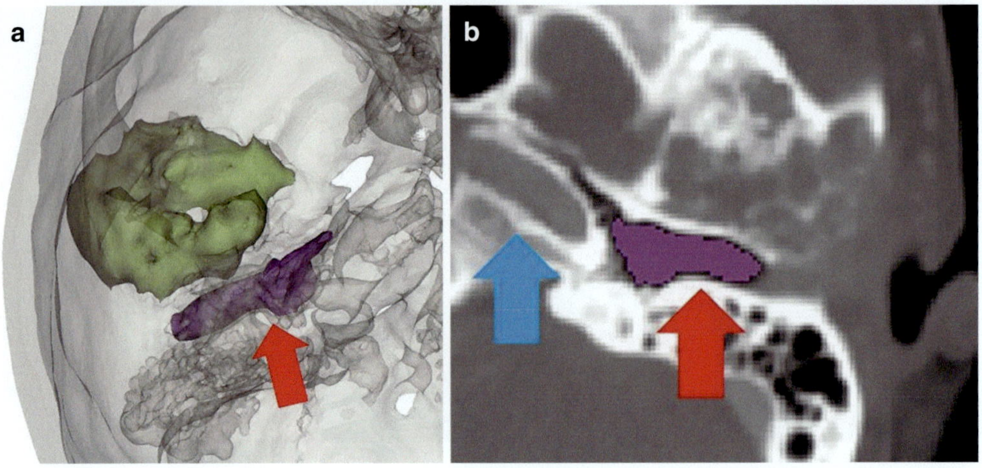

Fig. 6.57 Case M. Relationship of the tumor (green) to the ear canal (purple) and blood vessels. Red arrows point to the ear canal, and blue arrow points to the internal carotid artery and internal jugular vein. (**a**) CT reconstruction of the brain in face view. (**b**) Axial view

6.3.2 Case M. Diagnostic Imaging

6.3.3 Case M. Treatment Plan

6.3.3.1 Overall Treatment Option

Resection of the left TMJ-skull base tumor and prosthetic reconstruction utilizing a combined TMJ-skull base prosthesis with integrated fixation of the temporal bone window.

6.3.3.2 Surgical Resection Design

Resection extent design: resection of the tumor en bloc, removal of the diseased condyle (condylar head and subcondylar), and resection of the skull base (posterior border to the anterior wall of the external auditory canal, anterior border to the anterior margin of the tumor, and medial border to the foramen ovale); this case is a Class III defect.

6.3.4 Case M. Design and Processing of the Combined TMJ-Skull Base Prosthesis with Integrated Fixation of the Temporal Bone Window Opening and the Cutting Guides

Digital simulation surgery

- Temporal bone craniotomy: design the temporal bone squamosal window opening position (orange) (Fig. 6.58).
- Skull base osteotomies: anterior skull base osteotomy, posterior skull base osteotomy, and intraskull base osteotomy (brown), with care taken to protect the petrous part of the temporal bone (near the ear canal), the internal carotid artery, and the foramen ovale (Fig. 6.59).
- Subcondylar osteotomy: design the position of the subcondylar osteotomy (Fig. 6.60).
- Post-excision defect model: a model of a combined articular-skull base defect is created after excision of the lesion (Fig. 6.61).
- Design and processing of the combined TMJ-skull base prosthesis with integrated fixation of the temporal bone window

Design of an open-window bone-plate-fixed articulating-cranial-base joint prosthesis

Core components are imported to the design and positioned correctly: see Case L in this chapter (Fig. 6.62).

- Design of prosthesis extension components:
  Stress analysis of the normal whole head joint-craniomandibular stress distribution leads to extension of the skull base components with several wing plates, which serve the dual purpose of distributing the stresses while securing the temporal bone window opening block. The skull base component and the articulating socket component are connected by friction stir welding (Fig. 6.63).
  Mandibular extension component design, the same as described in Chap. 2 (Fig. 6.64).
- Screw hole depth measurement: the thickness of the bone at the squamous area of the temporal bone window opening (Fig. 6.65) and the depth of all screw holes to be used for the prothesis fixation (Fig. 6.66) are measured to determine the screw lengths to be used in intraoperative implantation.
- Prosthesis fabrication and fitting: the titanium skull base component was fabricated using a metal 3D printer, and the UHMWPE fossa component was fabricated using 5-axis finishing, with the two being joined using metallic and nonmetallic friction welding techniques. After machining, the prosthesis is test fitted on a resin mold to see if the prosthesis fits the bone surface and is stable (Fig. 6.67).

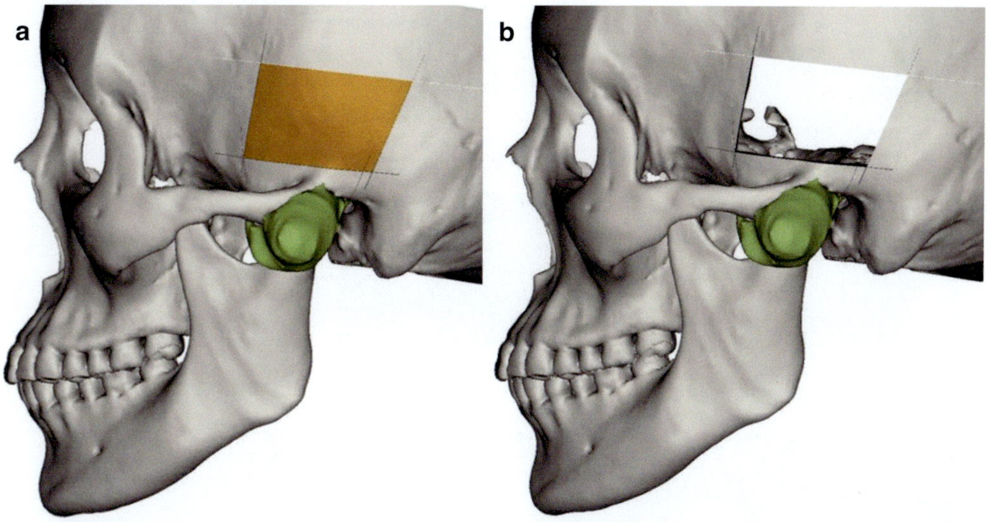

Fig. 6.58 Case M. Temporal bone window opening (orange). (**a**) Temporal bone osteotomy line design. (**b**) After the temporal bone opening

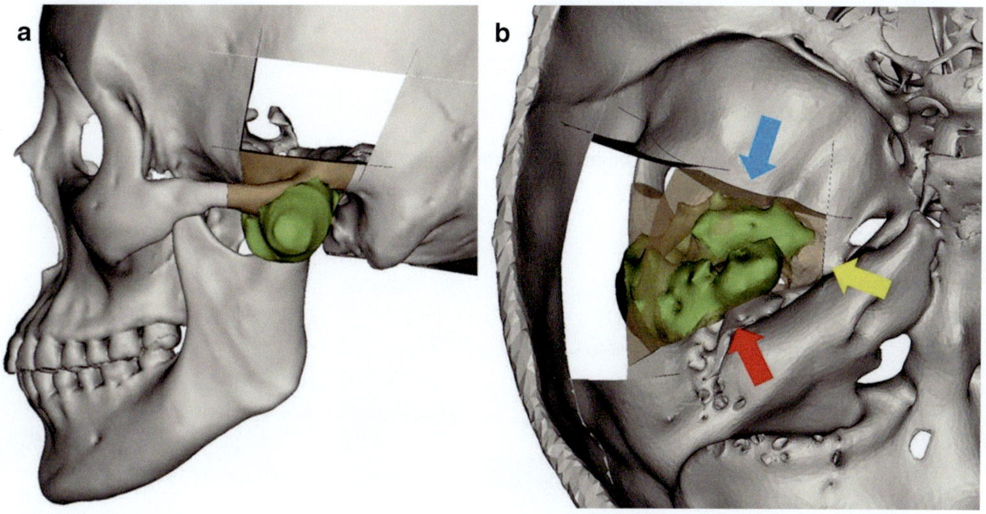

Fig. 6.59 Case M. Osteotomies at the skull base, with the tumor shown in green and the diseased bone to be removed from the skull base shown in brown. Anterior skull base osteotomy (blue arrow), posterior skull base osteotomy (red arrow), and intracranial skull base osteotomy (yellow arrow). (**a**) Lateral view, (**b**) Cerebrofacial view

- Digital design of the cutting guides for precise positioning

  Design of the zygomatic arch cutting guide: design the cutting guides along the zygomatic arch osteotomy line (Fig. 6.68).

Design of temporal bone window opening and skull base cutting guides: design the temporal bone window opening and skull base cutting guides along the temporal bone osteotomy lines (Fig. 6.69).

Design of the subcondylar osteotomy positioning guide: the cutting guide is designed along the subcondylar osteotomy line and the posterior border of the mandible (Fig. 6.70).

Screw hole position design: transfer the screw hole positions of the prothesis to the cutting guides to aid direct intraoperative positioning of the prosthesis (Fig. 6.71).

6.3.5 Case M. Surgical Procedures

Preoperative laboratory tests: the same as described in Sect. 3.2.5, Preoperative Laboratory Tests.

Preoperative preparation: see Sect. 6.2. Preoperative Preparation in (iv) Surgical Procedures in Case L of this chapter.

6.3.5.1 Steps of Surgical Procedure

1. Surgical approach: a modified auriculotemporal anterior incision and temporal incision to expose the temporal bone and the TMJ.
2. Installation of the cutting guide and temporary removal of the zygomatic arch: the zygomatic arch cutting guide is installed and used to assist in the temporary removal of the zygomatic arch and positioning of the prosthesis (Fig. 6.72).

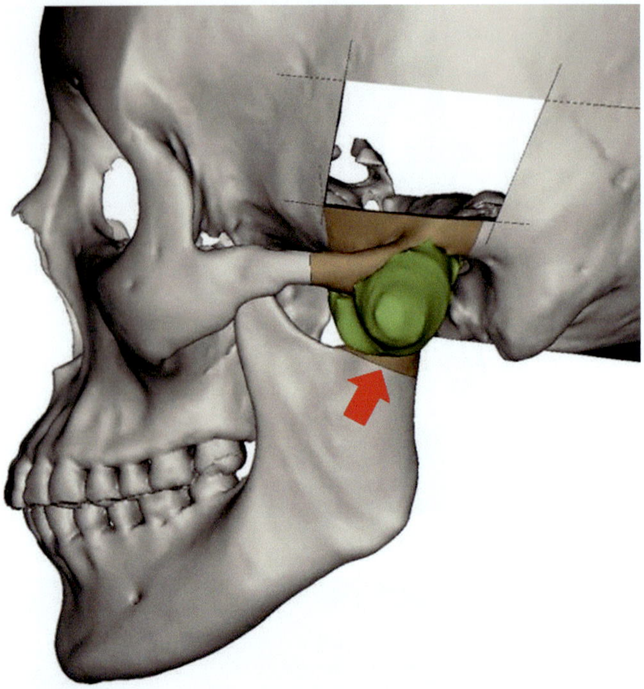

Fig. 6.60 Case M. Subcondylar osteotomy (red arrow points to the osteotomy line)

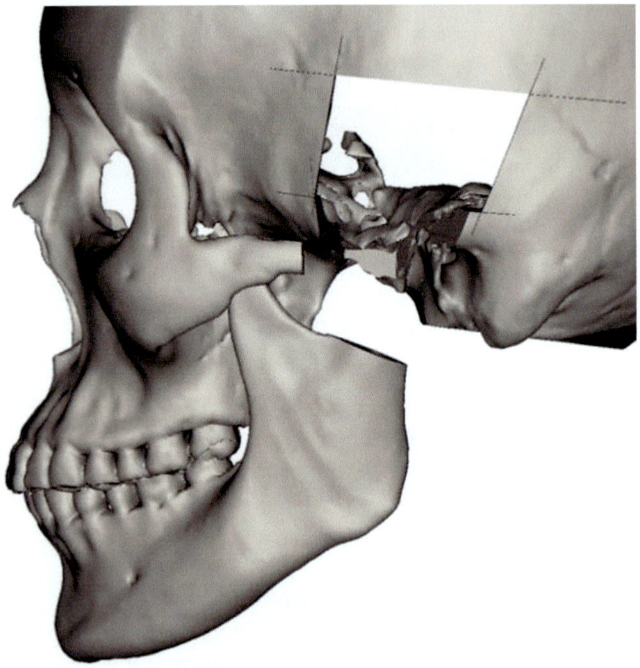

Fig. 6.61 Case M. Combined TMJ-skull base defect after resection

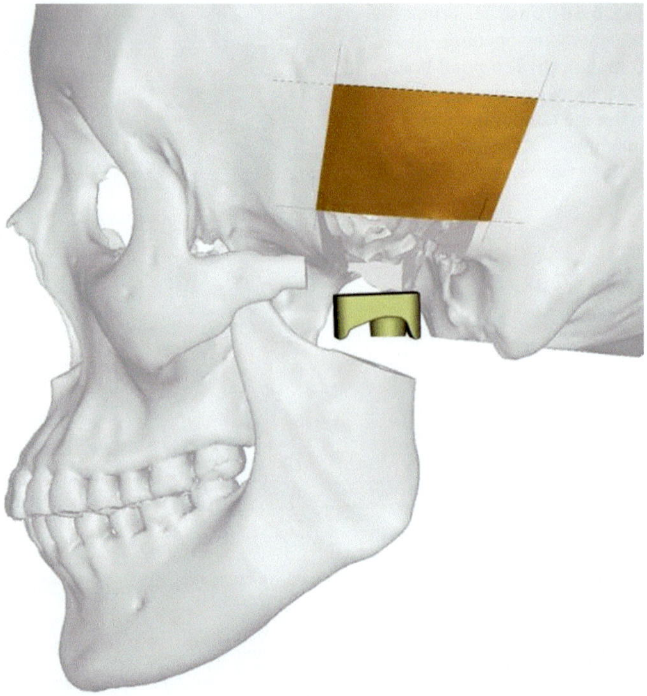

Fig. 6.62 Case M. Fossa core component (yellow) location placement

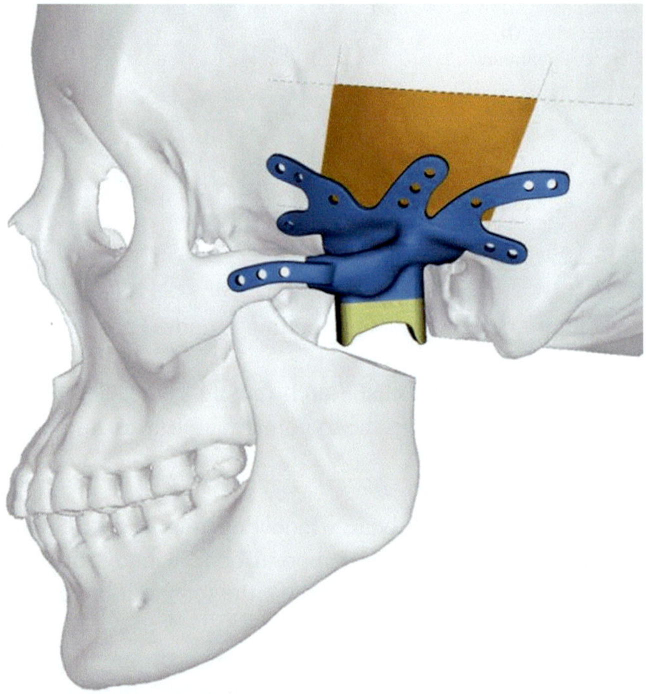

Fig. 6.63 Case M. Skull base extension component (blue) of the combined TMJ-skull base prosthesis with integrated fixation of the temporal bone window

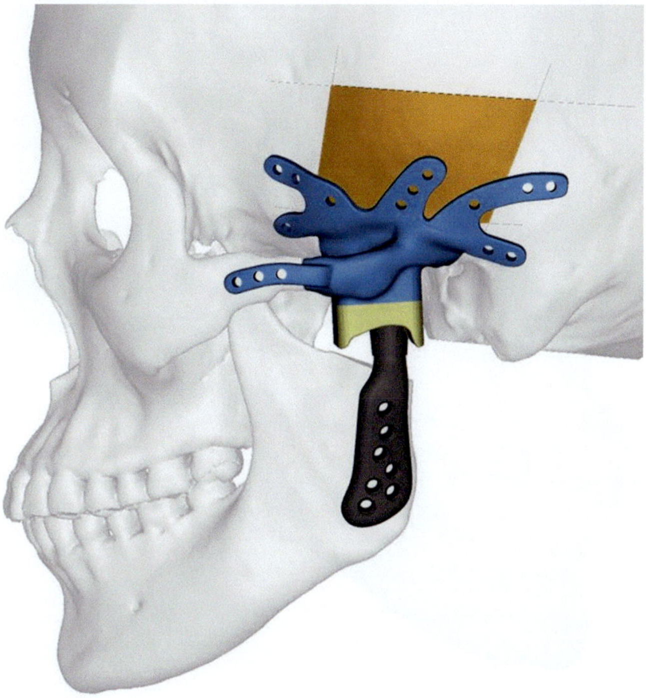

Fig. 6.64 Case M. Mandibular prosthesis extension component (dark gray) design for the combined TMJ-skull base prosthesis with integrated fixation of the temporal bone window

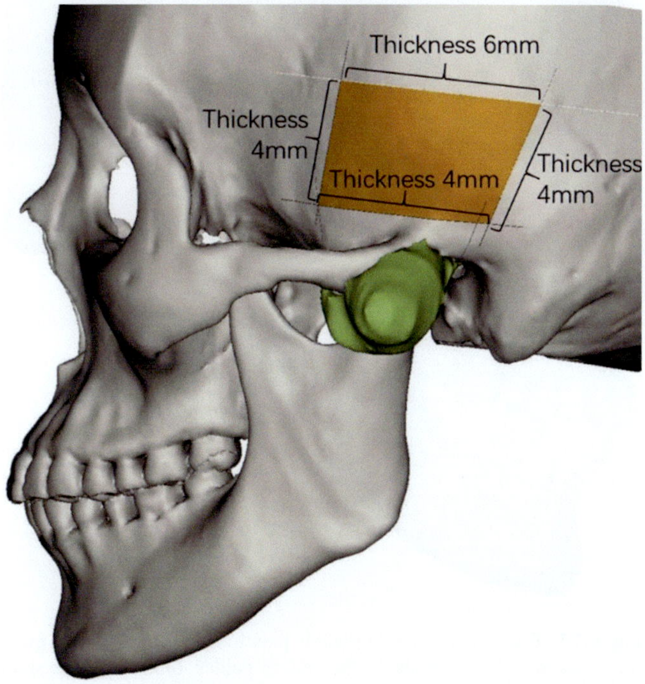

Fig. 6.65 Case M. Measurement of the thickness of the bone at the squamous area of the temporal bone window opening (orange)

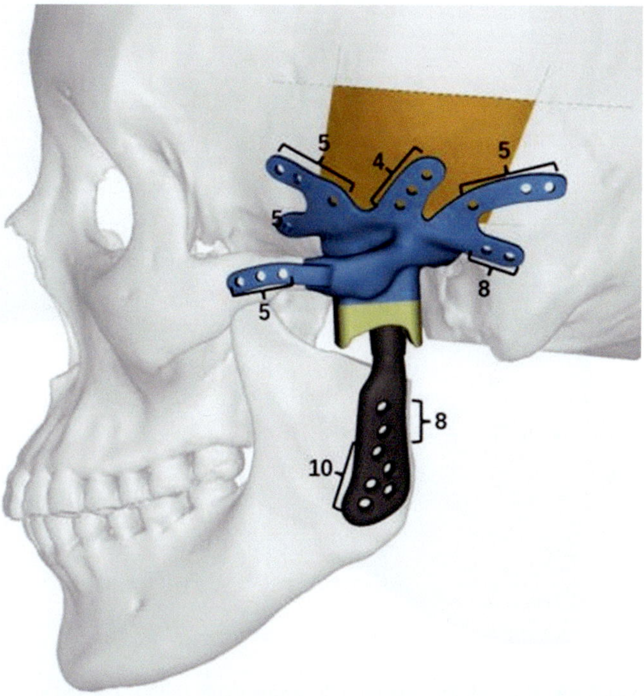

Fig. 6.66 Case M. Screw hole depth measurements: blue shows skull base extension component (in mm), dark gray shows the mandibular component of the prosthesis, and orange shows the temporal bone window

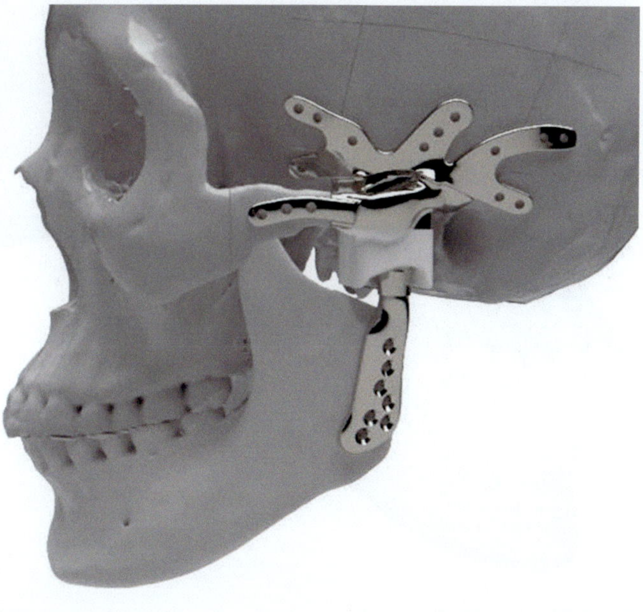

Fig. 6.67 Case M. Prosthesis fabrication and fitting on a resin mold

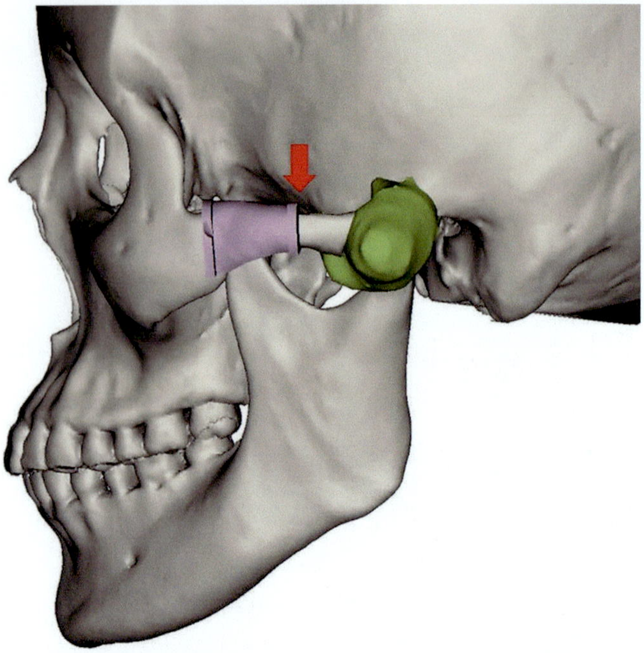

Fig. 6.68 Case M. Zygomatic arch cutting guide (pink). The red arrow points to the osteotomy line on the anterior edge of the tumor

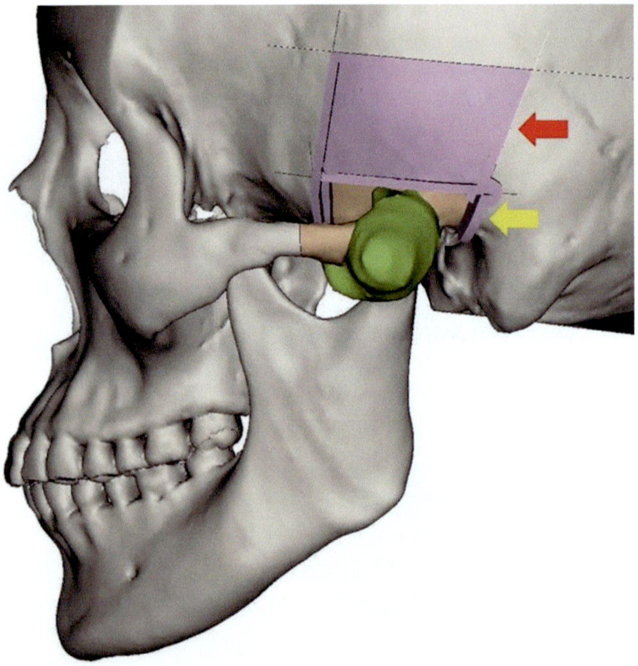

Fig. 6.69 Case M. Temporal bone window opening (red arrow) and skull base osteotomy (yellow arrow) positioning guides (pink)

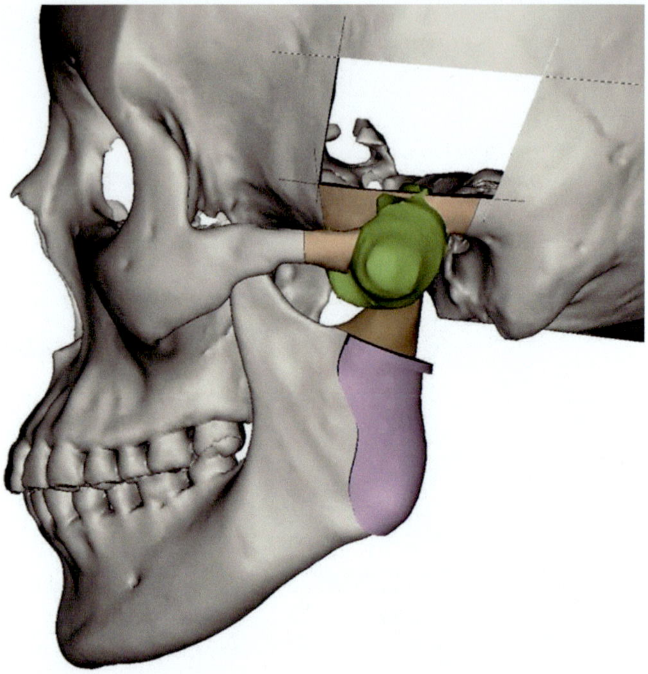

Fig. 6.70 Case M. Design of the subcondylar cutting guide (pink) for precise positioning

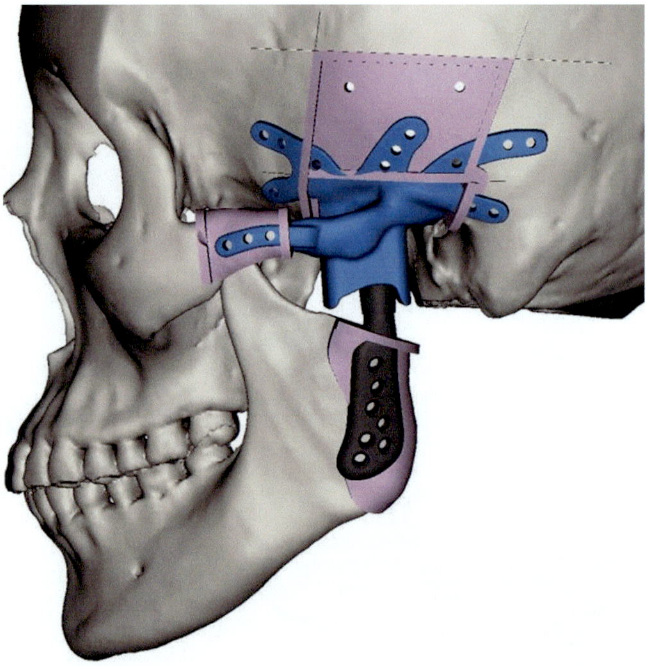

Fig. 6.71 Case M. The guide plate is positioned in line with the prosthesis screw holes. Pink shows the cutting guides, blue shows the skull base component of the prosthesis, and dark gray shows the mandibular component of the combined TMJ-skull base prosthesis with integrated fixation of the temporal bone window

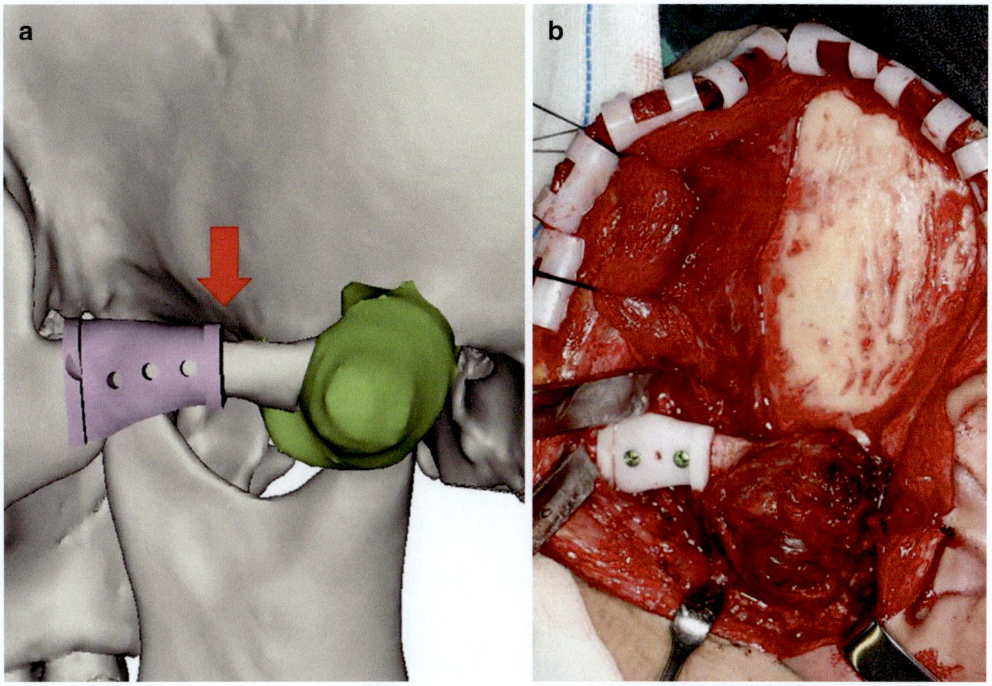

Fig. 6.72 Case M. Zygomatic arch cutting guides assist in zygomatic arch temporary removal and prosthesis positioning (red arrows). (**a**) Design. (**b**) Actual

3. Temporal bone window opening, skull base osteotomy, and prosthetic positioning: utilize the temporal bone and skull base cutting guides to assist with the craniotomy, skull base osteotomy, and prosthetic positioning (Fig. 6.73)
4. Subcondylar osteotomy: the subcondylar cutting guide is utilized to assist with condylar osteotomy and positioning of the prosthesis (Fig. 6.74).

Resection of the lesion: Complete resection of the tumor, joints, and skull base and, after resection, complete preservation of the dura (Fig. 6.75). In practice, the resection of the posterior margin of the tumor is insufficient, which requires further careful abrasion of the tumor and preservation of the bone of the anterior wall of the ear canal, due to the concern that the removal of the anterior wall of the ear canal may affect hearing by exposing the middle ear (which would require further treatment) (Fig. 6.76).

Repositioning of the temporal bone window, and implantation and fixation of the fossa component of the TMJ-skull base prosthesis with integrated fixation: the dura is lined with fat (taken from the periumbilical area) between the dura and the prosthesis. Then the temporal bone flap is repositioned, and the prosthesis component is implanted and fixated (Figs. 6.77 and 6.78).

Mandibular prosthesis component implantation and fixation: Implantation and fixation of the mandibular prosthesis component are performed using endoscopic assistance (Fig. 6.78).

6.3.6 Case M. Postoperative Analysis of Prosthesis Implantation Precision

Regular postoperative follow-ups were performed for appearance (facial shape), function (mouth opening degree, mouth shape), and prosthesis evaluation (safety, accuracy).

Immediately after surgery: The intraoperative guide plate was accurately seated and the prosthesis was fitted smoothly (Fig. 6.79), and a comparison between the preoperative design and the postoperative reconstruction showed that the prosthesis was accurately seated (Fig. 6.80). The analysis of the postoperative prosthesis fitting error showed that the error in the core component was 1.07 mm and the overall error in the combined prosthesis was 1.46 mm (Figs. 6.81 and 6.82).

6.3.7 Case M. Long-Term Follow-Up and Prognosis

6.3.7.1 Three-Year Postoperative Follow-Up

There was no recurrence of pre-existing disease, the face is in good shape with no abnormalities, and there is no redness, swelling, or other reactions in the operative area. The diet of the patient was normal (Fig. 6.83).

Improvement in preauricular pain, improvement in VAS pain score to 1 out of 19; joint-mandibular-occlusal-facial coordination, occlusal relationship stabilized.

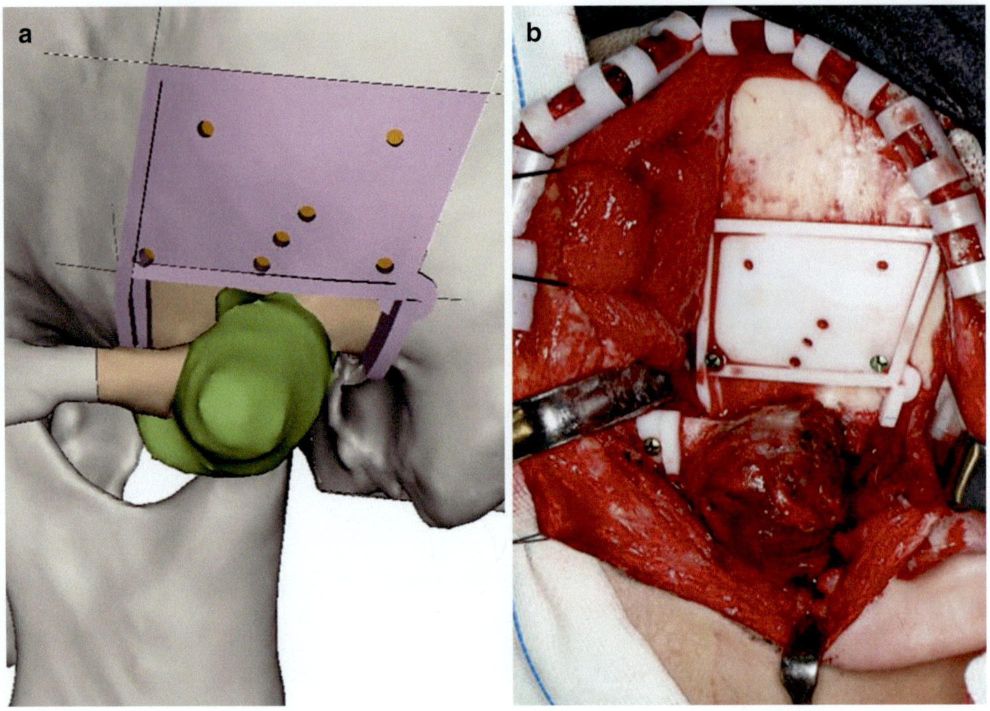

Fig. 6.73 Case M. Temporal bone window opening and skull base osteotomy cutting guides assist with temporal bone craniotomy and anterior and posterior osteotomy at the skull base. (**a**) Design. (**b**) Actual

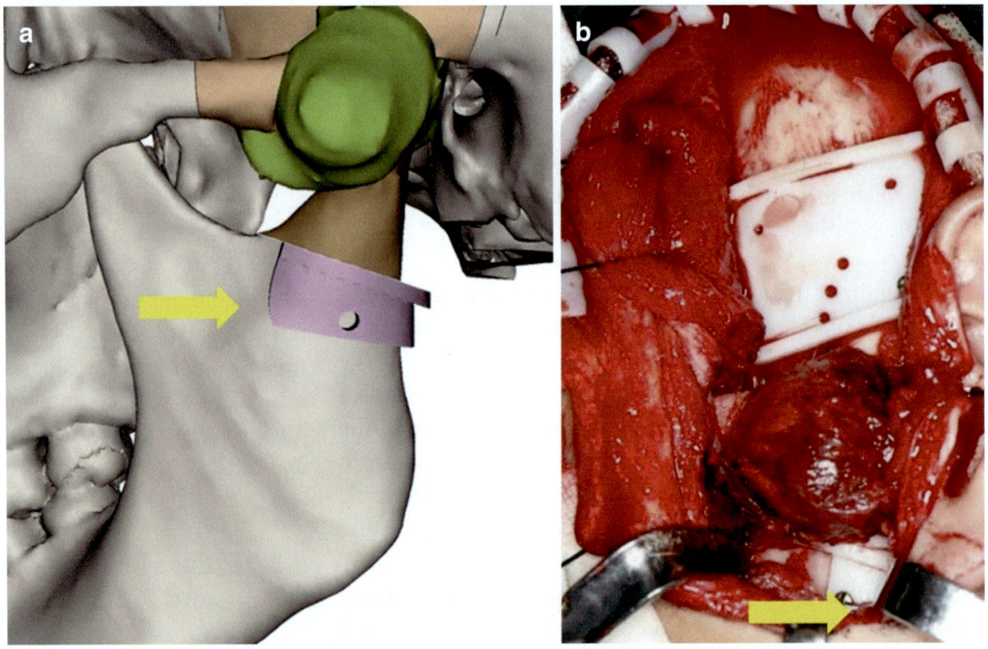

Fig. 6.74 Case M. Subcondylar cutting guide (yellow arrows) assists in truncating the condyle and positioning the prosthesis. (**a**) Design. (**b**) Actual

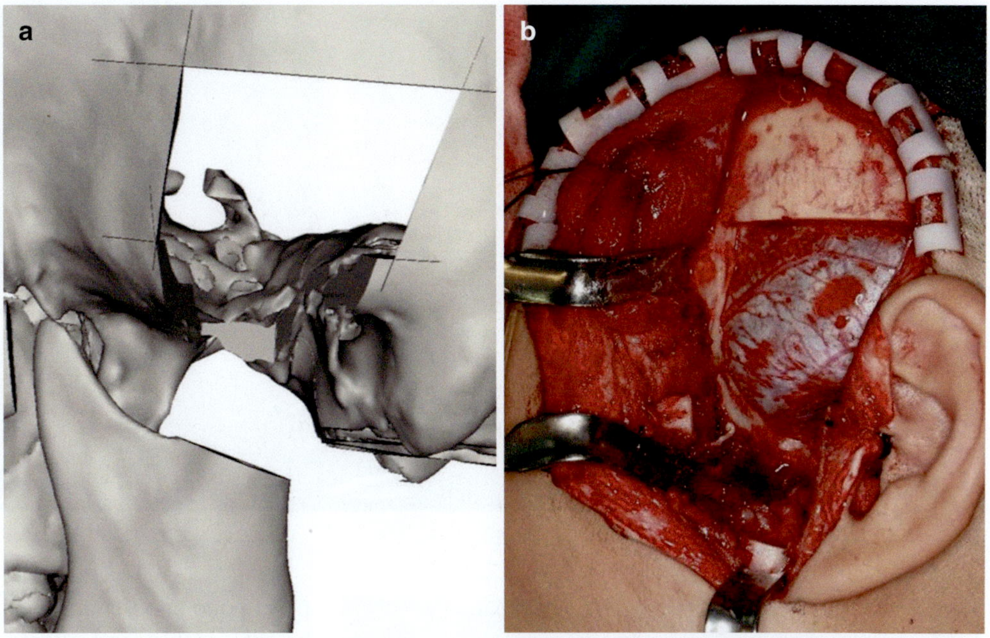

Fig. 6.75 Case M. Complete resection of the tumor. (**a**) Design. (**b**) Actual

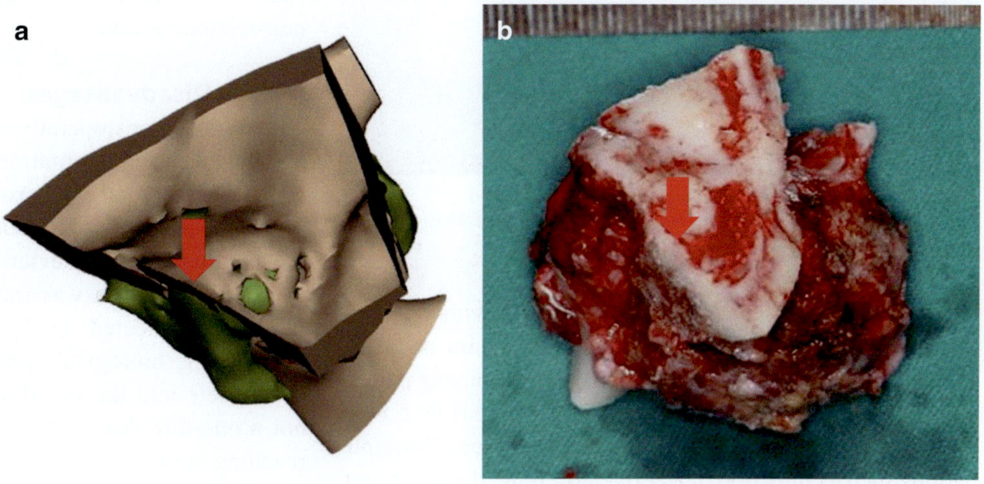

Fig. 6.76 Case M. Comparison of preoperative design and complete intraoperative resection of the tumor. Red arrows show the posterior margin of the tumor. (**a**) Design. (**b**) Actual

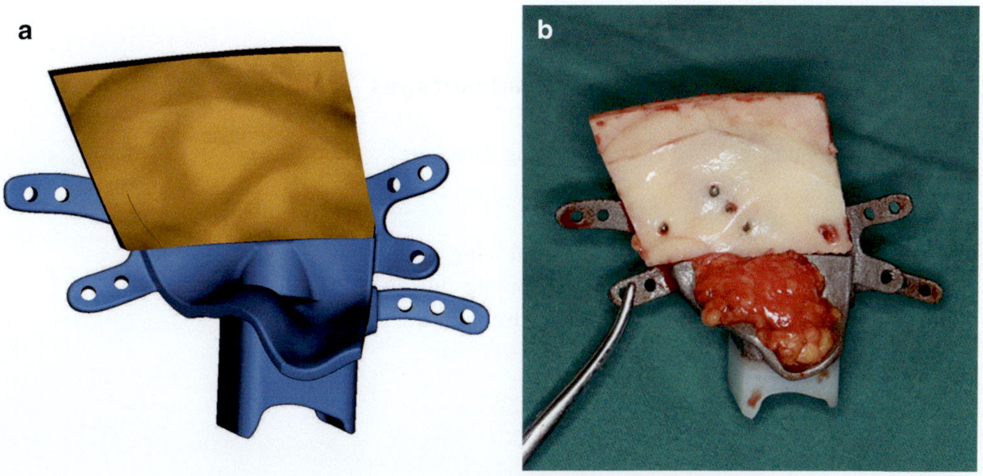

Fig. 6.77 Temporal bone flap affixed with screws to the articular fossa component of the TMJ-skull base prosthesis with integrated fixation. (**a**) Design. (**b**) Actual

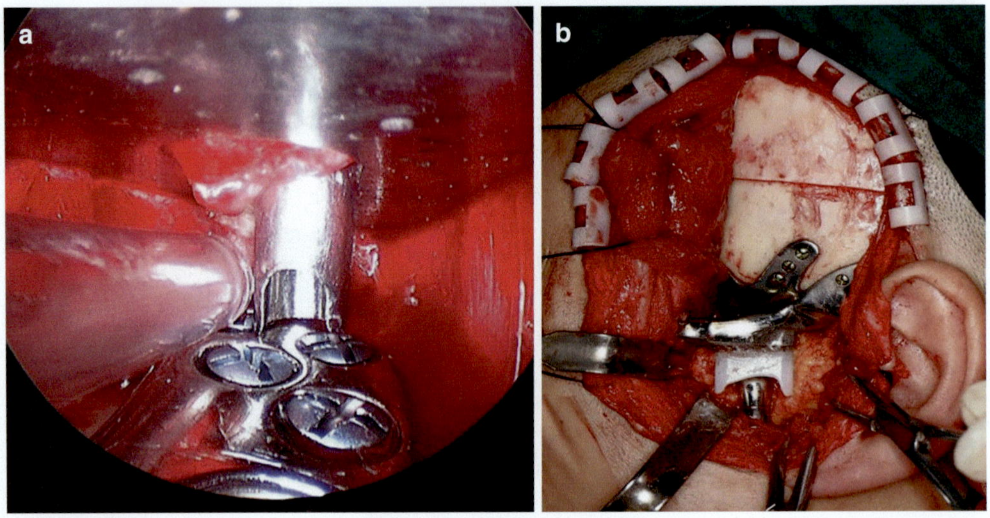

Fig. 6.78 Case M. Completion of endoscopically assisted mandibular prosthesis component implantation and fixation. (**a**) Endoscopic view. (**b**) Lateral view

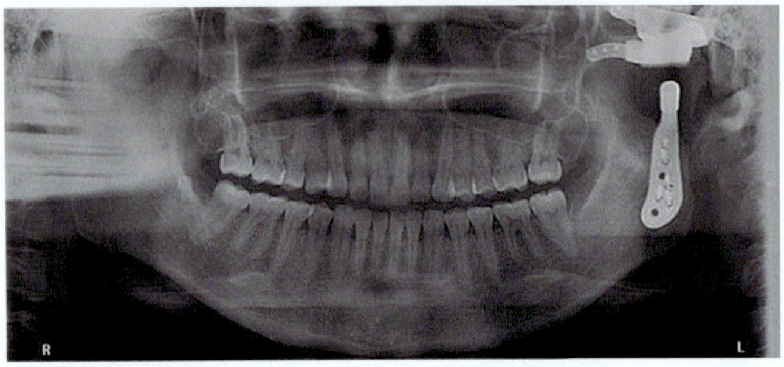

Fig. 6.79 Case M. Immediate postoperative panoramic film

The mouth opening improved to 30 mm, with 7 mm of lateral movement to the affected side and 5 mm of lateral movement to the healthy side, and the mouth opening pattern was deflected by 5 mm toward the affected side (Fig. 6.84).

Prosthesis evaluation: the prosthesis was free of complications such as infection, rejection, loosening, displacement, fracture, ectopic osteogenesis, or allergy (Figs. 6.85 and 6.86).

6.3.8 Case M. Advantages and Disadvantages

Chen Minjie, Zheng Jisi, Wu Hao, and Wang Zhaoyan

6.3.8.1 Advantages

The design goal was achieved, the temporal wing extension of the prosthesis made it easier to manipulate during the surgery, and at the same time, it could securely fix the temporal bone flap. After 3 years of follow-up, it was found to be safe, stable, and effective. The overall plan of precise resection and effective reconstruction has solved the drawbacks of traditional surgery, such as recurrence and non-reconstruction.

6.3.8.2 Disadvantages

Although the postoperative mouth opening of 30 mm was higher than the international standard of 25 mm to be achieved after total joint prosthesis implantation, it was still far less than the normal width of opening. The main reason for the mandibular deviation to the affected side when opening the mouth was that the lateral pterygoid muscle was not connected to the joint. Achieving this, which requires the biological connection between the tendon or the muscle and the metal surface (muscle attachment), is not a one-day task, but if it can be achieved this has far-reaching significance.

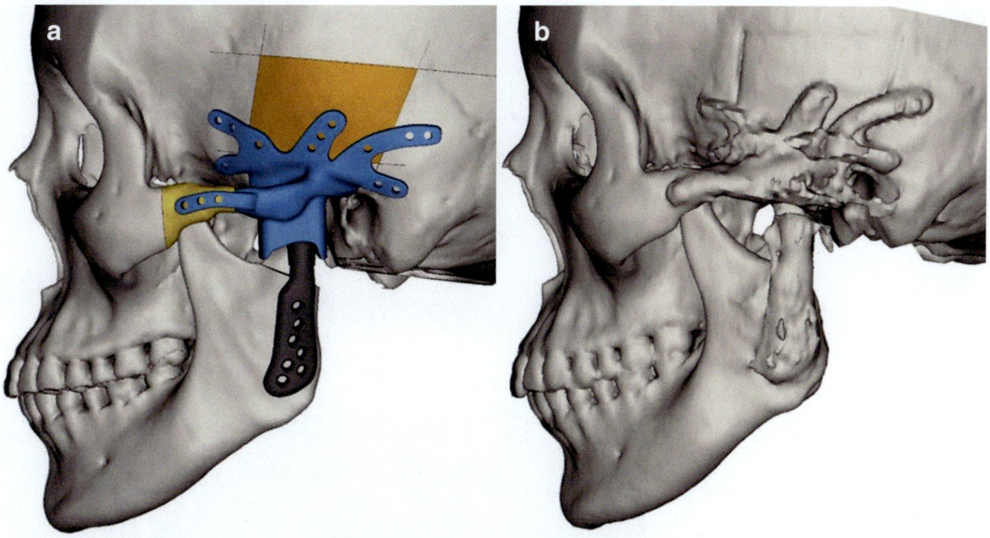

Fig. 6.80 Case M. Comparison of CT reconstructions showing precise prosthesis seating. (**a**) Preoperative design. (**b**) Immediate postoperative period

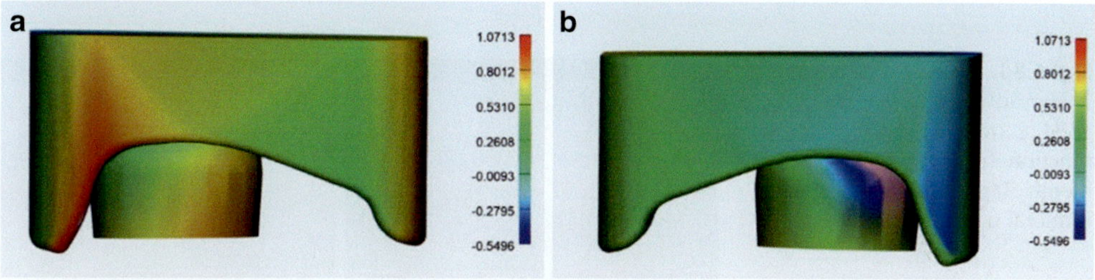

Fig. 6.81 Case M. Prosthetic core component error 1.07 mm. (**a**) Lateral error. (**b**) Medial error

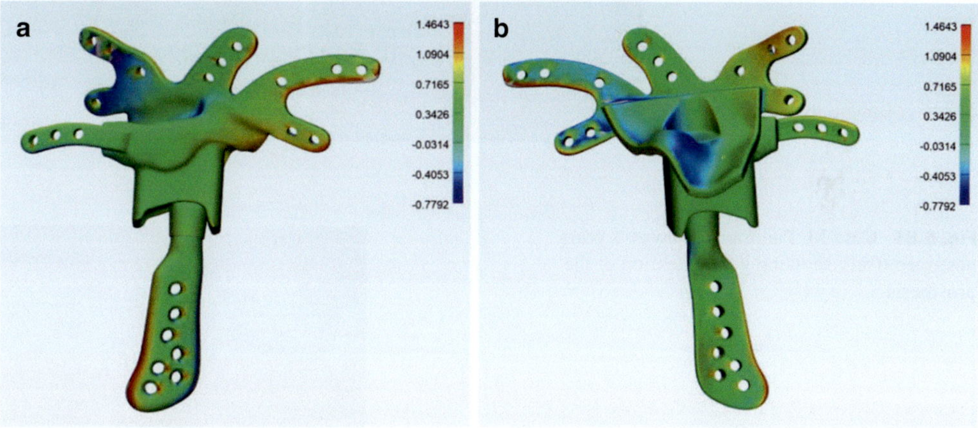

Fig. 6.82 Case M. Overall prosthesis error 1.46 mm. (**a**) Lateral error. (**b**) Medial error

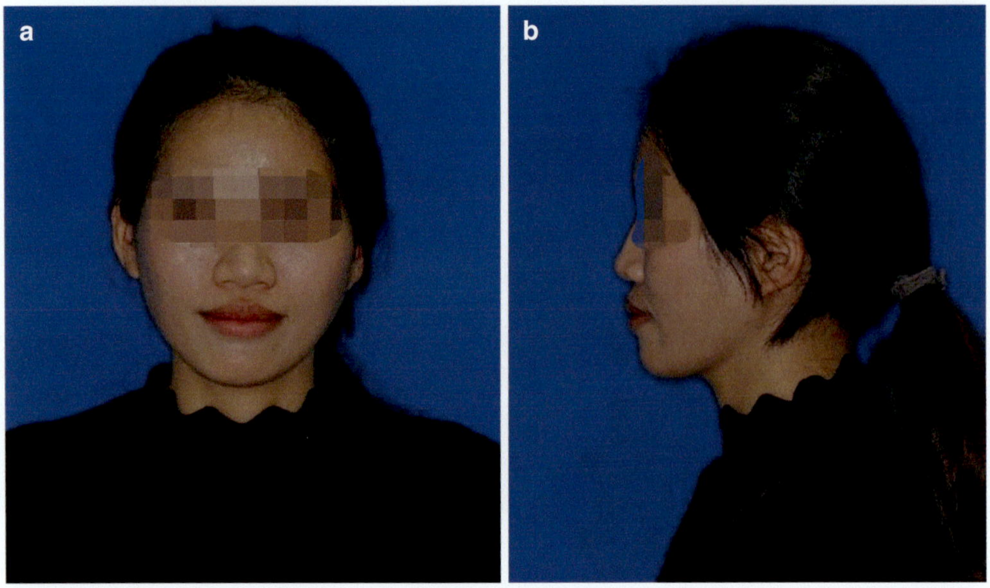

Fig. 6.83 Case M. Follow-up 3 years after surgery: good facial symmetry and no change in facial shape. (**a**) Frontal view. (**b**) Lateral view

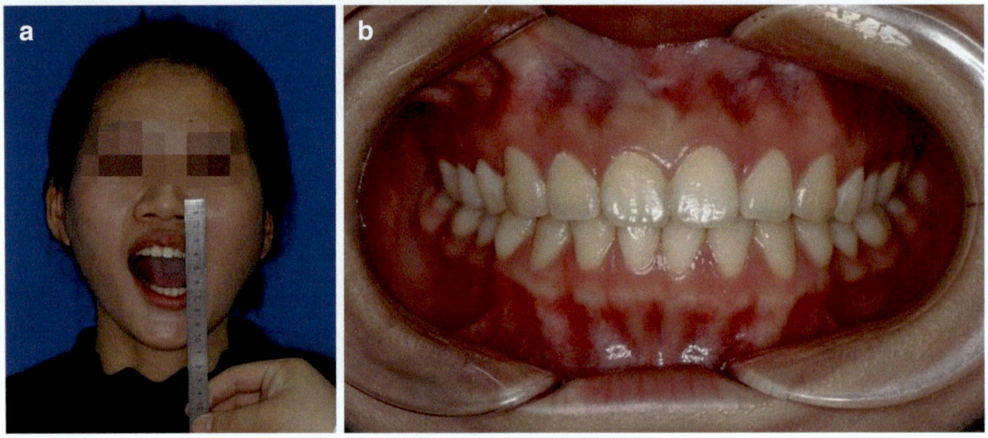

Fig. 6.84 Case M. Follow-up 3 years after surgery, with good recovery of joint function. (**a**) Opening of mouth 30 mm. (**b**) Stable intraoral occlusal relationship

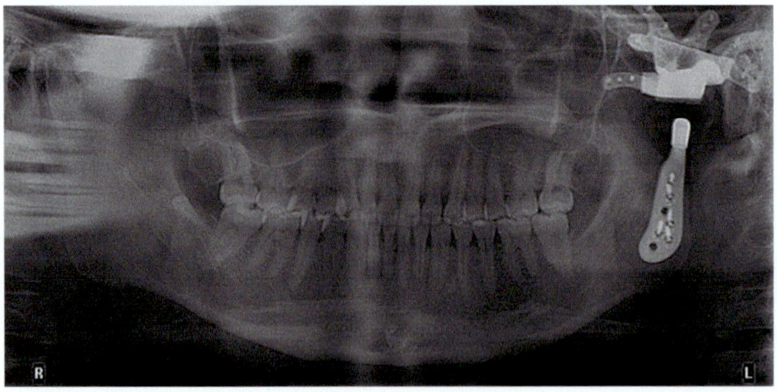

Fig. 6.85 Case M. Panoramic view at 3 years postoperatively showing good retention of the prosthesis

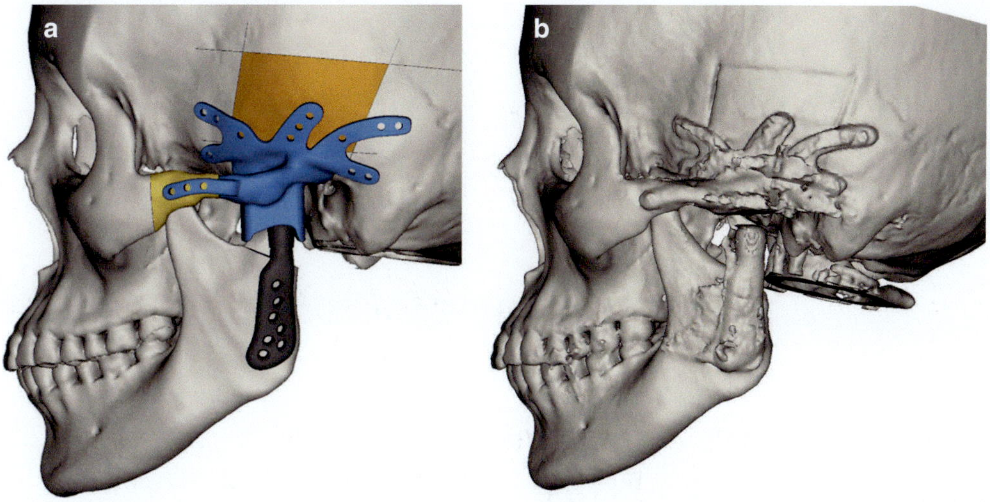

Fig. 6.86 Case M. Comparison of CT reconstruction showing precise prosthesis seating. (**a**) Preoperative design. (**b**) 3 years postoperatively

7 Reconstruction of Skull Base-Fossa Diseases, While Preserving the TMJ

Chi Yang, Minjie Chen, Zhilin Guo, and Jisi Zheng

This chapter focuses on Class I and Class II of Yang's new classification of combined TMJ-skull base lesions as defined in Chap. 6, i.e., lesions at the skull base with the articular fossa and/or the infratemporal fossa involved, and it discusses how the structures of the articular disc, condyle, and lateral pterygoid muscle can be preserved as much as possible when the lesion is resected. While designing and implementing complete resection of the lesion, every effort should be made to preserve the normal disc-articular-muscle complex and maximize the preservation of healthy joint tissue. So, in our practice, a personalized prosthesis is designed and manufactured according to the size of the defect and according to needs for the structural and functional reconstruction of the skull base and glenoid fossa. Such hemiarticular (skull base and articular fossa) prosthetic reconstruction should be particularly focused on:

1. Condylar non-resorption, i.e., adequate condylar blood supply and appropriate stress tolerance
2. Treatment of the articular disc so that it is not prone to adherence to the prosthesis, in order to ensure normal joint motion

For this reason, the author carried out a series of targeted prosthesis and surgical design innovations, and after clinical application and 5 years of follow-up, satisfactory results have been demonstrated. This chapter will be a detailed introduction to the reconstruction surgery of this prosthesis system.

7.1 Overview

This section summarizes the definition and classification of skull base-fossa diseases, reviews traditional prosthetic reconstruction methods and their shortcomings, and focuses on innovative prosthetic reconstruction methods and digital design processes for individualized skull base-fossa prostheses. The indications, contraindications, digital design, surgical points, and prosthesis design will be covered. The thinking behind skull base-fossa prosthesis reconstruction will be discussed as well. The introduction of this section will provide some theoretical knowledge on customized prosthetic repair and reconstruction techniques for skull base-fossa lesions.

7.1.1 Definition of Skull Base-Fossa Diseases

This refers to lesions in which the articular fossa, upper-articular cavity, and the skull base are involved simultaneously, and the tumor may also invade the infratemporal fossa and the ear, but the articular disc and condyle are not involved, or only the synovial membrane and capsule attached to the articular disc are invaded. These diseases are most commonly tumors. Clinically, the problem is usually manifested as swelling and pain in the preauricular and temporal regions and limited mouth opening; if it involves the ear canal, it may be accompanied by hearing impairment. Surgical excision is the preferred treatment, often requiring the collaboration of TMJ surgery, otorhinolaryngology, and neurosurgery. Opinions differ on whether reconstruction is necessary and how it should be performed.

7.1.2 Classification of Skull Base-Fossa Lesions

Skull base-fossa lesions include two types (see Fig. 7.1):

- Type I, in which the skull base and articular fossa are involved in the lesion and the articular disc and condyle are not involved and do not protrude into the infratemporal fossa, so there is no need to treat the condyle and the joint.

Chi Y. (✉) · Minjie C. · Zhilin G. · Jisi Z.
Shanghai Ninth People's Hospital, Shanghai Jiao Tong University School of Medicine, Shanghai, China

© People's Medical Publishing House, PR of China 2025
Chi Y. (ed.), *Atlas of Customized TMJ-Cranio-Jaw Prosthesis*, https://doi.org/10.1007/978-981-95-0611-8_7

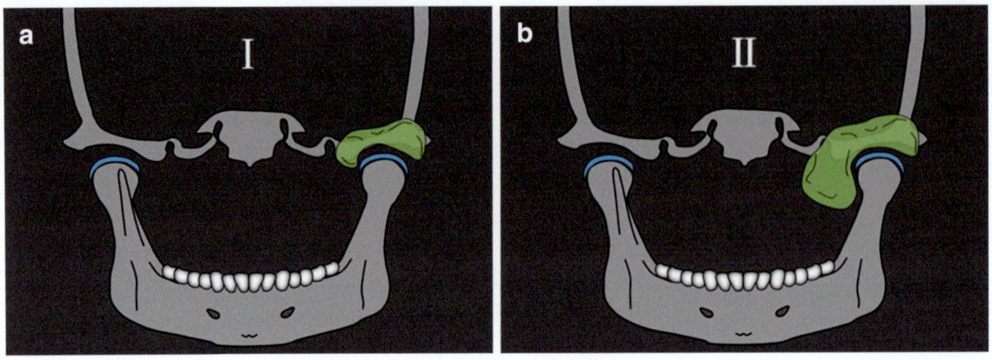

Fig. 7.1 Classification of skull base-fossa lesions, with the articular disc shown in blue and the lesion in green. (**a**) Type I shows involvement of the skull base and joint fossa without protrusion of the lesion into the infratemporal fossa, and condyles and articular discs are salvageable. (**b**) Type II shows involvement of the skull base and fossa with protrusion of the lesion into the infratemporal fossa, but condyles and articular discs are not affected, suggesting that they may be retained. In such cases, the infratemporal fossa lesions must be cleared after temporary detachment of the condyle

- Type II, in which the skull base and articular fossa are involved in the lesion, and it protrudes into the infratemporal fossa, but the condyle and articular disc are not yet involved, suggesting that the condyle and the articular disc may be preserved. But the condyle has to be temporarily detached before the infratemporal fossa lesion can be cleared, and then the condyle can be implanted back and secured with appropriate fixation plates.

This classification of the disease scope is illustrated in Fig. 7.1.

7.1.3 Traditional Methods of Repair and Reconstruction for Skull Base-Fossa Lesions

Traditional repair and reconstruction of skull base-fossa lesions include soft tissue flap filling, titanium mesh reconstruction, and autologous bone repair. These methods all have some shortcomings.

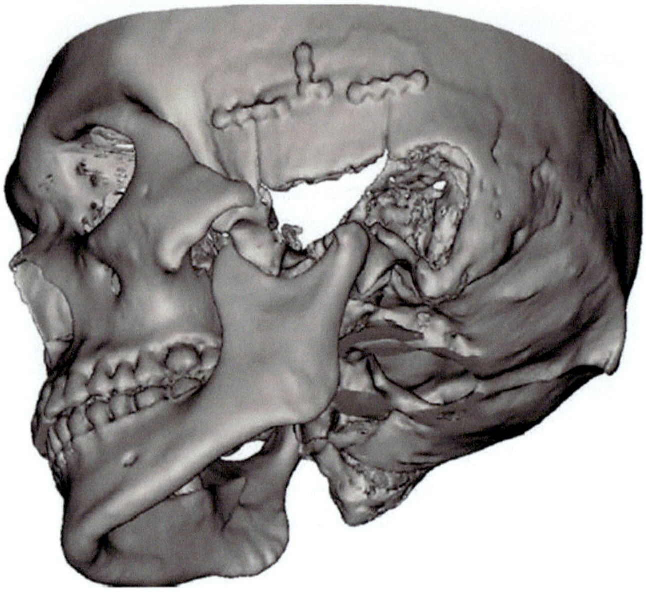

Fig. 7.2 After resection of a skull base-fossa lesion, the skull base defective bone tissue is not repaired or is only filled with a soft tissue flap

7.1.3.1 Filling with Soft Tissue Flaps

Both oral and maxillofacial surgery and otorhinolaryngology and neurosurgery commonly use temporal muscle flaps or fat flaps to fill in defects in the skull base and joint fossa. This method is the simplest and most used. However, the disadvantages are that the condyle does not fit smoothly into the joint fossa, which affects chewing efficiency, temporal depression deformities are common, and there is also a risk of malocclusion and occlusal disorders (Fig. 7.2).

7.1.3.2 Titanium Mesh Repair

Titanium mesh repair is also a relatively simple method for repairing skull base and joint fossa defects, and it can provide some support for restoring the shape. However, titanium mesh has limited bearing capacity for chewing forces; in addition, titanium mesh should not come into contact with the condyle or articular disc; otherwise, adhesion or condyle resorption may occur. There is also a risk of titanium plate exposure (Fig. 7.3).

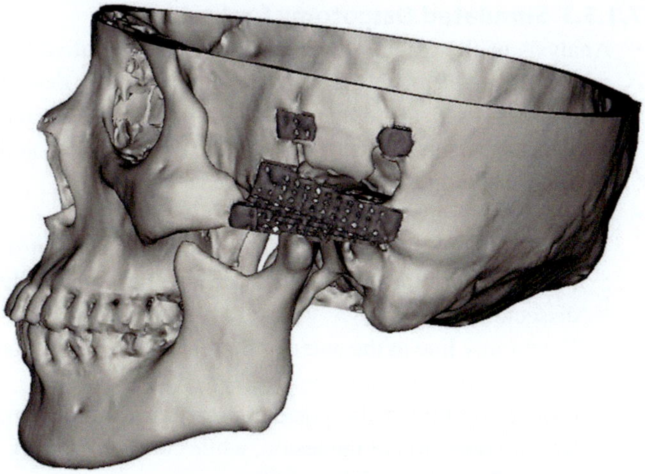

Fig. 7.3 Titanium mesh (dark gray) repair of skull base bone defect after resection of skull base-fossa lesion

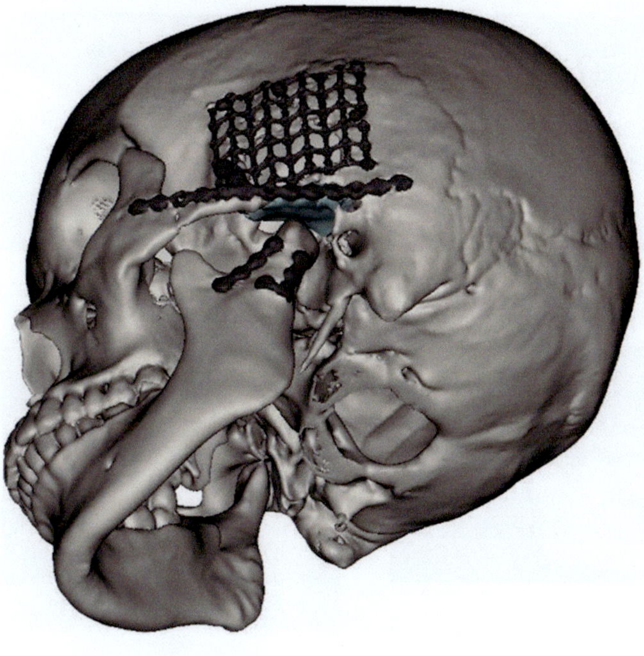

Fig. 7.4 Autologous temporal bone (light blue) repair of a skull base defect with titanium mesh (dark gray) after resection of a skull base-fossa lesion

7.1.3.3 Autogenous Bone Repair

The author at one time used free half-layer iliac bone or temporal bone to reconstruct the skull base (Fig. 7.4) and lesion and achieved good efficacy, but the iliac bone harvesting increased the trauma, and the defect of the temporal bone needed to be additionally repaired with titanium mesh and other repair materials. Moreover, free bone grafting is at risk of bone resorption.

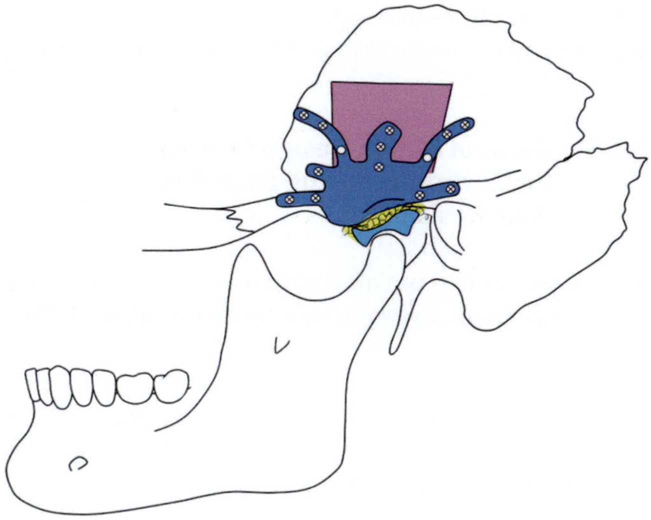

Fig. 7.5 Skull base-fossa prosthesis that does not include an articular fossa component because the articular disc is intact in this case. Bright blue shows the titanium skull base-joint fossa prosthesis, lighter blue shows the articular disc, and yellow shows the fat flap. Bright pink shows the temporal bone flap that provided intraoperative access to the inside of the cranium to remove the lesion

7.1.4 Innovative Repair and Reconstruction Methods with Customized Skull Base-Fossa Prostheses

In order to overcome the shortcomings of traditional repair methods, we have designed individualized prostheses to repair skull base-fossa defects, striving to make the repair method simple and easy to perform in surgery, as well as efficient and stable in outcome.

7.1.4.1 Types of Skull Base-Fossa Prosthesis Designs

Only one type of skull base-fossa prosthesis (Fig. 7.5) has been designed to reconstruct skull base-fossa defects while preserving the normal condyle, articular disc, and attached muscles.

7.1.4.2 Indications and Contraindications for Skull Base-Fossa Prostheses

7.1.4.2.1 Indications

This prosthesis is indicated for adults with skull base-fossa lesions, mainly benign or borderline tumors and tumorlike lesions, cases where malignant tumors are expected to be completely resected, quiescent inflammatory lesions, post-surgically acquired skull base-fossa defects, and osteolysis in the stable phase, provided that the condyles and articular discs have not been affected by the above-mentioned diseases.

7.1.4.2.2 Contraindications

See contraindications for TMJ-skull base prostheses in Chap. 6.

7.1.5 General Digital Design Process for Customized Skull Base-Fossa Prosthesis

This chapter focuses on types I and II (i.e., types in the extent of skull base-fossa lesions) within the classification of TMJ-skull base joint lesions, of which type II is more complex, so the general flow is exemplified by it (Fig. 7.6), and the general flow includes three aspects: simulated surgery of the osteotomies, prosthesis and cutting guide design, and the steps of the surgical procedure.

7.1.5.1 Simulated Osteotomy for Lesions

- Analysis of the extent of the lesion: the preoperative CT scan is received in DICOM format; the surgical design software is used to define the extent of the lesion, and important structures such as the middle ear, inner ear, and skull base should be labeled (Fig. 7.6a1).
- Design of osteotomy lines:
  - Zygomatic arch osteotomy line: for safe resection of the lesion, or if the zygomatic arch is to be temporarily dissected.
  - Osteotomy line at the anterior margin of the lesion: for safe resection of the lesion.
  - Osteotomy line at the posterior margin of the lesion: for safe resection of the lesion, while considering maximum. Protection of the middle ear structures.

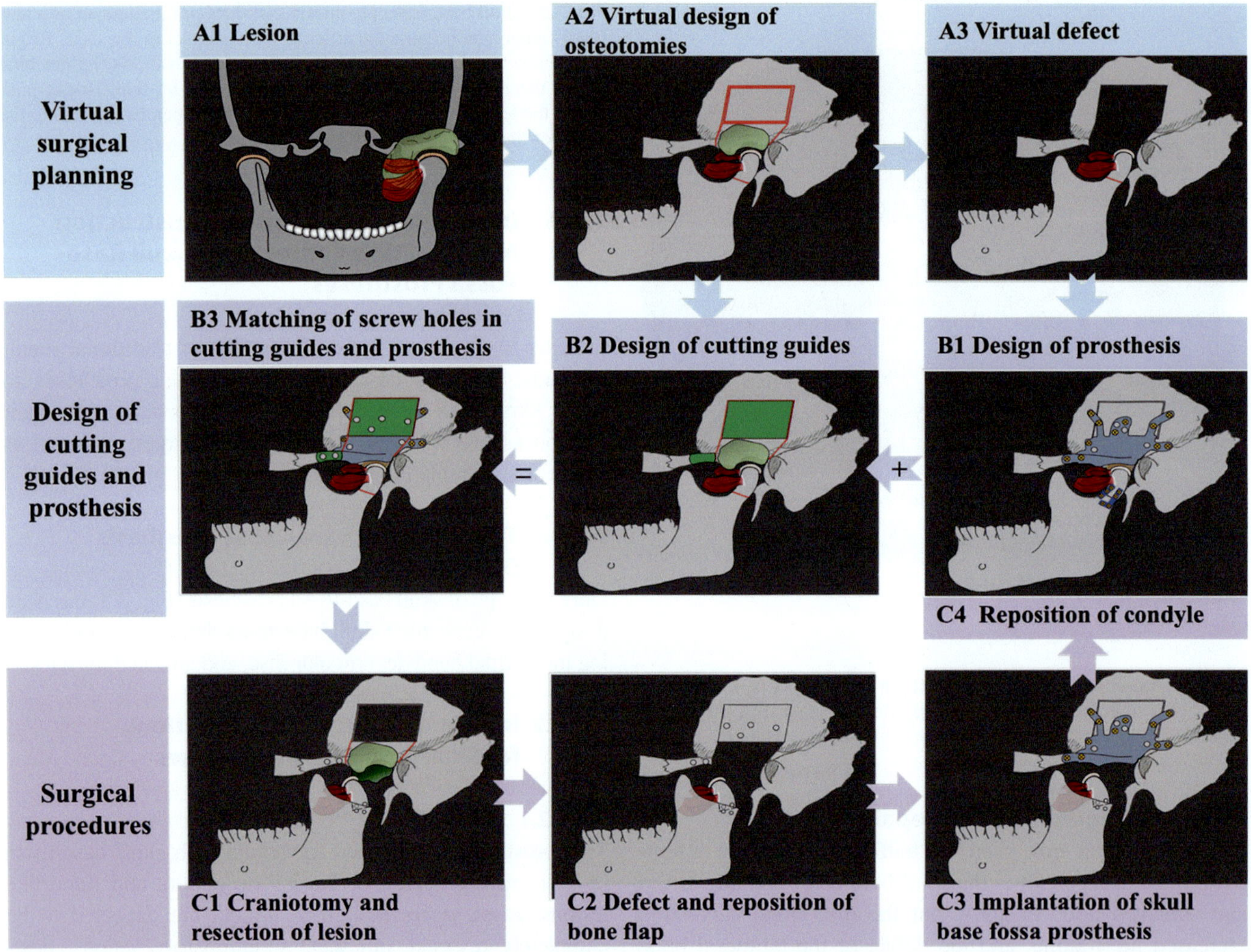

Fig. 7.6 Digital design of the skull base-fossa prosthesis: (**a1**) 3D reconstruction based on CT data, to define the scope of the lesion (green). (**a2**) Design of osteotomy line while assuring protection of the ear canal. (**a3**) Obtain a defect space model of the open space to be spanned by the prosthesis after osteotomy. (**b1**) Design of the prosthesis based on the defect model (blue). (**b2**) Design of the cutting guide based on the osteotomy line (green). (**b3**) Transfer the position of the prosthesis screw holes to the cutting guide. (**c1**) Osteotomy of the skull base-fossa lesion and osteotomy of the condylar neck according to the cutting guides, in order to expose the lesion. (**c2**) Re-implantation of the temporal bone flap after total resection of the lesion. (**c3**) Implantation of the skull base-fossa prosthesis. (**c4**) Reattachment of the condylar process and fixation with the pre-bent titanium plate

- Osteotomy line at the superior margin of the lesion: flush with the uppermost margin of the lesion.
- Temporal window osteotomy line: the anterior and posterior osteotomy lines are extensions of the anterior and posterior osteotomy lines of the lesion, respectively, and the superior osteotomy line is flexible according to the size of the intracranial portion of the lesion and the need for traction operations on the brain tissues.
- Mandibular osteotomy line: a flat mandibular osteotomy line is used to temporally dissect the condylar eminence, while preserving the lateral pterygoid muscle attachments (Fig. 7.6a2).

The above osteotomy lines will be used in the design of the cutting guides.

Defect space modeling: the lesion is removed at the osteotomy lines, and this defect space model will be used for prosthesis design (Fig. 7.6a3).

7.1.5.2 Prosthesis and Cutting Guide Design

- Skull base-fossa prosthesis design:
  Based on the defect space model (Fig. 7.6a3), a skull base-fossa prosthesis (Fig. 7.6b1) was designed. It contains two components, i.e., the cranial base component and the articular fossa component. Because of the potential for error between the defect space model and the actual surgical operation, especially due to the extent of the cranial base defect, the cranial base components should be designed to be slightly smaller than the defect space model for ease of seating, but should still be required to maximize the reconstruction of the skull base and should also be positioned higher than the plane of the normal skull base to accommodate the articular disc, the tipped mesial temporal fascial fat flap, and so on.
  The fixation components should be designed in at least three directions: anterior (zygomatic and temporal bones), posterior (above the ear canal), and superior (temporal bone), with at least two screw holes for fixation to the residual normal bone and screw holes for fixation of the temporal windowed bone block, so as to stabilize the fixation of the prosthesis to the zygomatic bone, to the prosthesis to the above the ear canal, to the prosthesis to the implanted temporal bone block, and to the prosthesis to the temporal bone.
- Osteotomy and positioning cutting guide design: the osteotomy cutting guide design is based on the design of the osteotomy lines (Fig. 7.6a2). Just a single guide plate, complex in structure, with slightly differing angles of cut around the curve of the cranium, but it can be 3D-printed, can be used to indicate and guide six osteotomy incisions: there are four lines around the temporal bone flap window opening, and the line at the lower margin of the temporal window and the line indicating the upper margin of the lesion on the skull base are the same line. There are two vertical osteotomy lines on the skull base, one each at the anterior and posterior margins of the lesion, and they may align with the right and left vertical edges of the temporal window above. (See Case N, Fig. 7.21 for an illustration of the cutting guide design.) The osteotomy lines at the anterior and posterior margins of the lesion should be labeled with the depth of the bone at that location and allowable depth of cut to avoid inadvertent injury to brain tissue (Fig. 7.6b2).
- Matching the guide plate to the prosthesis screw holes: transpose the images used in Figs. 7.6b1 and b2 by overlapping the images, in order to determine the screw hole positions for the guide plates based on the screw hole positions planned for the prosthesis, so that not only is the osteotomy accurate, but also the prosthesis installation can be precise, simple, and fast (Fig. 7.6b3).

7.1.5.3 Surgical Procedures

Yang Chi and Zheng Jisi

1. Surgical approach and exposure of the lesion: A modified preauriculotemporal anterior incision is used. A mesial temporal fascia fat flap is prepared for later use. The posterior superior temporalis muscle attachment is detached, turned up forward, and exposed forward to the zygomatic bone and lateral to the orbital wall, posterior to the final margin of the prosthesis mounting, upward to expose the upper margin of the temporal bone window, and downward to expose the mandibular incision. The aim is to fully expose the lesion.
2. Subcondylar osteotomy (Fig. 7.6c1): Two titanium plates are pre-bent to hold the condyle in place later when it is rejoined and re-implanted. The supracondylar cavity is opened, the neck of the condyle is cut off at the inferior margin of the mandibular notch, the anterosuperior and posterosuperior attachments of the articular disc are detached, and the attachment of the lateral pterygoid muscle is preserved. The condyle is pushed inward and downward together with the articular disc, away from the articular fossa, to fully expose the pathological tissue at the base of the skull.
3. Skull base and articular fossa osteotomy (Fig. 7.6c1): after affixing the cutting guide, the zygomatic arch osteotomy and temporal bone flap craniotomy are performed first; do complete removal of the temporal bone window bone block and put it in ice bucket. After traction and protection of the brain tissue, cut the anterior and posterior edges of the diseased temporal bone. At the posterior edge of the lesion, attention must be paid to follow the limited depth of the osteotomy according to the design, to avoid damage to the brain tissue. After com-

plete removal of the lesion, the medial edge of the skull base is trimmed to accommodate the prosthesis.

4. Prosthesis implantation and temporal bone flap replacement (Fig. 7.6c2): For fixation, first, select the spot with the most screw holes in contact with the residual bone tissue as the most stable position for initial fixation of the prosthesis. First, choose the screw holes originally prepared for the cutting guides, to ensure the greatest accuracy, before securing the other screw holes (Fig. 7.6c3).
5. Condylar replantation and fixation (Fig. 7.6c4): A pre-prepared mesial fascia fat flap is placed evenly spaced between the skull base-fossa prosthesis and the articular disc, and the condyle is reattached to the mandibular ramus and fixed in position with a pre-curved titanium plate.

7.2 Customized Skull Base-Fossa Prosthesis Repair and Reconstruction Techniques

This section describes a typical clinical case of a type II skull base-fossa disease, in which the tumor lesion involves the skull base and the articular fossa and protrudes into the infratemporal fossa. The tumor resection design, cutting guide manufacturing design, and simulated surgery design were carried out according to the digital design process in the first section of this chapter. The key point of the operation is to preserve the integrity of the disc-condyle-muscle complex. The crucial element of the design is the maintenance of a sufficient distance between the normal condyle and the prosthesis and the addition of a temporal mesial fascia fat flap to soften impact with the articular disc and to prevent condylar resorption and/or joint adhesion. Postoperative follow-up focuses on whether complications such as adhesion between the prosthesis and the articular disc, and condyle resorption will occur following prosthesis implantation, thereby affecting the preserved joint structure and function.

7.2.1 Case N. Design and Application of a Skull Base-Fossa Prosthesis That Preserves a Non-diseased Condyle

- Patient information: female, 53 years old.
- Complaint: pain in the right preauricular region with restriction of mouth opening for more than 6 months.
- History: the patient presented with right preauricular pressure and pain, limited mouth opening, but normal hearing, starting 6 months ago with no apparent cause.
- Past history: history of breast surgery 20 years ago, denied history of systemic diseases, and denied history of drug and food allergy.
- Clinical examination: facial symmetry, no obvious mass protruding (Fig. 7.7), mouth opening 13 mm., stable intraoral occlusion (Fig. 7.8). The pain in front of the ear had a VAS score of 5.
- Imaging examination: panoramic radiograph showed abnormal bone quality in the right joint area (Fig. 7.9). MRI of the joints showed abnormal soft tissue shadow of the right skull base and joint fossa and abnormal bone quality of the temporal bone, and the articular disc was

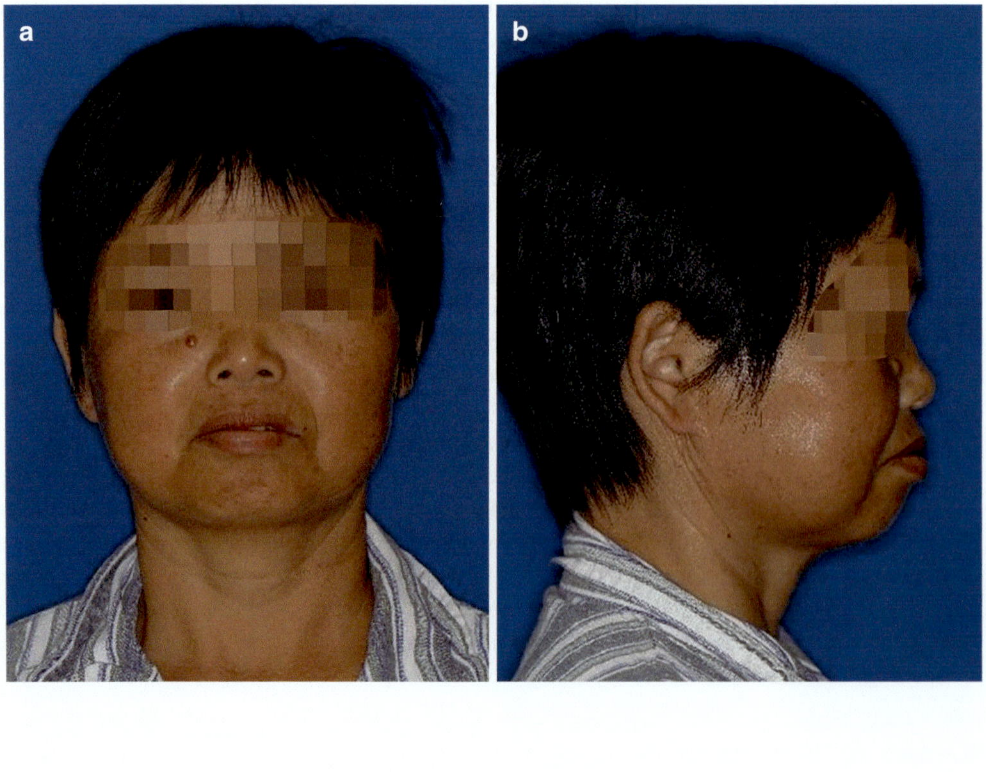

Fig. 7.7 Case N. Extraoral examination showed that the face was basically symmetrical and no obvious swelling was prominent. (**a**) Frontal view. (**b**) Lateral view

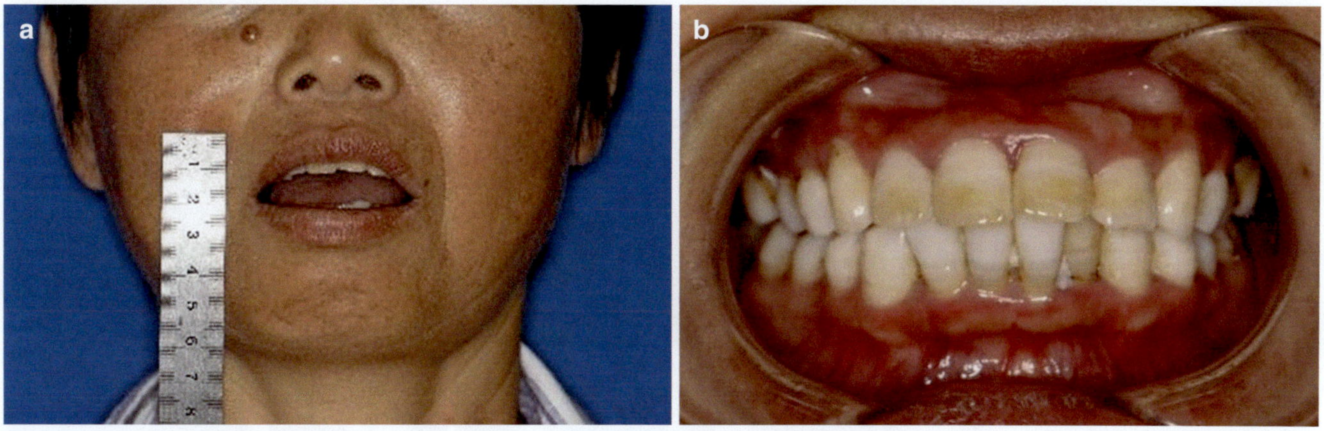

Fig. 7.8 Case N. Intraoral examination shows a 13 mm mouth opening and a stable intraoral occlusion. (**a**) Mouth opening. (**b**) Occlusal relation

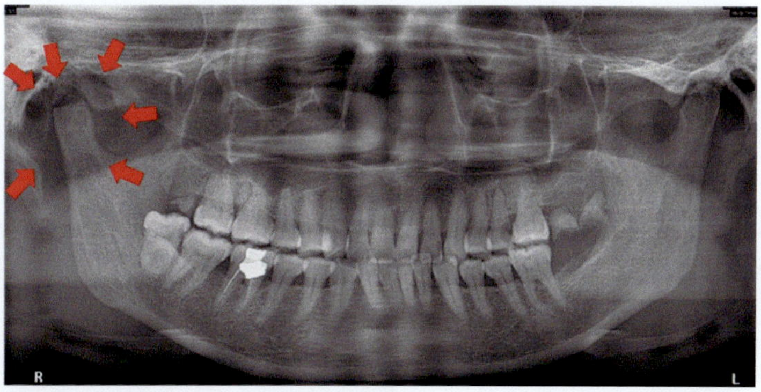

Fig. 7.9 Case N. Panoramic X-ray. The red arrows show a decrease in bone density in the right joint area, and the tip of the condyle is suspected to have been resorbed

not involved (Fig. 7.10). CT scan showed a lesion occupying the space in the right joint area, with the shadow of a soft tissue mass, measuring about 31 mm × 25 mm × 17 mm, and a CT value of about 50 HU in density, with clear boundaries, irregular morphology, and adjacent to the right temporal bone zygomatic process. The lesion was not clearly demarcated from the surrounding soft tissues, and it had a wider joint space than the opposite side; CT reconstruction showed that the lesion had not destroyed the condyle, and the inner part of the lesion had not damaged the condyle, although the joint gap was widened. The lesion was close to the foramen ovale on the medial side, and a 32 mm × 35 mm perforation was seen at the base of the skull, but the foramen ovale was not destroyed (Figs. 7.7 and 7.11), the ear canal was not involved, and the lesion did not involve the internal carotid artery (Fig. 7.12).

- Diagnosis: diffuse tenosynovial giant cell tumor of the right skull base-articular fossa.
- Postoperative pathology: microscopic description of a giant cell-rich lesion with mononuclear cell infiltration and ferritin deposits. Pathologic diagnosis: right fossa lesion consistent with diffuse giant cell tumor of the tendon sheath.

7.2.2 Case N. Diagnostic Imaging

7.2.3 Case N. Treatment Plan

- Overall treatment plan: it is a Type II defect. Resection of the right skull base-fossa lesion and customized skull base-fossa prosthetic repair and reconstruction.
- Surgical resection design
  - Design of resection scope: in order to expose the skull base-fossa lesion, the zygomatic arch and condylar process must be temporarily truncated during the operation. But try not to cut the attachment to the masseter muscle and the lateral pterygoid muscle when the articular disc is freed. Then, the skull base-fossa lesion is excised, and the prosthesis is implanted and fixed, and the condyle and the zygomatic arch are reset.

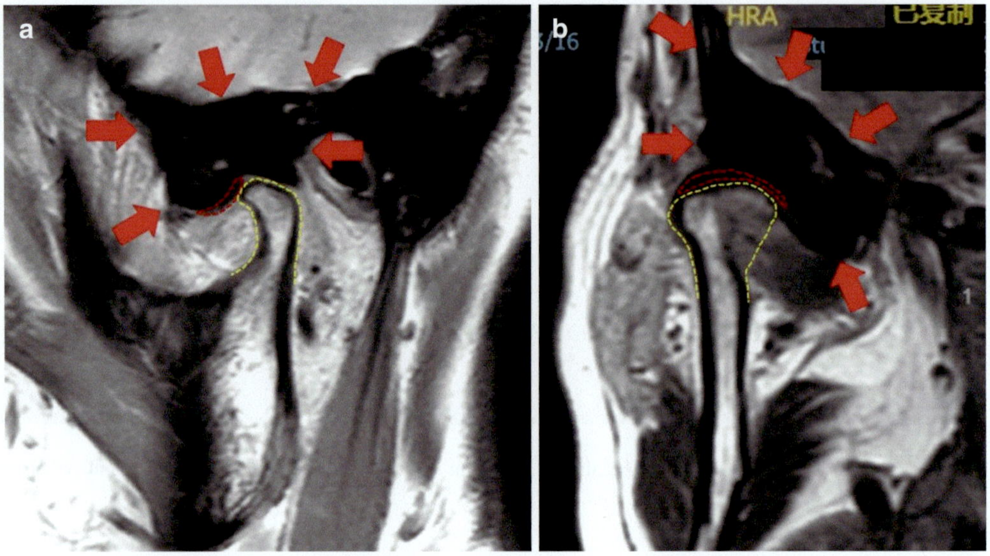

Fig. 7.10 Case N. MRI of joints. Red arrows show skull base-fossa low-signal shadows, red dotted lines show articular discs, and yellow dotted lines show condyles. (**a**) Sagittal view. (**b**) Coronal view

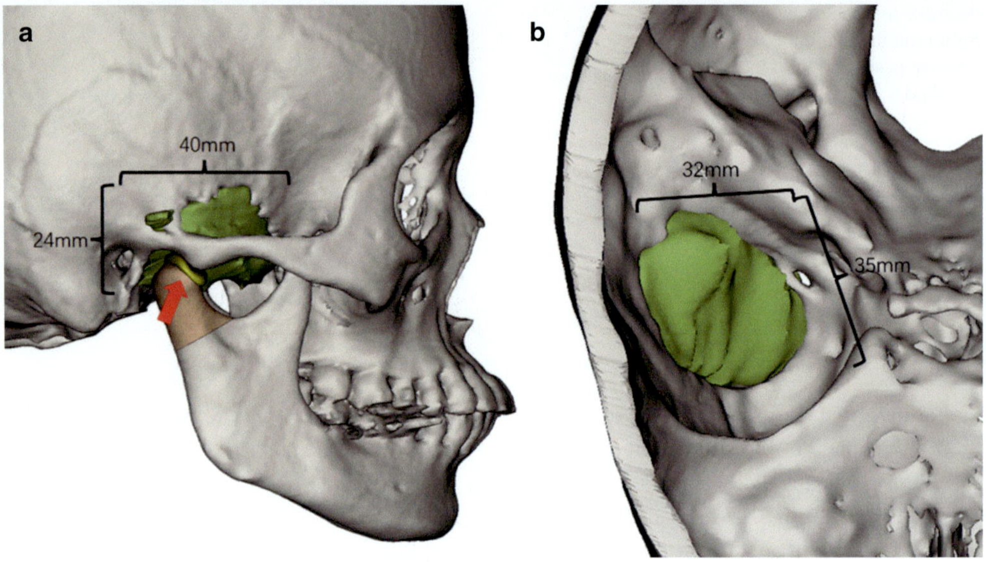

Fig. 7.11 Case N. 3D reconstruction of maxillofacial CT showing the extent of the mass (green) encroaching on the skull base-fossa (in mm). Red arrow points to the articular disc and brown color shows the condyle. (**a**) Lateral view. (**b**) Cerebrofacial view

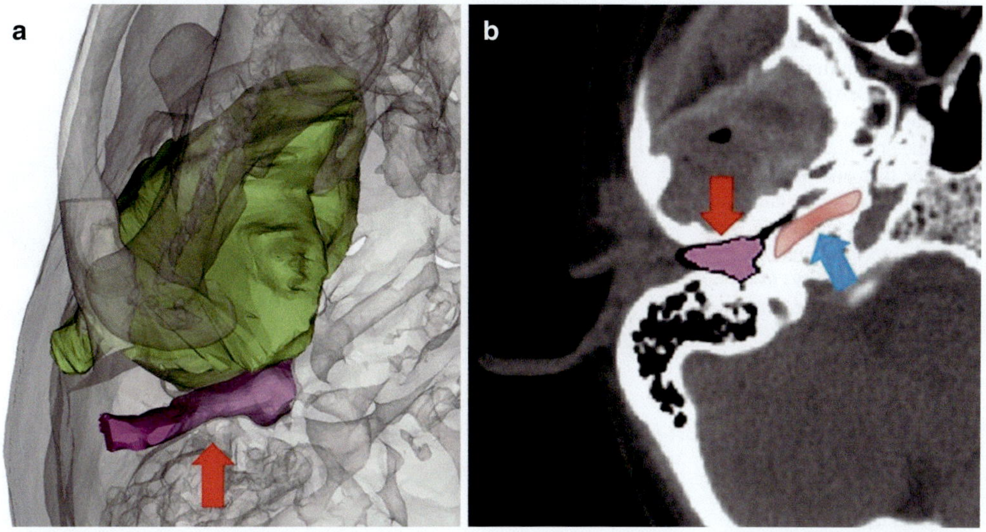

Fig. 7.12 Case N. Mass (green) in relation to the ear canal and internal carotid artery. Red arrows and bright pink color show the ear canal, and blue arrow and light pink color show the internal carotid artery. (**a**) CT 3D reconstruction of the skull base view. (**b**) Axial position CT

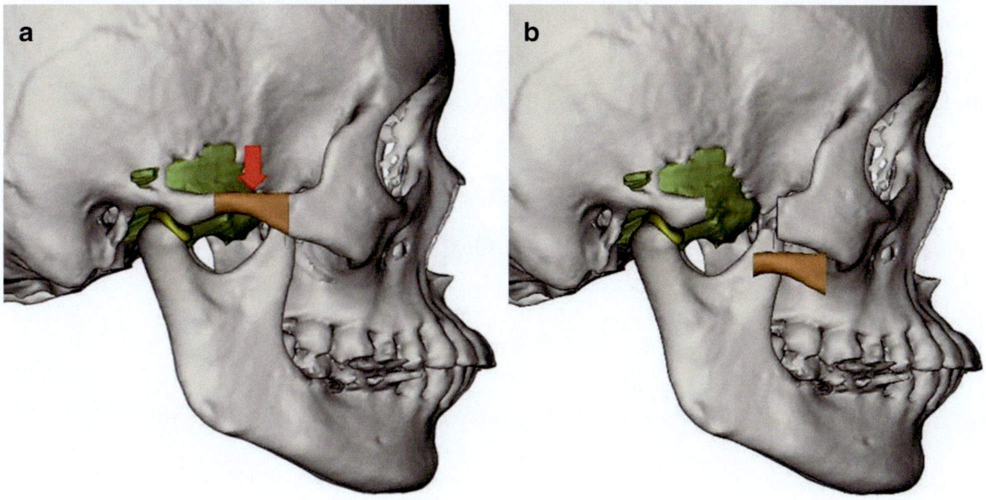

Fig. 7.13 Case N. Zygomatic arch osteotomies were carried out to free a segment of the bone (red arrow). The masseter muscle attachment was maintained to preserve the blood supply. The bone segment was pushed forward and down to expose the anterior border of the tumor. (**a**) Zygomatic arch osteotomy (red arrow). (**b**) Exposure of the anterior border of the lesion

- Digital simulation of surgery
  - Temporary osteotomy of the zygomatic arch: preserving the masseter muscle attachment, the zygomatic arch is pushed forward and down to expose the anterior border of the lesion (Fig. 7.13).
  - Subcondylar osteotomy: only the anterior superior and posterior superior attachments and lateral capsule of the articular disc are cut, and the anterior inferior and posterior inferior attachments and the attachment of the lateral pterygoid muscle are preserved. The condyle is pushed forward and downward, exposing the posterior border of the lesion (Fig. 7.14).
  - Craniotomy of the temporal bone window opening: the surface of the lesion overlying the brain is exposed, and the temporal bone flap is preserved in an ice bucket, to be implanted back later (Fig. 7.15).
  - Skull base osteotomies: anterior skull base osteotomies, posterior skull base osteotomies, and intracranial base osteotomies (brown), with care taken to protect the associated intra- and extracranial structures (Fig. 7.16).
  - Modeling of the defect after removal of the mass: the skull base-fossa defect is modeled after removal of the lesion, to prepare for design of the prosthesis (Fig. 7.17).

7.2.4 Case N. Design and Processing of the Skull Base-Fossa Prosthesis and Cutting Guides

- Skull base-fossa prosthesis design

  Skull base-fossa prosthesis design: after the design of the osteotomies of the condyle, zygomatic arch, and temporal window are set, the prosthesis is designed with the articulating surface of the prosthesis no less than 5 mm distance from the condylar head, allowing space reserved for the

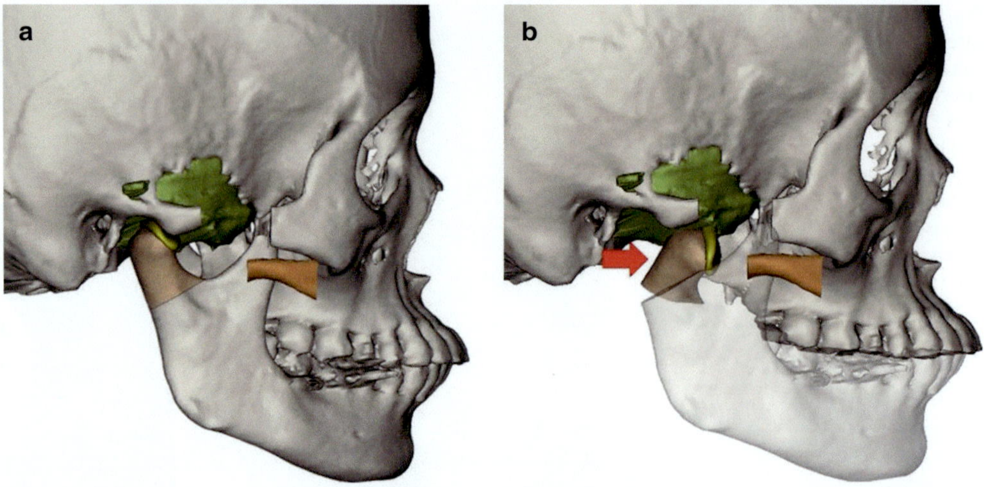

Fig. 7.14 Case N. Subcondylar osteotomy was carried out in the condylar neck. (**a**) The articular disc was detached from the articular fossa. (**b**) Both the disc and the lateral pterygoid muscle remained with the condyle while it was pushed anteriorly and inferiorly (red arrow) to expose the posterior border of the tumor

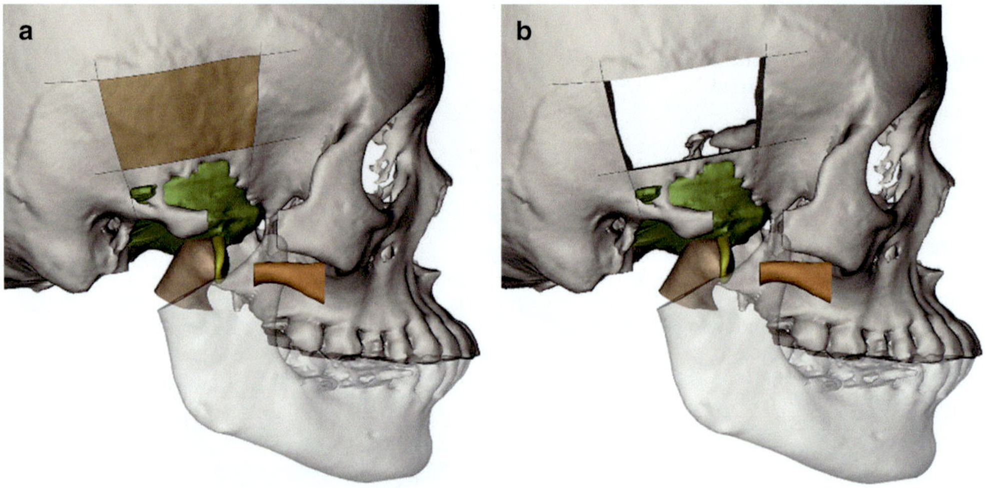

Fig. 7.15 Case N. Temporal bone window opening (brown) osteotomy. (**a**) Design of the osteotomy line. (**b**) Exposure of the surface of the lesion overlying the brain

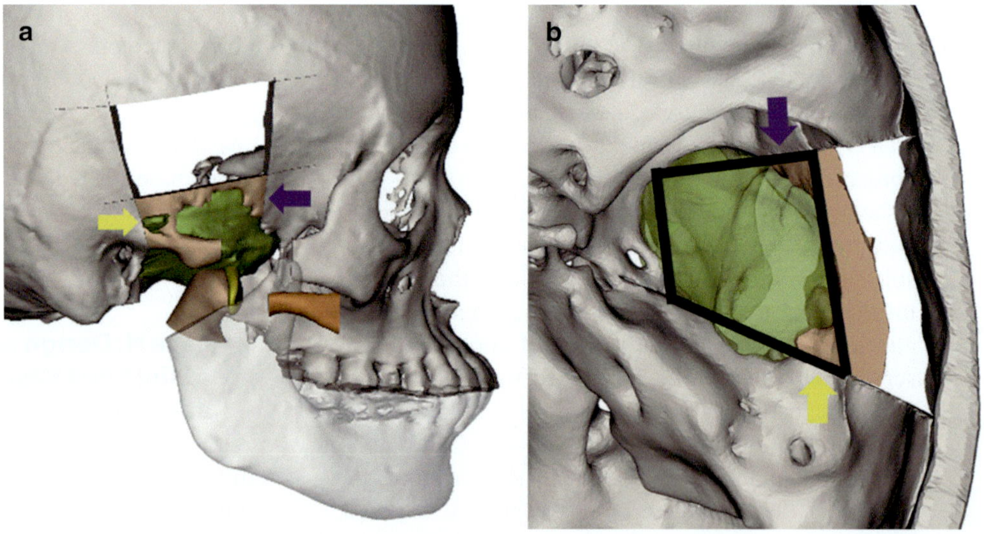

Fig. 7.16 Case N. Cranial base osteotomy. The purple arrows indicate the osteotomy line at the anterior boundary of the tumor, and the yellow arrows indicate the osteotomy line at the posterior boundary of the tumor. (**a**) Cranial base osteotomy line design in right lateral view. (**b**) Cranial base osteotomy line (black line) design in cranial cross section view, looking downward

articular disc, the mesial fascia fat flap, and the fat-filled space (Fig. 7.18).

- Measurement of temporal bone thickness and screw hole depth in the temporal bone window opening: intended to guide osteotomy to prevent damage to the dura mater (Fig. 7.19).
- Prosthesis fabrication and fitting: the cranial base-fossa prosthesis is made of titanium alloy and is fabricated using a metal 3D printer. After fabrication, the prosthesis is test fitted on a resin head mold to see if the prosthesis fits the bone surface and is stable (Fig. 7.20).

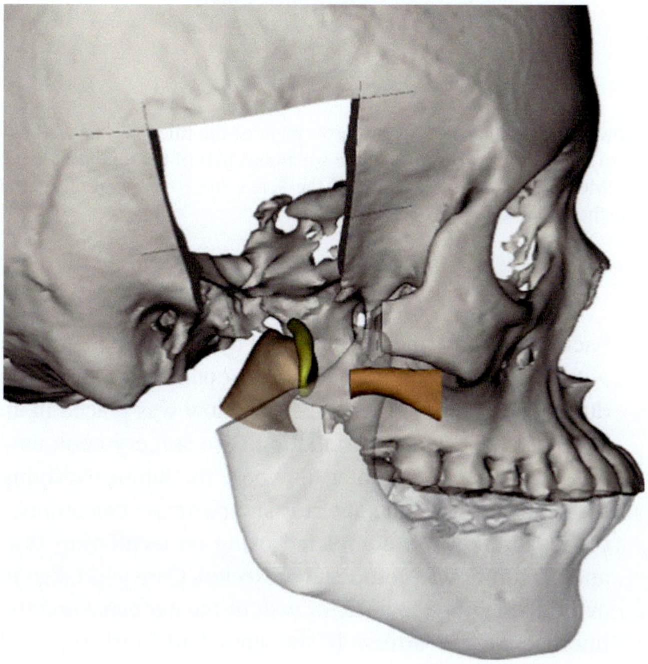

Fig. 7.17 Case N. Model of the skull base-fossa defect. Brown color shows the temporarily severed condyle displaced forward and downward, yellow color shows the articular disc, and orange color shows the temporarily severed zygomatic arch

- Digital cutting guide design: design of zygomatic arch cutting guide, temporal bone window, and skull base cutting guide for precise intraoperative osteotomy and direct positioning of the prosthesis (Fig. 7.21).

7.2.5 Case N. Surgical Procedure

Preoperative laboratory tests: the same as described in Sect. 3.2.5, Preoperative Laboratory Tests.

Preoperative preparation: the same as described in Case M.

Steps of the surgical procedure

1. Surgical approach: A modified auriculotemporal anterior incision was used to expose the surface of the temporalis muscle, the zygomatic arch bony surface, the lateral surface of the tumor, and the bony surface of the condylar neck. A mesial temporal fascia fat flap was prepared for later use in insulating the condylar head. The temporalis muscle was incised at the proximal temporalis muscle attachment to expose the temporal bone surface, and the temporalis muscle was pushed forward to fully expose the cranium at the upper border of the tumor.
2. Subcondylar osteotomy: Open the upper-articular cavity, separate the side of the capsule and the posterior superior and anterior superior disc attachments, suture and ligature of the posterior superior disc attachment to stop hemorrhage, and preserve the posterior inferior and anterior inferior disc attachments to the condylar head. Do not open the inferior cavity, to preserve the lateral pterygoid muscle attachments. The position of the subcondylar osteotomy was marked, and at the same time, the bone was marked with the position of the pre-bent titanium plate screw holes to be used in later resetting of the condyle. The titanium plate and titanium screws were

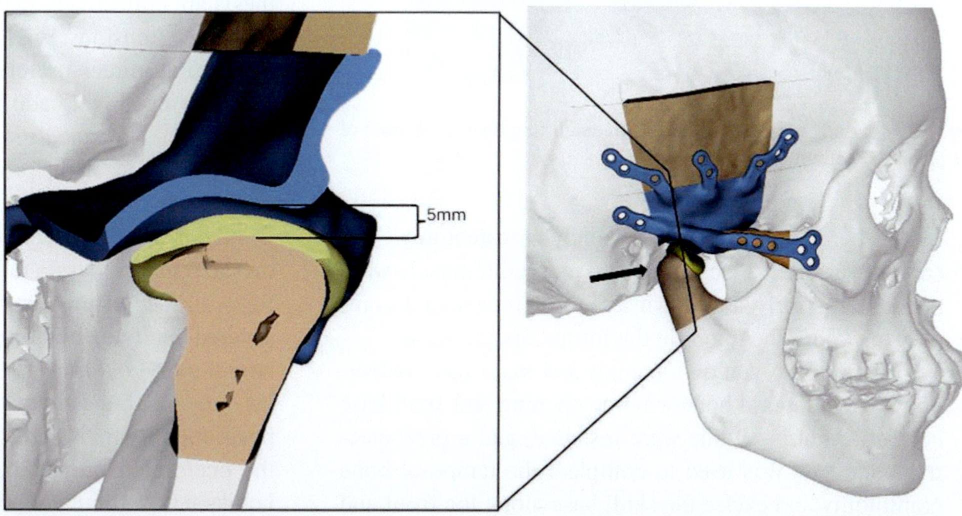

Fig. 7.18 Case N. Design of the skull base-fossa prosthesis. The skull base-fossa prosthesis is shown in blue, with the articular surface of the prosthesis not less than 5 mm from the condylar head (brown). The articular disc is shown in yellow, still attached to the condyle

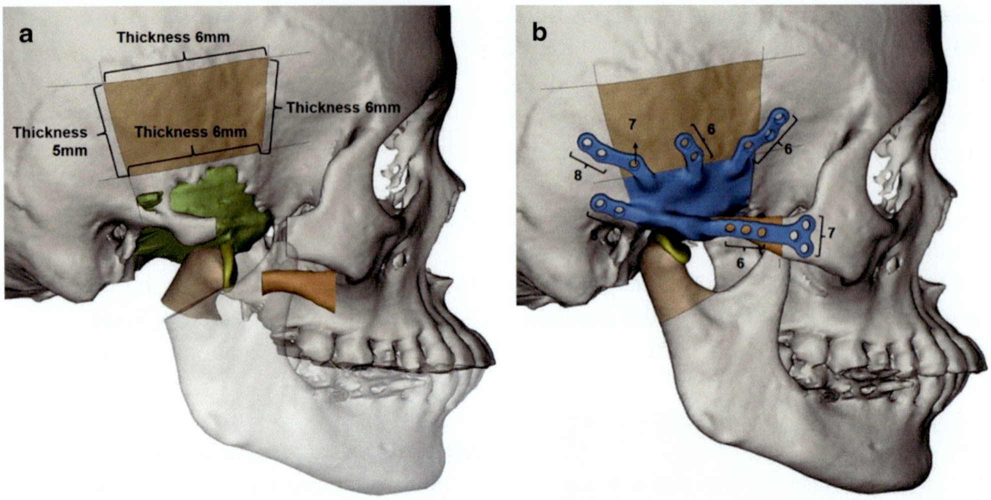

Fig. 7.19 Case N. Temporal bone thickness of the temporal bone opening and screw hole depth measurements (in mm). Green shows the mass, brown shows the temporal bone window opening and the temporarily removed condyle, orange shows the temporarily removed zygomatic arch, blue shows the skull base-fossa prosthesis, and yellow shows the articular disc. (**a**) Measurement of the thickness of the temporal bone window opening in the squamous part of the temporal bone. (**b**) Measurement of the depth of the screw holes for fixation of the prosthesis and the zygomatic arch

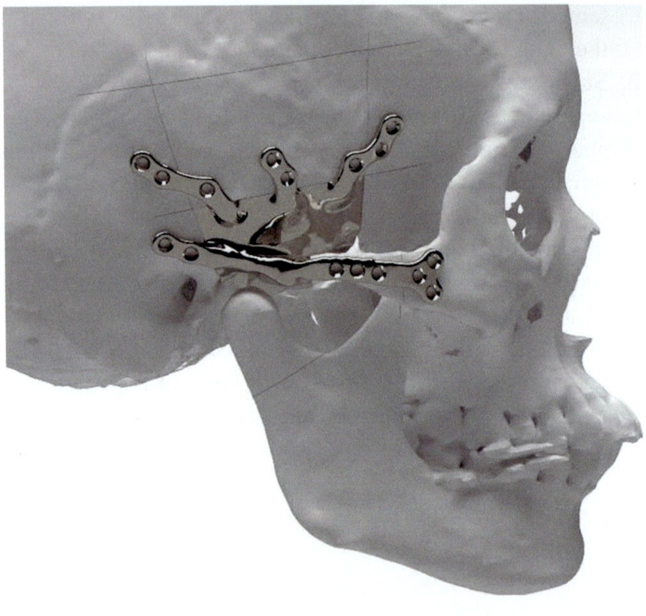

Fig. 7.20 Case N. Prosthesis fabrication and fitting on a resin mold of the patient's cranium

removed to complete the subcondylar osteotomy. The condyle, articular disc, and lateral pterygoid muscle were pushed anteriorly and down as an interconnected complex to expose the tumor in the infratemporal fossa.

3. Temporal bone window opening and skull base osteotomy: The temporal bone window opening and skull base combined cutting guide were installed, and a piezoelectric bone saw was used to complete the temporal bone craniotomy and excise the skull base along the front and back osteotomy lines as indicated by the guide plate. The window in the temporal bone was opened to expose the dura mater, and the bone block window was placed in an ice bucket for later reinstallation. The surgery continued to separate the dura mater to expose the tumor overlying the brain surface. The anterior and posterior osteotomies of the tumor were completed using an oscillating saw, and the tumor was completely resected. Care was taken to avoid damaging the anterior wall of the ear canal and the internal carotid artery. If the dura had been ruptured during the operation, it could be repaired by suture, fascia, or patching (Figs. 7.22 and 7.23).
4. Prosthesis implantation and fixation of the temporal bone and zygomatic arch blocks: The temporal bone flap, the zygomatic arch bone block, and the skull base-fossa prosthesis are collectively held in place by the prosthesis and its wing extensions, with the screw hole positions left by the cutting guides preferentially securing them all without the need for additional titanium plate fixation (Fig. 7.24). Note the need for a flat layer of free fat flap to be placed between the prosthesis and the dura, as was prepared early in the surgery.
5. Condylar fixation and joint space management: A tipped mesial temporal fascia fat flap was sutured to the articular fossa surface of the prosthesis, and then the temporarily severed condyle, including the attached articular disc and lateral pterygoid muscle, was reattached to the mandibular ramus with the aid of the two pre-bent titanium plates, positioned by their screw hole positions. After checking the occlusal relationship, a free fat flap was then filled between the articular disc and the tipped mesial temporal

Fig. 7.21 Case N. Design of zygomatic arch cutting guide, as well as temporal bone craniotomy and skull base cutting guides (pink). Note that a single guide plate with customized design can indicate the cuts for several osteotomies. (**a**) Design the guides according to the osteotomy lines. (**b**) The screw holes for the guides are in the same positions as the prosthesis screw holes

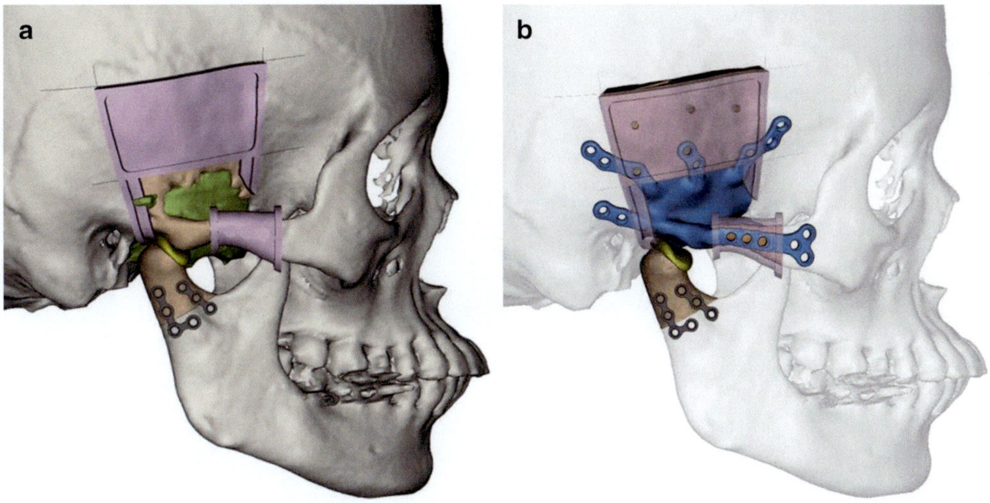

Fig. 7.22 Case N. Skull base osteotomy. Purple arrows show anterior margin osteotomy, yellow arrows show posterior margin osteotomy, and black arrows show preserved condyle and articular disc. (**a**) Design. (**b**) Actual

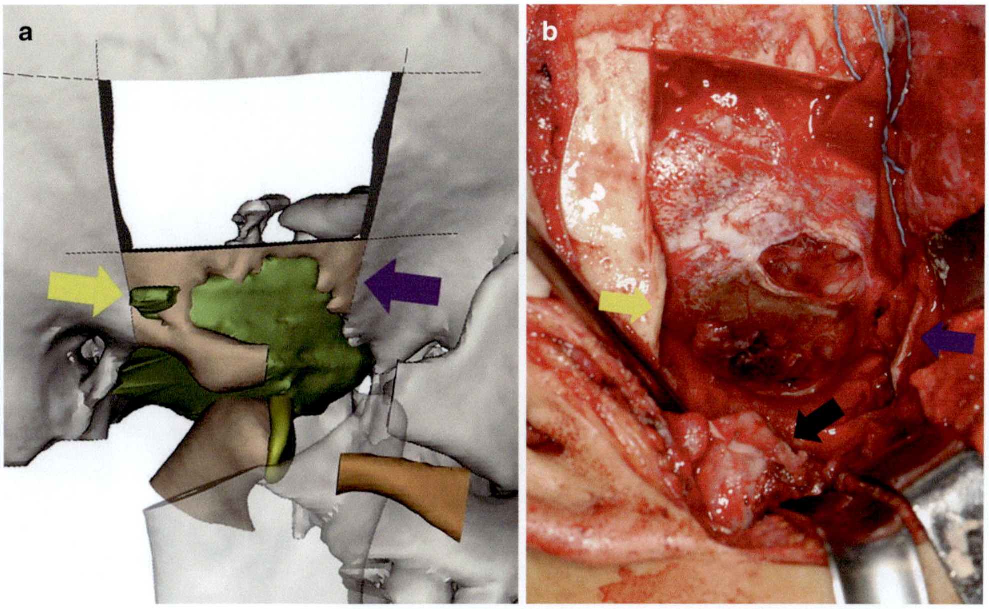

Fig. 7.23 Case N. Comparison of the design of the mass removal and the actual intraoperative osteotomy. The resected tumor is shown from the brain view, still attached to a piece of the skull base. Purple arrows show anterior margin osteotomies, and yellow arrows show posterior margin osteotomies. (**a**) Design. (**b**) Actual

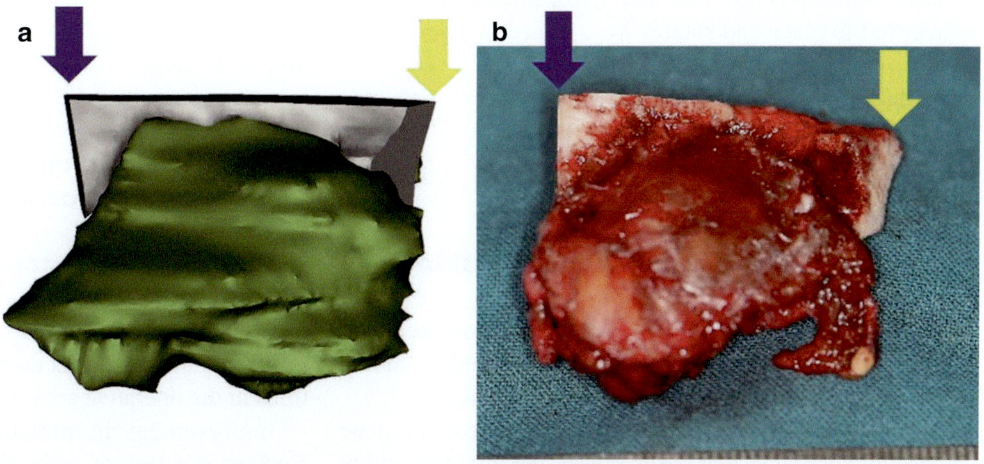

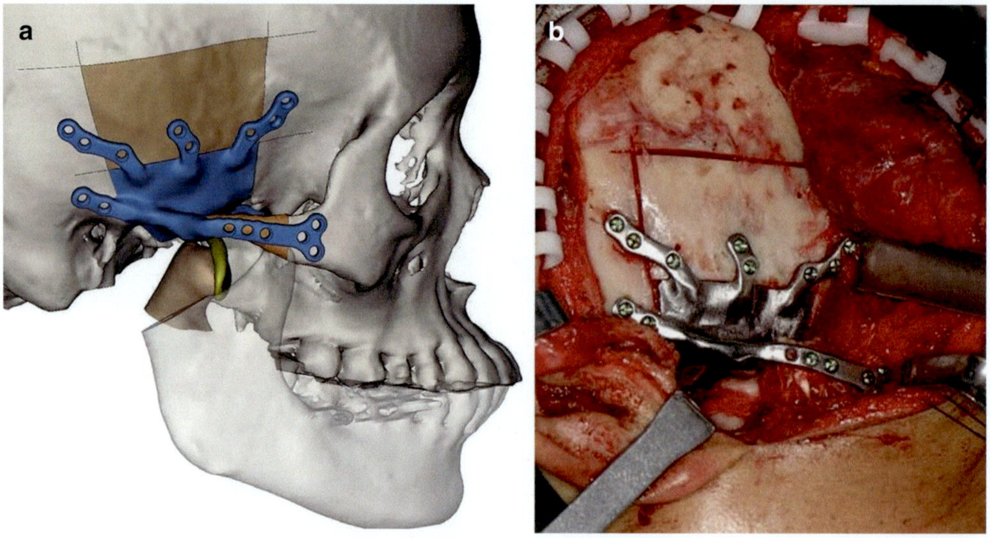

Fig. 7.24 Case N. Prosthesis installation, together with temporal bone and zygomatic arch bone block fixation. (**a**) Design. (**b**) Actual

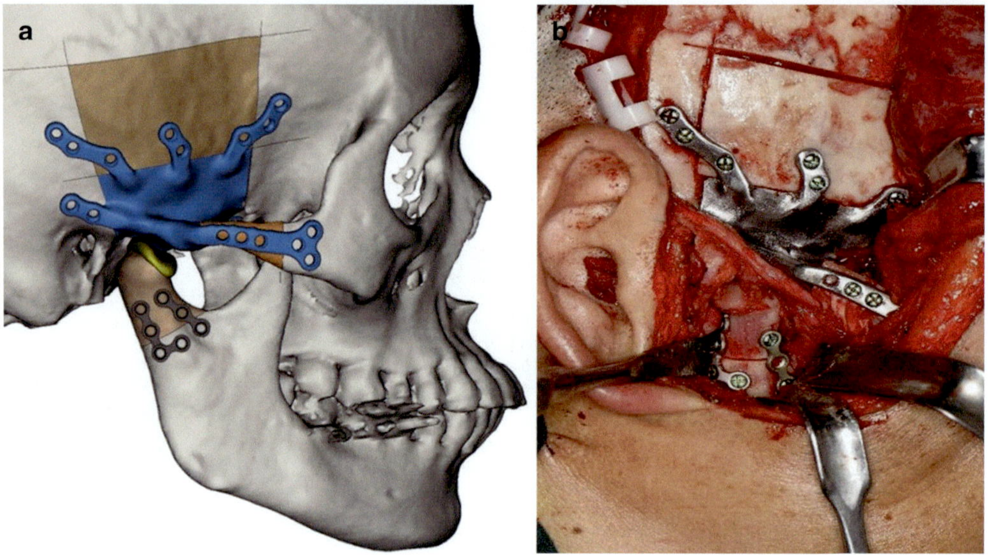

Fig. 7.25 Case N. Condylar fixation and joint space management. Condylar fixation was made simple because plates were previously adapted, and screw holes were pre-drilled. (**a**) Design. (**b**) Actual

fascia fat flap (Figs. 7.25 and 7.26). Finally, a drainage was left in place and sutures were placed in layers in the closing of the incision.

6. Surgical points: the relevant surgical points are shown in Fig. 7.27.

7.2.6 Case N. Postoperative Analysis of Prosthesis Implantation Precision

Regular postoperative follow-ups were performed for appearance (facial shape), function (mouth opening, mouth shape), and prosthesis evaluation (safety, accuracy).

Immediately after surgery: the intraoperative guide plate was accurately seated, and the prosthesis was fitted smoothly (Fig. 7.28); a comparison between the preoperative design and the postoperative reconstruction shows that the prosthesis was seated accurately (Fig. 7.29). The postoperative prosthesis error was 1.02 mm (Fig. 7.30), well within an allowable range.

7.2.7 Case N. Long-Term Follow-Up and Prognosis

7.2.7.1 One-Year Postoperative Follow-Up

There was no recurrence of previous disease, the face was in good shape with no abnormalities, the patient was eating normally, and there was no redness, swelling, or other reactions in the operative area (Fig. 7.31).

Improvement in preauricular pain, improvement in VAS to a score of only 1 out of 10, joint-mandibular-occlusal-facial coordination, and occlusal relationship stabilized.

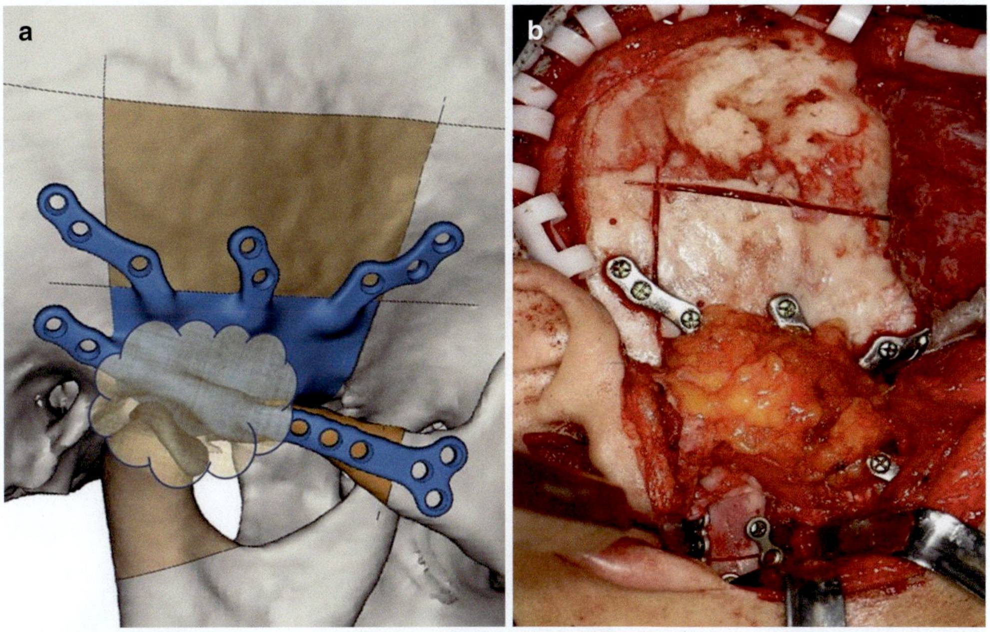

Fig. 7.26 Case N. The wound was irrigated, and an abdominal fat graft was used to fill the dead space around the prosthesis. A suction catheter was placed, and the incision was closed in layers. (**a**) Design. (**b**) Actual

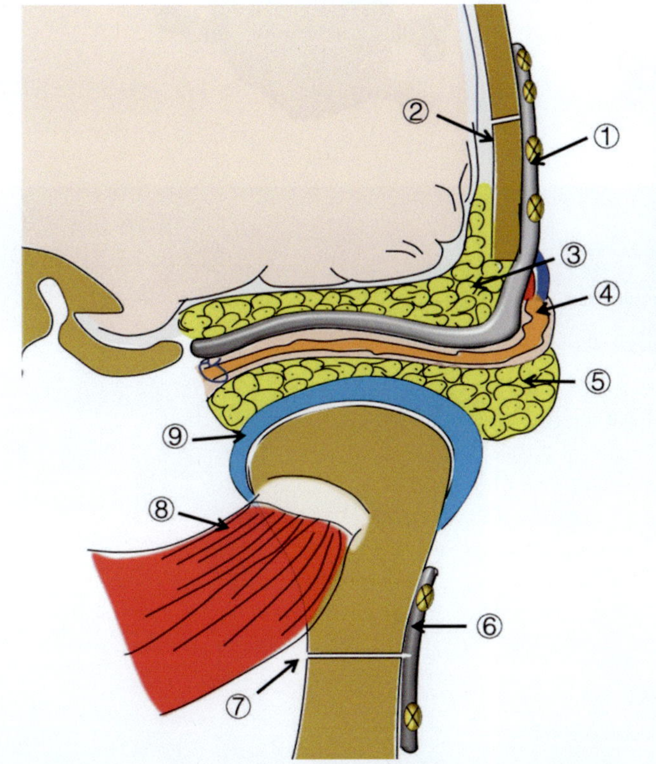

Fig. 7.27 Case N. Schematic diagram of the completed reconstruction. (1) Skull base, fossa prosthesis. (2) Bone flap returned to craniotomy. (3) Fat graft between the dura and prosthesis. (4) Temporalis fascia fat flap (with the middle temporal artery and vein at the tip). (5) Fat graft. (6) Condylar fixation plate. (7) Condylar osteotomy line. (8) External pterygoid muscle. (9) Articular disc of the TMJ

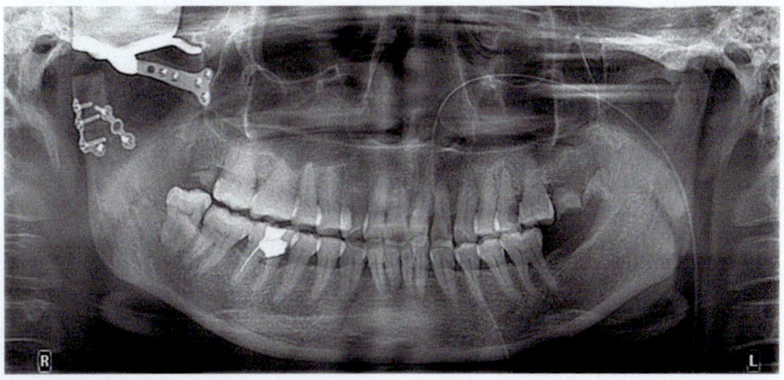

Fig. 7.28 Case N. The immediate postoperative panoramic X-ray shows that the prosthesis is in place and stable

The mouth opening improved to 38 mm, with 10 mm of lateral movement to the affected side and 7 mm of lateral movement to the healthy side, while the mouth opening pattern was deflected 3 mm toward the affected side (Fig. 7.32).

Prosthesis evaluation: no complications such as infection, rejection, loosening, displacement, fracture, ectopic osteogenesis, and allergy (Figs. 7.33 and 7.34).

Condylar evaluation: CT showed no resorption of the condyle, and the cortical bone was intact and well remodeled (Fig. 7.35).

Other: normal hearing.

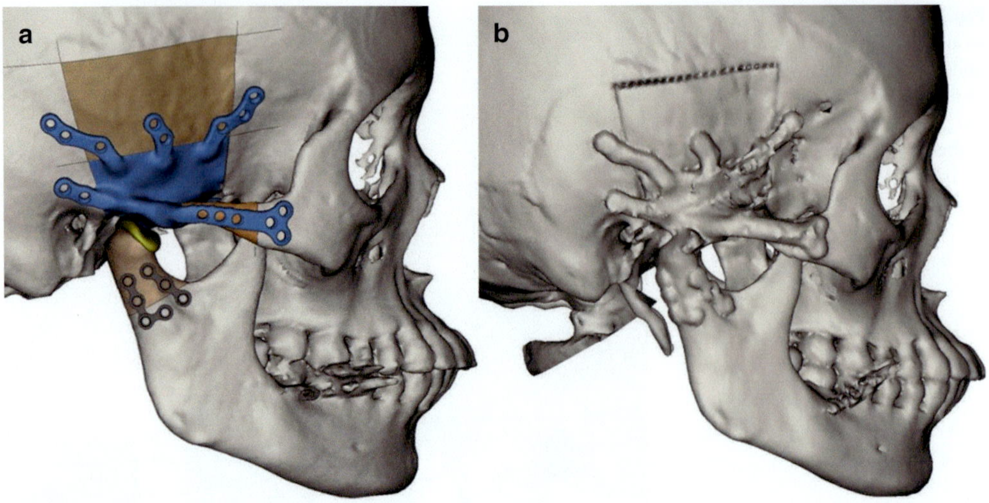

Fig. 7.29 Case N. CT reconstruction comparison showing precise prosthesis seating. (**a**) Preoperative design. (**b**) Immediate postoperative period

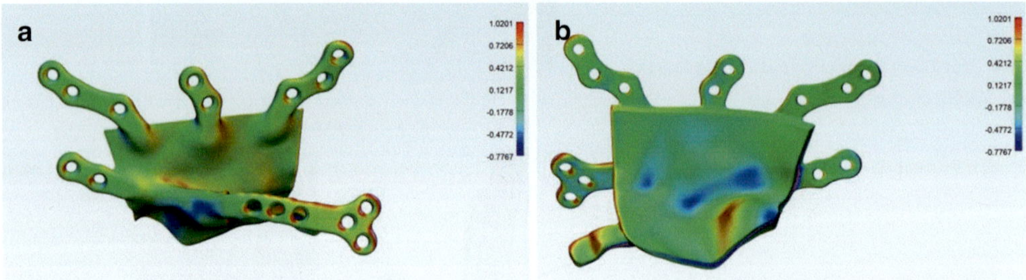

Fig. 7.30 Case N. Prosthetic error 1.02 mm. (**a**) Lateral error. (**b**) Medial error

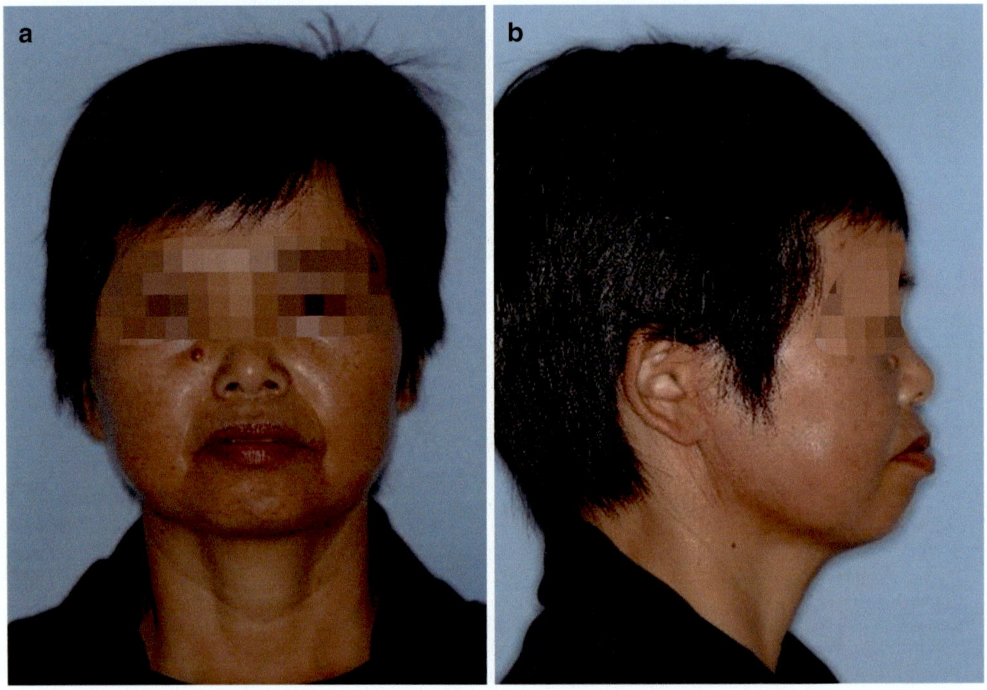

Fig. 7.31 Case N. No abnormalities in the facial shape at 1 year after surgery. There was no reaction such as redness or swelling in the surgical area. (**a**) Frontal view. (**b**) Lateral view

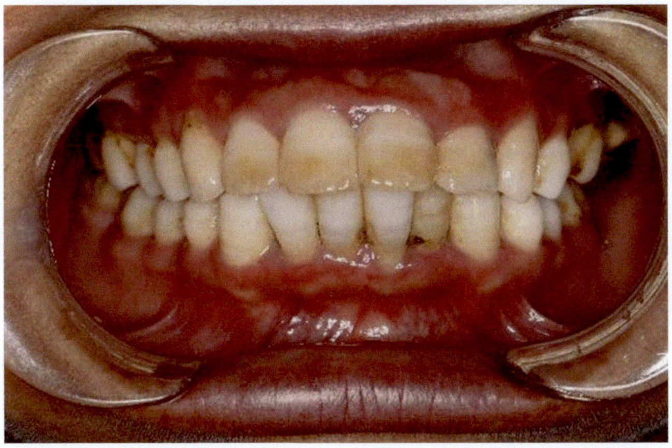

Fig. 7.32 Case N. Good recovery of joint function and stable intraoral occlusal relationship at 1 year after surgery

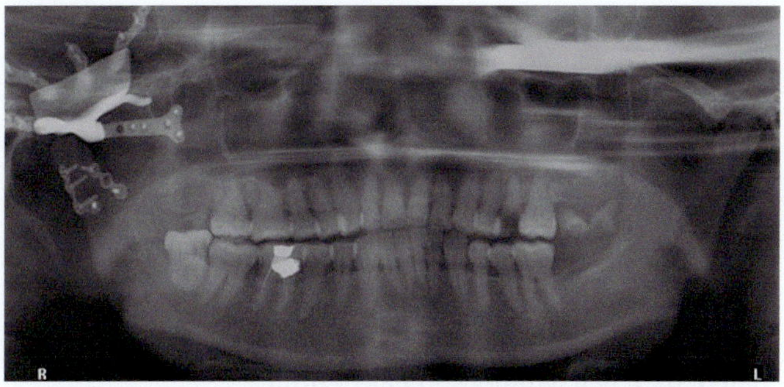

Fig. 7.33 Case N. One-year postoperative panoramic view showing no loosening, dislocation, migration, or fracture of the prosthesis

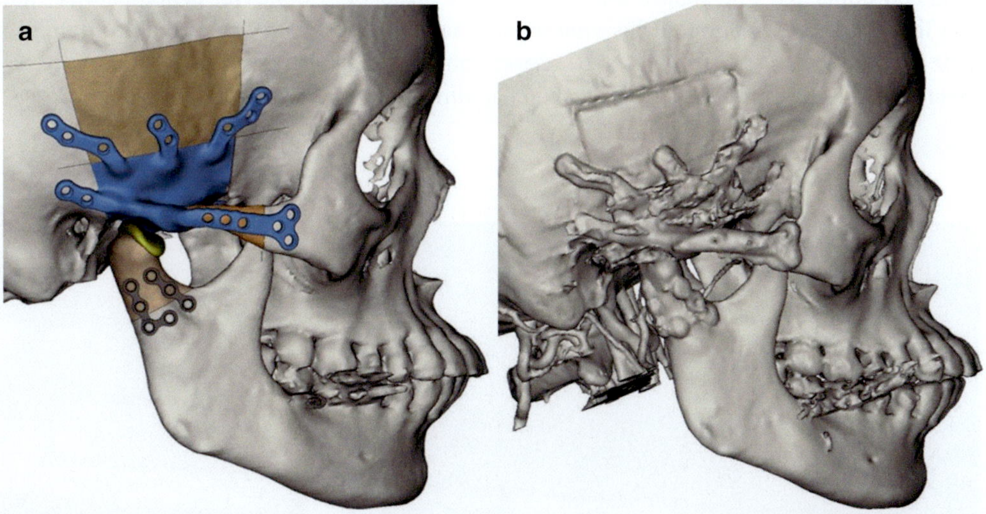

Fig. 7.34 Case N. Comparison of preoperative design with CT reconstruction at 1 year postoperatively, showing precise prosthesis seating. (**a**) Preoperative design. (**b**) 1 year postoperatively

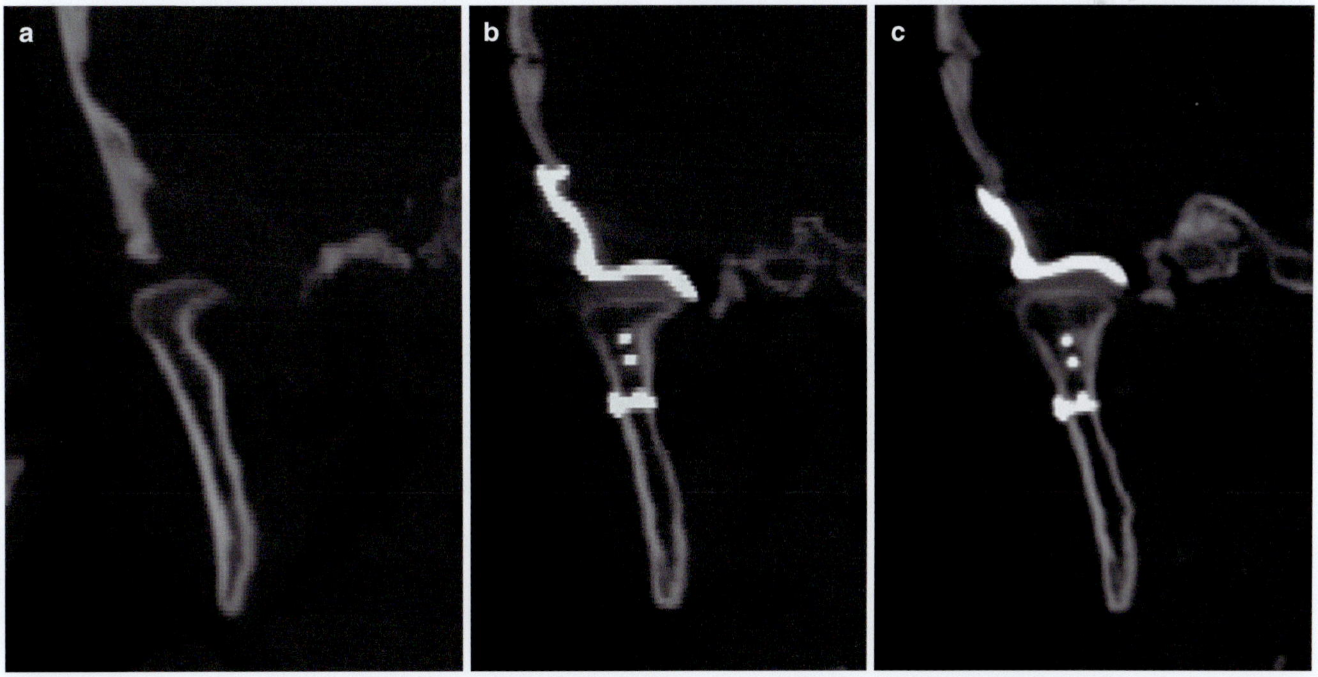

Fig. 7.35 Case N. Comparison of condylar status showing no resorption of the condyle and good remodeling after surgery. (**a**) Preoperative. (**b**) 6 months postoperatively. (**c**) 1 year postoperatively

7.2.7.2 Five-Year Postoperative Follow-Up

The mouth opening improved to 39 mm, and the preauricular pain VAS score improved to 0 (Figs. 7.36, 7.37, 7.38 and 7.39). The rest was the same as the 1-year postoperative follow-up.

7.2.8 Case N. Advantages and Disadvantages

Yang Chi, Chen Minjie, and Guo Zhilin

7.2.8.1 Advantages

This prosthesis is the first international design and application that has achieved its design goals, both in terms of innovative prosthesis design solutions and technological innovations in condylar preservation, which have been well validated clinically. The significance of condylar preservation lies in the preservation of this vital organ, making possible postoperative remodeling and restoration of joint function. The success of this case is attributed to three points:

- In the design and manufacture of the prosthesis, the design fully considered the condylar movement trajectory, and the careful manufacture of the articular surface made it as smooth as a mirror.
- The preservation of the articular disc assured that the condylar would not be subjected to excessive force, and preservation of the lateral pterygoid muscle attachment is a guarantee of the blood supply and the capacity for anterior movement.
- The joint space was enlarged and filled with a fat fascial flap, which, on the one hand, can cushion the force on the condylar-disc, and on the other hand, it can prevent adhesion between the disc and the fossa prosthesis.

Other advantages of this prosthesis can be found in Chap. 6.

Overall, the protocol not only preserves the normal condyle, articular disc, and lateral pterygoid muscle but also solves the problem of non-reconstruction of the skull base and articular fossa seen in traditional surgical protocols.

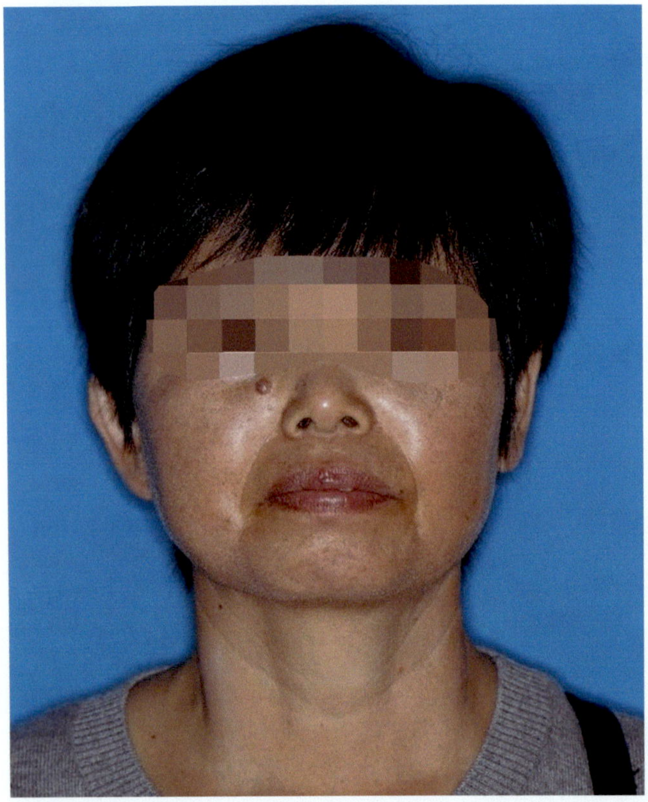

Fig. 7.36 Case N. Postoperative 5-year follow-up showed no change in facial morphology compared to 1-year follow-up

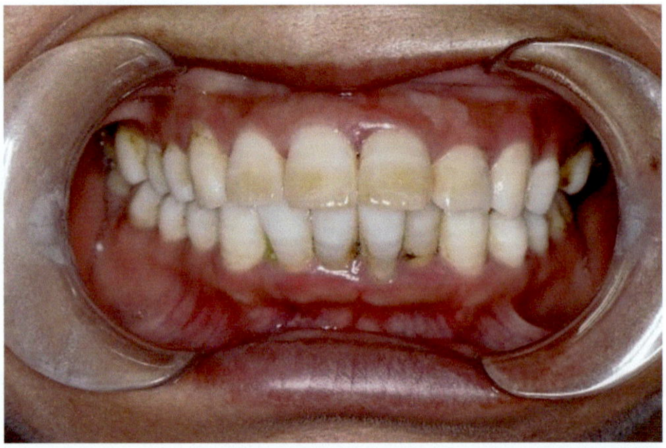

Fig. 7.37 Case N. Postoperative 5-year follow-up shows a stable intraoral occlusion relationship

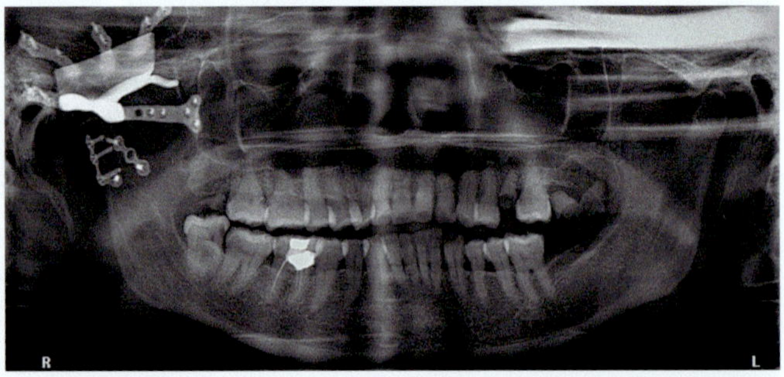

Fig. 7.38 Case N. 5-year postoperative panoramic view

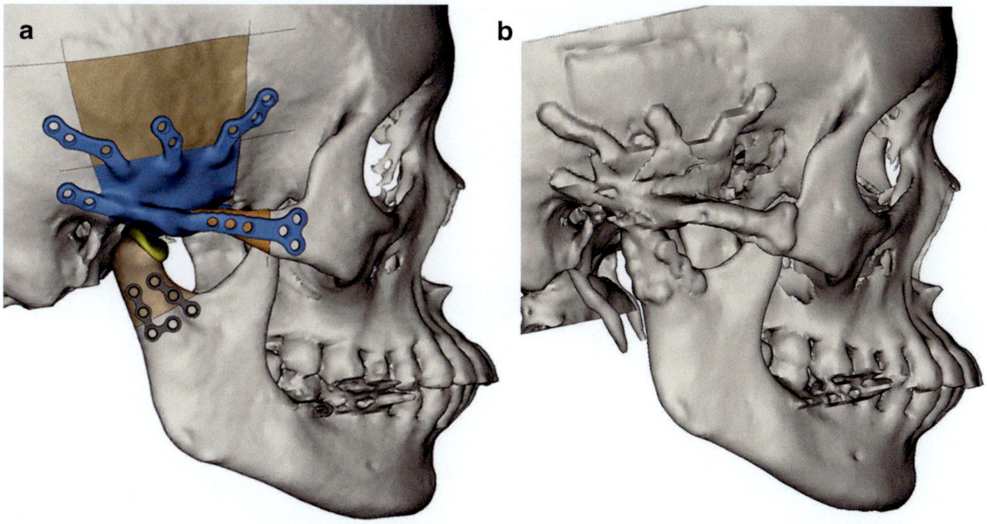

Fig. 7.39 Case N. Comparison of CT reconstruction at 5 years postoperatively showing precise prosthesis seating. (**a**) Preoperative design. (**b**) 5 years postoperatively

7.2.8.2 Disadvantages

Regarding the design, no specific optimization is envisioned currently. However, a preliminary idea is that a thin layer of wear-resistant, elastic material on the prosthetic articular surface might provide further advantages.

Prosthetic Reconstruction of Combined Temporomandibular Joint-Mandibular Diseases with Non-salvageable Joint

8

Chi Yang, Minjie Chen, Zixian Jiao, and Duohong Zou

This chapter is aimed at Class IV, the sub-Class IVa, of Yang's new classification, that is, temporomandibular joint (TMJ) diseases where the joint is non-salvageable. Whether the condylar primary lesion extends downward or the mandibular lesion invades upward, it will result in a TMJ and mandibular defect, the reconstruction of which is a formidable challenge in oral and maxillofacial surgery. The main difficulties include:

1. Precise restoration of the TMJ motion center in order to ensure good motor function.
2. Restoration of the TMJ-mandible shape, including the selection of donor bone and design of bone graft reconstruction.
3. Preservation of tissues including important structures such as the inferior alveolar neurovascular bundle.
4. Occlusal restoration, that is, to provide sufficient bone support for implantation or prosthodontic treatment.
5. Long-term efficacy, that is, to avoid various influencing factors such as implant exposure.

Recognizing these issues and based on our successful experience of total joint replacement in the previous period, the author's team focused on the above difficult problems and constructed a customized TMJ-mandibular joint prosthesis system which was gradually optimized and matured. We finally obtained stable long-term efficacy, observing up to a maximum of 8 years of clinical application and follow-up. This will be introduced in detail in this chapter on the reconstructive surgery performed with this prosthesis system.

Chi Y. (✉) · Minjie C. · Zixian J. · Duohong Z.
Shanghai Ninth People's Hospital, Shanghai Jiao Tong University School of Medicine, Shanghai, China

© People's Medical Publishing House, PR of China 2025
Chi Y. (ed.), *Atlas of Customized TMJ-Cranio-Jaw Prosthesis*, https://doi.org/10.1007/978-981-95-0611-8_8

8.1 Overview

Chi Yang and Minjie Chen

In this section, a definition of temporomandibular joint (TMJ) diseases where the condyle cannot be saved and a new classification of these diseases are proposed. Reviewing traditional prosthetic reconstruction methods, we have found problems. Therefore, an innovative prosthetic reconstruction method with a digital design process for customized TMJ-mandible combined prostheses is proposed, in preparation for continuing clinical application. In this chapter, innovative treatment modalities for TMJ-mandibular lesions will be introduced in detail.

8.1.1 Definition of Combined TMJ-Mandibular Diseases Where the TMJ Cannot Be Preserved

A lesion caused by tumors, inflammation, etc., that simultaneously involves the joint and other parts of the mandible is called a "TMJ-mandibular disease." It is confirmed as a case where the TMJ cannot be preserved through a comprehensive judgment of clinical manifestations, imaging evaluation, and pathological diagnosis and is then classified as "TMJ-mandibular disease with non-salvageable joint." Clinically, it is usually manifested as swelling and pain in the joint and mandible area. The preferred treatment is surgical removal of the condyle and mandibular lesions. There are many types of reconstruction, and there is no standardized protocol that has been universally agreed upon.

8.1.2 Classification of Combined TMJ-Mandibular Diseases Where the TMJ Cannot Be Preserved

The author has categorized TMJ-mandibular combined diseases in the following two ways, each of which has its own uses and merits: (1) classification according to the origin of the lesion and (2) classification according to the extent of the lesion.

8.1.2.1 Classification According to the Origin of the Lesion

The origin of the lesion can be categorized into two types, depending on whether the origin is outside of the TMJ but involves the condyle (Type I) or whether the origin is the condyle itself (Type II).

Type I is more common when the primary lesion from other parts of the mandible invades past the point of the mandibular notch and, furthermore, even involves the condylar head. This class can again be subdivided into two subgroups:

- Type Ia, the diseases involve only the condyle in the TMJ without destroying the articular disc and fossa structure, and it is commonly associated with benign or borderline tumors, cystic lesions, and congenital defects of mandibular origin (Fig. 8.1).
- Type Ib, the lesion involves the entire joint and results in ankylosis of the joint, such as disease due to osteomyelitis and osteoradionecrosis (Fig. 8.2).
- Type II cases, where the origin is the condyle itself, which is relatively rare, are primary joint diseases invading the mandibular ramus such as osteochondroma of the condyle and osteosarcoma (Fig. 8.3).

8.1.2.2 Classification According to the Extent of the Lesion (See Fig. 8.4)

There are five categories to describe the area of the extent of the lesion, from smallest to greatest extent:

- Class I is the area from the affected condyle to the plane of the mandibular foramen.
- Class II is the area from the affected condyle over the mandibular foramen to the posterior region of the ipsilateral molar.
- Class III is the area from the affected condyle over the posterior region of the molar to the midline of the mandible.
- Class IV is the area from the affected condyle over the midline of the mandible to the subcondylar area of the contralateral condyle, with the requirement that healthy condylar tissue on the contralateral side should be at least 10 mm.
- Class V is the area covering the entire mandible and bilateral condyles.

8.1.3 Traditional Prosthetic Reconstruction of Combined TMJ-Mandibular Diseases Where the TMJ Cannot Be Preserved

The traditional prosthetic reconstructive surgical approaches for combined TMJ-mandibular diseases include autogenous tissue reconstruction (bone flap, soft tissue flap) and artificial material reconstruction (titanium plate, etc.), but both have their own limitations, which are mainly reflected in the following aspects.

Resection without repair: this is used more commonly for malignant tumors or those with large soft tissue defects. It often leads to malformations such as mandibular deviation affecting the lower third of the face, deformity with facial depressions, occlusal disorders, inefficient mastication, and even breathing disorders if the defect extends beyond the midline of the mandible, such as narrowed airway (Fig. 8.5).

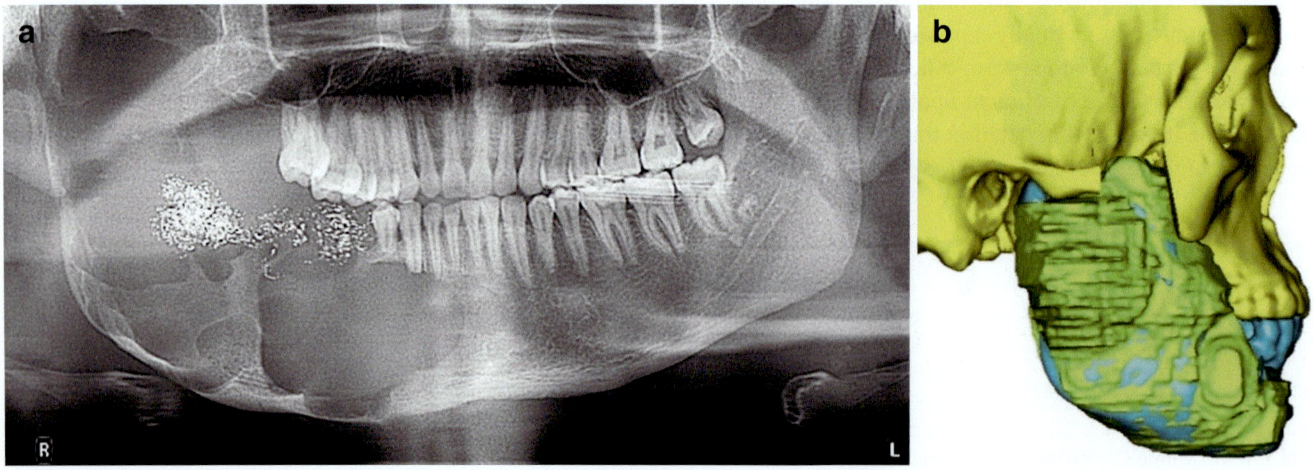

Fig. 8.1 Ameloblastoma of the mandible involving only the right condyle but not the articular disc (Type Ia). (**a**) Panoramic view. (**b**) Three-dimensional reconstruction

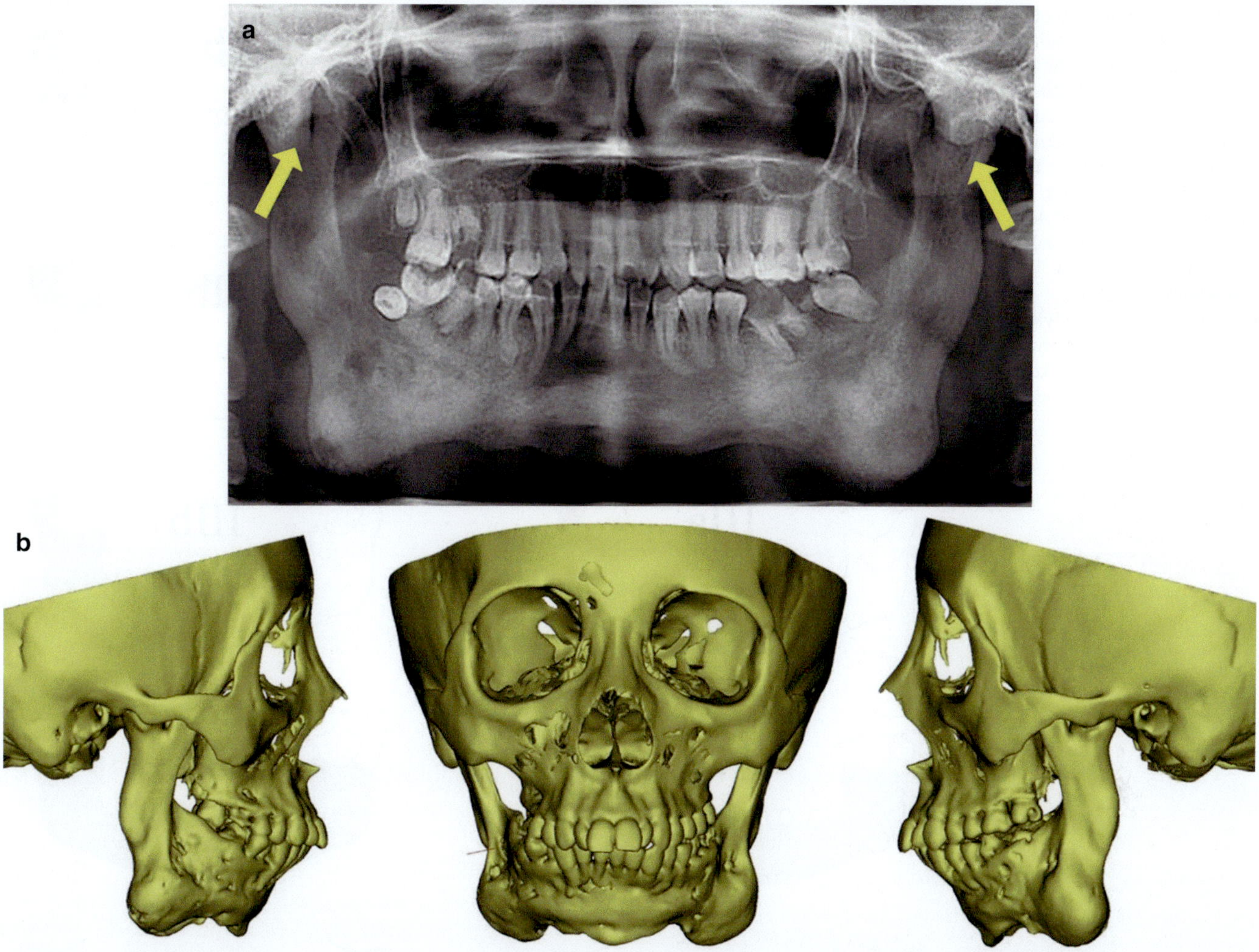

Fig. 8.2 Mandibular fibrous dysplasia resulting in bilateral joint ankylosis (Type Ib, the lesion involves the entire joint). (**a**) Panoramic film with yellow arrows showing joint ankylosis. (**b**) Three-dimensional reconstruction (right, frontal, and left views, respectively)

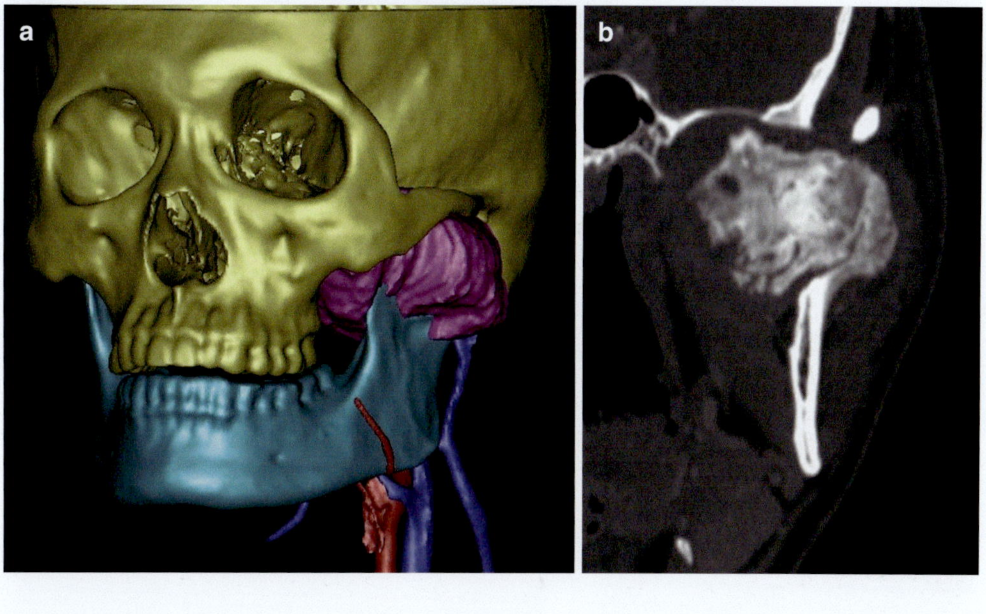

Fig. 8.3 Condylar osteosarcoma involving the plane of the mandibular foramen (Type II, the lesion origin is the condyle itself). (**a**) Three-dimensional reconstruction showing the tumor (pink) originating from the joint and reaching downward to the plane of the mandibular foramen. (**b**) CT coronal view

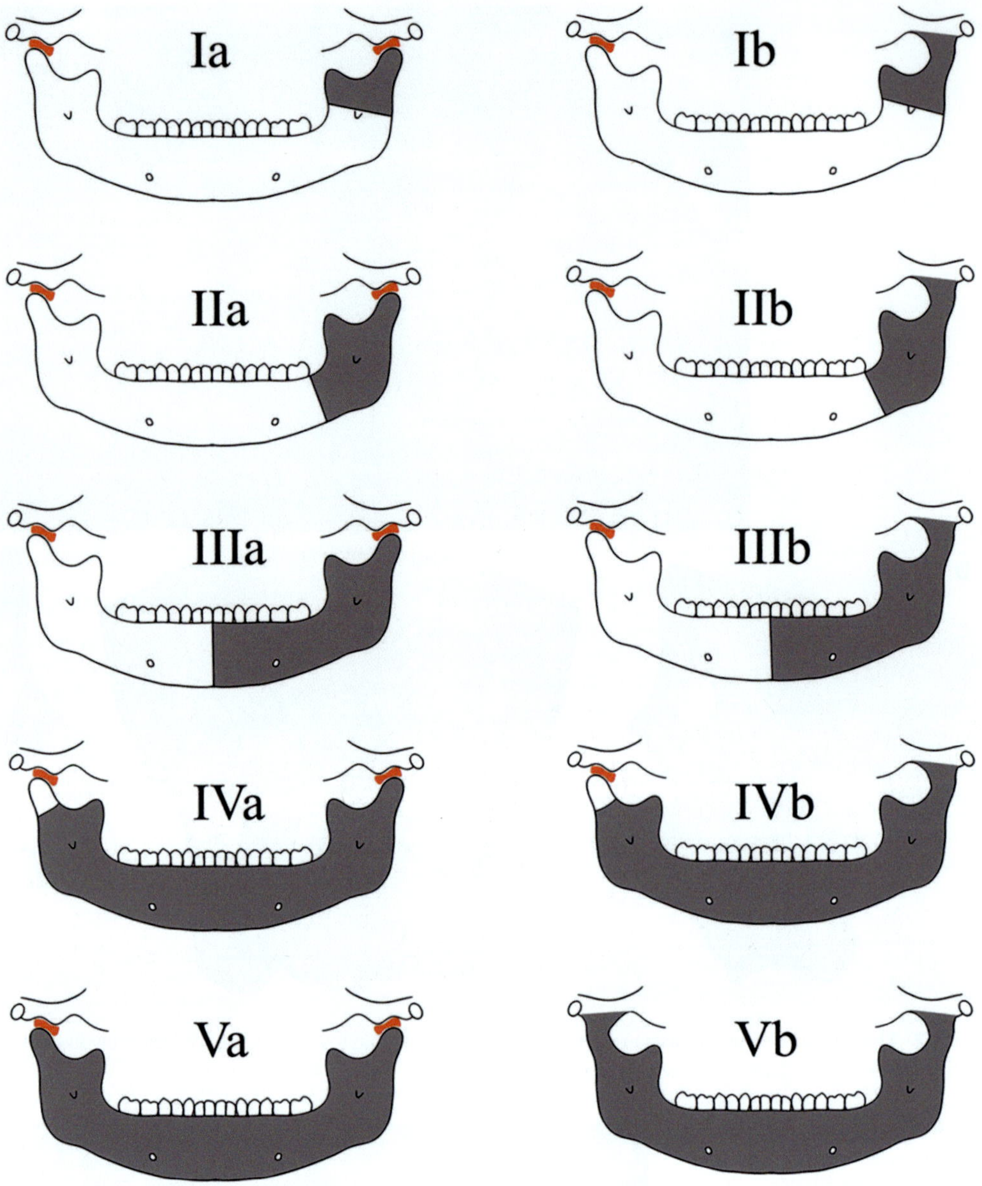

Fig. 8.4 Classification of combined TMJ-mandibular diseases according to the extent of the lesion. White is healthy tissue, orange is the intact articular disc, and dark gray is diseased tissue. Class I, condyle to mandibular foramen; Class II, condyle to distal middle of ipsilateral second molar; Class III, condyle to mandibular midline; Class IV, condyle to contralateral condylar neck; and Class V, lesion covering the total mandible, including two condyles

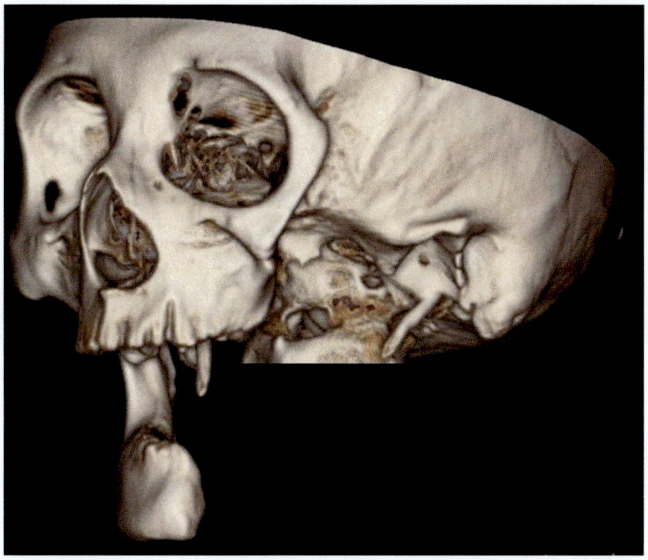

Fig. 8.5 Combined TMJ-mandibular lesion resected without reconstruction

Titanium plate restorations generally only play a purely supportive role, because they are unable to restore bone and dental support after the lesion is removed; after long-term implantation, the titanium plate may suffer displacement, fracture, or exposure (Fig. 8.6).

Prosthetic restoration of the semi-articular joint is mostly used when there is still residual dentition with a stable occlusal relationship; although the articular joint head is restored, the operation does not restore joint stability and function, and there is a risk that the metal articular joint head might protrude into the base of the skull (Fig. 8.7).

Vascularized or nonvascularized autogenous bone flap restoration: although there have been successful cases of hemi-mandibular reconstruction with long ribs, the vascularized fibular flap is still the dominant method of restoration, with better restoration of the mandibular shape. But dislocation often occurs when the fibular head is used in place of the condyle (Fig. 8.8). Both the rib and fibula are limited in length, not long enough to restore larger joint-mandible

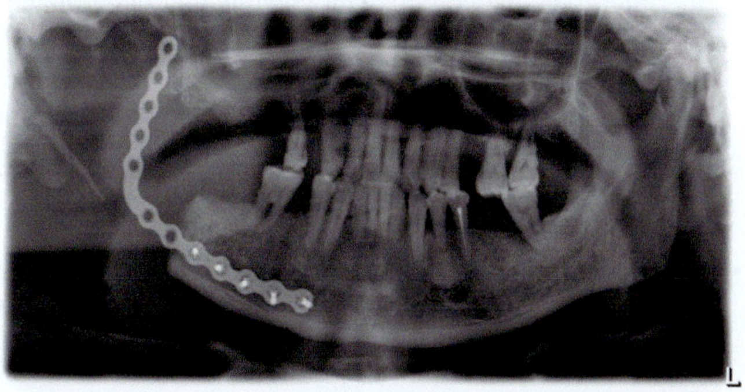

Fig. 8.6 Displacement after titanium plate-only restoration of a combined TMJ-mandibular lesion

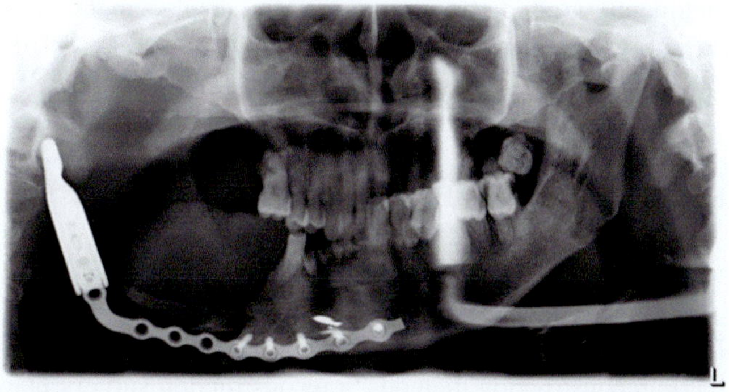

Fig. 8.7 Prosthetic dislocation after repair of combined TMJ-mandibular lesion

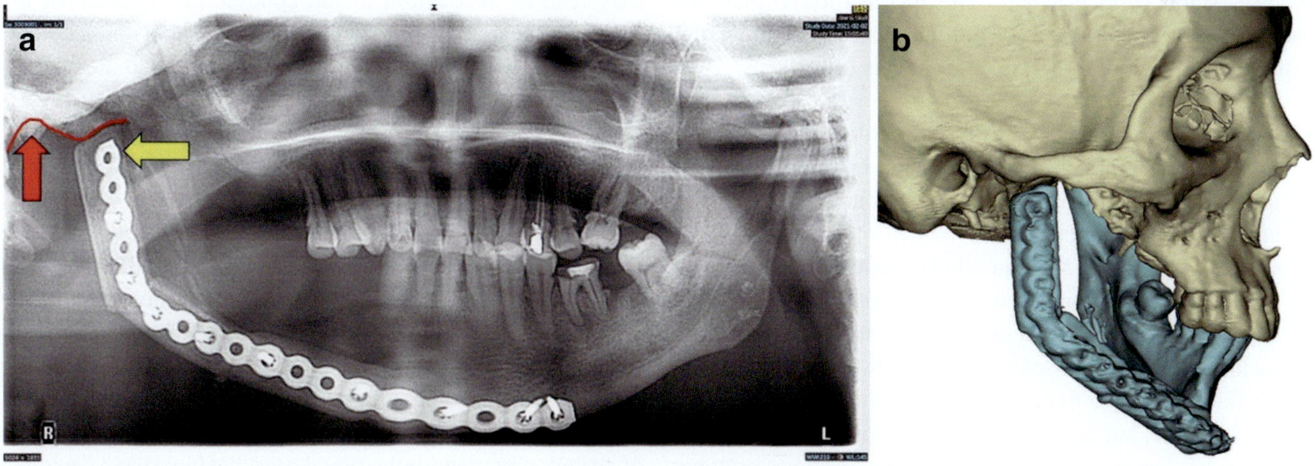

Fig. 8.8 Anterior dislocation of the condylar process after fibular grafting. (**a**) The red arrow with the red contour line shows the articular fossa and eminence, and the yellow arrow highlights the grafted fibular flap, which can be seen anteriorly and below the articular eminence. (**b**) Three-dimensional reconstruction

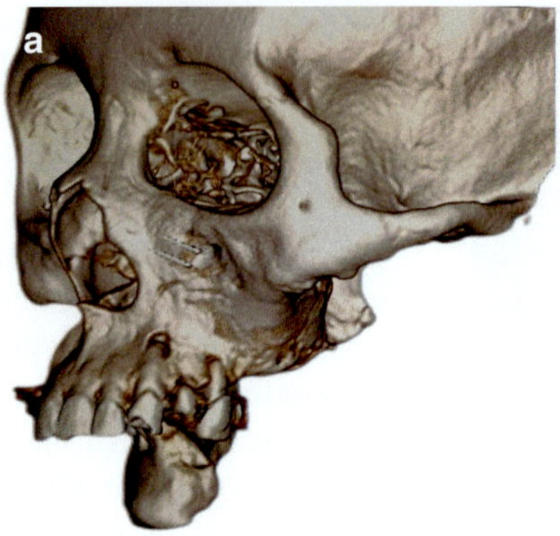

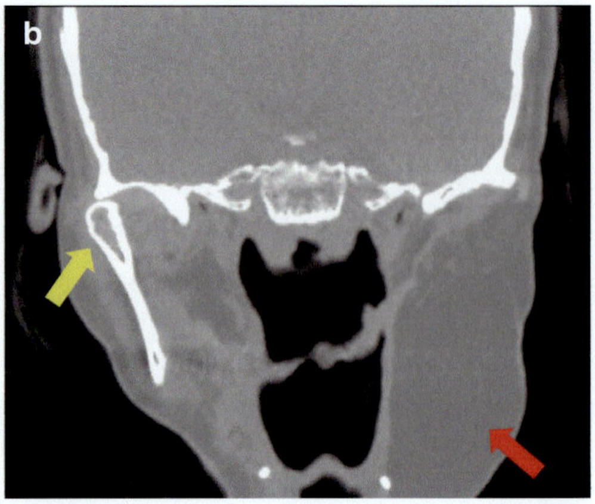

Fig. 8.9 Condition of the patient 19 years after resection of a combined joint-mandible lesion, resulting in dislocation of the condylar process on the healthy side (yellow arrow), with only a residual fat flap repair on the affected side (red arrow), and loss of muscle tissue, such as the masseter muscle and the internal pterygoid muscle. (**a**) Three-dimensional reconstruction of the CT. (**b**) CT coronal view

combined diseases, and a single bone flap is usually not wide enough to support dental implants.

Staged reconstruction: only the lesion is resected in Stage 1, and the mandible and articular structures are reconstructed in Stage 2. Stage 2 reconstruction suffers from muscle atrophy, resulting in a severe lack of soft tissues for muscle reattachment, grafted tissues prone to displacement, and difficulty in determining the correct jaw-maxilla relationship due to long-term occlusal loss. (Fig. 8.9).

8.1.4 Innovative Prosthetic Reconstruction with Customized Combined TMJ-Mandibular Prosthesis

In order to overcome the shortcomings of traditional prosthetic reconstruction methods, a reconstruction surgery plan utilizing a customized combined joint-mandible prosthesis together with autogenous bone is proposed, with the aim of making this type of complex reconstruction surgery simple, precise, stable, and efficient. The reconstructive plan for each class of lesion, listed according to the extent of the lesion as shown in Fig. 8.4, is described as follows:

- Class I diseases: total joint replacement is preferred, involving the reattachment of the lateral pterygoid muscle to preserve the functions of mandibular anterior extension and wide mouth opening.
- Class II diseases: TMJ-mandibular simultaneous restoration is appropriate, involving the preservation or removal of the inferior alveolar neurovascular bundle and the reattachment of the masseter muscle and medial pterygoid muscle in addition to the reattachment of the lateral pterygoid muscle, but not the dental restoration.
- Class III diseases: TMJ-mandibular-occlusal restorations are preferred, that is, the embodiment of the "TMJ-mandibular-occlusal complex" concept, which involves the preservation or resection of the inferior alveolar neurovascular bundle and the reattachment of the lateral pterygoid muscle, masseter muscle, and medial pterygoid muscle, as well as the reattachment of not only the lateral pterygoid, masseter, and medial pterygoid muscles but also the mylohyoid muscle, partial genioglossus muscle, geniohyoid muscle, and digastric muscle.
- Class IV diseases: TMJ-mandibular-occlusal restoration that preserves the contralateral condyle and other attachments of the joint is preferred; free condyle reimplantation is not advocated, as it is very likely to result in resorption, but it involves the preservation or excision of the bilateral inferior alveolar neurovascular bundles, and it involves the reattachment of the bilateral mandible-related muscles except the contralateral lateral pterygoid muscle.
- Class V diseases: these are rare, and the nerves, muscles, and occlusion as described above need to be considered, with simultaneous reconstruction being the most challenging.

In the simultaneous reconstruction of Class IV and V diseases, the lack of mandible-related muscle attachment and the weight of the customized prosthesis and the bone graft may lead to dislocation of the condyle or exposure of the grafted bone, and intraoperative fascial suspension and other methods of fixation are required to obtain immediate postoperative condylar and mandibular stabilization.

8.1.4.1 Types of Combined Temporomandibular TMJ-Mandibular Prostheses

A customized TMJ-mandibular prosthesis is a reconstructive prosthesis that is digitally designed, 3D printed, and 5-axis machined to be individualized according to the extent of the lesion and the patient's needs, considering both jaw reconstruction (block restoration) and occlusal reconstruction (including dental implantation).

There are three types (but potentially not limited to three) of articulating mandibular prostheses that have been designed by our team. These are differentiated by the shape of the mandibular body, designed to address different needs. The cases in this chapter focus on the second and third types of prostheses described below.

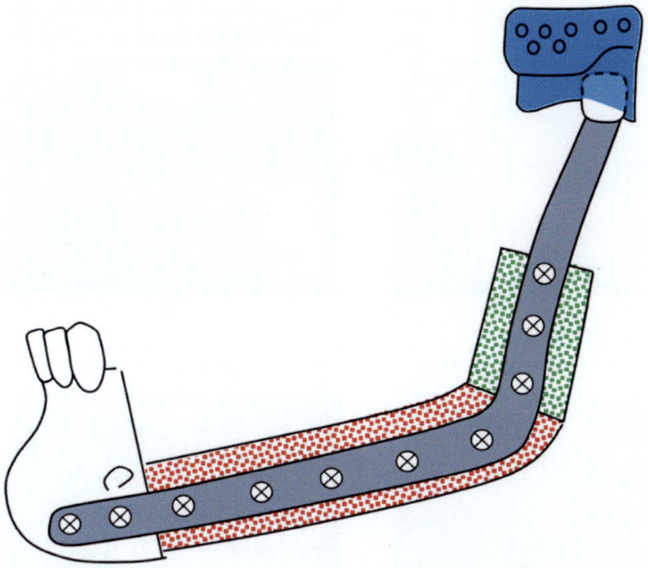

Fig. 8.10 Reconstruction plate-type combined TMJ-mandibular prosthesis. The prosthesis body (gray, mandible component; blue, articular fossa component) resembles a mandibular reconstruction plate for fixation of the autogenous bone graft blocks (red and green), restoring the contour of the mandible

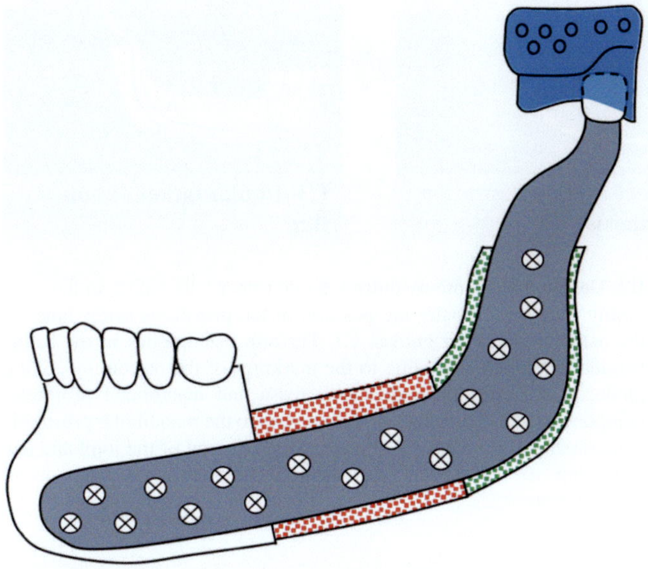

Fig. 8.11 Wide-type reconstruction plate combined TMJ-mandibular prosthesis. The mandibular prosthesis body (gray) is wider and designed with a double row of screw holes, which are fixed to the grafted bone flap (red and green). Blue is the articular fossa component of the prosthesis

1. Reconstruction plate-type combined TMJ-mandibular prosthesis (Fig. 8.10), secured to the grafted bone with a single row of screws, is indicated for combination with autogenous bone grafts for Class III and advanced cases without the need for dental implants.

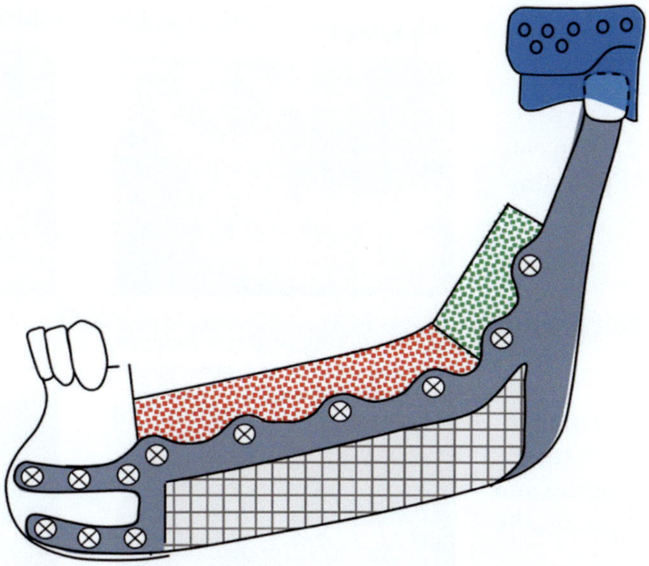

Fig. 8.12 Mandibular body augmentation-type combined TMJ-mandibular prosthesis. The mandibular prosthesis morphology (gray) is divided into a solid portion and a porous portion, with the solid portion elevating and securing the grafted bone block (red and green). Blue is the articular fossa component of the prosthesis

2. Wide-type reconstruction plate combined TMJ-mandibular prosthesis (Fig. 8.11), fixed to the grafted bone with double rows of screws, should be used for iliac bone graft for Class II and Class III diseases, which can be completed with second-stage dental implantation.
3. Mandibular body augmentation-type combined TMJ-mandibular prosthesis (Fig. 8.12), with a porous structure in the lower half to support the graft and reduce weight and a single-row screw fixation to the graft in the upper half, is indicated for autogenous bone grafts of Class III and higher. It can be supplemented with second-stage dental implantation.

- Indications and contraindications for implanting a combined temporomandibular TMJ-mandibular prostheses
  - Indications

  This prosthesis is indicated for a wide range of TMJ-mandibular diseases in adults, mainly benign or borderline tumors and tumorlike lesions, quiescent inflammatory lesions, fibrous dysplasia, congenital TMJ-mandibular underdevelopment, acquired TMJ-mandibular diseases caused by tumors or trauma, etc.
  - Contraindications

  Acute phase of secondary infection (e.g., acute osteomyelitis or other lesions) and cases with incomplete resection of malignant tumors. Use with caution in: osteoradionecrosis, adolescents in the growth and development stage, and cases with insufficient soft tissue to cover the graft area.

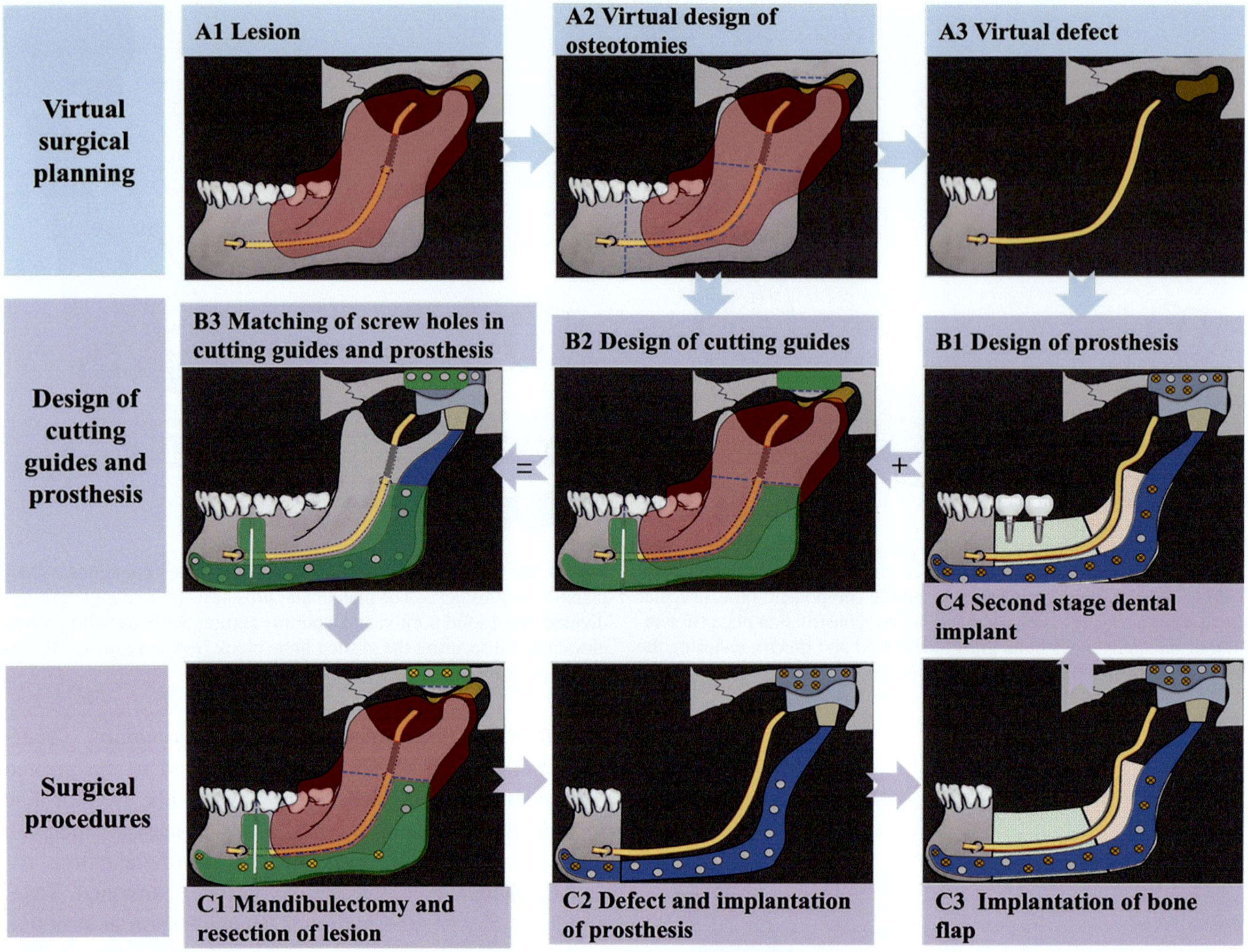

Fig. 8.13 Digital design of the combined joint-mandible prosthesis, including articulating fossa: A1. 3D reconstruction based on CT data to define the extent of the joint lesion (red) and to mark the course of the inferior alveolar neurovascular bundle (yellow). A2. Design of the osteotomy line with protection of the inferior alveolar neurovascular bundle. A3. Obtaining the defect model expected after osteotomy with preservation of the articular disc (brown). B1. Design of the graft bone flap (light green and light pink) and the prosthesis form (blue) according to the defect model and simulation of the dental implantation site. B2. Design the osteotomy cutting guide (green) according to the osteotomy line. B3. Transfer the position of the prosthesis screw holes to the osteotomy cutting guides. C1. Perform osteotomies in the actual surgical operation according to the markings of the osteotomy cutting guides. C2. Install the articulating fossa and mandibular prosthesis components. C3. Secure the graft bone flap to the mandibular prosthesis component with screws. C4. Finish reconstruction of the joint and jaw according to the design, and then accomplish with later dental implantation

8.1.5 Total Digital Design Process for Customized Combined TMJ-Mandibular Prosthesis

In the case of a Class III lesion (benign or borderline), for example, the total process consists of three aspects (Fig. 8.13): lesion osteotomy simulation, prosthesis and cutting guide design, and surgical procedure.

8.1.5.1 Simulated Osteotomy for Lesions

Lesion scope analysis: the computed tomography (CT) is received in DICOM format, and through the surgical design software, the extent of the lesion is reconstructed, and the inferior alveolar neurovascular bundle is labeled at the same time (Fig. 8.13, A1).

Design of osteotomy lines:

- Anterior osteotomy line: ensures safe resection of the lesion.
- Mandibular foramen osteotomy line: facilitates mandibular segmentation and isolation of the inferior alveolar neurovascular bundle. The superior segment (condyle and coronoid process) is extracted via the preauricular approach.
- Inferior alveolar neurovascular bundle osteotomy line: designed to mobilize the neurovascular bundle.
- Articular eminence osteotomy line: required in cases of ankylosis, articular eminence pathology, or excessive steepness to ensure complete lesion removal and stable placement of the glenoid fossa prosthesis (Fig. 8.13, A2).

These osteotomy lines serve as the basis for designing the osteotomy cutting guide.

The defect is modeled: the diseased bone is removed at the osteotomy line, and the inferior alveolar neurovascular bundle is preserved. This model will be used for prosthesis design (Fig. 8.13, A3).

8.1.5.2 Prosthesis and Osteotomy Cutting Guide Design

- Design of the TMJ-mandibular prosthesis:

The design of the TMJ-mandibular prosthesis (Fig. 8.13, B1), which is derived from the defect model (Fig. 8.13, A3), requires a two-pronged approach. We might say that this is figuratively "Grasping both ends while taking care of the center," if we want to humorously apply an old Chinese political slogan to this medical explanation. "Grasping both ends" refers to judging the accurate ideal position of the artificial joint (the head component should be in the center of the posterior portion of the fossa component when the mouth is closed and in contact with the retaining plate of the fossa component) and assures the occlusal stability of the residual natural dentition. We have repeatedly emphasized the need to balance the three parts, the TMJ-mandibular-occlusal complex. "Taking care of the center" refers to the design of the dental implants and the corresponding bone grafts, with the contralateral teeth as the reference for planned implant placement. The "center" refers to the occlusion, which is achieved through design of the dental implant and the corresponding bone graft, which is needed both for the dental implant and to ensure the reattachment of the masticatory muscles.

This part of the design reflects the functional surgical plan of the "TMJ-mandibular-occlusal" relationship reconstruction. If the iliac bone is chosen for the bone graft, the implant bone flap can be grooved to incorporate the preserved inferior alveolar neurovascular bundle.

The final design of the prosthesis screw holes allows for stable fixation of the articulating fossa prosthesis component to the temporal bone, the mandibular prosthesis component to the residual mandible, and the mandibular prosthesis to the grafted bone, while it avoids the locations of the reserved implant screws. The TMJ-mandibular prosthesis implantation and bone grafts were completed simultaneously, and dental implants were performed in phase II.

- Design of the osteotomy cutting guides:

Based on the design of the osteotomy lines (Fig. 8.13, A2), the osteotomy cutting guides are designed for precise positioning.

1. Mandibular osteotomy cutting guide design: one cutting guide is designed to serve for three osteotomy lines, which are the mandibular foramen plane osteotomy line, the inferior alveolar neurovascular bundle osteotomy line, and the anterior osteotomy line of the lesion, respectively. In addition, the cutting guide also sets the anterior extension for the transfer of the screw holes for the mandibular prosthesis fixation; this is planned to be similar in shape to the fixation pattern of the mandibular prosthesis when applied to normal bone tissue. If this part of the cutting guide is too long for convenient production, then to prevent deformation and positioning difficulties in the process of processing and sterilization, it can also be divided into two parts for production, that is, two parts located, respectively, in the angle of the jaw and chin.
2. Articular eminence osteotomy cutting guide design: the same as in total joint replacement, see Chap. 3 (Fig. 8.13, B2).
3. Matching the cutting guide screw holes to the prosthesis screw holes: overlap the images prepared for the processes in Fig. 8.13, B1 and B2 to set the screw holes of the cutting guide according to the screw holes of the prosthesis, so that not only the osteotomy is accurate, but also the prosthesis can be fitted accurately, easily, and quickly without the need for intermaxillary ligation (Fig. 8.13, B3).
4. In addition, the design of the bone grafting guide should be carried out at this time. According to the length and shape of the defect, the appropriate bone graft should be selected, and the guide should be designed to harvest the bone graft so that it is suitable for the defect repair.

8.1.6 Surgical Procedures

- Mandibular and articular eminence osteotomies (Fig. 8.13, C1):
  1. Mandibular osteotomy: after fixation of the osteotomy plate, sequential osteotomy of the plane of the mandibular foramen, the neurovascular bundles, and the anterior end of the lesion is carried out, and only a single corticotomy is carried out for the neurovascular bundles of the inferior alveolar nerve. Then the osteotomy plate is removed, and the bone chisel cuts along the osteotomy line to remove the bone below the level of the mandibular foramen, in pieces.
  2. Osteotomy of the articular eminence on the zygomatic arch, the same as for total joint replacement.
  3. Preauricular-temporal incision to separate the lateral pterygoid muscle and temporalis muscle attachments, and remove the bone mass above the level of the mandibular foramen.
- Prosthesis installation:
  1. Installation of the articular fossa prosthesis, prioritize the fixation of the two screw holes left by the osteotomy cutting guide of the articular tubercle to ensure accuracy, and then fix the other screw holes three to four pieces.

2. Install the mandibular prosthesis, prioritize the fixation of the two screw holes left by the mandibular osteotomy cutting guide, and check that the articulating head parts are in place and the occlusal relationship is normal, to ensure that the position is accurate. If the screw holes are correct, affix two to four other screws (Fig. 8.13, C2).
   - Bone graft installation: bone is harvested and shaped with the guidance of a cutting guide, and the grafted bone block is seated and secured as designed and embedded with the inferior alveolar neurovascular bundle (Fig. 8.13, C3).
   - Occlusal reconstruction: mostly restored with dental implants (Fig. 8.13, C4).

8.2 Customized TMJ-Mandible Combined Prosthesis Reconstruction Techniques

Following the exposition on classifications of defects and types of prostheses in Sect. 8.1, the subsequent sections will illustrate the application of the prostheses in a series of clinical cases. The design considerations and efficacy of each type of prosthesis are presented in the form of specific clinical case.

Case O in Sect. 8.2 is the case of a patient with a mandibular Class IIa lesion that was reconstructed with a wide-type TMJ-mandibular prosthesis, using free iliac bone flap to restore joint structure and function and to preserve or improve dentofacial morphology.

Case P in Sect. 8.3 is the case of a patient with a mandibular Class IIa lesion, in which the inferior alveolar neurovascular bundle was preserved by osteotomy of the mandible in pieces. Reconstruction was performed at the same time with a wide-type TMJ-mandibular prosthesis and iliac bone flap and was later completed with dental implant restoration.

Case Q in Sect. 8.4 is the case of a patient with a mandibular Class IIIa lesion, and the design of the prosthesis was further optimized by using a mandibular body augmentation-type TMJ-mandibular prosthesis with a fibula flap for reconstruction, which embodied the prosthetic requirements of tissue preservation, morphology, and function in a balanced manner.

8.2.1 Case O. Design and Application of a Wide-Type Combined TMJ-Mandible Prosthesis

- Patient information: male, 34 years old.
- Complaint: recurrent swelling and pain in the right lower jaw for 25 years.
- History: at the age of 9 years, the patient underwent right mandibular mass curettage at a local hospital due to right mandibular swelling and pain, after which he developed numbness of the right lower lip. At 20 years of age, the swelling recurred, and he underwent mandibular mass curettage again, with an unclear pathologic diagnosis. In the past 2 years, he came to the hospital with progressive swelling of the right side of his face and occasional pain.
- Past history: history of systemic disease was denied.
- Clinical examination: the right parotid occlusal area was slightly swollen, with no tenderness, the right lower lip was dull to the touch, the right submandibular scar was visible, the mouth opening degree was 40 mm, and the mouth opening type was slightly leftward. The intraoral occlusal relationship was stable, and the periodontal and dental conditions were good (Figs. 8.14 and 8.15).
- Imaging examination: CT of the maxillofacial region showed that the right mandibular body, angle, and ascending ramus of the bone were swollen, with reduced density and soft tissue-like changes, expanding buccolingually, with multiple bony septations within the cyst, thinning of the peripheral wall of the lesion, interruption of local continuity, and a clear demarcation from the surrounding soft tissues (Fig. 8.16).
- Laboratory tests: refined preoperative tests were applied to rule out contraindications to surgery.
- Diagnosis: possible odontogenic keratocyst.
- Postoperative pathology: microscopically, fibrous cyst wall-like tissue lined with incompletely keratinized squamous epithelium with a fenestrated arrangement of cells in the basal layer was seen. Pathologic diagnosis was mandibular odontogenic keratocyst, with hyperplastic odontogenic epithelial masses and cyst formation seen within the cyst wall.

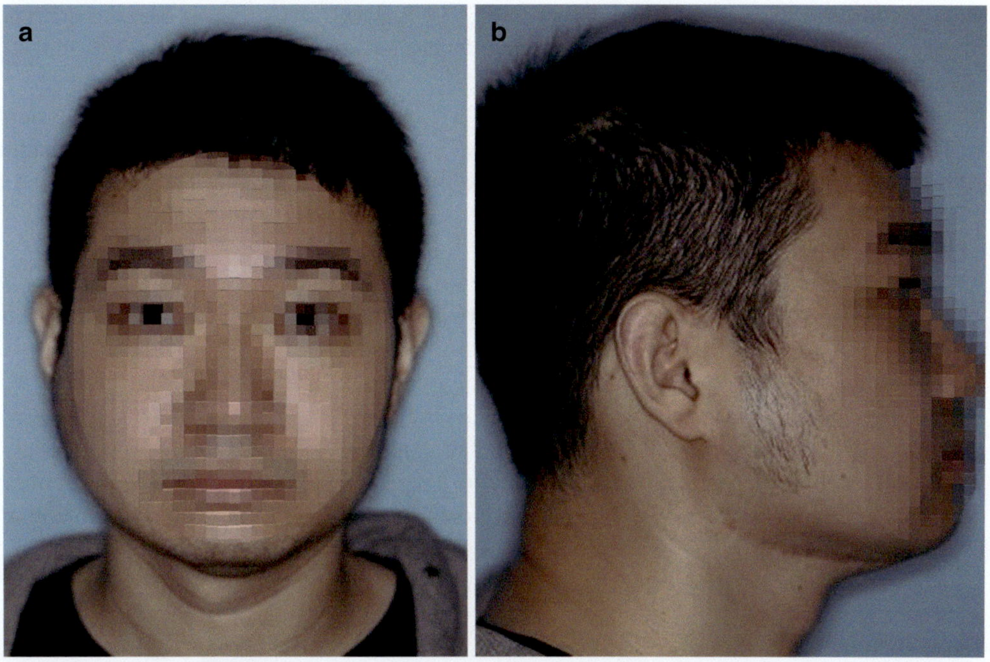

Fig. 8.14 Case O. Extraoral examination. Swelling of the right parotid occlusal area with no localized tenderness, dull tenderness of the right lower lip, and submandibular scarring from previous surgery visible. (**a**) Frontal view. (**b**) Lateral view

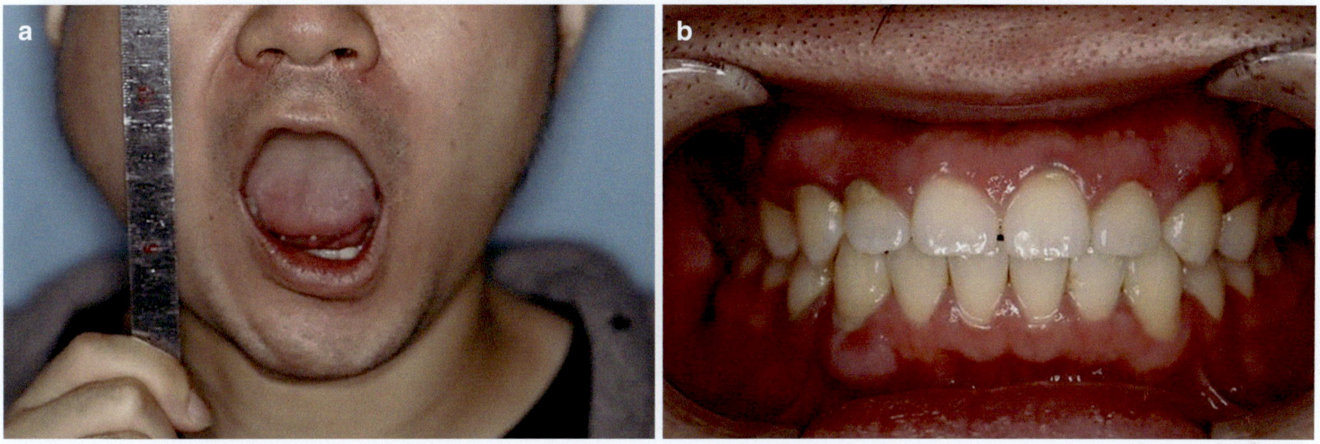

Fig. 8.15 Case O. Intraoral examination. (**a**) Mouth opening 40 mm. (**b**) Stable occlusal relationship

8.2.2 Case O. Diagnostic Imaging (Fig. 8.16)

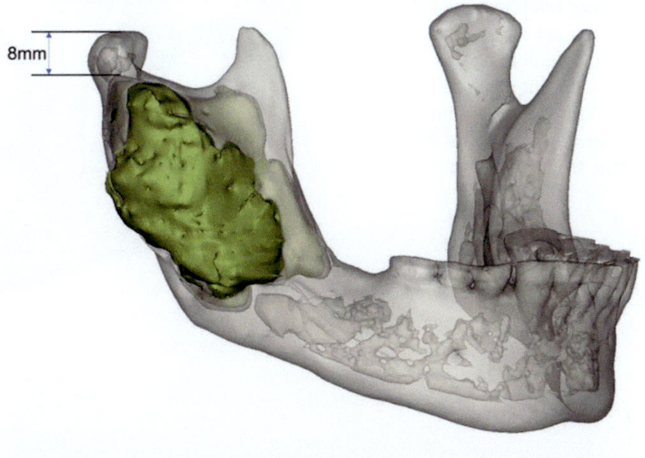

Fig. 8.16 Case O. CT reconstruction showing the mass (green) in relation to the condyle (40% transparency). Right mandibular ramus and angular lesion with buccolingual bulge, just 8 mm below the highest point of the condylar surface, suggesting that condylar preservation is not possible or very difficult

8.2.3 Case O. Treatment Program

- Overall treatment plan

The right TMJ-mandibular mass is to be resected and prosthetic reconstruction performed with a wide-type combined TMJ-mandible prosthesis.

- Surgical resection design

Resection design: condyle to the distal of the right second molar, a Class II combined lesion with low retention value due to the presence of signs of inferior alveolar nerve damage.

Digital simulation of the procedure: an osteotomy line (yellow arrow) is designed 10 mm in front of the anterior margin of the mass (green), and the extent of resection (brown) is marked, and a model of the defect after osteotomy is obtained (Fig. 8.17).

- Design of surgical procedure: in this case, taking a free iliac bone flap to be incorporated into a wide-type joint-mandible prosthesis was proposed for prosthetic reconstruction.
- Design of graft bone harvesting: considering the contour of the inferior and posterior margins of the mandible on the affected side (red line), it seems that the contour of the inferior and posterior margins of the ipsilateral iliac block is the best match, and so the iliac bone is used as the donor area for the reconstruction of the mandible. The extent of the defect does not involve the dentition, and therefore, the upper front iliac edge is used to repair the contour of the mandible; the main purpose of grafting the bone is to reconstruct the muscular attachments (Fig. 8.18).

Graft bone trimming design: trim the graft bone (yellow bone block) along the contour line of the mandible to complete the iliac bone design and design the prosthesis form with this shape (Fig. 8.19).

8.2.4 Case O. Design and Processing of Wide-Type Joint-Mandible Combined Prosthesis and Osteotomy Cutting Guides

Wide-type TMJ-mandibular joint prosthesis design.

Import and placement of core components: import and place the articular fossa core component (yellow) and the

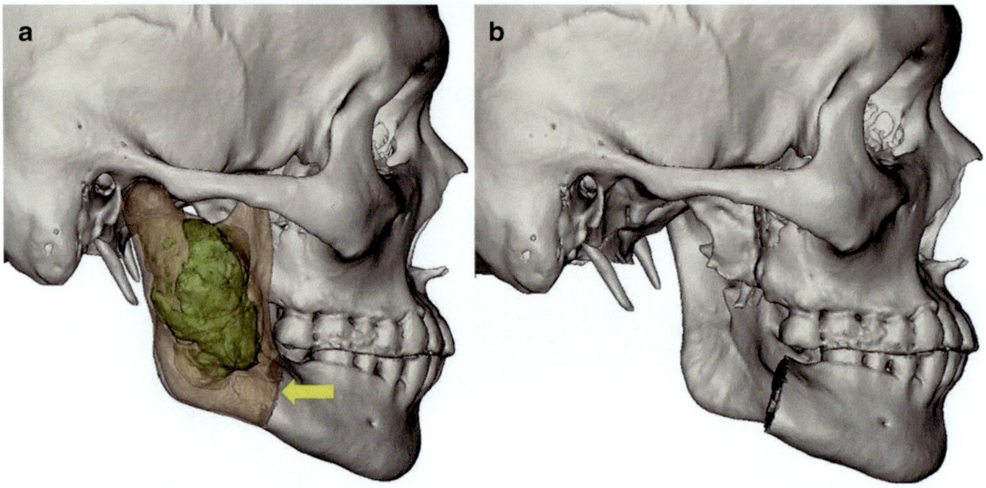

Fig. 8.17 Case O. Design of osteotomy line and defect model acquisition. A. Mandibular osteotomy line (yellow arrow) proposed to be designed 10 mm anterior to the anterior margin of the mass (green). B. A model of the TMJ-mandibular defect after completion of the osteotomy was obtained

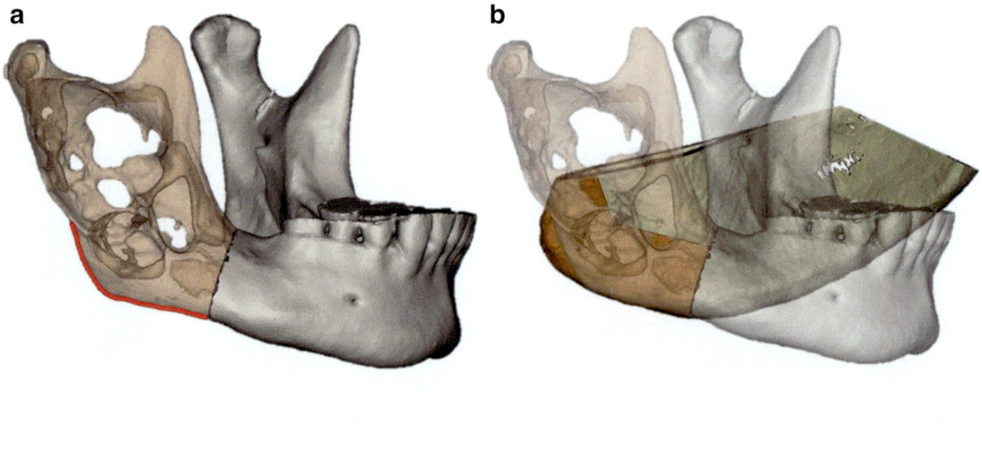

Fig. 8.18 Case O. Planning for graft bone harvesting. (**a**) Contour reference line of the inferior and posterior margins of the mandible on the affected right side (red line). (**b**) Mandibular contour restoration plan using the upper front iliac edge

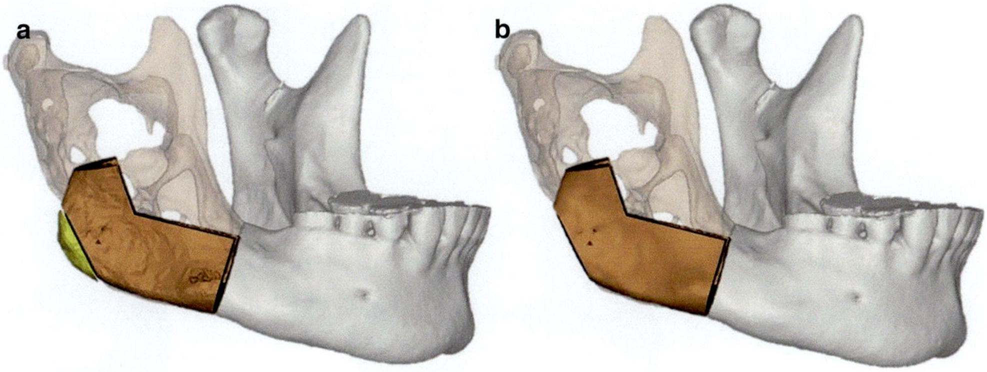

Fig. 8.19 Case O. Planning for graft bone trimming. A. Trim the graft bone block (yellow part of the bone block) to the posterior mandibular margin. B. Complete the iliac bone flap design

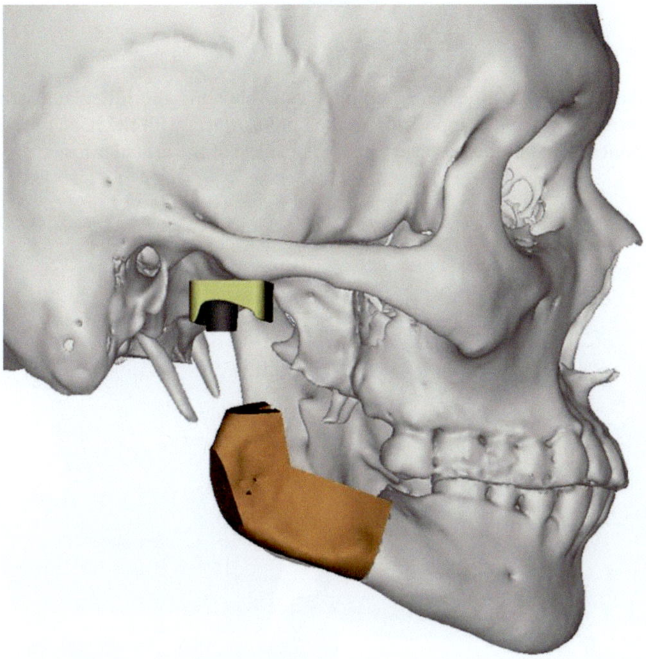

Fig. 8.20 Case O. The core component is positioned, because the articular eminence is flat, and the bone is normal so that it does not need to be treated. The articular fossa component is shown in yellow, the articular head component in dark gray, and the grafted iliac bone flap in light brown

articular head core component (dark grey, see Chap. 2), positioning of the core components (Fig. 8.20).

Design of joint fossa and mandibular extension components: design principles are described in Chap. 2 (Fig. 8.21).

Screw hole depth measurement: measure the thickness of the prosthesis and graft bone flap to determine the depth of the screw holes at each site (Fig. 8.22a).

Prosthesis fabrication and fitting: the fabrication process is described in Chap. 2 (Fig. 8.22b).

Digital Osteotomy Cutting Guide Design

Mandibular osteotomy cutting guide design: design the osteotomy cutting guide (pink) along the osteotomy line and the inferior border of the mandible and transfer the prosthetic screw position to the cutting guides (Fig. 8.23).

Autogenous free iliac osteotomy cutting guide design: design the iliac osteotomy cutting guide (pink) according to the range of the iliac block osteotomy and transfer the prosthetic screw position to the osteotomy cutting guide (Fig. 8.24). After all guides are designed, they are printed with a resin 3D printer.

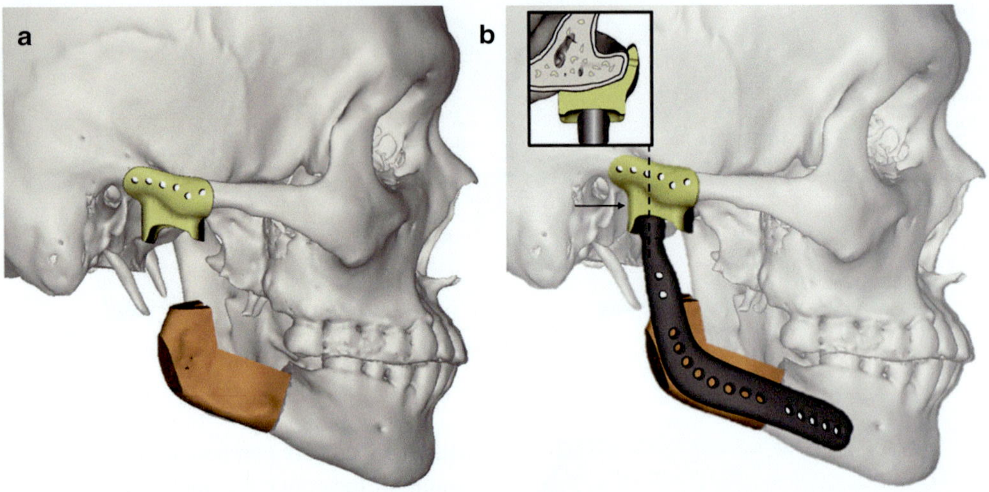

Fig. 8.21 Case O. Articular fossa prosthesis and mandibular prosthesis extension design. The articular fossa prosthesis is shown in yellow, the mandibular prosthesis in dark gray, and the grafted iliac bone flap in light brown. (**a**) Design of the articular fossa prosthesis; (**b**) Design of the mandibular prosthesis, coronal view showing the articular fossa prosthesis in close apposition to the bony surface, with the head of the joint located in the posterior median position of the articular fossa

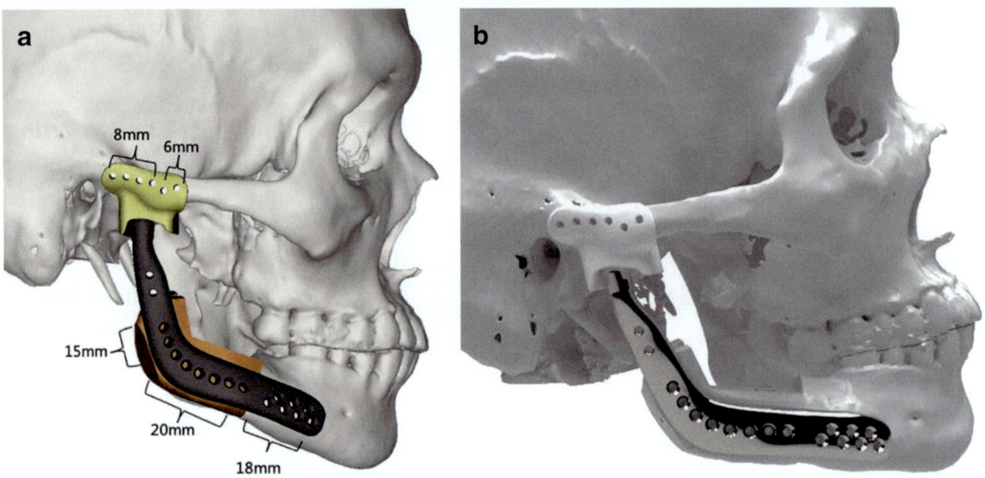

Fig. 8.22 Case O. Completion of design and production. (**a**) Screw hole depth measurement (in mm). (**b**) Prosthesis fitting

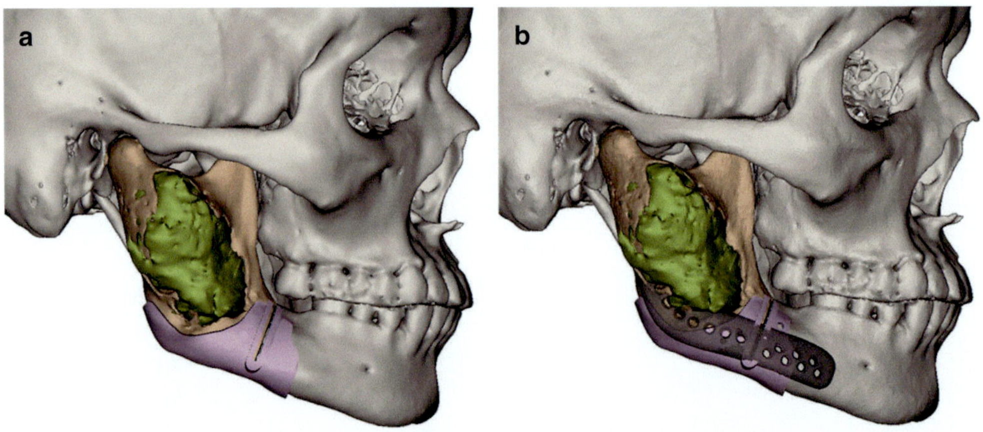

Fig. 8.23 Case O. Design of mandibular osteotomy cutting guides. (**a**) Design of osteotomy guides according to the mandibular osteotomy line. (**b**) Determination of cutting guide screw holes by prosthesis screw holes

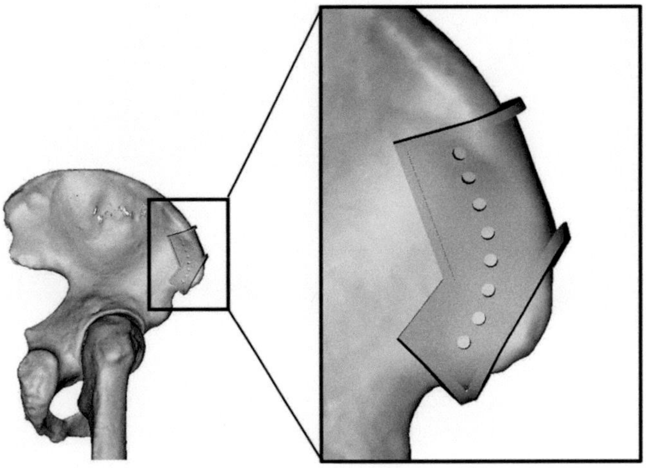

Fig. 8.24 Case O. Autogenous free iliac bone harvesting guide. The cutting guide (pink) screw holes also serve as prosthetic screw holes, thus defining the intraoperative iliac bone flap location

8.2.5 Case O. Surgical Procedures

Preoperative laboratory tests: the same as described in Sect. 3.2.5.

Preoperative preparation: skin preparation of the affected periauricular and submandibular regions, blood preparation of 400 mL, and the rest of the preoperative preparations are described in Sect. 3.2.5.

Steps of the Surgical Procedure

Surgical approach: an anterior auriculotemporal incision combined with a submandibular incision was used.

Mandibular osteotomy: install the mandibular osteotomy cutting guide (pink) and perform mandibular osteotomy (Figs. 8.25 and 8.26).

Preparation of the free iliac block: install the iliac osteotomy cutting guide (pink) to harvest the iliac bone flap (Fig. 8.27).

Articular disc management: release the anterior articular disc attachment, cut and suture the bilaminar zone, and rotate the articular disc (green arrow) medially to line the medial aspect of the articular fossa prosthesis (Fig. 8.28).

The articular prosthesis is implanted, and the graft block is secured (Figs. 8.29, 8.30 and 8.31).

Treatment of the operative area: free fat flap prepared from a submandibular incision and filled in the neck of the prosthesis; see Chap. 3.

Actual surgical modification: intermaxillary ligation was performed to ensure accurate seating of the prosthesis, and after the prosthesis was fitted, it was confirmed that the osteotomy guides and locating screw holes were accurately designed, and at this point, no intermaxillary ligation was required in subsequent cases.

- Postoperative orders and nursing care: see Sect. 3.2.5.

8.2.6 Case O. Postoperative Analysis of Prosthesis Implantation Precision

Regular postoperative follow-ups were performed for appearance (facial shape), function (mouth opening, mouth shape), and prosthesis evaluation (safety, accuracy).

Immediately after surgery: the intraoperative cutting guide was accurately seated and the prosthesis was fitted smoothly (Fig. 8.32), and a comparison between the preoperative design and the postoperative reconstruction showed that the prosthesis was accurately seated (Fig. 8.33). Postoperative prosthesis installation error analysis showed that the error of the core component was 0.5 mm and the overall error of the combined prosthesis was 1.5 mm (Fig. 8.34 and Fig. 8.35).

8.2.7 Case O. Long-Term Follow-Up and Prognosis

- 1-year postoperative follow-up

No recurrence of facial swelling or pain, no pain or discomfort in the joint area, and no other complications.

The facial shape was good (Fig. 8.36), the joint function was well restored, the TMJ-mandibular-occlusal-facial coordination was stable, the mouth opening was 38 mm, the

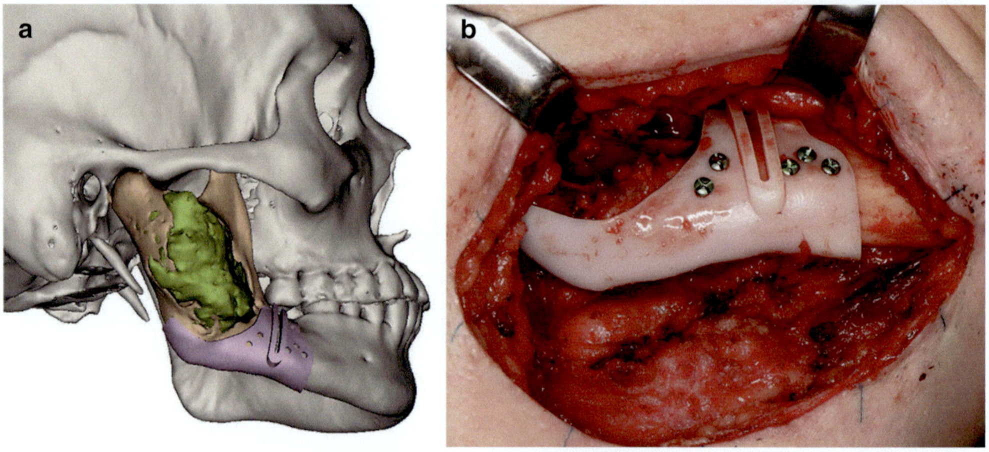

Fig. 8.25 Case O. Submandibular approach to expose the diseased mandible. (**a**) Design. (**b**) Placement of the cutting guide (white), identification of the prosthetic screw holes, and mandibular osteotomy

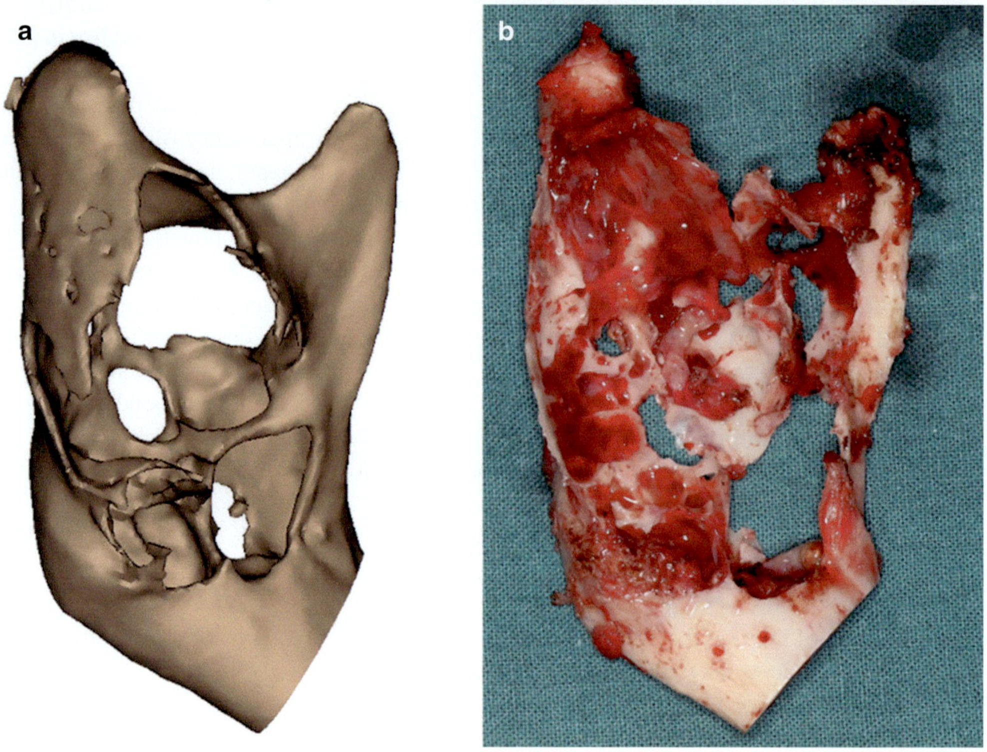

Fig. 8.26 Case O. Precision resection of diseased mandible. (**a**) Design. (**b**) Actual

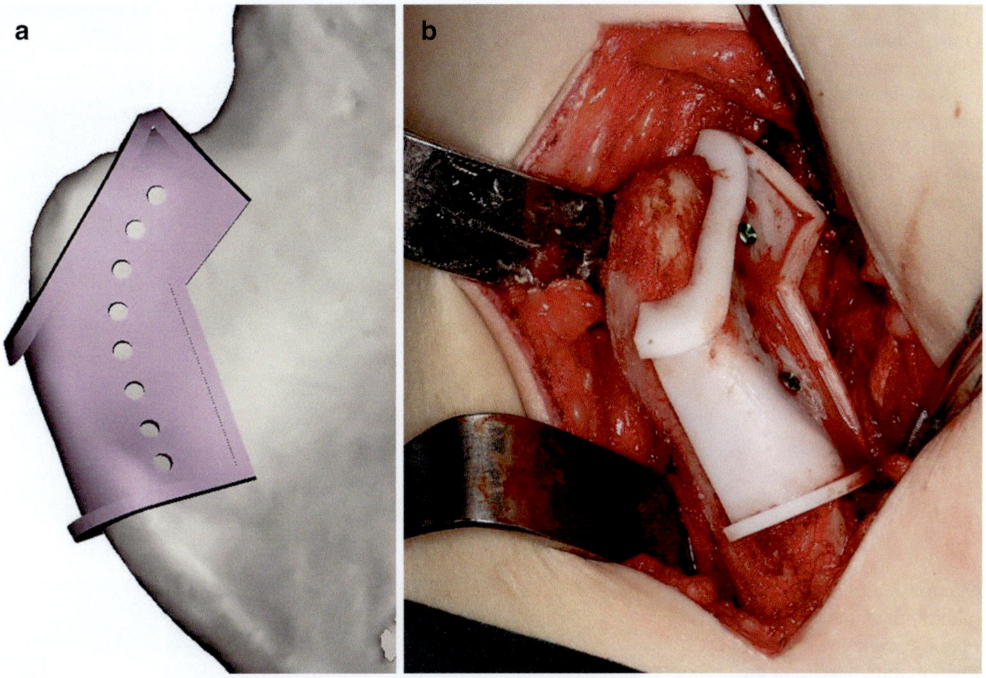

Fig. 8.27 Case O. Taking the right iliac bone flap. (**a**) Design. (**b**) Actual

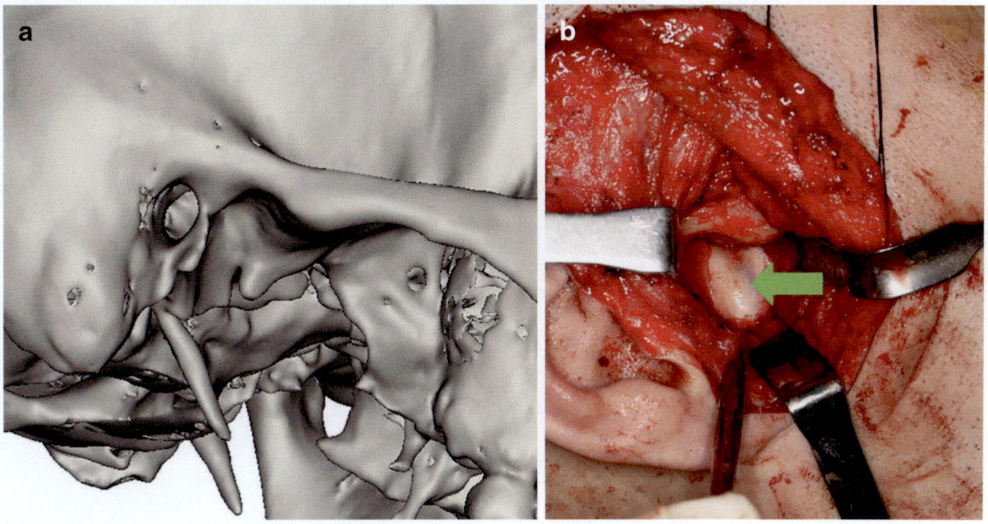

Fig. 8.28 Case O. Preimplantation preparation of an articular fossa prosthesis. (**a**) Schematic. (**b**) Preservation of the articular disc (green arrow), rotate the disc medially to the prosthesis

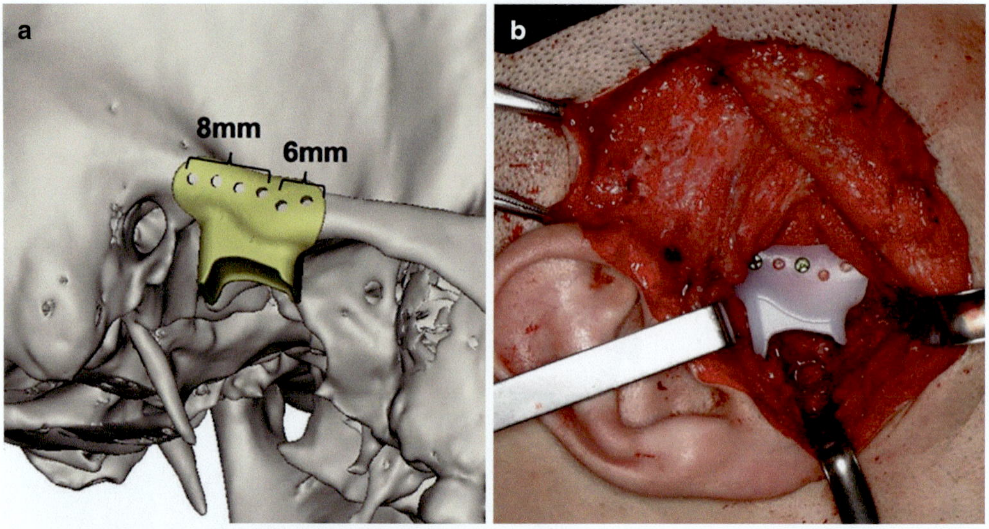

Fig. 8.29 Case O. Installation of articular fossa prosthesis (unit: mm): (**a**) Measurement of preoperative screw hole depth. (**b**) Prosthesis is fitted into position primarily with 2 screws and then fixed with 5 to 6 screws

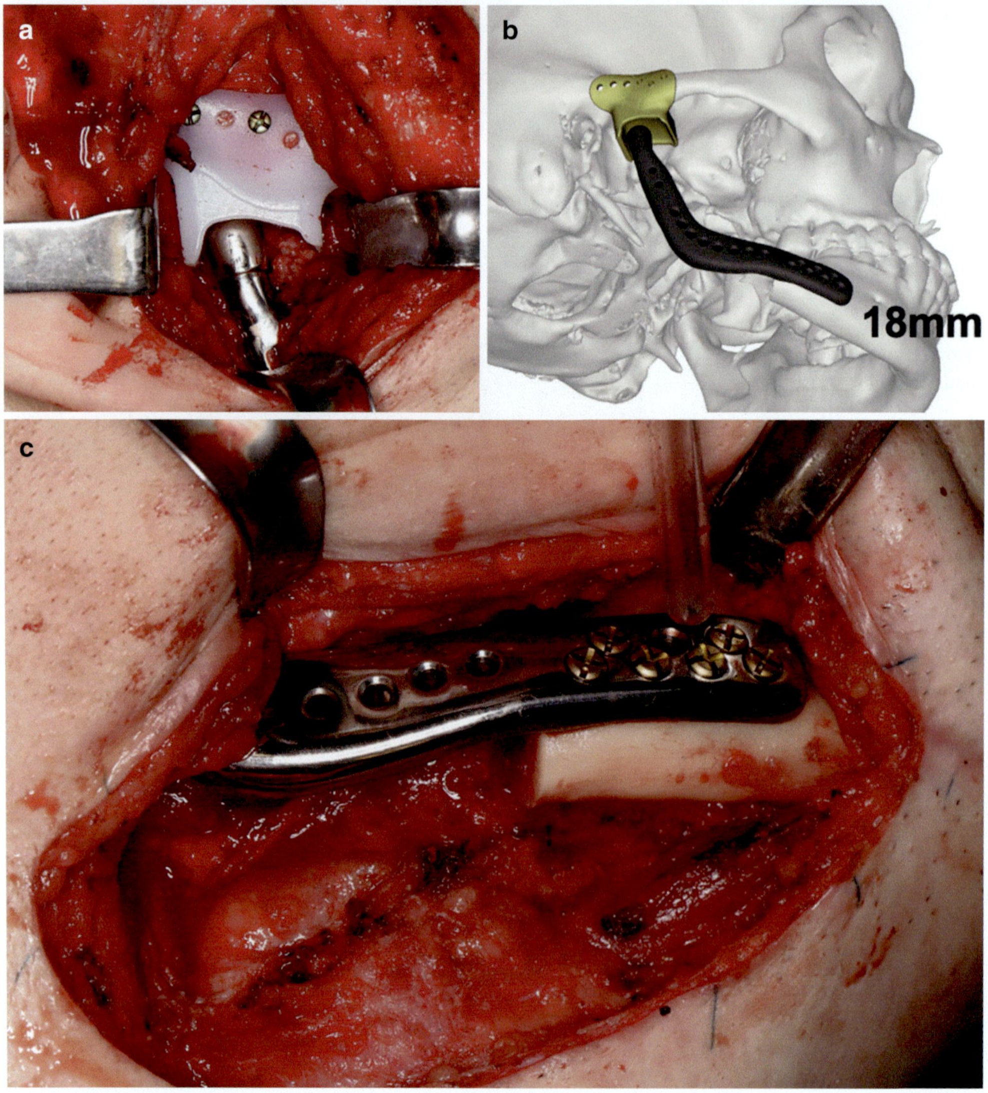

Fig. 8.30 Case O. TMJ-mandibular Combination Prosthesis mounted to ensure that the joint head is in the posterior median position of the articular fossa. (**a**) The joint head component is ideally positioned; (**b**) Design; (**c**) Fixation of mandibular prosthesis

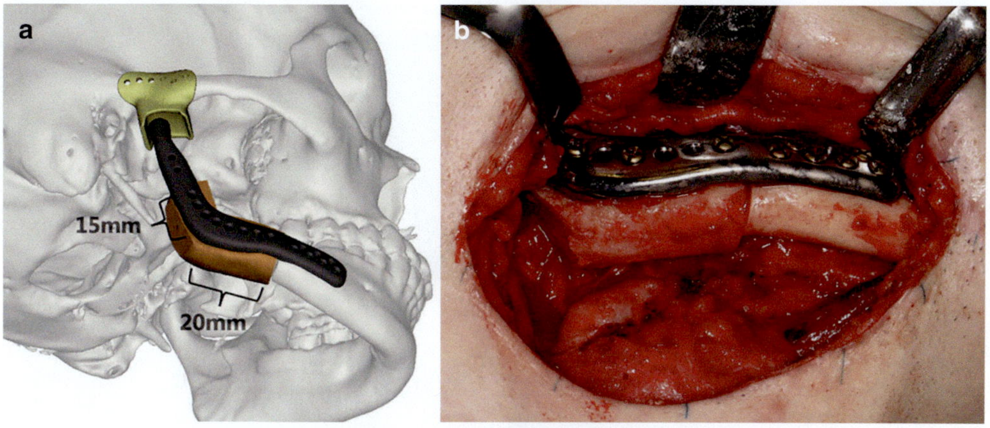

Fig. 8.31 Case O. Fixation of the iliac bone flap according to the designed screw hole depth (in mm). (**a**) Design. (**b**) Actual

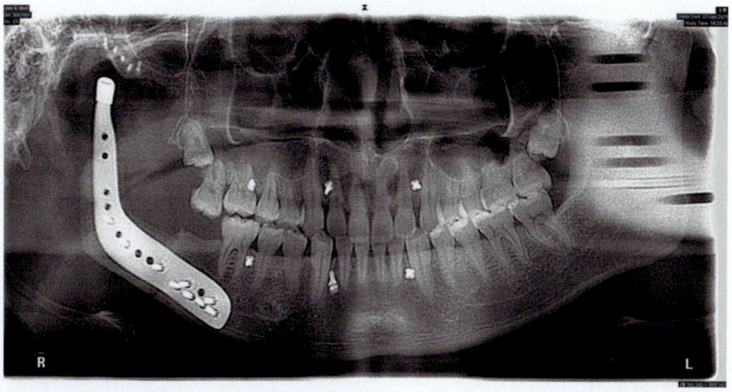

Fig. 8.32 Case O. Immediate post-operative panoramic film

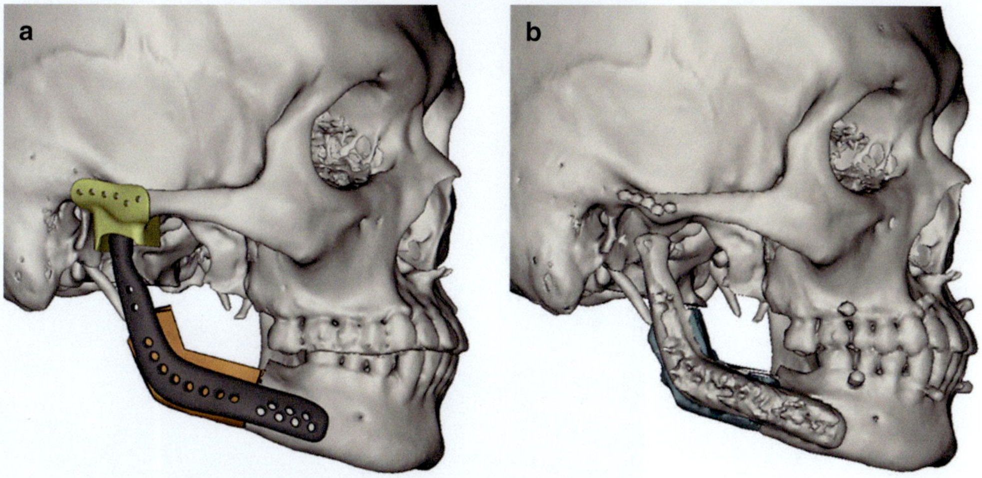

Fig. 8.33 Case O. Comparison of CT reconstruction showing precise prosthesis installation. (**a**) Preoperative design. (**b**) Immediate postoperative CT

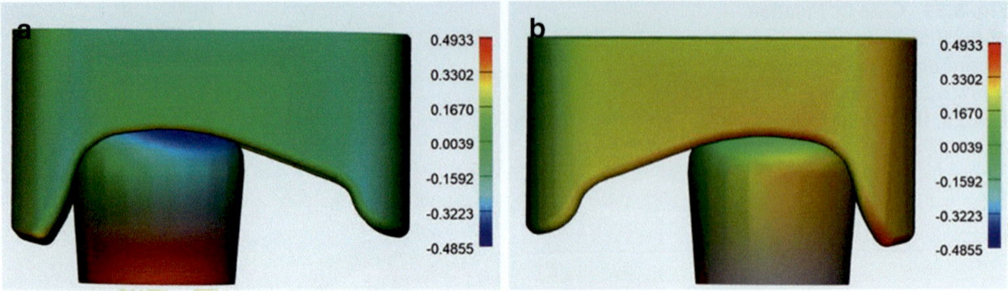

Fig. 8.34 Case O. Prosthetic core error 0.5 mm. (**a**) Lateral error. (**b**) Medial error

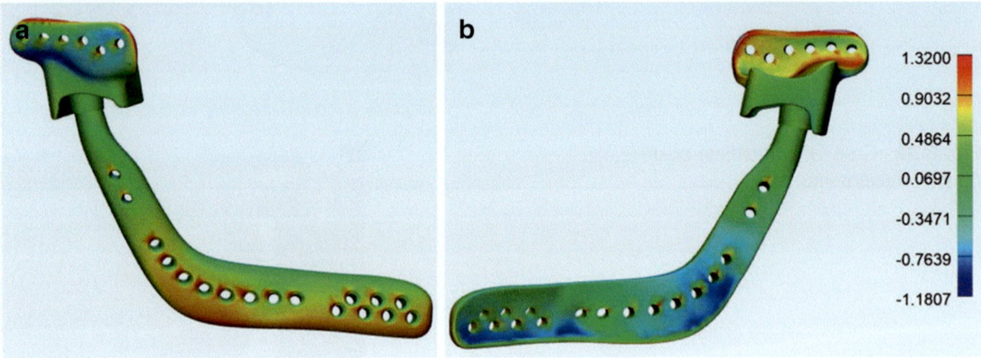

Fig. 8.35 Case O. TMJ-mandibular coalition prosthesis with an overall error of 1.5 mm. (**a**) lateral error. (**b**) medial error

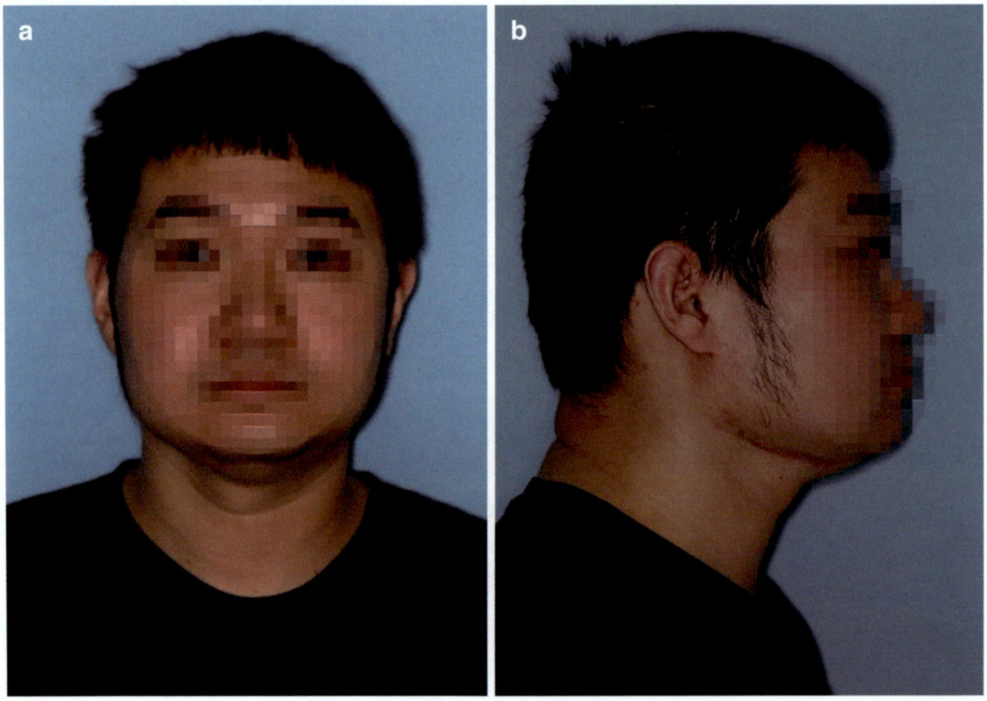

Fig. 8.36 Case O. Follow-up 1 year after surgery with no change in facial shape. (**a**) frontal view. (**b**) lateral view

mouth opening was centered, and the occlusal relationship was stable (Fig. 8.37).

Evaluation of the grafted bone and prosthesis: immediately postoperatively, the volume of the bone block was 10657.44 mm^3, and at 1 year postoperatively, the volume of the bone block was 8174.74 mm^3. There were no complications such as prosthetic infections, rejection, loosening, breakage, ectopic osteogenesis, or material allergy (Fig. 8.38).

- 3-year postoperative follow-up

The mouth opening improved to 33 mm, the occlusal relationship was stable, and the graft was well remodeled to the mandible (Figs. 8.39, 8.40 and 8.41).

8.2.8 Case O. Advantages and Disadvantages

- Advantages

Stability, compared with the simple fibular flap commonly used in the past, the TMJ-mandibular joint prosthesis restores the structure and function of the jaws and joints during the same period, and the joint fossa-joint head relationship is stable, which avoids the common complication of dislocation of the fibular head and ensures the stability of the occlusion.

Masticatory muscle attachment, the masticatory muscle is the power source of jaw movement, and restoration of muscle attachment is one of the purposes of bone grafting; in addition, rebuilding the muscle attachment can also effectively prevent the prosthesis from being exposed.

- Disadvantages

Intermaxillary fixation, theoretically, can be done with cutting guides without intermaxillary ligation, which is used for insurance purposes since this is an early case, and should be considered not to be used in the future.

Infected lesions, most do not use this method (free bone grafting).

Lateral pterygoid muscle attachment is not yet considered.

Bone grafting, and the possibility of avoiding the implantation of autogenous bone blocks and replacing them with tissue-engineered or bioprinted bone, is a future endeavor.

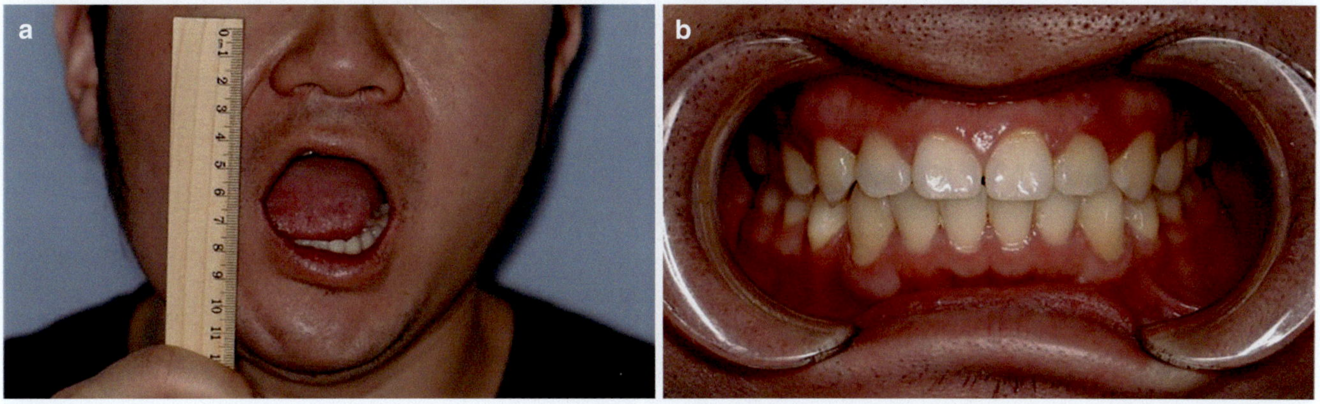

Fig. 8.37 Case O. Intraoral examination. Good recovery of joint function (**a**) Mouth opening 38 mm. (**b**) Stable occlusal relationship

Fig. 8.38 Case O. Graft bone volume changes. (**a**) Immediately postoperatively, bone mass volume was 10657.44 mm^3. (**b**) 1 year postoperatively, bone mass volume 8174.74 mm^3

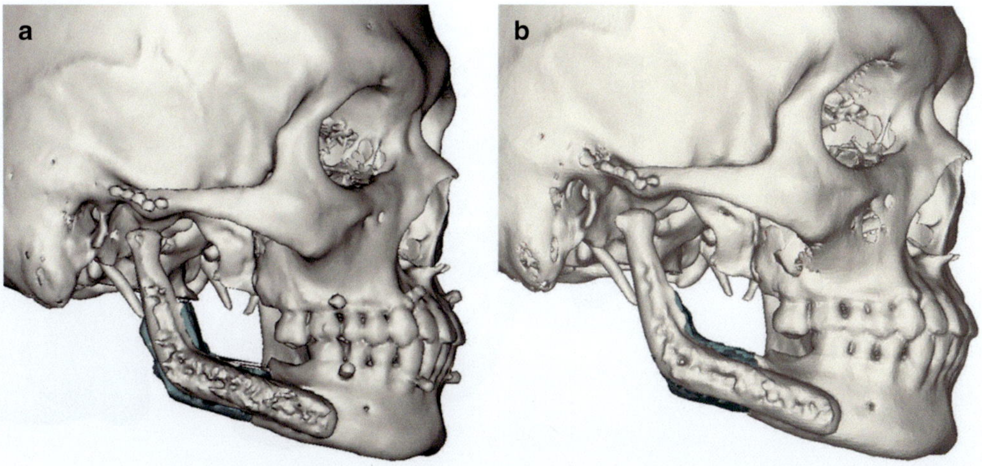

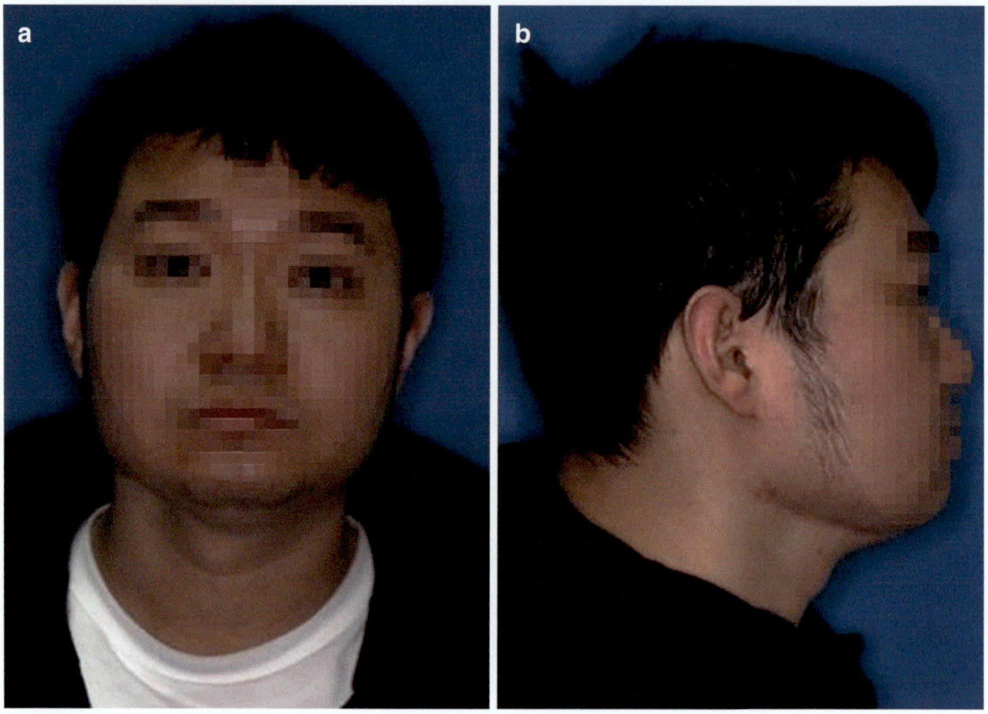

Fig. 8.39 Case O. Good facial shape at 3-year postoperative follow-up. (**a**) Frontal view. (**b**) Lateral view

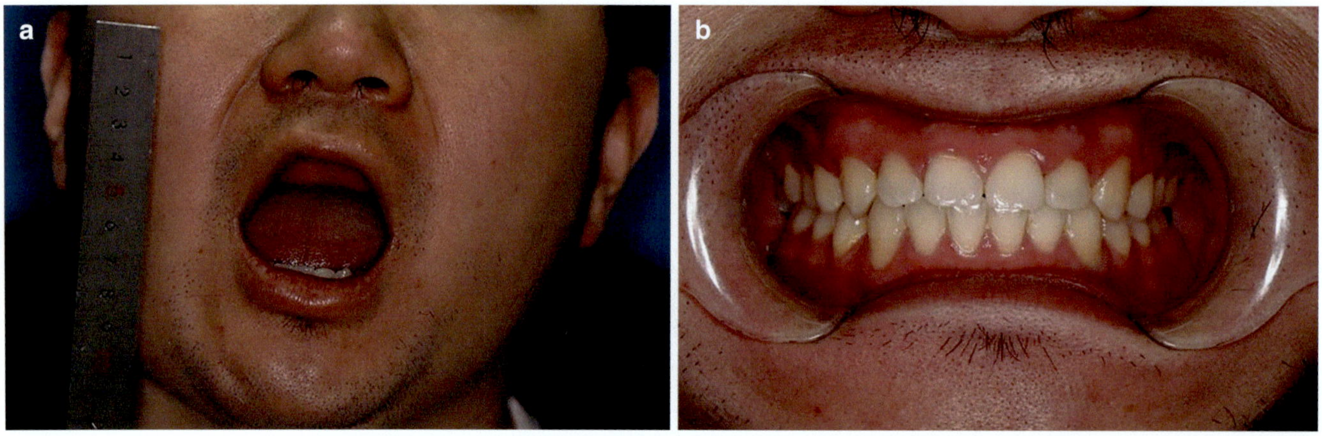

Fig. 8.40 Case O. Intraoral examination. Good recovery of joint function at 3 years after surgery. (**a**) Mouth opening of 37 mm. (**b**) Stable occlusal relationship

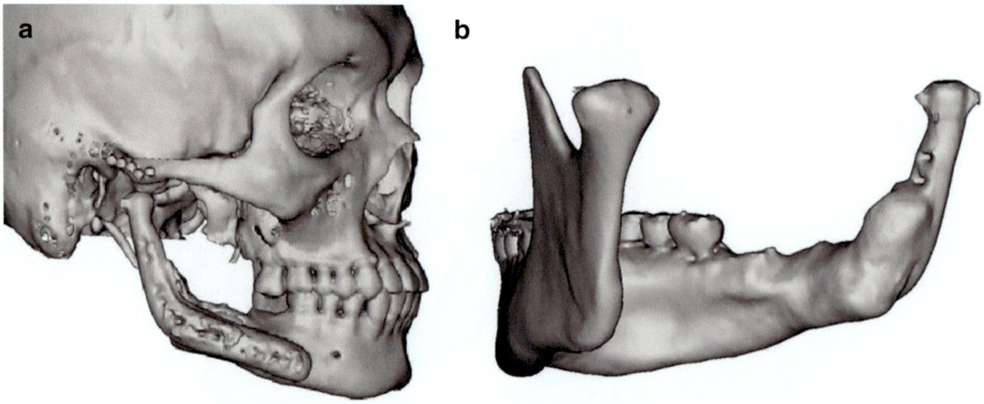

Fig. 8.41 Case O. CT 3 years postoperatively showing stable prosthesis position and good graft-to-mandibular remodeling. (**a**) Lateral view. (**b**) Medial view

8.3 Design and Application of a Wide-Type Temporomandibular TMJ-Mandibular Combined Prosthesis Combined with Dental Implants

Case P in Sect. 8.3 is the case of a patient with a mandibular Class IIa lesion, in which the inferior alveolar neurovascular bundle was preserved by fractional osteotomy, and reconstruction was performed with a wide-type mandibular prosthesis and iliac bone flap, and dental implant restoration was completed.

8.3.1 Case P. Wide-Type Temporomandibular TMJ-Mandibular Prosthesis Combined with Dental Implants

Patient information: male, 23-year-old.

Complaint: progressive swelling in the right submandibular region for more than 6 months.

History: the patient presented with swelling in the right submandibular region 6 months ago with no apparent cause, no spontaneous pain, and no restriction of mouth opening.

Specialized examination: the right mandibular angle is slightly bulging compared with the opposite side, hard, with localized light pressure pain, and bilateral lower lip tenderness is symmetrical. There were permanent teeth in the mouth, the occlusal relationship was stable, and the mouth opening was 30 mm (Figs. 8.42 and 8.43).

Ancillary examination: maxillofacial CT showed a well-defined multicompartmental translucency image of the right mandibular molar region and mandibular ramus, containing the right lower third molar (Figs. 8.44 and 8.45).

Diagnosis: possible odontogenic keratocystic tumor of the right mandible.

Postoperative pathology: odontogenic keratocystic neoplasm of the right mandible with mild abnormal proliferation of the lining epithelium. Immunohistochemical findings: CKH, CKpan, p63 (+); CK14, CK19, Ki-67 partial (+); Vim, S-100 (−).

8.3.2 Case P. Diagnostic Imaging

8.3.3 Case P. Treatment Plan

- Overall treatment plan: resection of the right TMJ-mandibular mass, prosthetic reconstruction with a combined TMJ-mandibular prosthesis, wide type, and dental implants in a second stage.
- Surgical resection design
  The extent of resection was designed: from the condyle to the distal of the right lower second premolar, a Class III combined lesion. This case is a benign mandibular lesion with no signs of inferior alveolar nerve involvement, so the nerve should be preserved.
  – Digital simulation of the procedure: the osteotomy line (yellow arrow) is designed 10 mm anterior to the

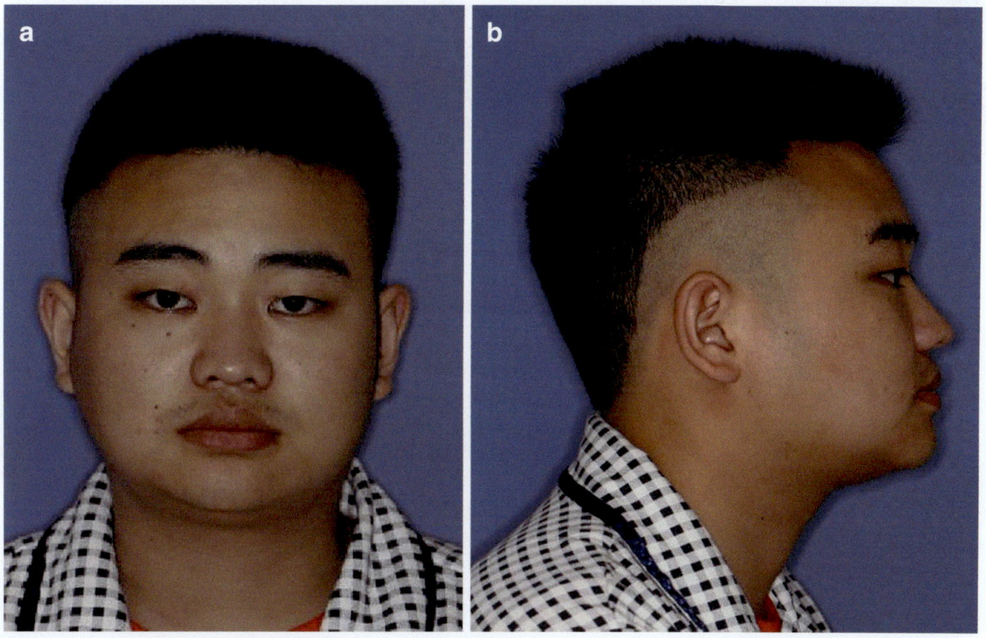

Fig. 8.42 Case P. Extraoral examination. Slight swelling of the right mandibular parotid occlusal area without tenderness and symmetrical sensation of the lower lip bilaterally. (**a**) Frontal view. (**b**) Lateral view

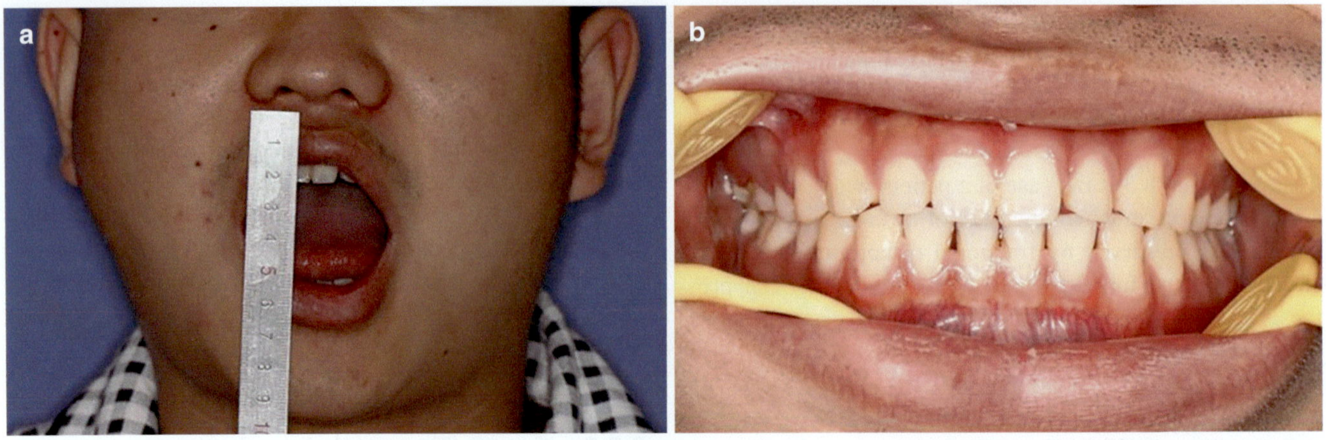

Fig. 8.43 Case P. Intraoral examination: (**a**) Mouth opening of 30 mm. (**b**) No fistulae in the mouth and stable occlusal relationship

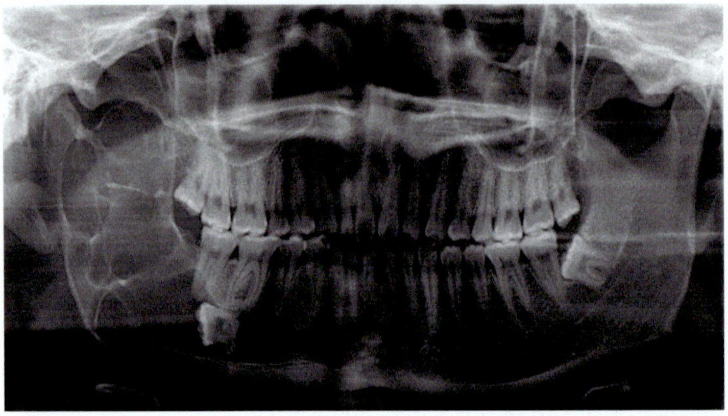

Fig. 8.44 Case P. Panoramic view. Multi-housed hypodense shadows are seen from the right lower second molar to the condyle, with interosseous septa and teeth seen within the capsule

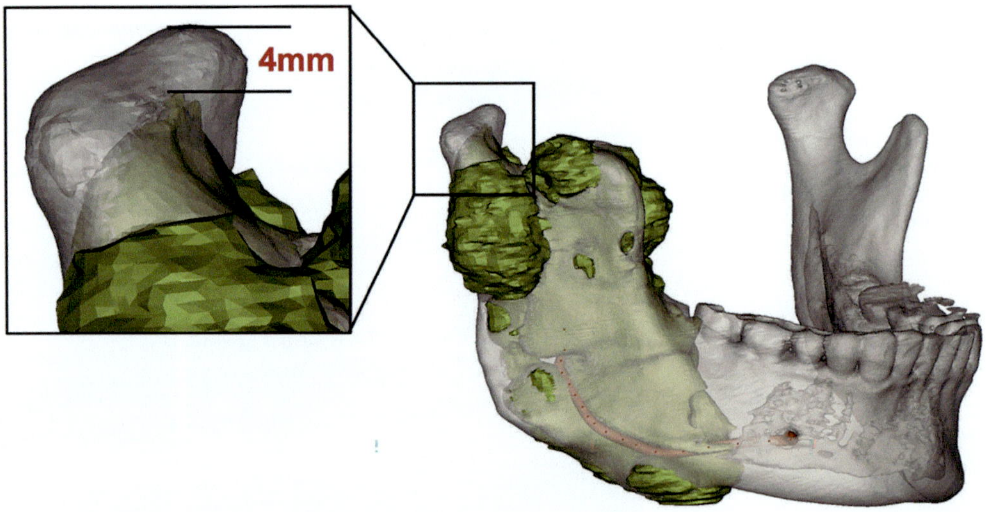

Fig. 8.45 Case P. CT reconstruction (40% transparency) shows that the upper border of the mass (green) is 4 mm from the apex of the condyle, suggesting that the condyle cannot be preserved, and the channel of the inferior alveolar nerve vascular bundle is clearly visible, suggesting that it can be preserved

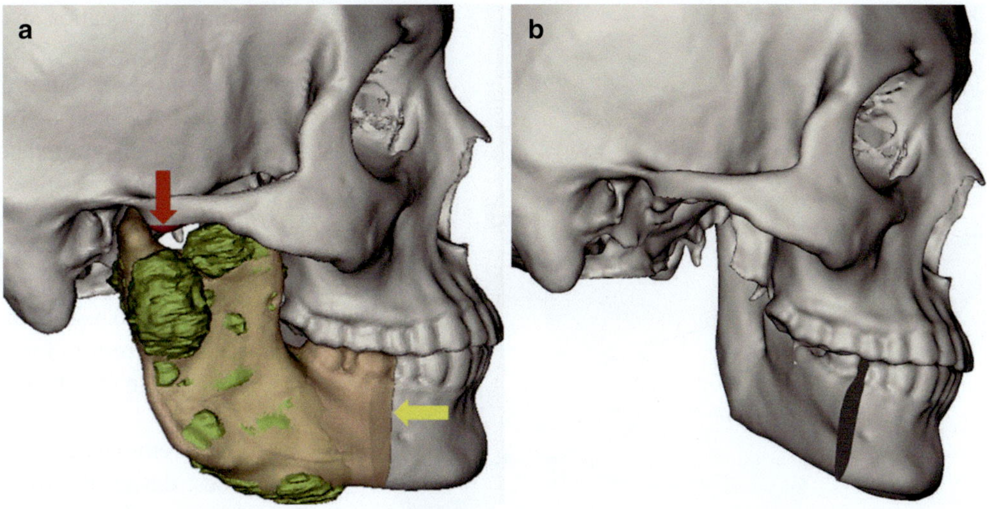

Fig. 8.46 Case P. Design of osteotomy lines. (**a**) Articular eminence osteotomy line (red arrow), to allow implantation of articular fossa prosthesis component, and anterior mandibular osteotomy line (yellow arrow), with brown showing the diseased mandible to be removed. (**b**) Model of the combined TMJ-mandibular defect obtained after resection of the mass

anterior margin of the mass (green), the extent of resection is marked (brown), and the osteotomy line (red arrow) is designed for the articular eminence; the defect model after osteotomy is obtained (Fig. 8.46).

- Surgical prosthetic program design
- In this case, a wide-type TMJ-mandibular prosthesis with a free iliac bone flap was proposed for prosthetic reconstruction, and later dental implant restoration was considered.

  Design of graft bone harvesting: the iliac bone restoration should be designed to meet the primary goal of the later implant restoration, while considering the restoration of the mandibular contour. After determining the location and number of bone segments that will be required for harvesting and grafting, the prosthesis form can be designed accordingly. In this case, the right free iliac bone flap is designed to mirror the contralateral healthy mandible, to replace the affected mandibular contour and occlusal relationship (Fig. 8.47).
- Graft bone flap design: use the anterior top edge of the ilium to repair the posterior mandibular angle and rebuild the muscle attachment. The rounded cortical edge of the iliac bone flap, placed facing downward, is compatible with the contour of the posterior edge of the mirror image mandible; this autogenous bone graft will rebuild the right posterior mandible to the distal of lower second molar. The anterior bone flap design is that the rounded cortical bone edge will face upward like the alveolar ridge, facilitating the later dental implantation. The top of this new alveolar ridge is to be set approximately 5 mm below the future gum line, to allow suturing of the intraoral wound at the end of surgery. Protruding edges of the bone graft must be shaved away in preparation. The iliac bone flap design is finalized to simulate the dental implant site and orientation (Fig. 8.48).
- Graft trimming: trim the graft to match the mandibular profile to complete the iliac bone flap design and incorporate the shape to design the prosthesis (Fig. 8.49).

8.3.4 Case P. Design and Processing of the Wide-Type TMJ-Mandibular Prosthesis and Osteotomy Cutting Guides

8.3.4.1 Core Component Sizing and Prosthesis Design: See Chapter 2

- Core component (articular fossa) placement and extension component design (Fig. 8.50).
- Screw hole depth measurement: measure the thickness of the prosthesis and graft bone flap to determine the depth of the screw holes at each site (Figure 8.51a).

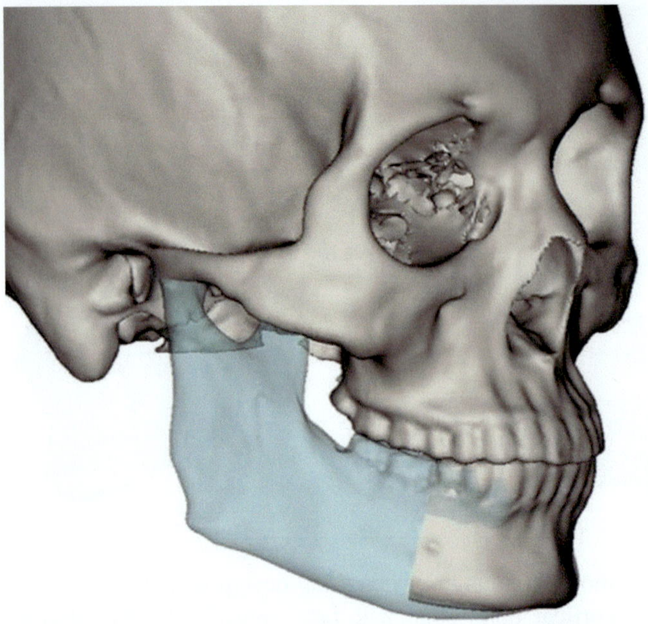

Fig. 8.47 Case P. Planning for graft bone harvesting. Mirror the healthy mandible on the left to determine the contour of the bone to be grafted to the affected right side (light blue)

- Prosthesis fabrication and fitting are the same as described in Chap. 2 (Figure 8.51b).
- Second-stage dental implantation design: to facilitate intraoperative suturing of the intraoral mucosa and avoid exposure of the grafted bone and prosthesis, the height of the iliac bone block should be reduced by 5 mm compared with the original alveolar ridge height. Considering the problem of postoperative resorption of free bone grafting, it is proposed to design the tent peg bone grafting in a second stage to restore the height of the alveolar ridge for implantation restoration (Fig. 8.52).
- Digital design of osteotomy cutting guide

Articular eminence and mandibular osteotomy positioning guides: design the osteotomy cutting guides along the line of the articular eminence osteotomy and the mandibular osteotomy line, and transfer the prosthesis screw holes to the cutting guides (Fig. 8.53).

Inferior alveolar neurovascular bundle preservation osteotomy cutting guide: design the cutting guide (pink) in alignment with the inferior alveolar neurovascular bundle,

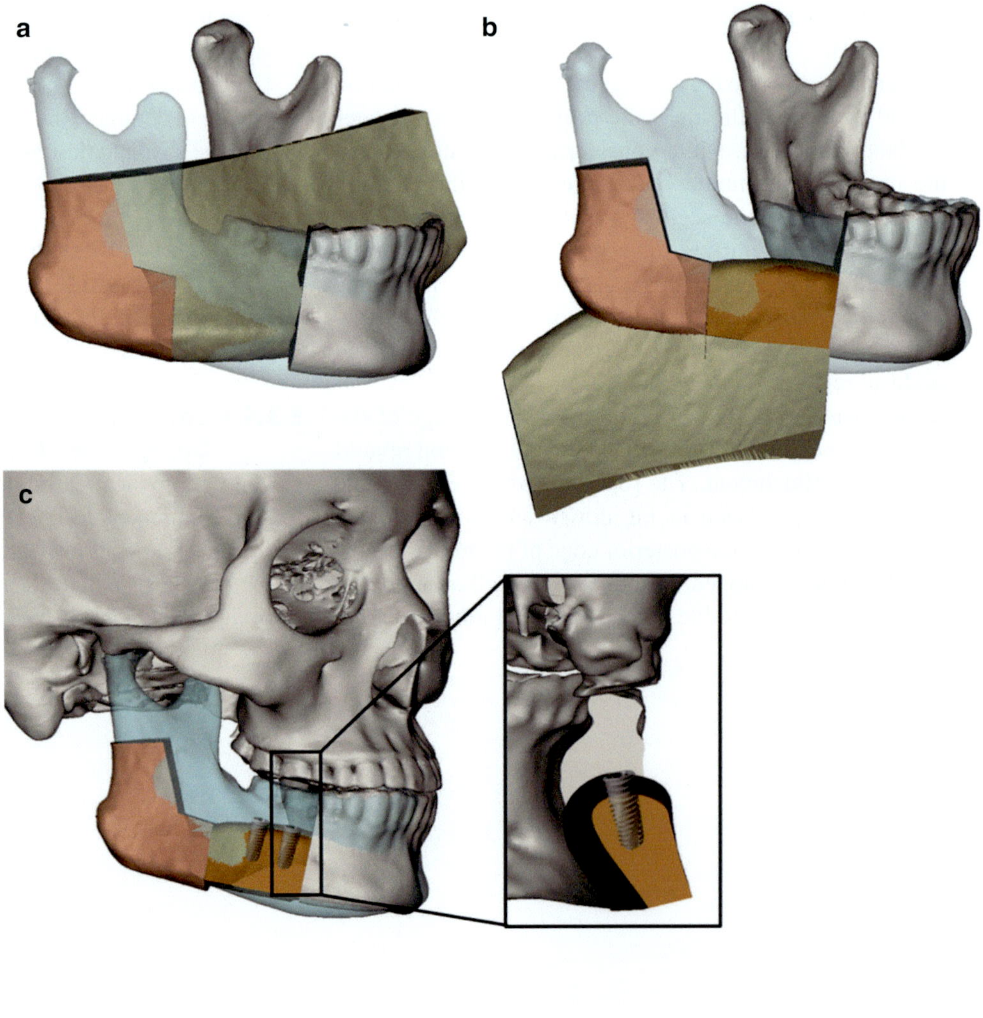

Fig. 8.48 Case P. Graft bone flap design based on the mirror image of the healthy mandible (light blue). (**a**) Posterior mandible position iliac bone flap design, with the cortical bone facing down (light brown), restores the back edge of the jaw, that is, the right mandibular angle to the lower mid-distal region. (**b**) Anterior mandible position, iliac bone flap design, with the cortical bone facing up (dark brown), with the top to be set approximately 5 mm from the top of the future alveolar ridge. (**c**) Completion of the iliac flap design, simulating the alveolar ridge implant site and orientation

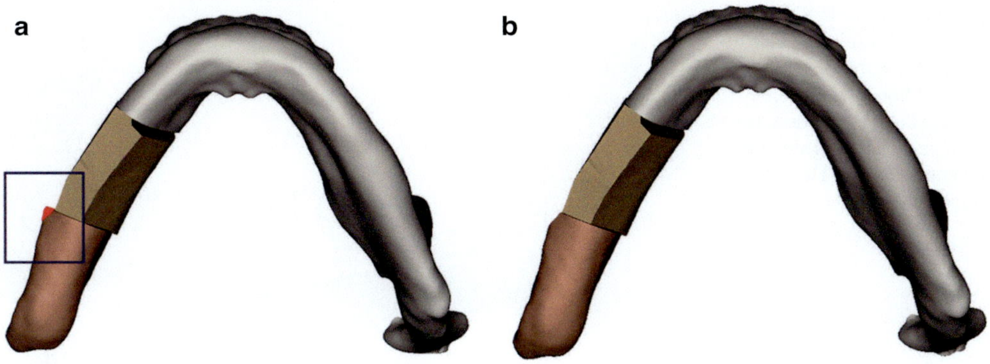

Fig. 8.49 Case P. Trimming bone block steps to facilitate prosthesis design. (**a**) Box showing trimmed bone block (red). (**b**) Trimmed profile is smooth and flat

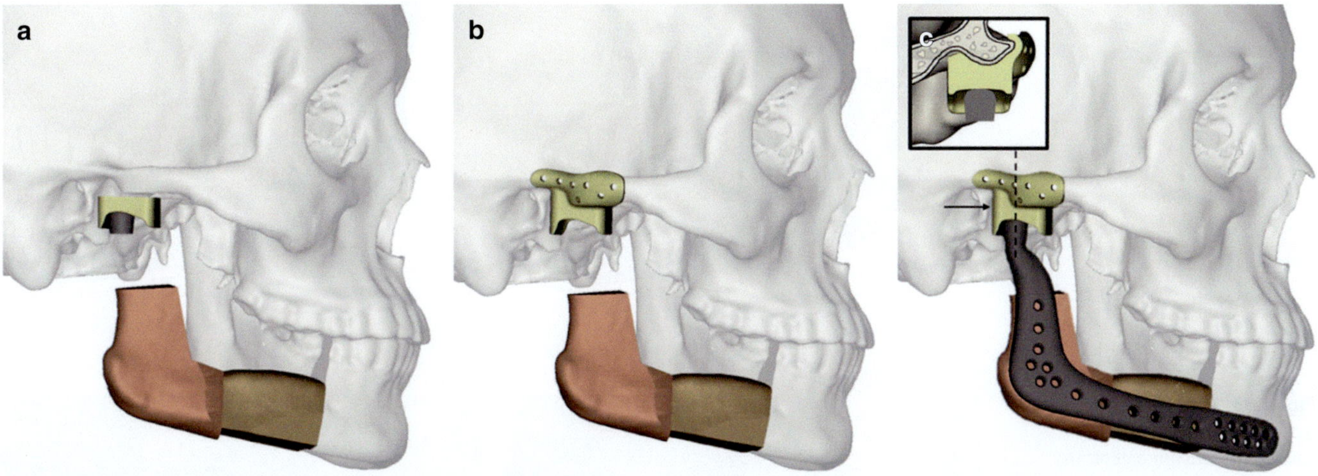

Fig. 8.50 Case P. Articular fossa prosthesis and mandibular extension component prosthesis design. The articular fossa component is shown in yellow, the articular head component in dark gray, and the grafted iliac flap in light and dark brown. (**a**) Determination of core component location. (**b**) Articular fossa prosthesis design. (**c**) Mandibular extension prosthesis design

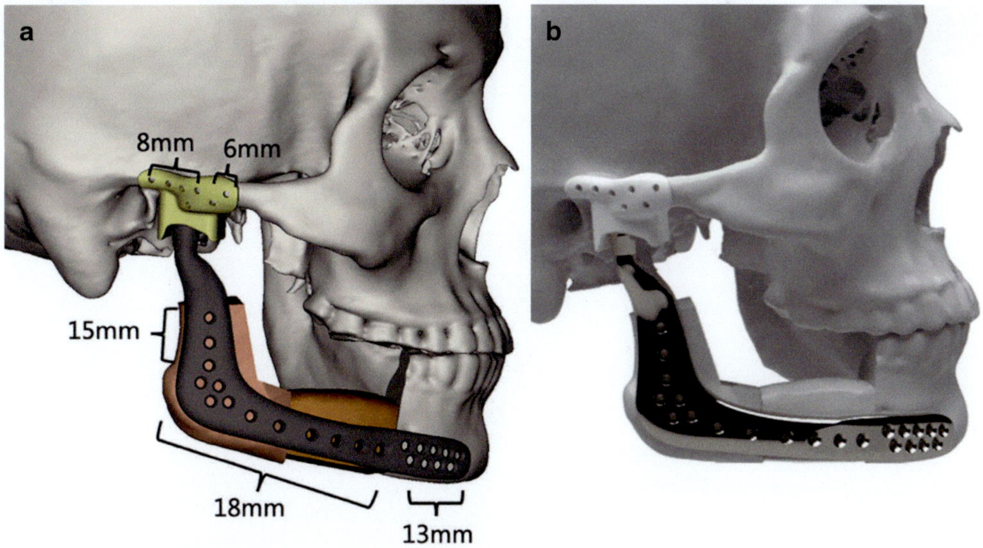

Fig. 8.51 Case P. Completion of design and production. (**a**) Screw hole depth measurement (in mm). (**b**) Prosthesis fitting

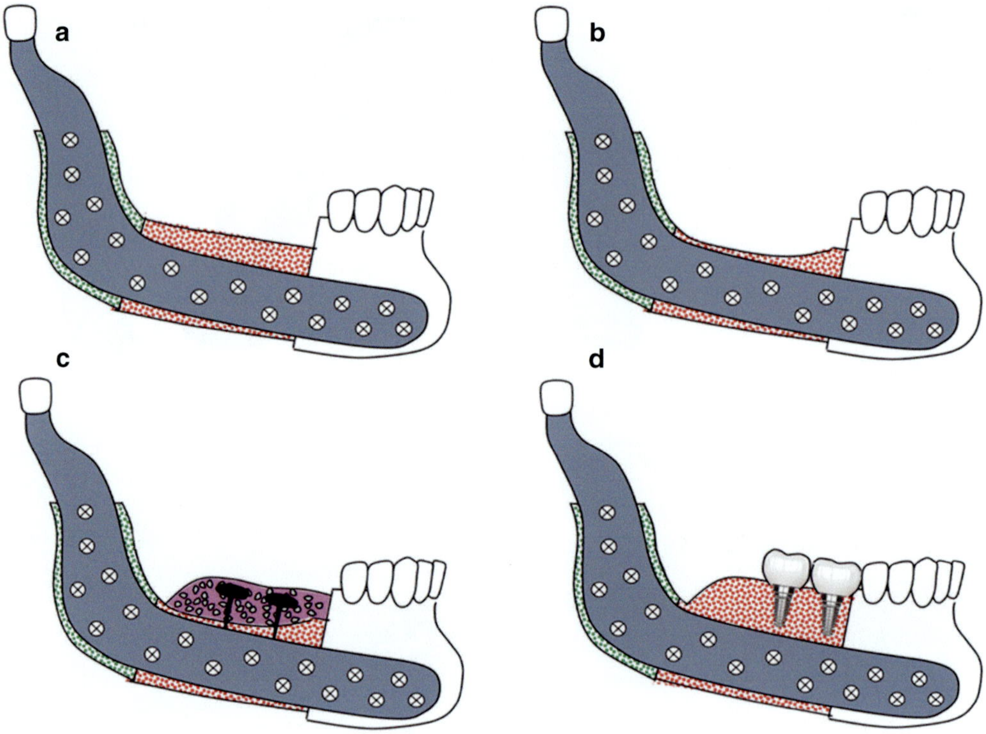

Fig. 8.52 Case P. Schematic diagram of a second stage of implant restoration. (**a**) Grafted bone. (**b**) Possible grafted bone resorption. (**c**) Tent peg-assisted guided bone regeneration. (**d**) Dental implantation

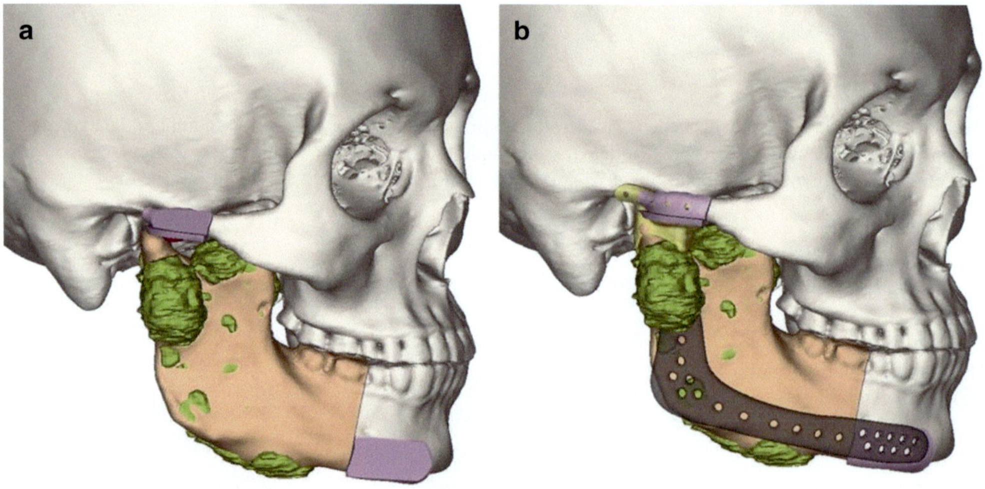

Fig. 8.53 Case P. Design of osteotomy cutting guides (pink). (**a**) Design osteotomy cutting guides according to the osteotomy line. (**b**) Guides in line with the prosthesis screw holes

and measure the distance of the inferior alveolar neurovascular bundle from the buccal aspect of the mandible (Fig. 8.54).

- Iliac osteotomy cutting guides were designed and printed with a resin 3D printer (Fig. 8.55).

8.3.5 Case P. Surgical Procedures

Preoperative laboratory tests: the same as described in Sect. 3.2.5.

Preoperative preparation: the same as described in Case O of this chapter.

Steps of the Surgical Procedure

Surgical approach: see Case O of this chapter. The submandibular incision is extended forward with care taken to protect the chin nerve.

Mandibular osteotomy: the mandibular osteotomy cutting guide is installed, and the mandibular osteotomy is performed (Figs. 8.56, 8.57 and 8.58).

Preparation of the free iliac bone flap: install the iliac osteotomy cutting guide to harvest the iliac flap (Fig. 8.59).

Articular eminence osteotomy and articular disc management: see Case O in this chapter. Surgical sequence: release the anterior attachment of the articular disc and turn the disc inward to serve as a medial liner for the articular fossa prosthesis (Fig. 8.60).

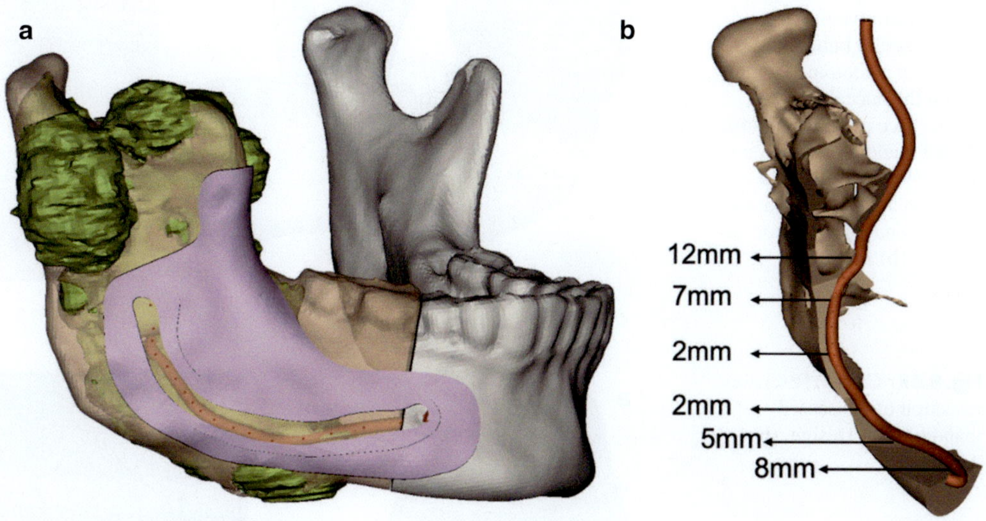

Fig. 8.54 Case P. Design of the osteotomy cutting guide (pink) to preserve the inferior alveolar neurovascular bundle (in mm). (**a**) Mark the course of the inferior alveolar neurovascular bundle (small red dots) and design the osteotomy cutting guides. (**b**) Measure the buccal osteotomy depth

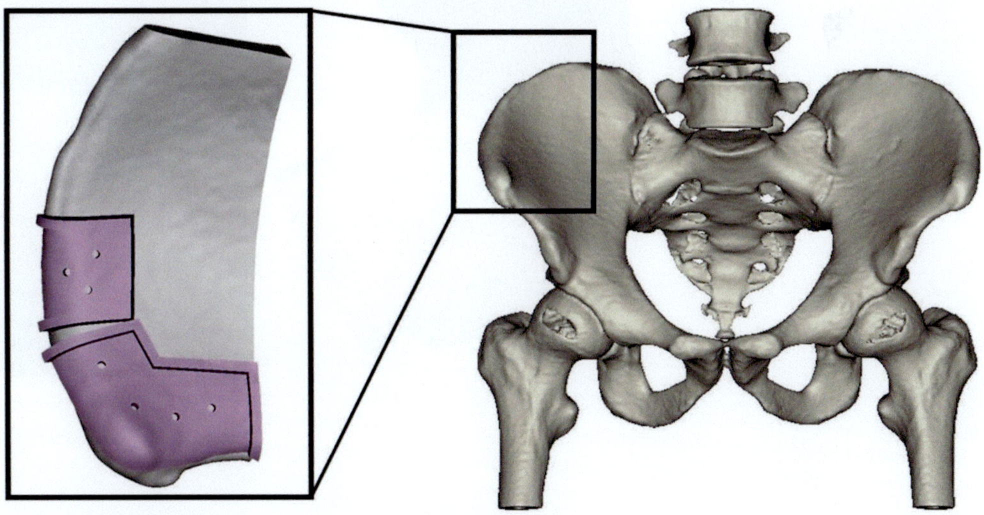

Fig. 8.55 Case P. Design of the iliac osteotomy cutting guide (pink)

Fig. 8.56 Case P. Freeing the inferior alveolar neurovascular bundle. (**a**) Design of the osteotomy guide (pink). (**b**) Placement of the cutting guide (white), at the designed depth, with an oscillating saw and piezoelectric osteotomy (a safer instrument to use in the proximity of the mental nerve), performing a buccal cortical osteotomy

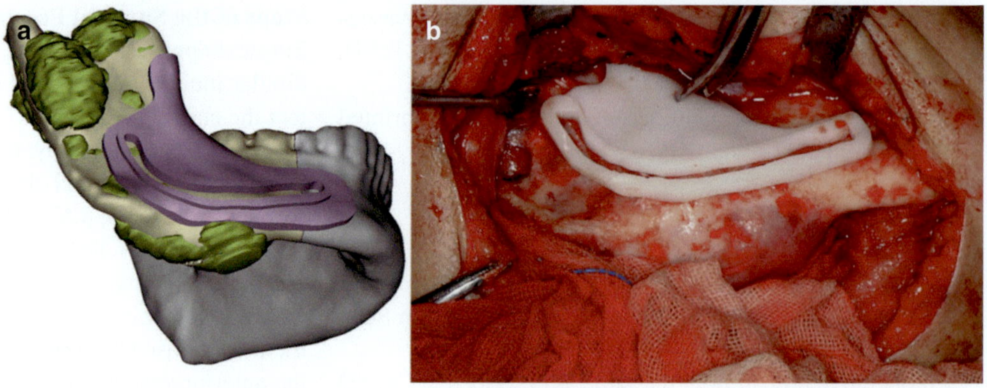

Fig. 8.57 Case P. Order of osteotomies to remove the diseased jaw part in segments. (1) Inferior alveolar neurovascular bundle trajectory osteotomy (shallow cut on the buccal cortical surface, see previous figure), (2) flat mandibular foramen osteotomy, and (3) distal mandibular osteotomy at the anterior end of the tumor. (**a**) Design. (**b**) Actual

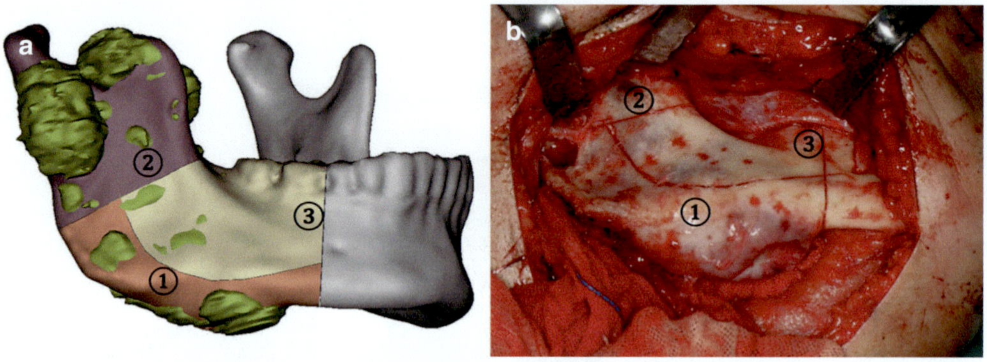

Fig. 8.58 Case P. Precision resection of a diseased mandible. (**a**) Design. (**b**) Actual

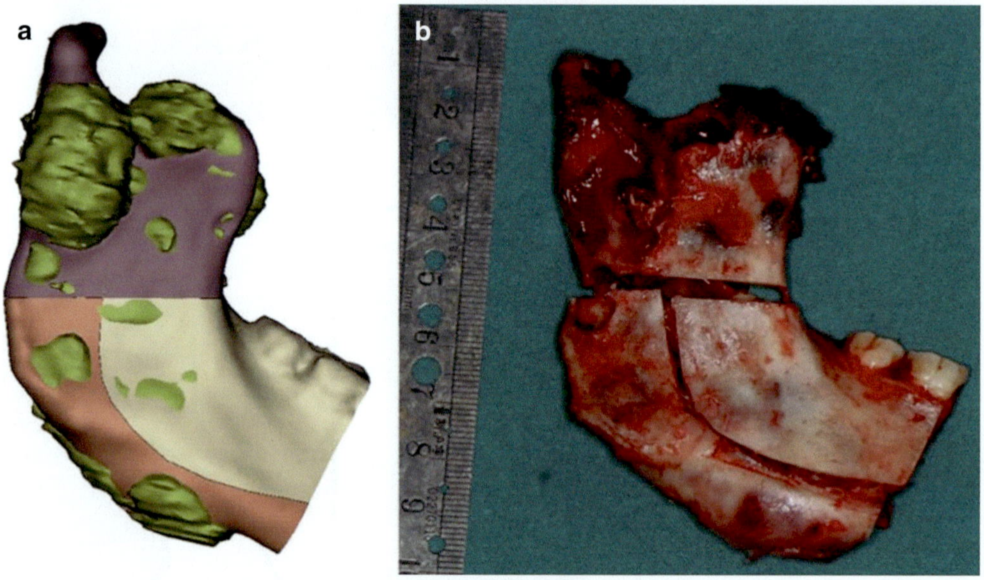

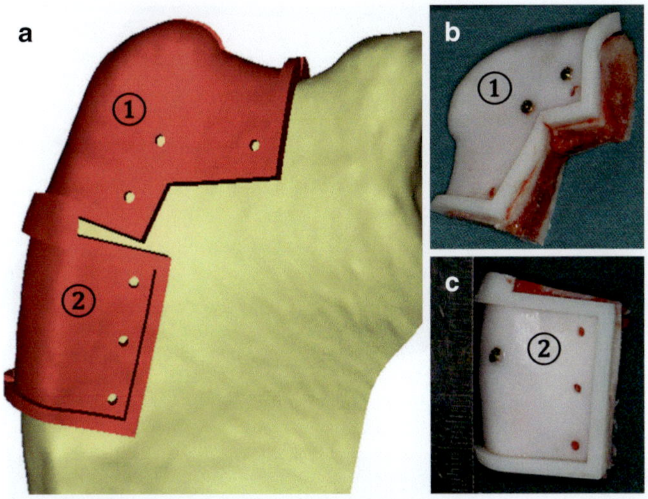

Fig. 8.59 Case P. Harvesting of the right iliac bone flap. The iliac osteotomy positioning cutting guide is shown in red. (1) Bone block for the posterior edge of the mandible. (2) Bone block for the anterior portion of the mandible. (**a**) Design. (**b**, **c**) Actual

The TMJ-mandibular prosthesis, wide type, was fitted and the bone flap was secured (Figs. 8.61 and 8.62).

Fat flap filling: a free fat flap from the submandibular region was obtained and used to fill around the neck of the mandibular prosthesis (Fig. 8.63).

Actual surgical modification: to facilitate suturing of the oral mucosa and to avoid exposure of the implant block, the second premolar was extracted during the operation. Because there was no lesion involved in the bone at the designed osteotomy line, the actual osteotomy range was moved back by 2 mm, and the anterior iliac bone was trimmed accordingly to facilitate fitting the prosthesis in place.

Postoperative medical advice and care: postoperative nasal feeding for 1 week, daily observation of intraoral wounds, and attention to oral care.

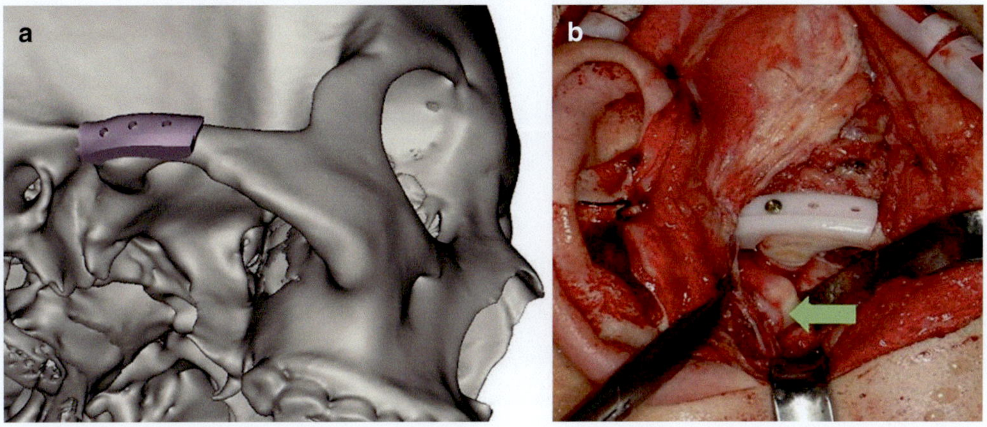

Fig. 8.60 Case P. Articular eminence osteotomy positioning and articular disc handling. (**a**) Design, placement of the articular eminence osteotomy cutting guide (pink). (**b**) Actual, the anterior attachment of the articular disc was released, and the articular disc (green arrow) was pushed medially to serve as a liner for the prosthesis fossa component; then fixation of the guide, oscillating saw osteotomy, and trimming of the bony surface

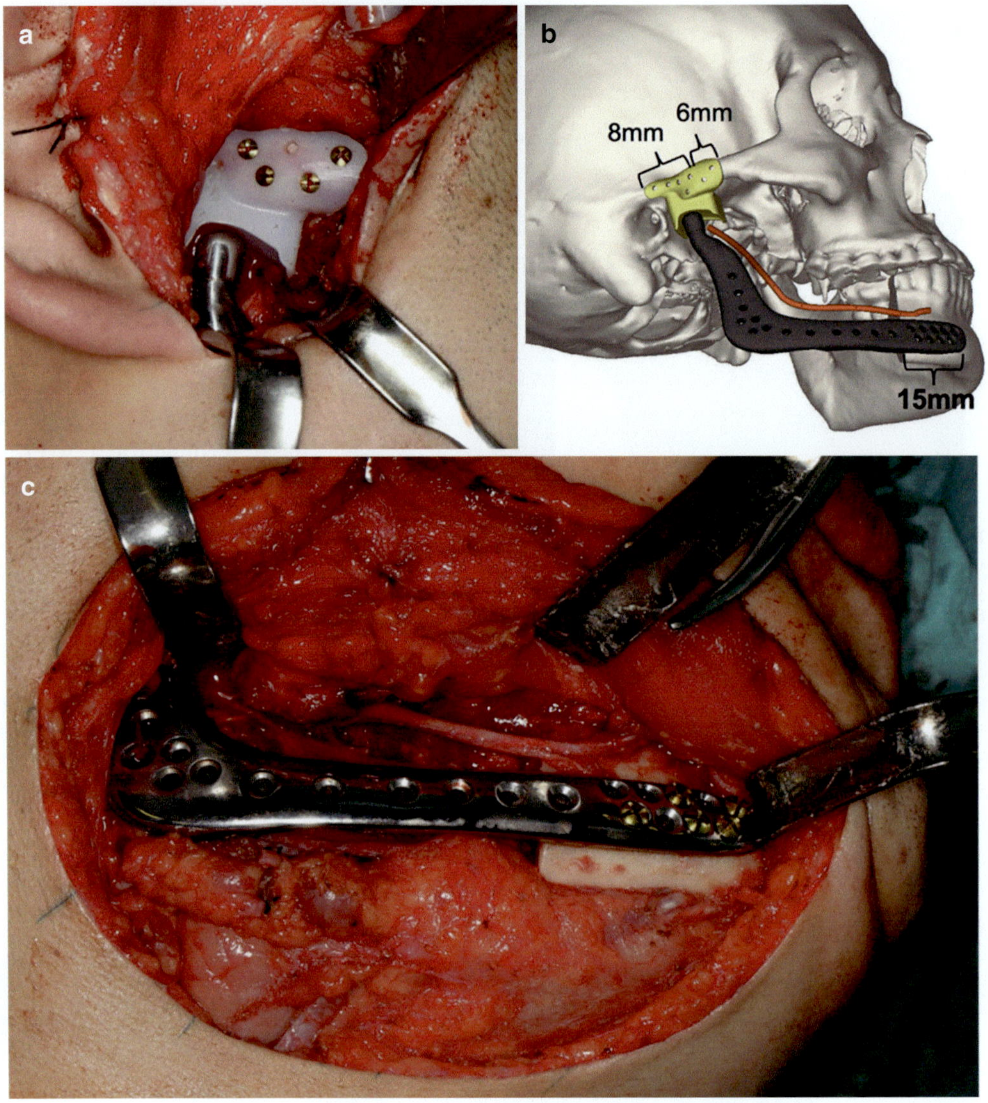

Fig. 8.61 Case P. Installation of the prosthesis. (**a**) When installing the articular fossa component, make sure that the articular head component is fitted into the posterior median position of the articular fossa, the normal position for the closed mouth. (**b**) According to the design, two screw holes identified by the cutting guide should be fixed first, and then the remaining screws should be fixed, for a total of five to six screws attachment. (**c**) Installation of the mandibular component of the prosthesis

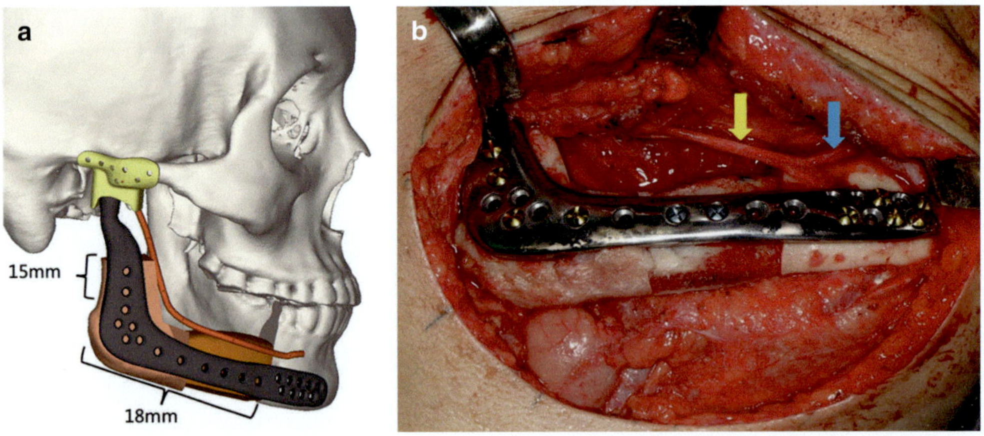

Fig. 8.62 Case P. Fixed iliac bone blocks (dark yellow and orange blocks) (in mm). Yellow arrow shows the inferior alveolar neurovascular bundle, and blue arrows show the mental nerve. (**a**) Design. (**b**) Actual

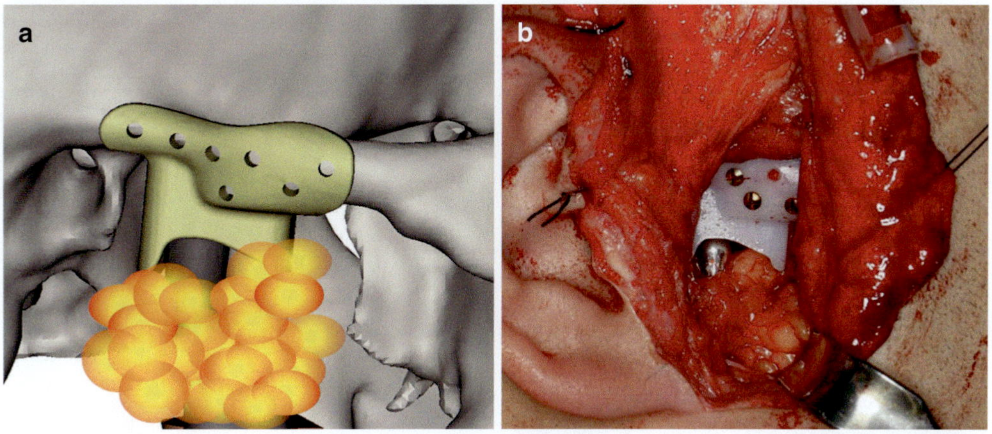

Fig. 8.63 Case P. Fat flap filling. (**a**) Schematic. (**b**) A fat flap was taken from around the submandibular incision and placed around the neck of the prosthesis to prevent ectopic osteogenesis and scar formation

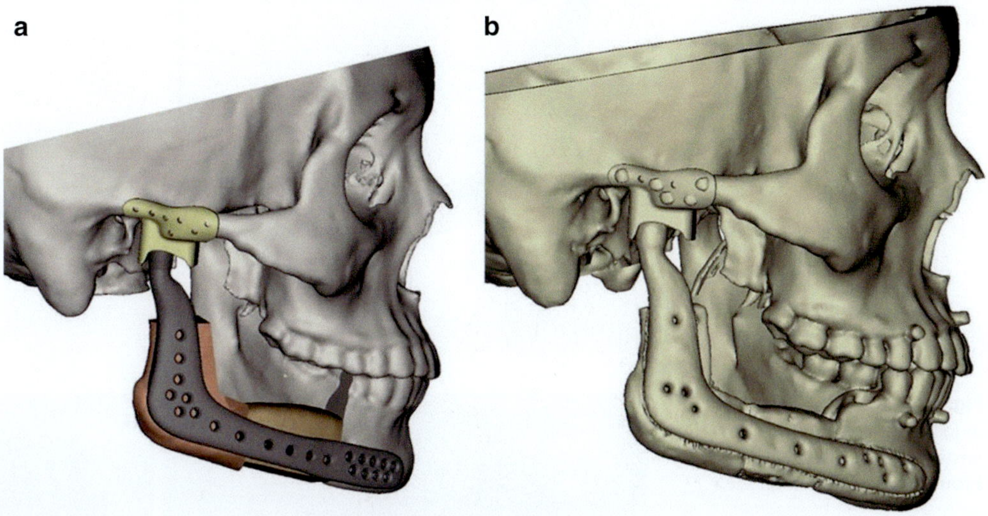

Fig. 8.64 Case P. Comparison of CT reconstructions showing precise prosthesis installation. (**a**) Preoperative design. (**b**) Immediate postoperative CT

8.3.6 Case P. Postoperative Analysis of Prosthesis Implantation Precision

Regular postoperative follow-ups were performed for appearance (facial shape), function (mouth opening, mouth shape), and prosthesis evaluation (safety, accuracy).

Immediately after surgery: the intraoperative cutting guides were accurately seated, the prosthesis was fitted smoothly, and a comparison between the preoperative design and the postoperative reconstruction showed that the prosthesis was accurately seated (Fig. 8.64). Postoperative prosthesis installation error analysis showed a core component error <1 mm, overall error 1.5 mm (Figs. 8.65 and 8.66). There were no complications such as prosthesis infection, rejection, ectopic osteogenesis, material allergy, loosening, and fracture.

8.3.7 Case P. Long-Term Follow-Up and Prognosis

- One-year postoperative follow-up

No recurrence of facial swelling or pain, no pain or discomfort in the joint area, and no other complications.

Good facial shape (Fig. 8.67), good recovery of joint function, no pain or discomfort in the joint area.

Facial pattern was harmonized and stable, mouth opening increased to 40 mm, and occlusal relationship was stable (Fig. 8.68).

Evaluation of the grafted bone and prosthesis: CT at 1 year postoperatively showed a stable grafted bone flap (Fig. 8.69 and Table 8.1).

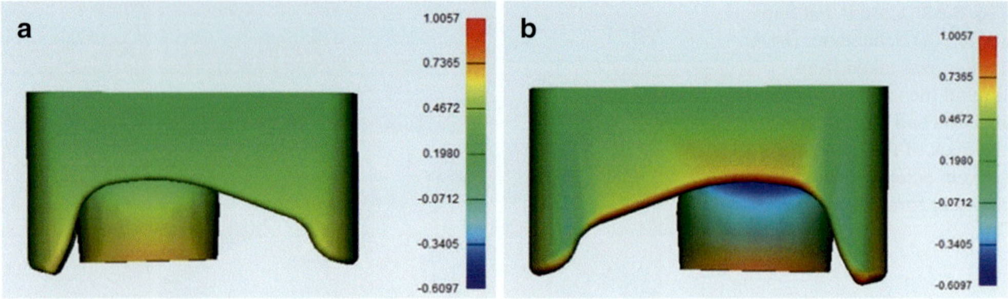

Fig. 8.65 Case P. Prosthetic core component error is about 1 mm. (**a**) Lateral error. (**b**) Medial error

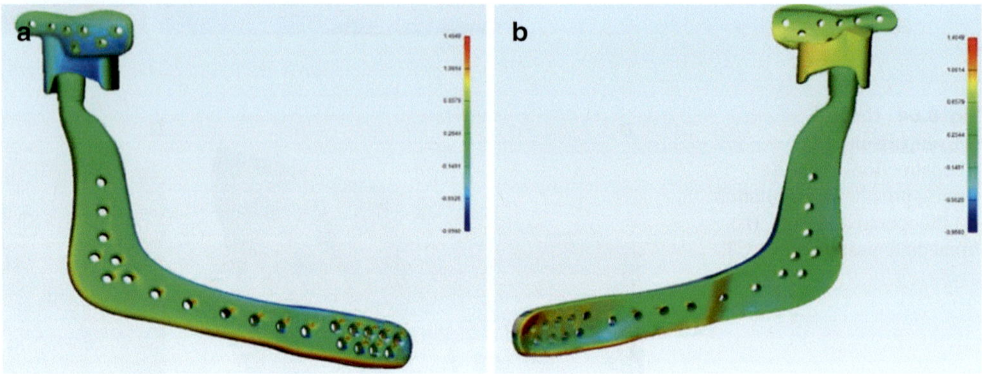

Fig. 8.66 Case P. TMJ-mandibular prosthesis was installed with an overall error of 1.5 mm. (**a**) Lateral error. (**b**) Medial error

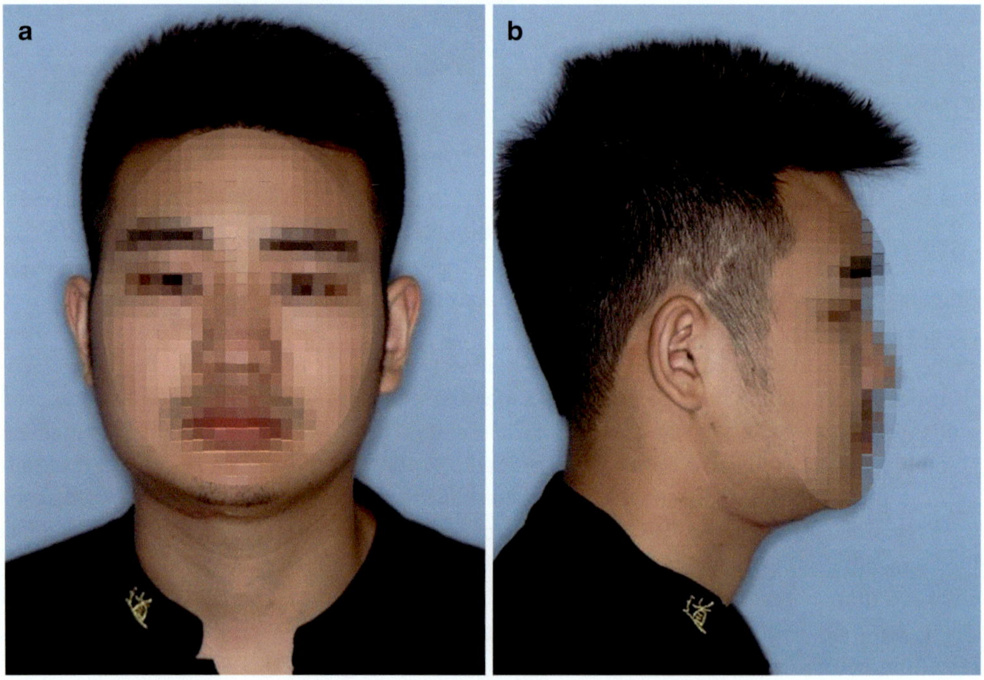

Fig. 8.67 Case P. No change in facial shape at 1-year postoperative follow-up. (**a**) Frontal view. (**b**) Lateral view

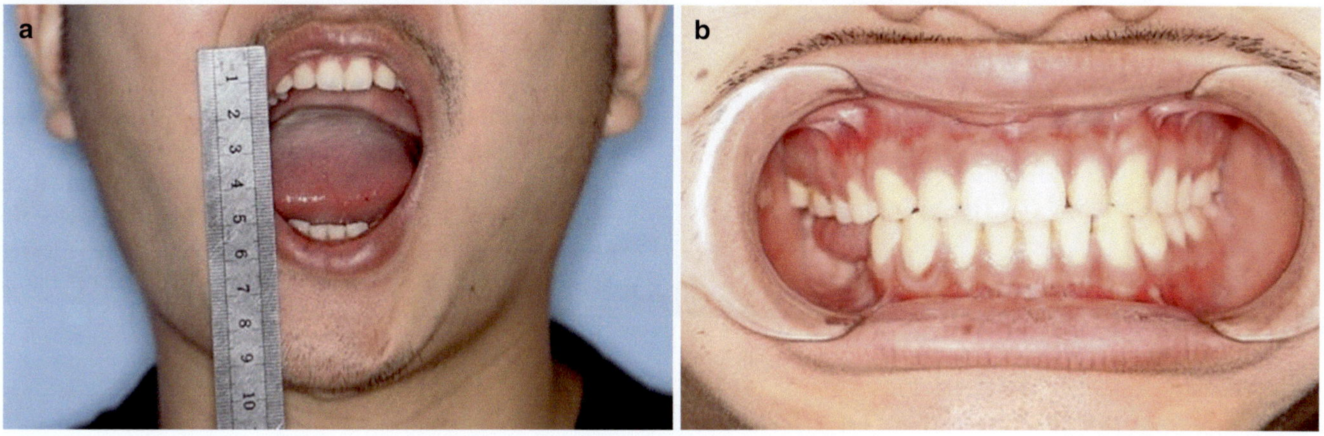

Fig. 8.68 Case P. Good recovery of joint function 1 year after surgery. (**a**) Open mouth of 40 mm. (**b**) Stable occlusal relationship

Fig. 8.69 Case P. Bone block volume changes. (**a**) Immediate postoperative. (**b**) One year postoperative

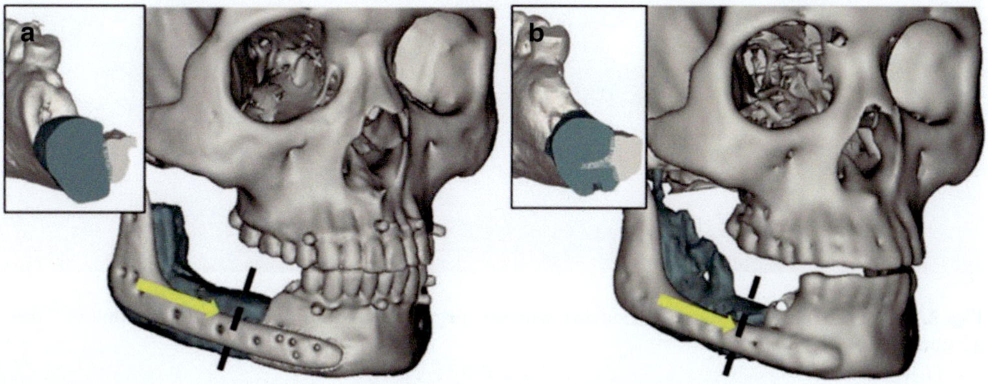

Table 8.1 Changes in bone mass volume, surface area, height, and width at each follow-up time point

Evaluation indicators	Time	
	Immediately after surgery	One year after surgery
Bone block height	17.33	16.36
Bony block width	16.56	15.83
Bone mass volume	22,556.81	19,591.92
Surface area of bone block	6354.12	6887.11

Volume in mm^3, surface area in mm^2, length in mm

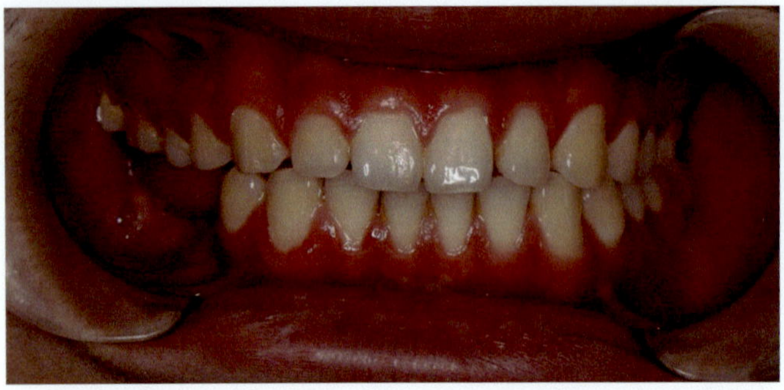

Fig. 8.70 Case P. Follow-up 3 years after surgery with a stable occlusal relationship

Implant restoration: at the 3-year postoperative follow-up, the top of the alveolar ridge was in good shape, but the bone height at the implant site was insufficient (Fig. 8.70), so tent peg bone grafting was performed (Figs. 8.71 and 8.72), and the dental implantation was completed (Fig. 8.73).

(6) Lower lip sensory function examination: quantitative sensory nerve testing showed no difference in lower lip sensation bilaterally (Table 8.2). Although there is lower sensitivity on the reconstructed side, patient still has a functional sense of feeling and no impairment.

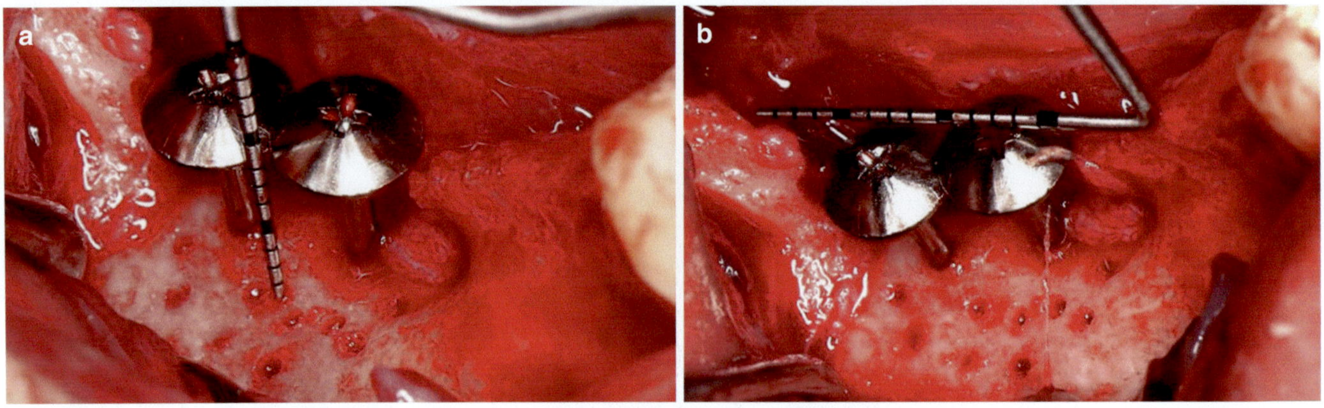

Fig. 8.71 Case P. Bone augmentation surgery with tent peg placement. (a) Vertical augmentation of 7 mm. (b) Proximal-distal-medial length of 12 mm

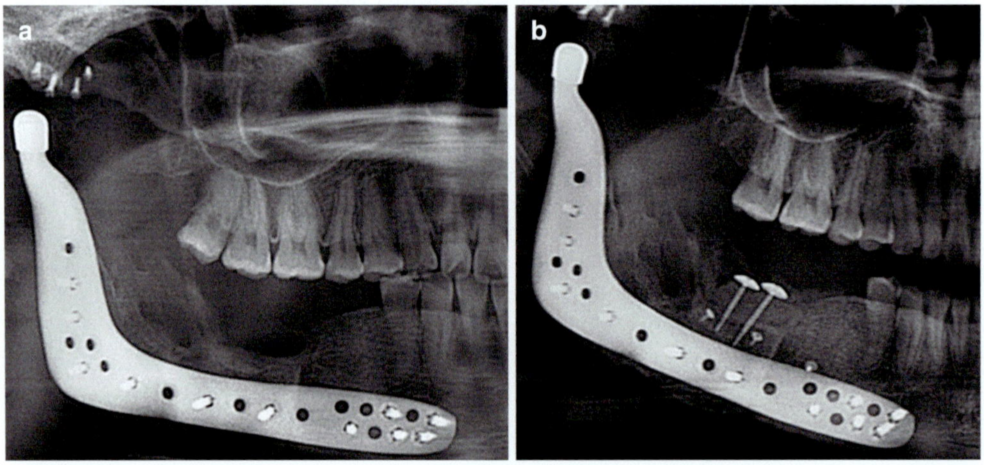

Fig. 8.72 Case P. Before and after tent peg bone grafting. (a) Insufficient height before bone grafting. (b) After bone augmentation, the bone height in the implant area is flush with the top of the alveolar ridge

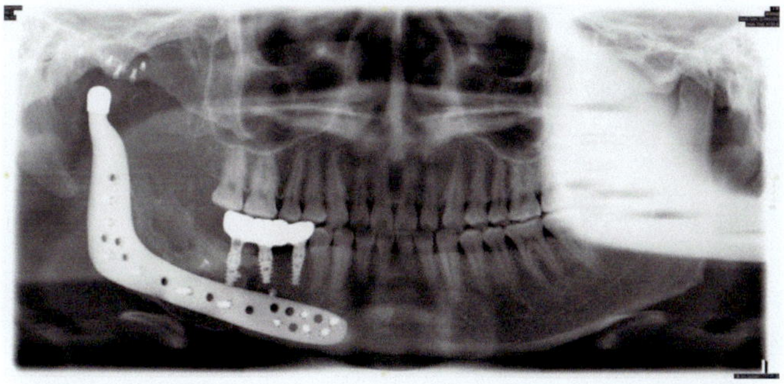

Fig. 8.73 Case P. Completing the dental implantation

Table 8.2 Sensory nerve quantitative test results Frequency unit: Hz

	Inspection area					
Testing program	Right lower lip			Left lower lip		
Stimulation frequency	2000	250	5	2000	250	5
Test score	70	9.5	9	95	19	11
Damage level	0.00			0.00		

- Follow-up 8 years after surgery

The TMJ-mandibular-occlusal-facial shape remained harmonized and stable, and the rest was the same as the one-year postoperative follow-up (Figs. 8.74, 8.75 and 8.76).

8.3.8 Case P. Advantages and Disadvantages

- Advantages

The safety and stability of the prosthesis have been proven to be successful and reliable with no adverse reactions or complications after a maximum of 8 years of follow-up.

The design concept is more advanced in achieving structural and functional restoration as well as balance of TMJ-mandibular-occlusal-facial reconstruction.

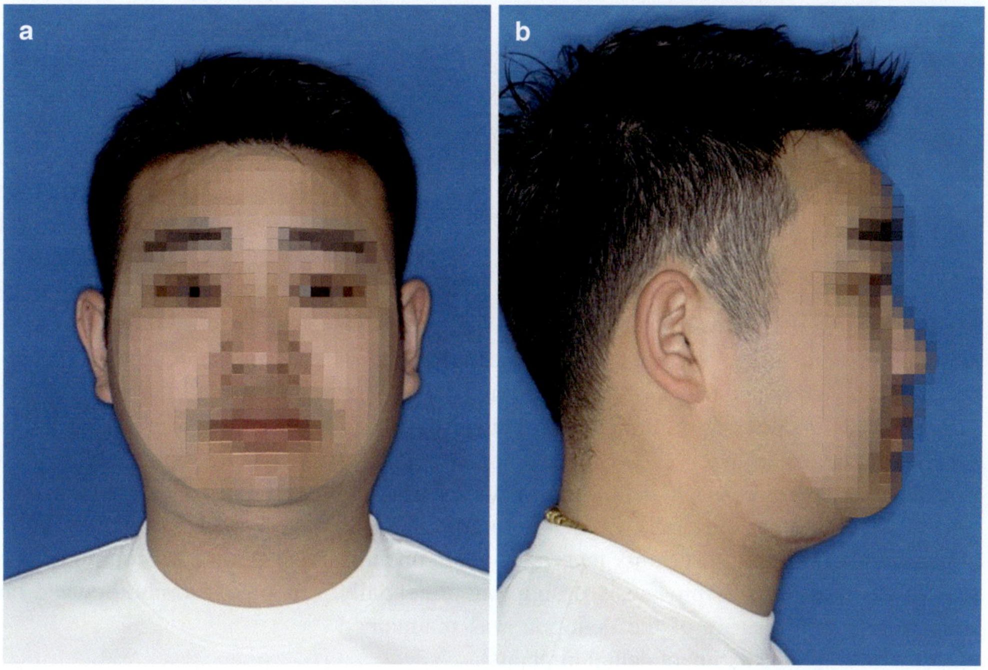

Fig. 8.74 Case P. Follow-up 8 years after surgery with good facial shape. (**a**) Frontal view. (**b**) Lateral view

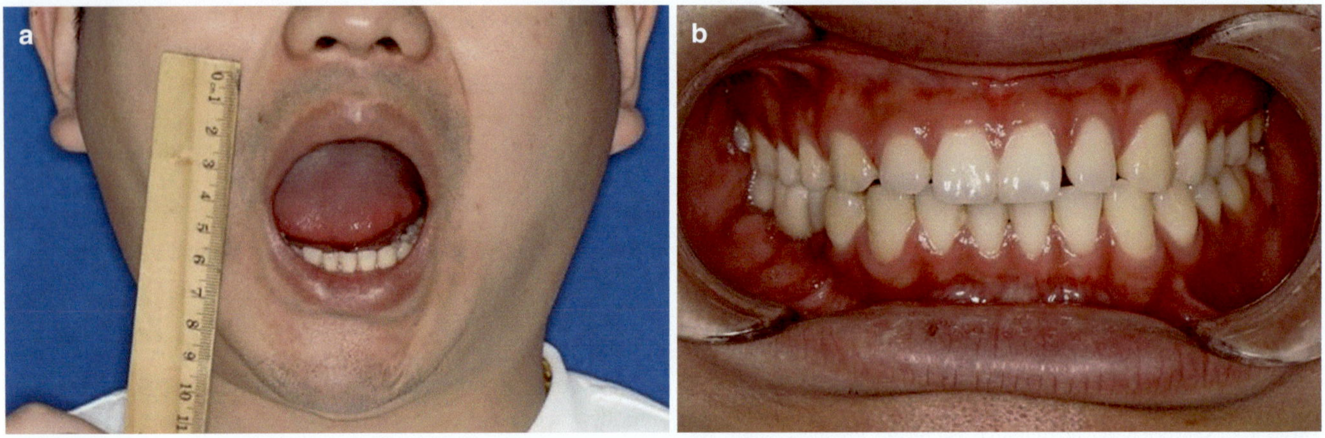

Fig. 8.75 Case P. Stabilized joint function. (**a**) Mouth opening 39 mm. (**b**) Stabilized occlusal relationship

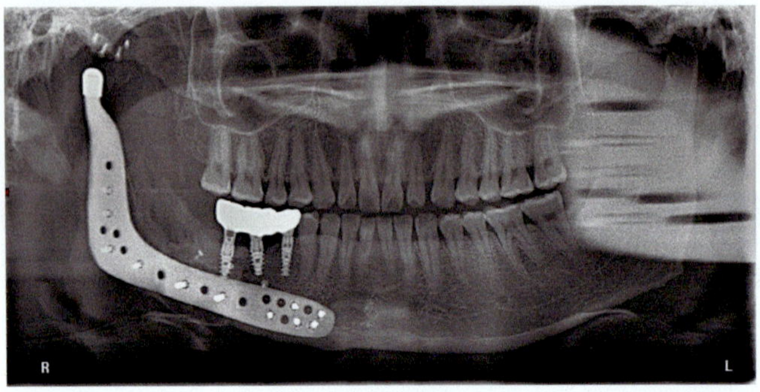

Fig. 8.76 Case P. Stable position of grafted bone and prosthesis at 8-year follow-up

Highly digitized and precise, digital design controlled the entire process, including osteotomy, graft bone harvest, prosthesis design and manufacture, and installation.

Important functions were maintained, including sensory function of the lower lip (because of preservation of the inferior alveolar neurovascular bundle), masticatory force was essentially consistent bilaterally (grafted bone provided an attachment bed for the masticatory muscles), mouth opening was essentially normal (prosthesis design was essentially sound), and the integrity of the dentition was maintained (successful implementation of dental implants).

- Disadvantages

The design of the prosthesis (mandibular prosthesis) is slightly awkward and should be combined with individualized masticatory muscle force measurements to design the prosthesis form based on the obtained stress parameters and distribution.

Bone grafting problems were encountered. Free iliac bone has controllable plasticity and good postoperative shape, but there was the disadvantage of bone resorption in the implant area, which then required a second-stage bone grafting before implantation of teeth. If a vascularized iliac muscle flap is used, there are problems such as excessive volume and postoperative facial bloating; if a fibula flap is used, there is insufficient height for dental implantation.

Free bone grafting is not indicated for infected lesions.

This bone flap design cannot be used in overly long mandibular defects.

The above deficiencies are issues that need to be addressed in future R&D.

8.4 Design and Application of a Combined Temporomandibular TMJ-Mandibular Prosthesis with Mandibular Body Augmentation

Minjie Chen, ZixianJiao , and Duohong Zou

Case Q in Sect. 8.4 is the case of a patient with a mandibular Class IIIa lesion, and the design of the prosthesis was further optimized by using a mandibular body augmentation prosthesis with a fibula flap for reconstruction, which embodied the prosthetic requirements of tissue preservation, and restoration of morphology and function in a balanced manner.

8.4.1 Case Q. Application of a Combined Temporomandibular TMJ-Mandibular Prosthesis with Mandibular Body Augmentation

- Patient information: female, 28 years old.
- Complaint: recurrent swelling and pain in the left mandible for more than 4 years.
- History: the patient came to the clinic because of recurrent swelling and pain in the left mandible for more than 4 years. Four years ago, she underwent mandibular cyst opening and extraction of the affected tooth, and the

pathology examination after the operation confirmed a diagnosis of "odontogenic keratocyst." Two years after the operation, she underwent three scraping treatments of mandibular masses because of recurrent swelling and pain in the left cheek, but the results were not good after the operation, and the swelling and pain continued to recur about 1–2 times/month.

- Clinical examination: the left cheek and mandibular ramus were swollen and hard, with high local skin temperature and obvious tenderness. Permanent teeth in the mouth, stable occlusal relationship, mouth opening of 17 mm, left deviation of mouth opening, left lower first and second molars missing, and the fistula seen in the posterior area of the left molar (Figs. 8.77 and 8.78).
- Imaging examination: the left mandibular body and mandibular ramus had swelling and bone changes, plus uneven density of the medullary cavity, partly increased density, partly soft-tissue density shadow. A group of elliptical low-density shadows could be seen in the left condyle (Figs. 8.79 and 8.80).
- Diagnosis: possible odontogenic keratocyst of the left mandible with secondary infection.
- Postoperative pathology: microscopically, it could be seen that there was an inflammatory fibrous cystic wall tissue lined with incompletely keratinized complex squamous epithelium and focal cystic wall infiltrated with inflammatory cells. Pathologic diagnosis was left mandibular odontogenic keratinizing cyst with secondary infection.

8.4.2 Case Q. Diagnostic Imaging

8.4.3 Case Q. Treatment Plan

- Overall treatment plan: resection of the left TMJ-mandibular mass, prosthetic reconstruction with a combined TMJ-mandibular prosthesis (mandibular body augmentation type), and consideration of a phase II dental implantation.
- Surgical resection design.

The scope of resection was designed from the condyle of the affected side to the left lower second incisor, which is a Class IIIa lesion. This case is a benign mandibular lesion without symptoms of inferior alveolar nerve involvement, so it should be preserved.

- Digital simulation of the surgery

See surgical resection design in Case O of this chapter.

Surgical resection design: design the osteotomy line at the anterior margin of the mass and mark the extent of the resection. After the osteotomy, obtain a model of the defect and mirror the healthy mandible to the affected side, and use this to design the grafting flap and the prosthesis (Fig. 8.81).

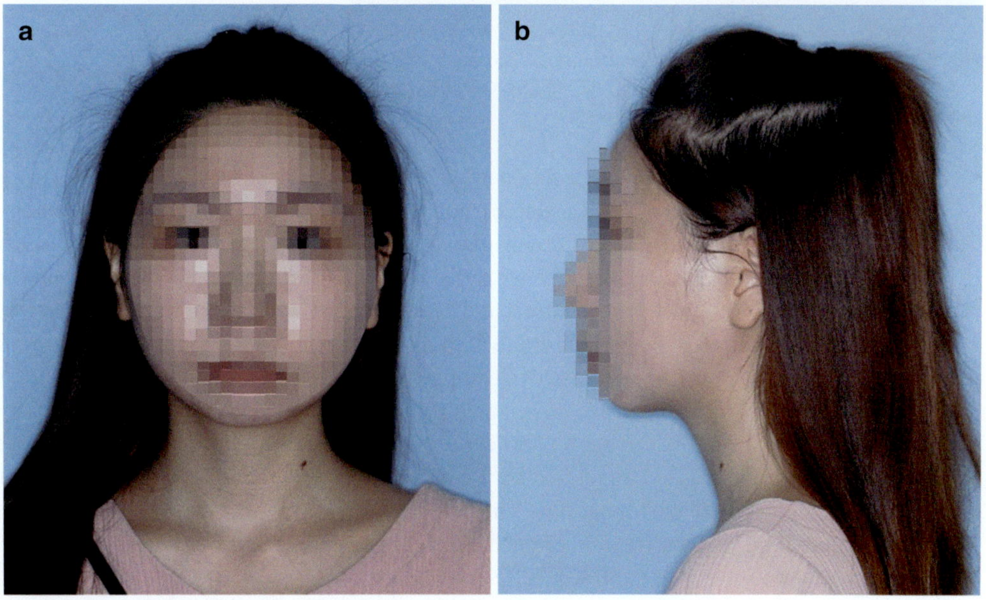

Fig. 8.77 Case Q. Clinical examination. Swelling of the left side of the face, mild tenderness in the left mandibular angle and preauricular region, and symmetrical bilateral sensations of the lower lip. (**a**) Frontal view. (**b**) Lateral view

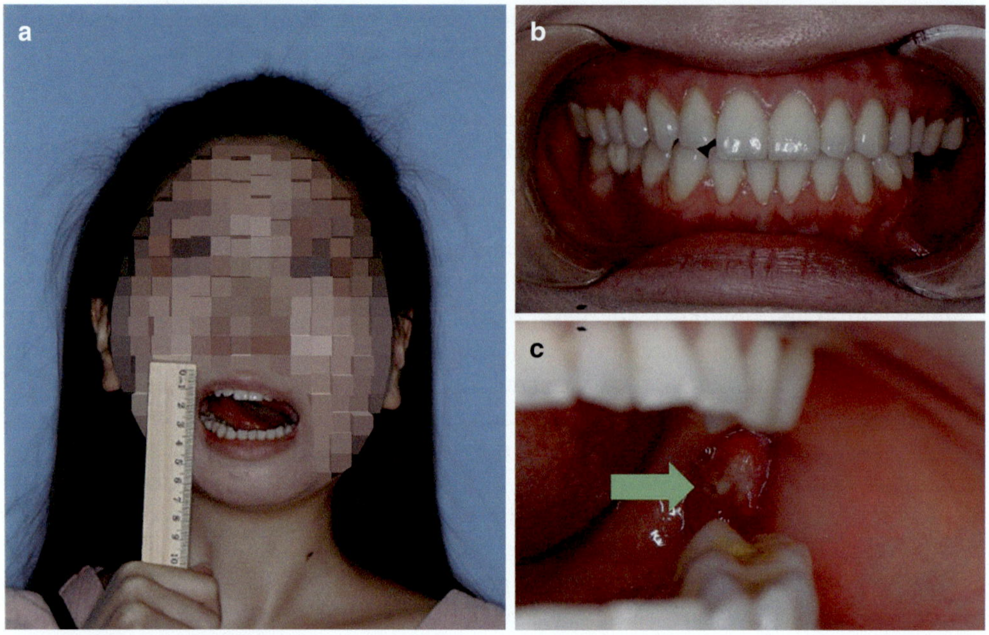

Fig. 8.78 Case Q. Clinical examination: (**a**) mouth opening of 17 mm, left deviation of mouth opening; (**b**) intraoral permanent dentition mostly good, lower incisors 2 mm to the left of the midline, left lower first and second molars were missing, stable occlusion; (**c**) fistulae visible in the posterior region of the left distal molar region (green arrows)

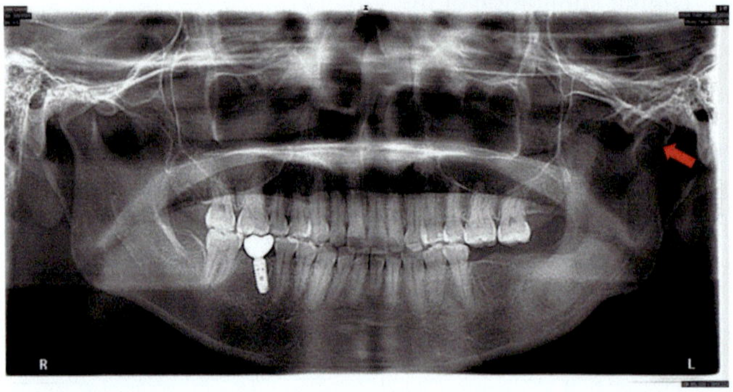

Fig. 8.79 Case Q. Panoramic film. Uneven bone density in the body and mandibular ramus of the left mandible, and an ovoid hypodense shadow (red arrow) is seen in the left condyle

- Design of the graft and prosthesis: a fibula myocutaneous flap is used to repair the mandibular defect, and the harvesting of the fibula is designed to reconstruct the mandibular body in three blocks, together with the titanium prosthesis that will augment the contour and volume of the new left mandible. The fibular bone flap is to be designed to meet the primary purpose of dental implantation, so the fibular graft is to be positioned somewhat above the jaw line, and the shape of the contour of the lower mandibular edge is to be restored by the prosthesis, which will extend below the fibular flap. The first segment of the fibular flap restores the mandible from the distal lower left second incisor to the lower left second premolar, the second segment from the lower second premolar to the mandibular angle, and the third segment from the posterior mandibular angle to the mandibular foramen plane. The graft fibular flap design is completed, designed to simulate the profile of the mandible at the dental implant site, and the prosthesis is designed with this profile (Fig. 8.82).

- Design and processing of the TMJ-mandibular prosthesis, mandibular body augmentation type, and osteotomy cutting guides.
  - Design of the TMJ-mandibular prosthesis, mandibular body augmentation type:

  Import and placement of core components: see Chap. 2, positioning of the core components (Fig. 8.83).

- Design of the articular fossa component and the mandibular extension component of the prosthesis.

The design principles are described in Chap. 2, Sect. 2.1.2.

Design of the extension component: the design of the extension is presented in a new design form, in which the cross-section of the mandibular prosthesis is designed as a layered structure. The overlap with the fibular flap is designed to be a solid part for stable fixation of the grafted bone flap, while the lower edge of the prosthesis is also a solid part to enhance its mechanical properties in serving as the rounded lower edge of the mandible, but the middle layer is porous to facilitate overall weight reduction and muscle attachment (Fig. 8.84).

- Prosthesis fabrication and fitting: see Chap. 2 (Fig. 8.85).
- Design of the osteotomy cutting guides for positioning during surgery

Mandibular anterior osteotomy cutting guide design: the cutting guide is designed along the anterior mandibular oste-

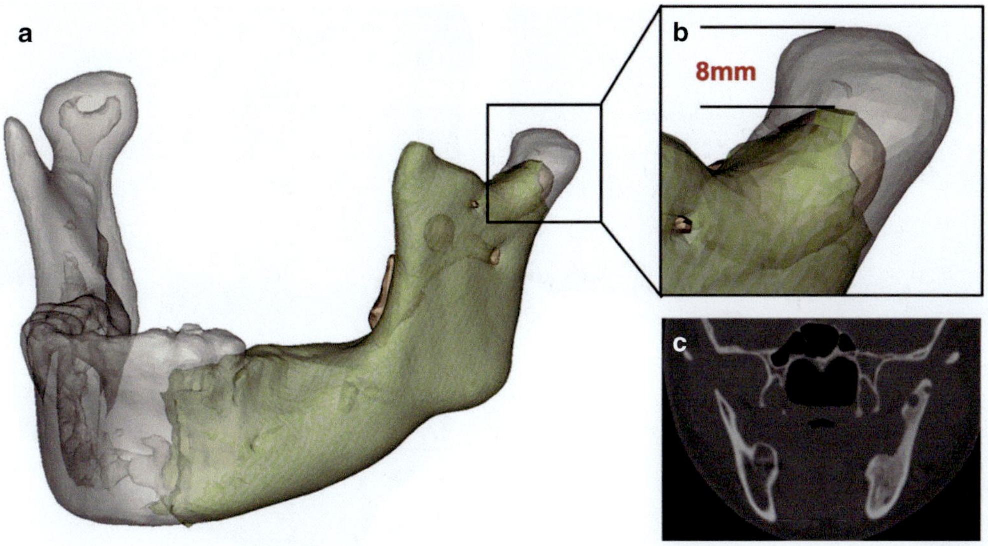

Fig. 8.80 Case Q. Extent of the mandibular lesion (40% transparency). The left mandibular body and mandibular ramus have swelling and extensive bone changes with uneven density in the medullary cavity, some with increased density and some with soft tissue density shadows, suggesting chronic osteomyelitis of the mandible. A group of elliptical low-density shadows was seen in the left condyle, and the upper boundary of the abnormal mass was 8 mm from the tip of the condyle, suggesting that the condyle cannot be preserved. (**a**) CT 3D reconstruction of the whole mandible. (**b**) Condyle detail. C. Coronal CT

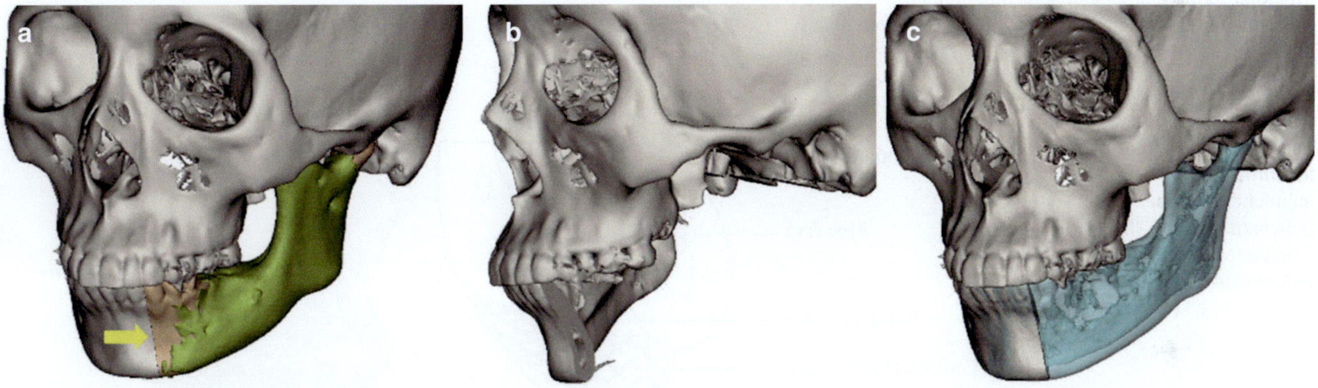

Fig. 8.81 Case Q. Digital simulation of resection of mass and defect model acquisition. The mass is shown in green, the extent of resection is shown in brown, and the healthy mandible is mirrored in light blue to plan for restoration of the diseased side. (**a**) The mandibular osteotomy line was designed to be at the lower second incisor of the left side (yellow arrows). (**b**) Resection of the mass resulted in a large joint-mandibular defect. (**c**) Mirroring of the healthy mandible projects the occlusal relationship and the contour of the healthy side onto the affected side and provides a model for reconstruction

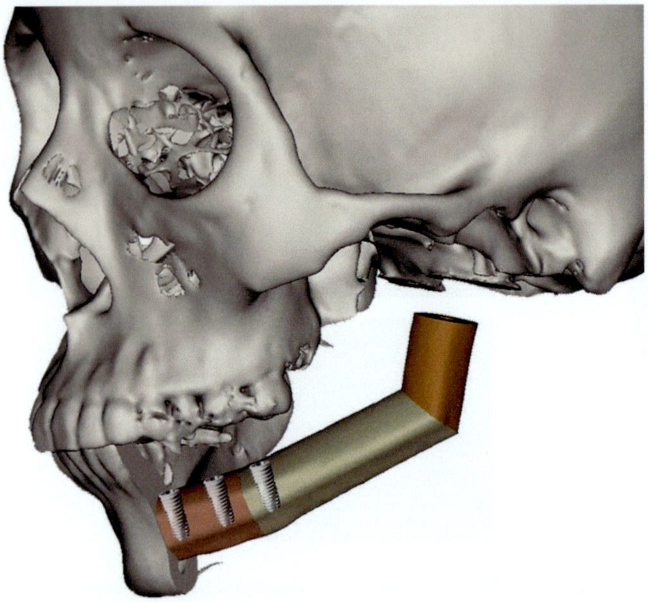

Fig. 8.82 Case Q. Planning for graft bone harvesting to simulate the profile of the mandible at the dental implant site and designing the prosthetic from this profile. The first segment (from anterior to posterior) of the fibular flap restores the mandible from the lower left second incisor to the second premolar, the second segment from the lower left second premolar to the mandibular angle, and the third segment from the posterior mandibular angle to the mandibular foramen plane

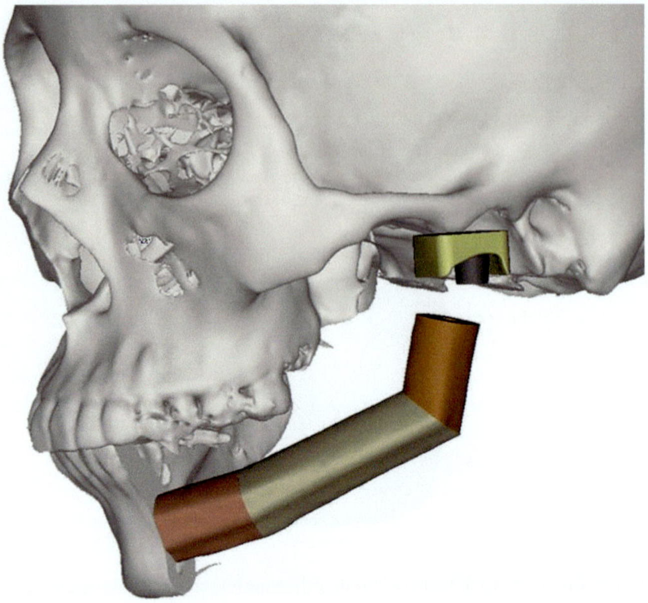

Fig. 8.83 Case Q. Design of the TMJ-mandibular prosthesis, mandibular body augmentation type: prosthetic core component placement. The articular fossa component is shown in yellow, and the articular head component is shown in dark gray

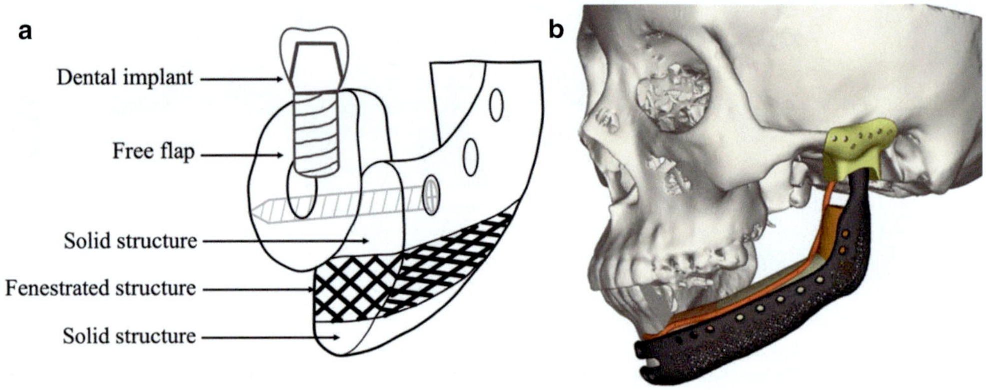

Fig. 8.84 Case Q. Cross-sectional design of the TMJ-mandibular prosthesis, mandibular body augmentation type. (**a**) Schematic design. (**b**) Completed articular fossa component and mandibular component prosthesis design

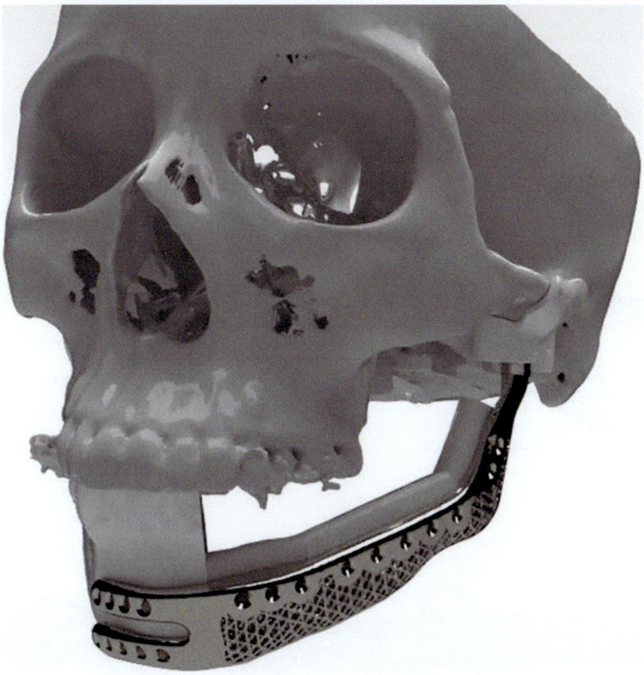

Fig. 8.85 Case Q. Mandibular body augmentation type of TMJ-mandibular prosthesis, showing trial fitting on a resin model, with also planned grafted bone models, to examine stability and fit of the prosthesis

otomy line to excise all the diseased bone, in this case close to the incisors, and the prosthetic screw hole positions are transferred to the cutting guide (Fig. 8.86).

Mandibular body osteotomy cutting guide design: the inferior alveolar neurovascular bundle is dissected from the mandible and preserved by the design of this osteotomy cutting guide (Fig. 8.87).

- Fibular osteotomy cutting guide design (Fig. 8.88). After all cutting guides are designed, they are machined and fabricated using a resin 3D printer.

8.4.4 Case Q. Surgical Procedure

Preoperative laboratory tests: the same as described in Sect. 3.2.5. Add a sentinel ultrasound examination of the tibiofibular trunk and peroneal artery of the right lower leg.

Preoperative preparation: skin preparation of the affected periauricular and submandibular regions, blood preparation of 400 mL. Add a sentinel ultrasound examination of the tibiofibular trunk and peroneal artery of the right lower leg.

Fig. 8.86 Case Q. Design of the anterior mandibular osteotomy cutting guide (pink). (**a**) Design of osteotomy cutting guides based on osteotomy lines. (**b**) Design of osteotomy cutting guide screw holes based on prosthesis screw holes

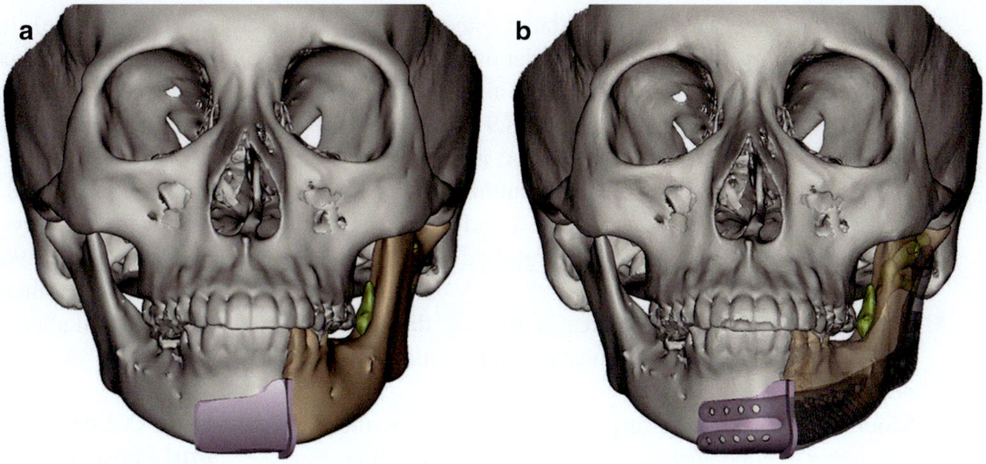

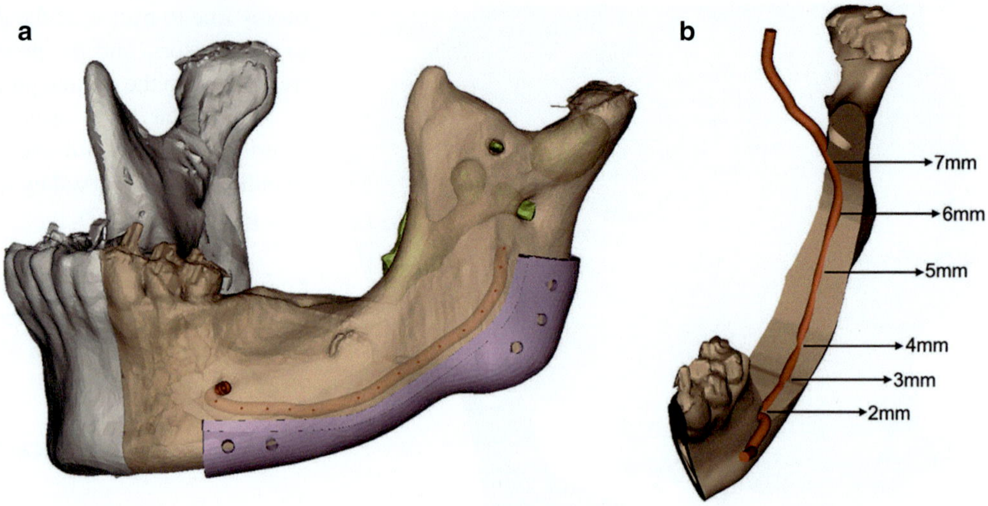

Fig. 8.87 Case Q. Design of osteotomy cutting guide (pink) for preservation of the inferior alveolar neurovascular bundle (unit: mm). (**a**) Mark the channel of the inferior alveolar neurovascular bundle, just above the upper edge of the osteotomy cutting guide, so that it does not get cut intraoperatively. (**b**) Measure the depth of the neural canal from the buccal bone cortex and accurately remove the partial bone according to the measured depth to extract and preserve the nerve during the operation

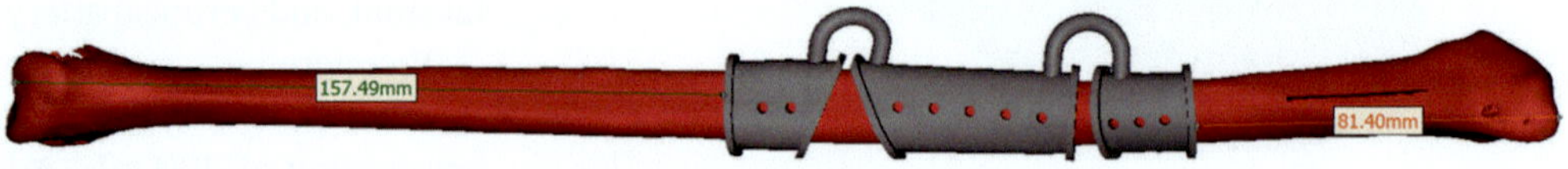

Fig. 8.88 Case Q. Osteotomy cutting guide design (gray) for fibula (red)

- Steps of the surgical procedure
  1. Surgical approach: see Case O, the submandibular incision is extended anteriorly to the midline with care taken to protect the mental nerve.
  2. Mandibular osteotomy: the mandibular osteotomy was begun by first installing the mandibular osteotomy cutting guide for preserving the inferior alveolar neurovascular bundle (Figs. 8.89, 8.90 and 8.91).
  3. Vascularized fibular flap fabrication and grafting, installation of the fibular osteotomy cutting guide, and fabrication of the bone flap (Figs. 8.92 and 8.93).
  4. The prosthesis is implanted, and the grafted bone block is fixed (Fig. 8.94).
  5. Treatment of the operative area: a free fat flap was taken through the submandibular incision to fill in the neck of the prosthesis.
  6. Modifications in actual surgery: intraoperatively, the left lower second incisor was extracted to facilitate suturing of the oral mucosa and to avoid exposure of the graft bone flap and prosthesis.
     - Postoperative medical advice and care: postoperative nasal feeding for 1 week, attention to daily observation of the intraoral flap, and oral care; see the rest in Case P.

8.4.5 Case Q. Postoperative Analysis of Prosthesis Implantation Precision

Regular postoperative follow-ups were performed for appearance (facial shape), function (mouth opening, mouth shape), and prosthesis evaluation (safety, accuracy).

Immediately after surgery: the intraoperative cutting guide was accurately seated, the prosthesis was installed smoothly, and the preoperative design was compared with the postoperative reconstruction (Fig. 8.95). The error of the core part of the prosthesis after surgery was 0.38 mm, and the overall error was 1.3 mm (Figs. 8.96 and 8.97). There were no complications such as prosthesis infection, rejection, ectopic osteogenesis, material allergy, loosening, or fracture.

8.4.6 Case Q. Long-Term Follow-Up and Prognosis

- Postoperative 6-month follow-up

The swelling and pain experienced before the operation disappeared, and diagnostic imaging follow-up showed no recurrence of the tumor.

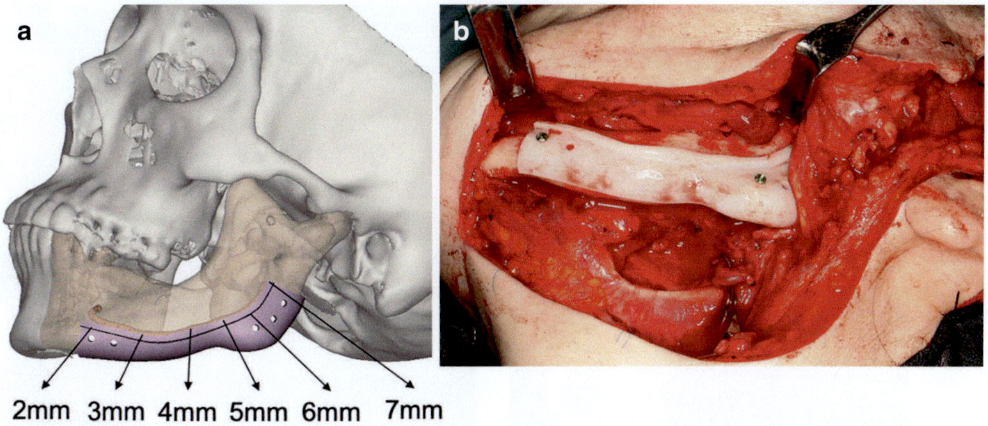

Fig. 8.89 Case Q. Freeing the inferior alveolar neurovascular bundle (unit: mm). (**a**) Schematic diagram of the design of the inferior alveolar neurovascular bundle preservation osteotomy and cutting guide (pink). (**b**) Actual placement of the cutting guide (white). Piezoelectric saw was used to remove buccal bone at the upper edge of the guide to the planned depth. An oscillating saw was used to cut the bone at the anterior and posterior edges of the guide

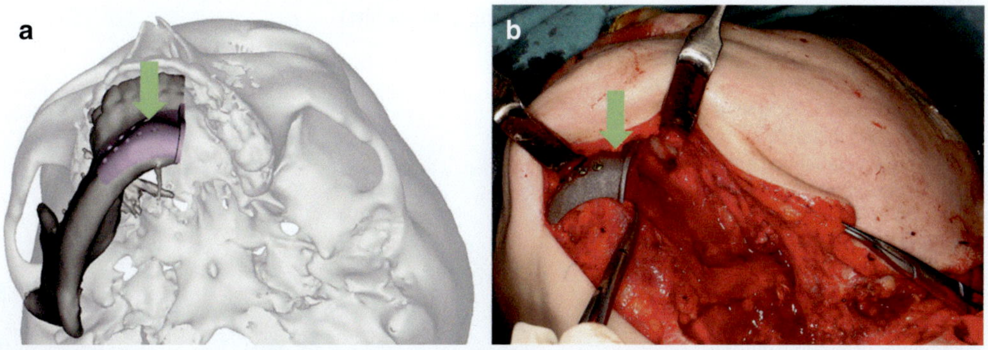

Fig. 8.90 Case Q. Anterior resection margin. After the cutting guide (green arrow) was placed, the mandibular osteotomy was cut. Screw holes in the guide were used later for precise placement of the mandibular prosthesis. (**a**) Placement of mandibular osteotomy cutting guide. (**b**) Actual

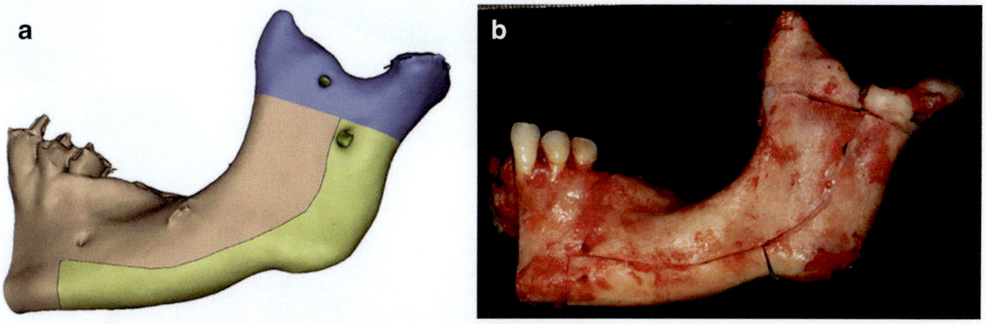

Fig. 8.91 Case Q. Precision resection of the diseased mandible in segments, with preservation of the inferior alveolar neurovascular bundle. (**a**) Design. (**b**) Actual

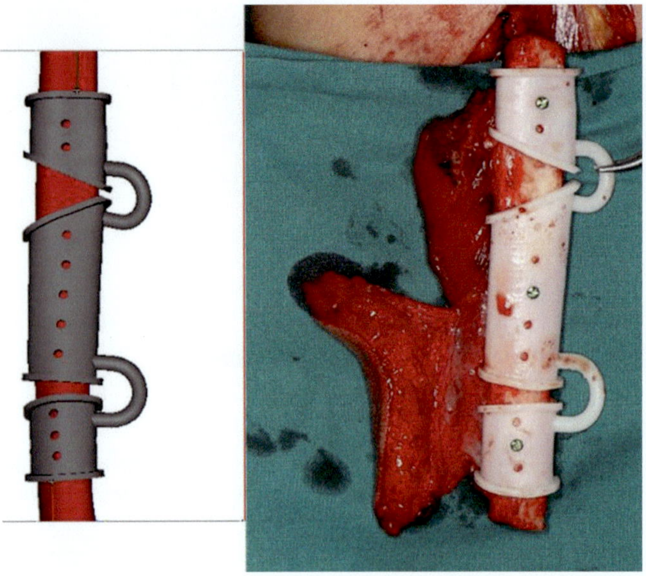

Fig. 8.92 Case Q. Cutting guide assists in fibular contouring. (a) Design of cutting guide (gray). (b) Installation of cutting guide (white) and fabrication of fibular flap

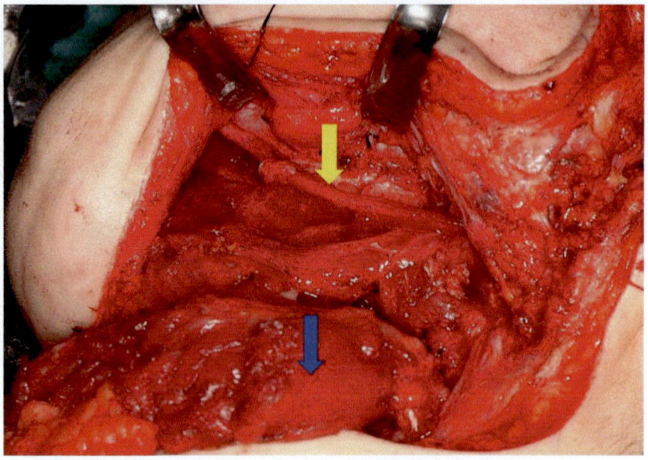

Fig. 8.93 Case Q. After resection of the diseased mandible, the inferior alveolar neurovascular bundle (yellow arrow) is preserved intact, and vascular anastomosis of the fibular flap (blue arrow) is completed

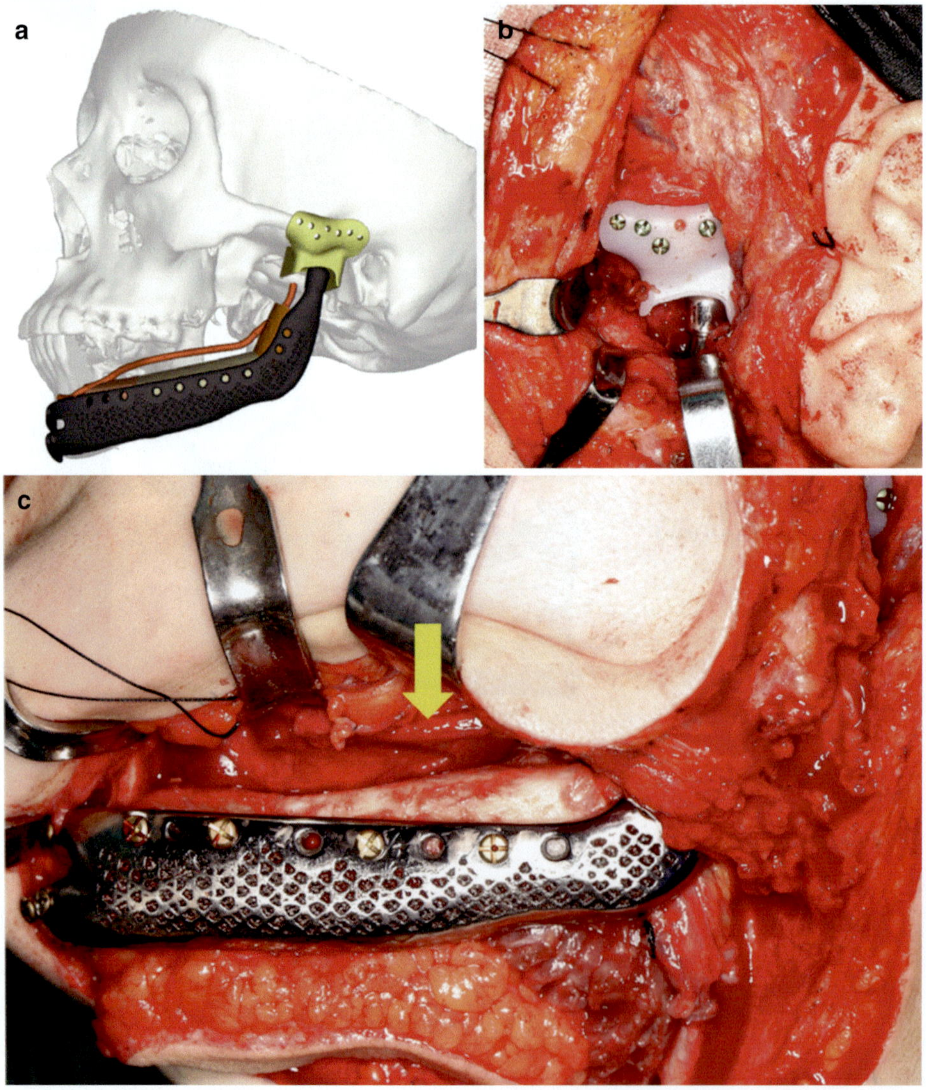

Fig. 8.94 Case Q. Prosthesis and bone graft installation. (a) Design. (b) Installation of the articular fossa prosthesis with five or six screws at the designed depth. (c) Installation of the mandibular prosthesis. Fix the screw holes identified by the mandibular osteotomy cutting guide; then fix the remaining screws to secure the fibular bone block to the prosthesis. The screws should be carefully placed to avoid the later dental implant sites, and the surgeon should make sure intraoperatively that the articular head component is correctly positioned in the posterior median position of the articular fossa component when the mouth is closed

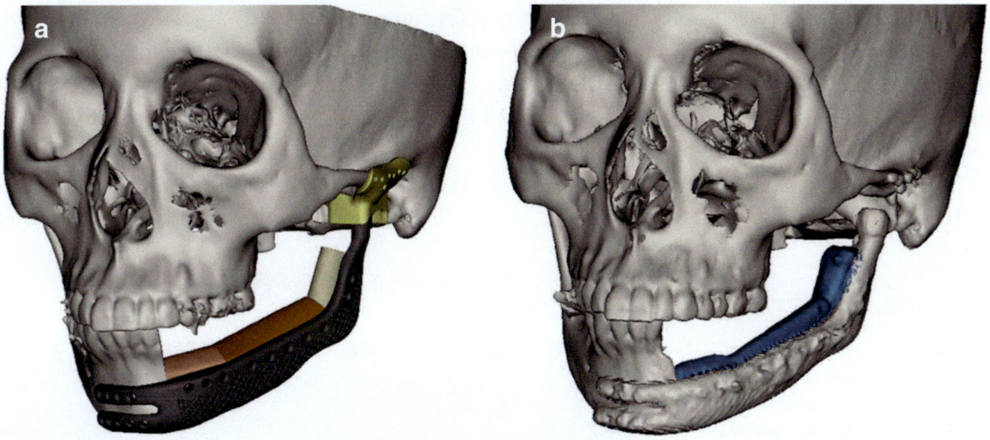

Fig. 8.95 Case Q. Comparison of CT reconstruction showing precise prosthesis seating. (**a**) Preoperative design. (**b**) Immediate postoperative period

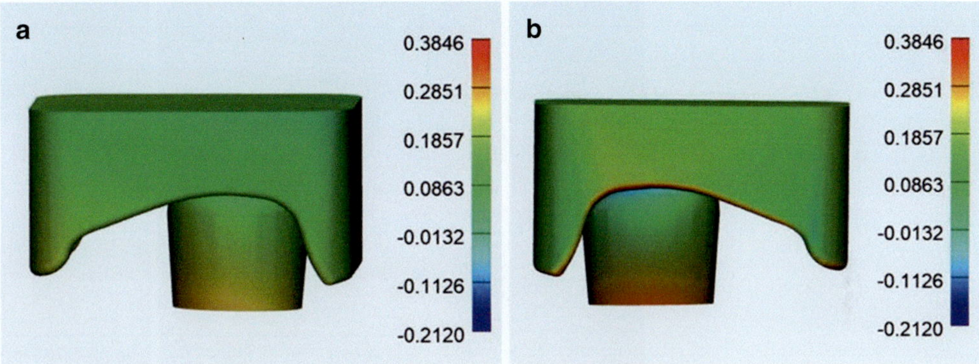

Fig. 8.96 Case Q. Prosthetic core component error 0.38 mm. (**a**) Lateral error. (**b**) Medial error

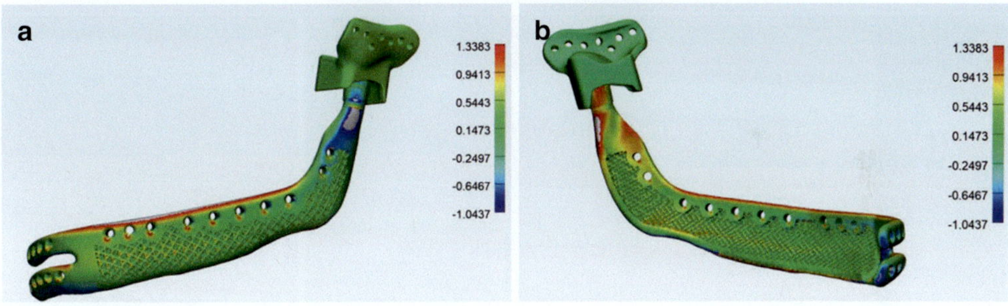

Fig. 8.97 Case Q. TMJ-mandibular coalition prosthesis with an overall error of 1.3 mm. (**a**) Lateral error. (**b**) Medial error

The facial shape was good (Fig. 8.98), the joint function was well restored, there was no pain or discomfort in the joint area, the TMJ-mandibular-occlusal-facial coordination was stable, the mouth opening improved to 25 mm, and the occlusal relationship was stable (Fig. 8.99).

Evaluation of grafted bone and prosthesis (Figs. 8.100, 8.101, and Table 8.3).

- At 2-year postoperative follow-up, dental implant-restorative treatment was proposed, starting with tent peg bone augmentation (Fig. 8.102).
- 3-year postoperative follow-up results.

At the 3-year postoperative follow-up, the facial shape was good, the occlusion was stable, the mouth opening had

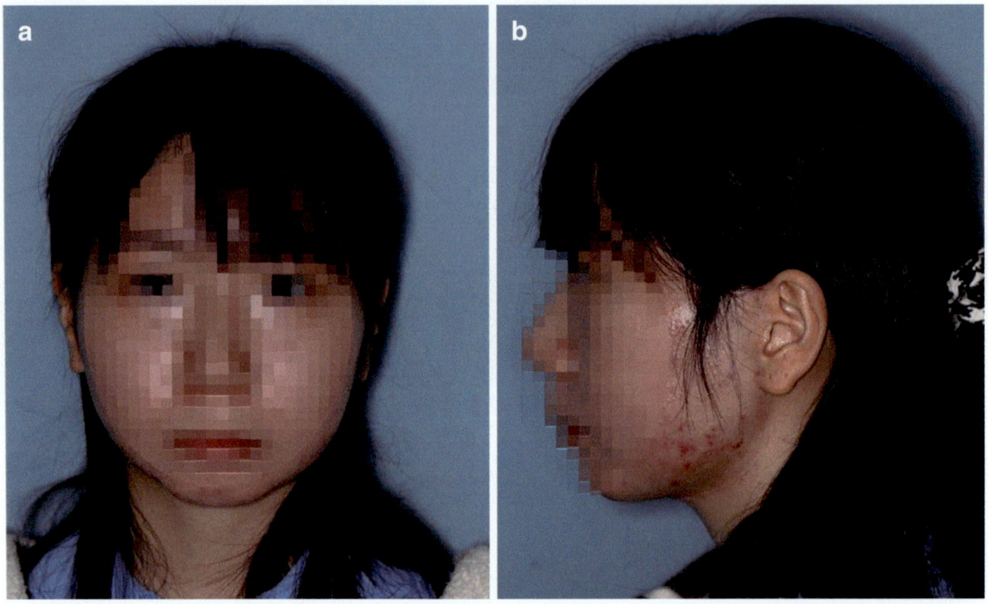

Fig. 8.98 Case Q. Six-month postoperative follow-up with slight fullness on the left side. (**a**) Frontal view. (**b**) Lateral view

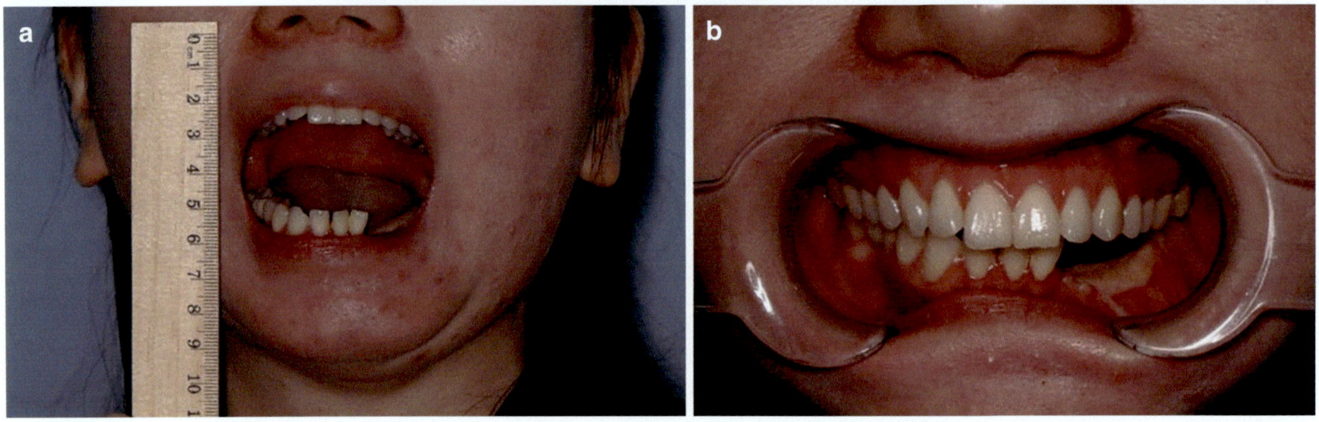

Fig. 8.99 Case Q. Joint function. (**a**) Mouth opening of 25 mm, slightly leftward. (**b**) Stable intraoral occlusion, lower incisors 3 mm to the left of the midline (an increase of 1 mm from the preoperative period), and good alveolar ridge morphology

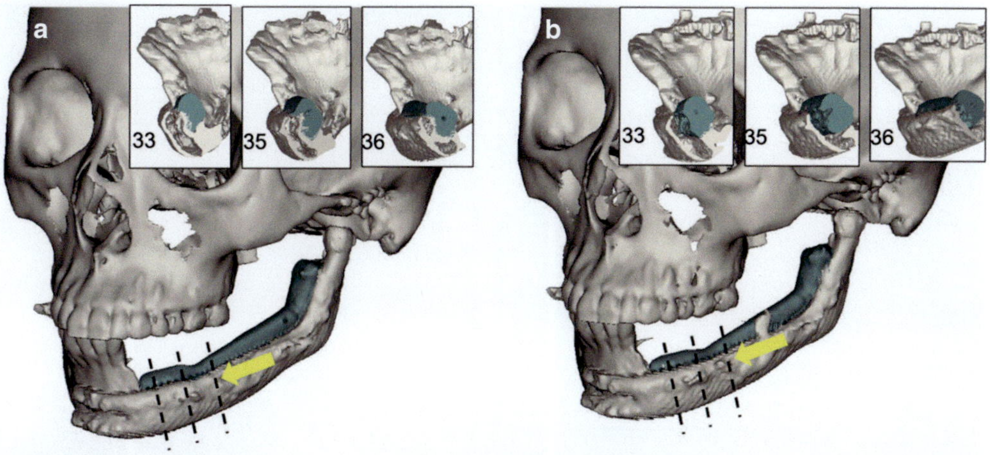

Fig. 8.100 Case Q. Grafted bone block volume and cross-section changes, showing some resorption of grafted bone, but sufficient alveolar ridge height to plan dental implants. (**a**) Immediately postoperatively, the grafted bone volume was 10,057 mm^3. (**b**) At 6 months postoperatively, the grafted bone volume was 9833.92 mm^3. See Table 8.3 for more details

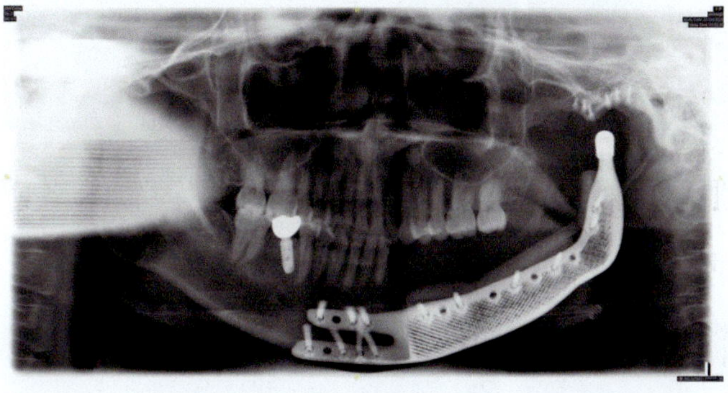

Fig. 8.101 Case Q. Six-month postoperative panoramic X-ray

Table 8.3 Case Q. Changes in mandibular grafted bone mass volume and cross-section measurements, immediately after surgery and six months after surgery

Evaluation indicators	Time: immediately after surgery		Time: six months after surgery	
	Height	Width	Height	Width
Bone block Lower left 3 position	22.9 mm	7.83	23.1	7.74
Bone block Lower left 5 position	22.3 mm	9.29	21.9	8.70
Bone block Lower left 6 position	21.5 mm	9.84	21.2	8.90
Bone mass volume	10,057		9833.92	

Volume in mm^3, surface area in mm^2, length in mm

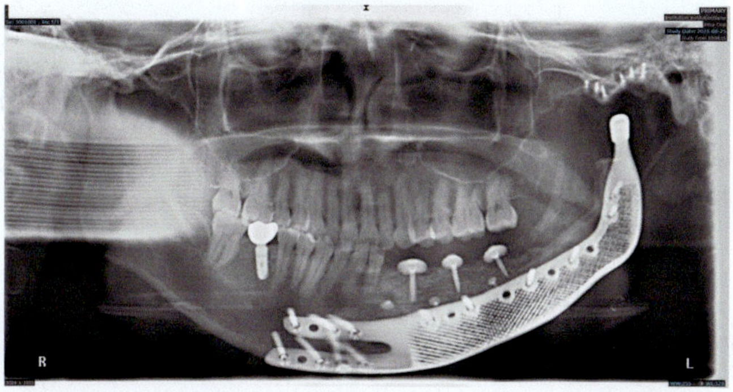

Fig. 8.102 Case Q. Tent peg bone grafting; after bone augmentation, the bone height in the planned dental implant area became flush with the top of the right alveolar ridge

improved to 30 mm (Fig. 8.103), dental implantation was completed (Fig. 8.104), and the grafted bone was well remodeled and integrated with the prosthesis, and the prosthesis was stable in position (Fig. 8.105). The rest of the case was not different from the 1-year postoperative follow-up.

8.4.7 Case Q. Advantages and Disadvantages

- Advantages

In the traditional method, to compensate for the lack of fibula height, another free fibula needs to be inserted in parallel to increase the height of the alveolar ridge. Zhang

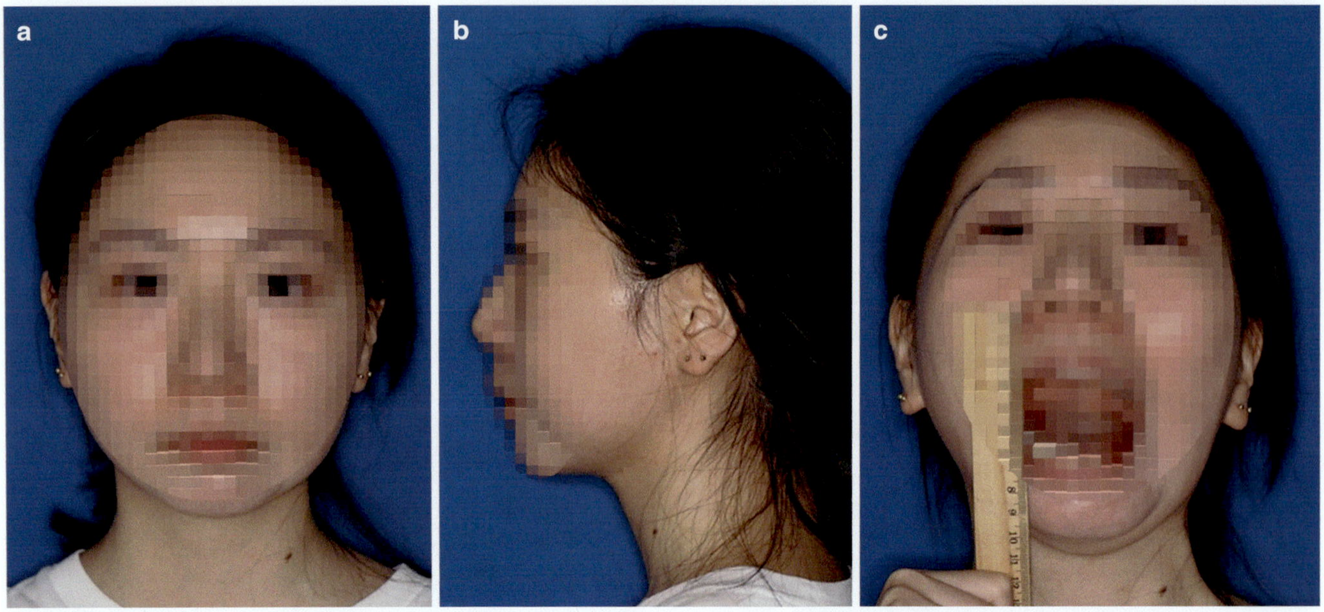

Fig. 8.103 Case Q. Three-year postoperative follow-up with good facial appearance and joint function. (**a**) Frontal view. (**b**) Lateral view. (**c**) Mouth opening improved to 30 mm

Fig. 8.104 Case Q. Complete dental implantation

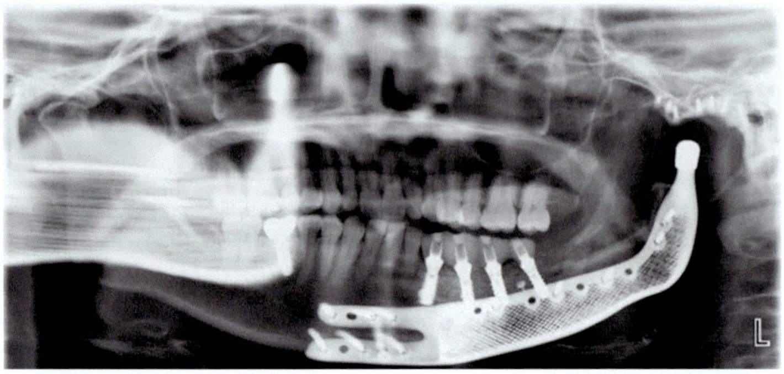

Fig. 8.105 Case Q. CT scan 3 years postoperatively showed a stable prosthesis position and good graft-to-mandibular prosthesis remodeling. (**a**) Lateral view. (**b**) Medial view

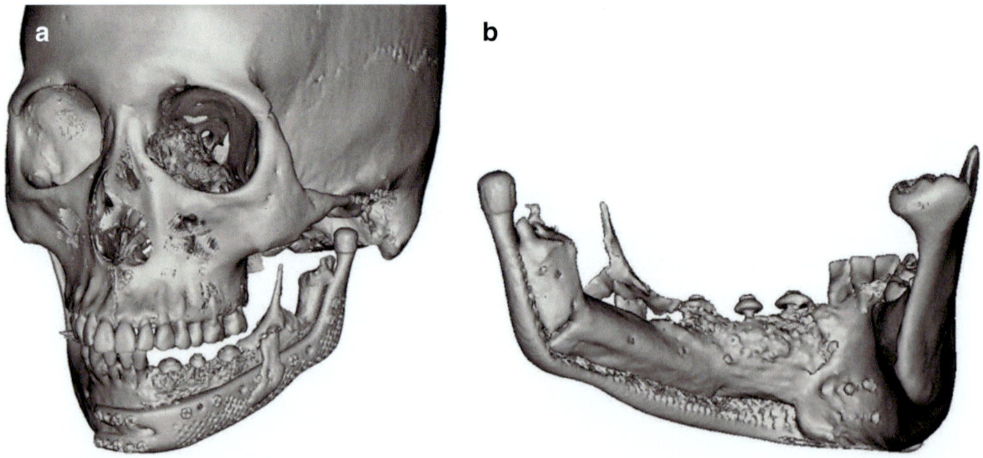

Chenping and others creatively integrated traction osteogenesis with dental implants to solve the problem of dental restoration. However, this method is difficult to operationalize and requires high precision. In this case, Case Q, the TMJ-mandibular prosthesis was innovatively optimized, and for the purpose of restoring the facial shape and joint function, the fibula bone flap was moved upward to serve to repair the top of the alveolar ridge, laying the foundation for the later implant restoration; at the same time, the lower portion of the mandibular prosthesis was increased in height, so as to maintain the overall height of the prosthesis and the alveolar ridge, as well as facial symmetry.

The contour of the prosthesis was good, and a good shape was obtained. Thanks to the mesh structure, prosthetic weight was reduced, and tissue attachment was facilitated. Most importantly, the design addresses the root cause of common mandibular-condylar reconstruction complications and poor restorations.

- Disadvantages

This case is a joint-mandible repair of an extensive lesion, and there is a risk of dislocation of the prosthetic condylar head because the earlier muscle power has not been restored. Further studies are needed to ensure the stability of the prosthesis in initial implantation.

9 Reconstruction of Mandibular Diseases with Salvageable Joint

Chi Yang, Minjie Chen, and Jisi Zheng

This chapter is aimed at Class IVb of Yang's new classification, that is, mandibular diseases in which the temporomandibular joint (TMJ) (namely, the condyle) can be preserved. This preservation calls for careful surgical planning and the customized design of a prosthesis, as will be discussed in this chapter.

Primary lesions of the mandible, such as cystic lesions and borderline lesions, often invade the proximity of the condyle. This is a common disease in oral and maxillofacial-head and neck oncology, and it calls for surgical resolution. But the deficiencies of traditional surgery for this condition are not paying attention to the preservation of the condyle, which is often removed altogether. Or the unattached condyle is reimplanted, and so it becomes prone to bone resorption and so on. How to effectively preserve the condyle and articular disc to maintain or restore normal TMJ morphology and function is a matter of concern.

In this chapter, we discuss the feasibility of using customized prostheses in reconstruction to solve the above problems with the goal of condylar preservation, joint stability, and occlusal restoration, applying implant design with advanced digital technology. The results of our innovative reconstruction system, after 5 years of clinical application and follow-up, are encouraging, and the design and application of this reconstruction plate reconstruction system will be described in detail in this chapter.

9.1 Overview

Chi Yang and Minjie Chen

In this introductory section of this chapter, we first propose a definition of mandibular diseases in which the temporomandibular joint (TMJ) (condyle) can be preserved, and a new categorization thereof will be made, one that relates to the types of prostheses that can be applied. A review of traditional prosthetic reconstruction methods and their less-than-ideal outcomes reveals the problems. An innovative prosthetic reconstruction method and a digital design process for customized condyle-preserving mandibular reconstruction plates are proposed, laying the foundation for subsequent clinical applications.

9.1.1 Definition of Mandibular Diseases with Salvageable Joint

When diseases such as tumors, tumorlike diseases, and osteomyelitis that occur in the mandible invade the mandibular notch to the condyle, and when the height of the healthy condyle is $\geq$10 mm or the disease is located outside the joint capsule, it is suggested to consider preserving the condyle. These lesions can be called subarticular mandibular lesions (Fig. 9.1). They usually present clinically with swelling and pain in the affected mandibular region, as well as restriction of mouth opening. There are many types of surgical resection and repair and reconstruction, and there is no standardized protocol that has been universally agreed upon.

9.1.2 Classification of Mandibular Diseases with Salvageable Joint

The classification of mandibular lesions is divided into two categories based on whether the mandible has a salvageable posterior lower edge, that is, the back angle of the jaw, which provides a block of bone to support all functions. Class I is a mandibular lesion with a salvageable posterior lower edge (Fig. 9.2); Class II is a mandibular lesion with a non-salvageable posterior lower edge (Fig. 9.3).

Chi Y. (✉) · Minjie C. · Jisi Z.
Shanghai Ninth People's Hospital, Shanghai Jiao Tong University School of Medicine, Shanghai, China

© People's Medical Publishing House, PR of China 2025
Chi Y. (ed.), *Atlas of Customized TMJ-Cranio-Jaw Prosthesis*, https://doi.org/10.1007/978-981-95-0611-8_9

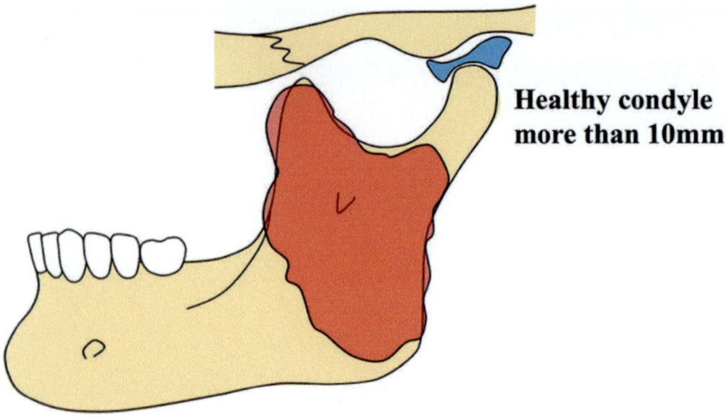

Fig. 9.1 Definition of subarticular mandibular lesions near the joint. Blue represents the articular disc. Red represents the extent of lesions. Condylar height ≥10 mm of normal tissue with the disease located outside the joint capsule suggests that it can be preserved

9.1.3 Traditional Methods of Prosthetic Reconstruction for Mandibular Diseases with Salvageable Joint

There are many shortcomings in the traditional repair and reconstruction surgery of mandibular lesions near the joint, which are mainly experienced as follows:

1. The condyle that can be preserved is removed, resulting in occlusal and facial deviation.
2. The detached condyle is implanted back and fixed in place, but resorption or displacement occurs in the post-operative period.
3. The detached condyle is implanted back, but does not achieve stability due to lack of attachment to the lateral

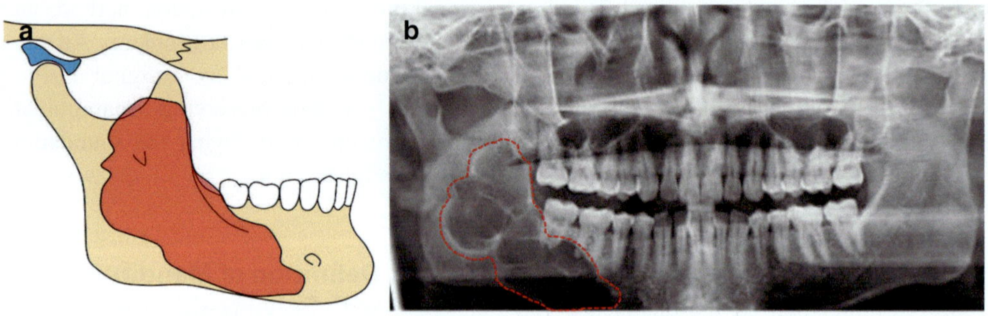

Fig. 9.2 Subarticular mandibular lesion (Class I, mandible with a salvageable posterior lower edge). (**a**) Schematic diagram, blue represents the articular disc, and red represents the extent of the lesion. (**b**) Panoramic view showing the right abnormal mass (red dotted line) not extending to the posterior edge of the mandible

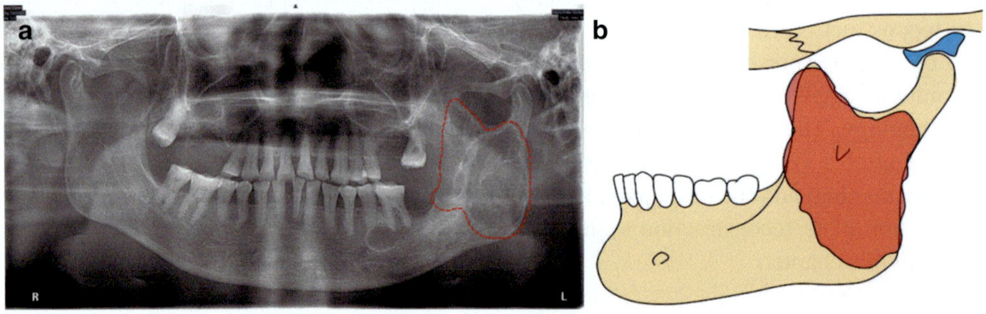

Fig. 9.3 Subarticular mandibular lesion (Class II, mandible lacking a salvageable posterior lower edge). (**a**) Panoramic view showing left abnormal mandibular mass (red dotted line). (**b**) Schematic diagram, blue represents the articular disc, and red represents a lesion extending all the way to the posterior edge of the mandible

pterygoid muscle, joint capsule, and ligaments and is prone to dislocation.
4. The method of fixation with preformed titanium plates without free movement of the condyle results in problems such as poor positioning and fixation and, thus, the tendency to displacement of the condyle.

Each of these will be discussed below, with clinical examples and diagnostic images.

- Salvageable condyles removed: the condyle and its attachments (articular disc, joint capsule, and lateral pterygoid muscles) are extremely important to the stability of the preserved condyle, and no bone graft can reconstruct the periarticular accessory structures to allow for complete joint function (Fig. 9.4).
- Resorption of the detached condyle after replantation: The conventional submandibular incision has the defect of being unable to fully expose the condyle. Even if the surgeon wants to preserve the condyle, due to the limited field of view and operating space, the condyle can only be pulled out along with the diseased mandible, and then the condyle is excised from the diseased mandible and fixed to the top of the grafted bone. In the long term, a condyle that has lost its attachment to the lateral pterygoid muscle is prone to problems such as resorption due to lack of blood supply or secondary osteoarthritis (Fig. 9.5).
- Condylar dislocation: condylar implantation or in situ fixation may result in condylar dislocation due to the following reasons:
  1. The conventional submandibular incision does not provide easy observation of the disc-condyle alignment of the implanted bone, and if there is no anterior auriculotemporal incision to provide a clear exposure of the joint, the reimplanted condyle or retained condyle may not be accurately positioned, that is, it is not returned to the joint fossa during the operation.
  2. The reimplanted condyle lacks control by the lateral pterygoid muscle, joint capsule, and ligaments, and so it is difficult for the position of the condyle to be stabilized in the joint fossa. Commonly, the condyle is anteriorly and medially dislocated, resulting in facial deviation and loss of dental occlusion (Fig. 9.6).

- Fixation with prefabricated titanium plates: For a salvageable condyle, a combined posterior submandibular incision and anterior auriculotemporal incision is needed to fully expose the condyle without damaging the joint capsule, as well as to preserve the attachment of the lateral pterygoid muscle. Moreover, even if the titanium plate is prefabricated using computer-aided design (CAD) and computer-aided manufacturing (CAM) technology, the

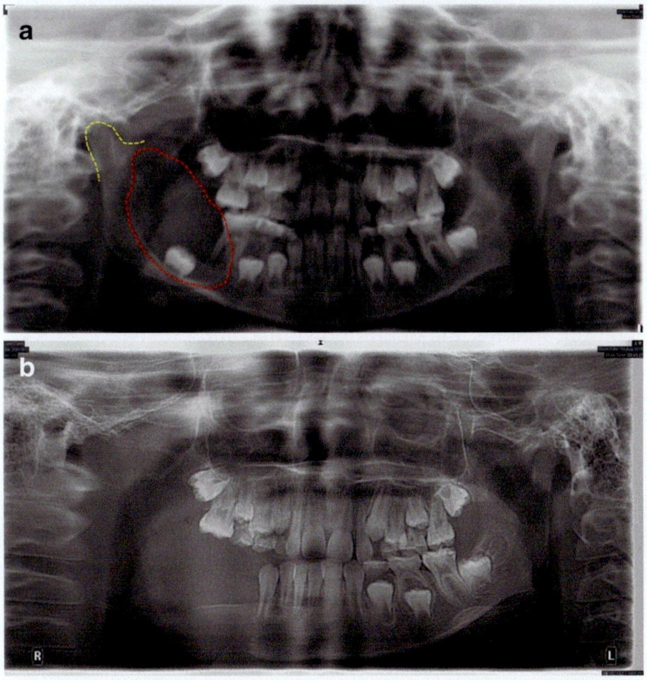

Fig. 9.4 Salvageable condyle excised. (**a**) Preoperative panoramic view showing the right mandibular mass (red dotted line) up to the level of the mandibular notch, with the condyle (yellow dotted line) uninvolved. (**b**) Postoperative panoramic view showing condylar removal

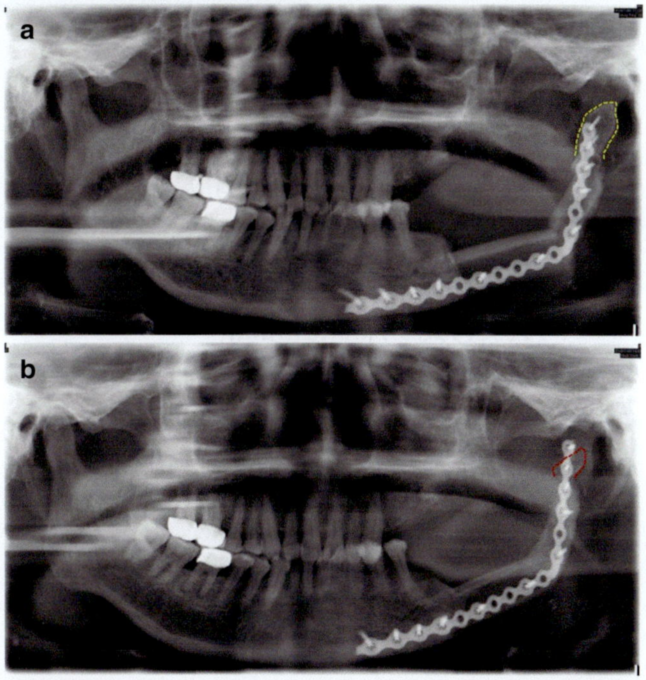

Fig. 9.5 Implantation of excised condyle. (**a**) One-week postoperative panoramic view showing the implanted condyle in good shape (yellow dotted line). (**b**) One-year postoperative panoramic view showing condylar resorption (red dotted line)

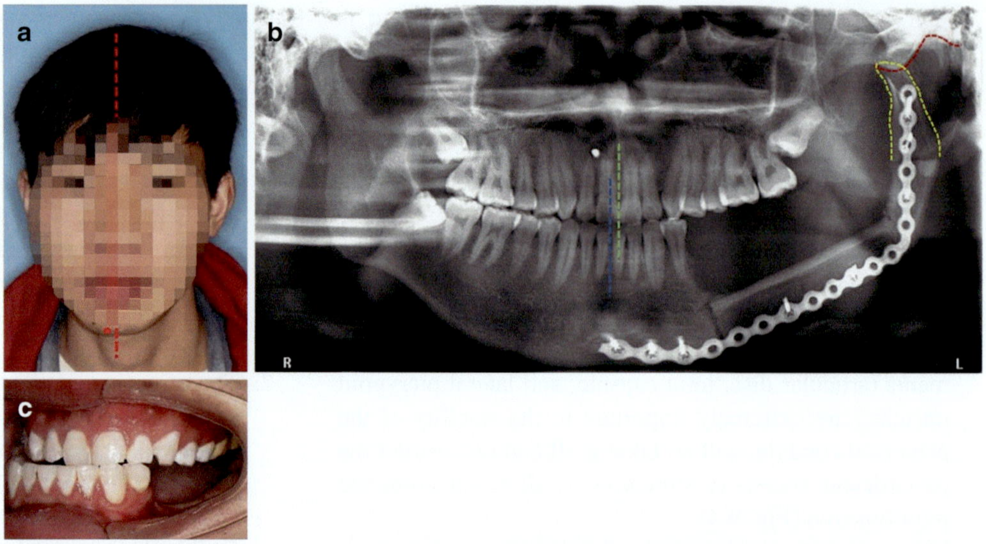

Fig. 9.6 Traditional condylar preservation combined with fibular reconstruction. (**a**) Frontal view of right deviation of the chin point. (**b**) Intraoral occlusal disorder with right deviation of the mandibular midline. (**c**) Panoramic view showing anterior dislocation of the condyle (yellow dashed line shows condyle, red dashed line shows articular fossa) and right deviation of the mandibular midline (blue dashed line) compared to the maxillary midline (green dashed line)

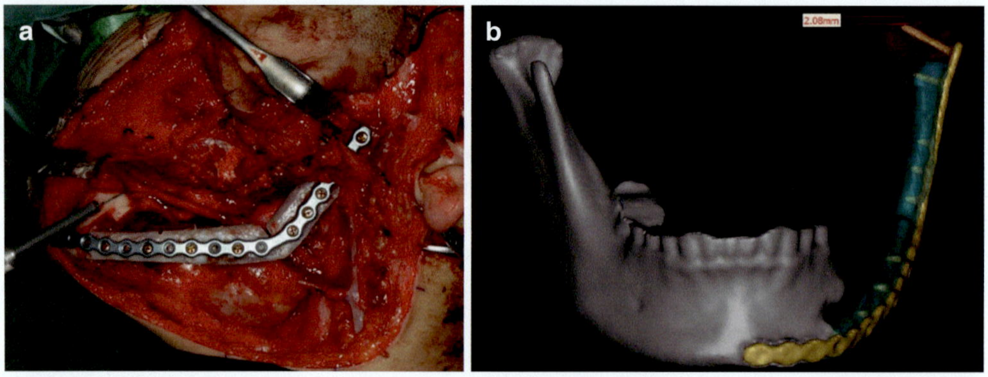

Fig. 9.7 Mandibular reconstruction with preservation of the condyle and articular attachments. (**a**) Intraoperative exposure of the joint was adequate to stabilize the joint position in the articular fossa. (**b**) Postoperative CT demonstrated that the preserved condyle was well positioned with stable retention

intraoperative shaping of the grafted bone is complicated, and it is difficult to achieve stable fixation with plates that do not closely fit the bone (Fig. 9.7).

9.1.4 Innovative Prosthetic Reconstruction Methods for Customized Condylar Preservation Mandibular Reconstruction Plate

To solve the above four problems, the authors have proposed a new reconstruction plan that should achieve joint preservation, precise positioning, and solid fixation, so as to achieve precise reconstruction of the mandibular occlusion and long-term stability. The proposed solution is to digitally design the osteotomy scope and autogenous graft bone contouring before the surgery and then design a customized mandibular prosthesis consistent with these.

Moreover, the surgical procedure should use a modified anterior auriculotemporal incision to achieve the preservation of the condylar-articular disc-lateral pterygoid muscle complex and, intraoperatively, use the customized mandibular prosthesis as the reference for placement and fixation of the grafted bone.

This serves to accurately align and connect the proximal condyle to the distal condyle. That is, the mandibular stump is connected to the condyle near the heart and the mandibular stump far from the heart. There is no need for intermaxillary ligation, making the operation simple and precise.

- Types of design for customized mandibular reconstruction prostheses with condylar preservation.
  The types of mandibular reconstruction plates that have been designed to the present are of two types (but not limited to two types for the future), and these differ in the presence or absence of the posterior lower edge of the mandible.
  - Mandibular reconstruction prosthesis that preserves the condyle and the lower posterior margin of the mandible. The position and shape of the grafted bone should consider the planned subsequent implant restoration (Fig. 9.8).

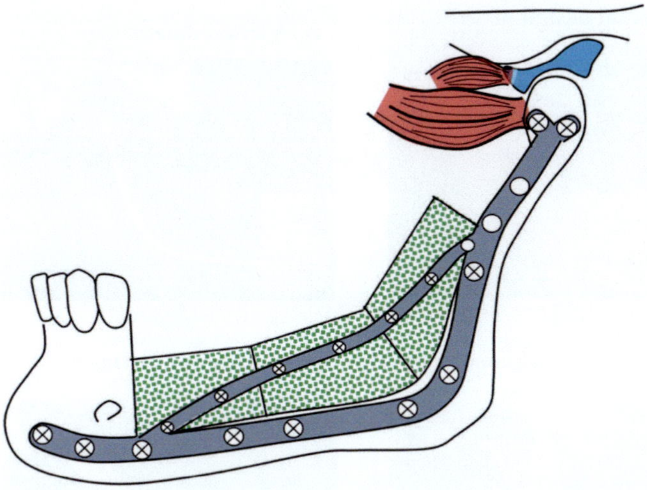

Fig. 9.8 Schematic diagram of a mandibular reconstruction prosthesis that preserves the condyle and the lower posterior margin of the mandible (Class I). Gray shows the mandibular reconstruction plate, green shows the autogenous graft bone blocks, blue shows the articular disc, and red shows the lateral pterygoid muscle. The condyle is attached to the original mandibular bone

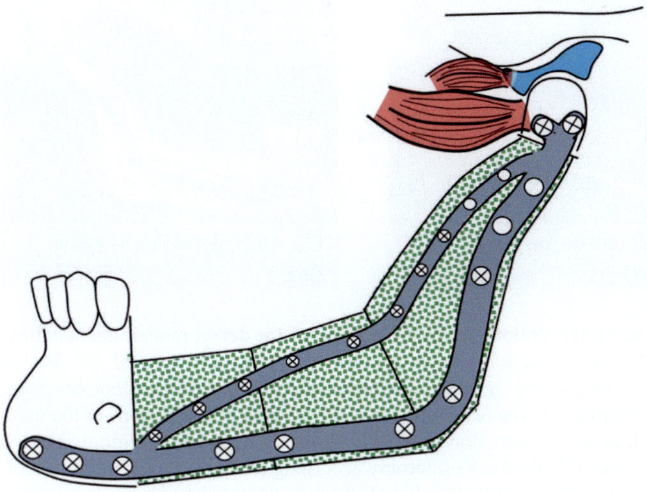

Fig. 9.9 Schematic diagram of a mandibular reconstruction prosthesis that preserves only the condyle (Class II). Gray shows the mandibular reconstruction plate, green shows the autogenous graft bone blocks, blue shows the articular disc, and red shows the lateral pterygoid muscle. The condyle is grafted to the autogenous graft bone

– Mandibular reconstruction prosthesis that preserves only the condyle. This mandibular reconstruction prosthesis is indicated for mandibular reconstruction where the posterior lower border of the mandible is discontinuous and repair of the alveolar ridge bone along with the posterior lower edge of the mandible (i.e., the back of the jaw) is required (Fig. 9.9).

9.1.4.1 Indications and Contraindications for Mandibular Reconstruction Prostheses

Indications

Application of a mandibular reconstruction prosthesis is suitable for a variety of adult diseases of the mandible or mandibular ramus, with the condition that at least 10 mm of the condyle is not affected. Mainly includes benign, borderline, or tumorlike diseases of the mandible, quiescent inflammatory diseases, etc.

Contraindications

See "Contraindications to the Combined TMJ-Mandibular Prosthesis" in Chap. 8.

9.1.5 General Digital Design Process for Customized Mandibular Reconstruction Prostheses Where the Condyle Is Preserved

The total process of digital design and surgical planning for installation of the prosthesis consists of three aspects (shown schematically in Fig. 9.10): simulated osteotomy of the diseased bone and removal of the lesion, design of the reconstruction prosthesis and osteotomy cutting guides, and the plan of the surgical procedure. The example given in Fig. 9.10 is that of a Class II case where the lower back of the jaw cannot be preserved, and the condyle, detached in the osteotomy to remove the diseased mass, is grafted directly to the autogenous graft bone.

- Simulated osteotomy of lesions in cases where the condyle is to be preserved.
  – Analysis of the scope of the lesion: preoperative CT is received in DICOM format, and the surgical design software is used to analyze the extent of the lesion and to mark the inferior alveolar neurovascular bundle (Fig. 9.10, A1).

The osteotomy lines are designed as follows:

1. Proximal osteotomy line: for safe resection of the lesion and preservation of the condyle and appendages
2. Mandibular foramen osteotomy lines: for mandibular dissection with shallow cortical cuts to facilitate the separation of the inferior alveolar neurovascular bundle (see specifications and considerations in Chap. 8, Fig. 8.13);
3. Inferior alveolar neurovascular bundle osteotomy lines marked on the mandible: for freeing and preserving the

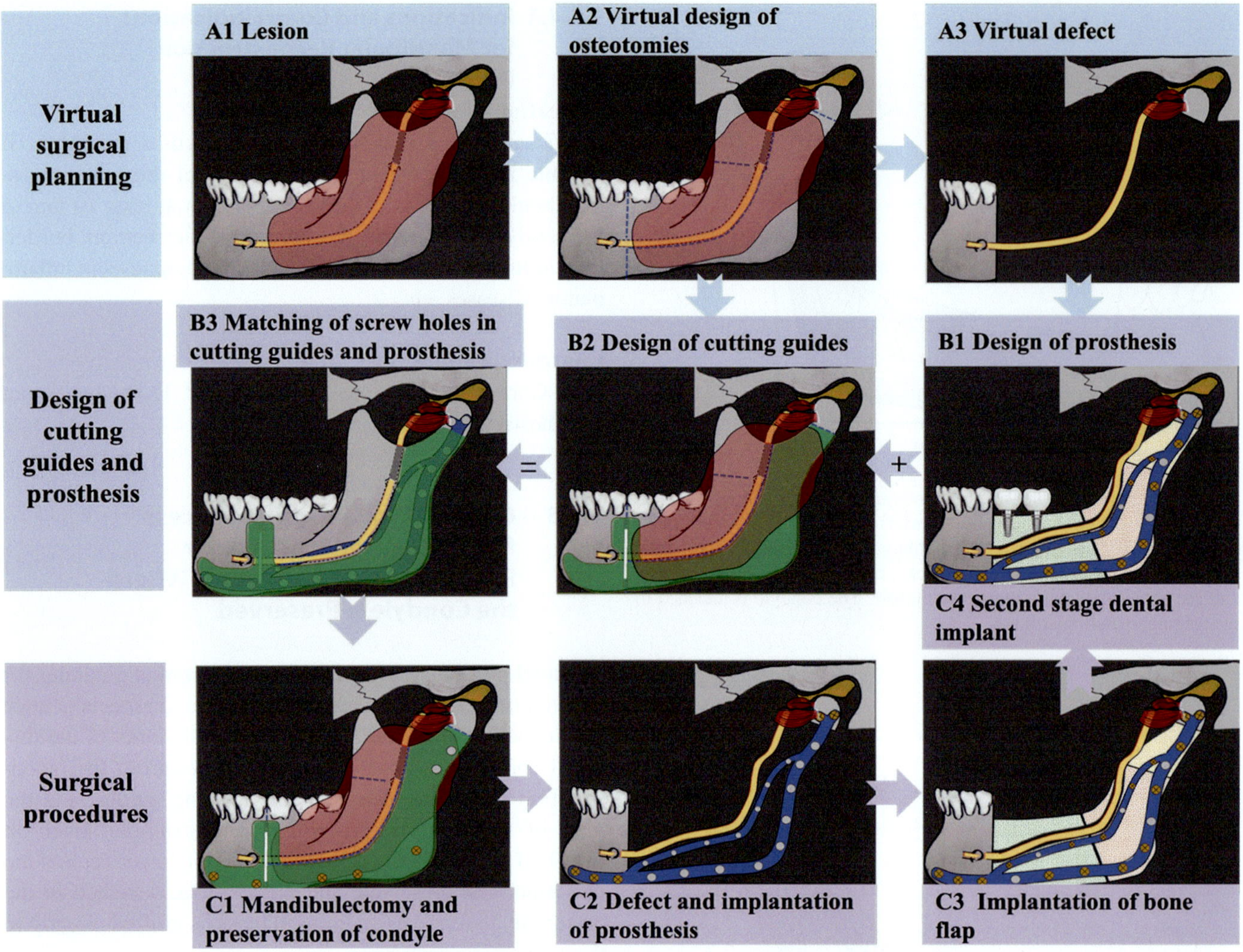

Fig. 9.10 Digital design of a customized mandibular reconstruction prosthesis. A1. Use CT 3D reconstruction to define the extent of the lesion (transparent red), and mark the course of the inferior alveolar neurovascular bundle within the mandible (yellow). A2. In designing the osteotomy lines, plan to retain the inferior alveolar neurovascular bundle by shallowly excising the cortical bone along its edges, and preserve the healthy joint attachments such as the lateral pterygoid muscle and the articular disc. A3. In simulated osteotomy to obtain the defect space model, plan to retain the condyle (the end of the mandibular ramus), the articular disc (brown), and the lateral pterygoid muscle (red). B1. Following the dimensions of the defect model, the mandibular reconstruction prosthesis is designed and manufactured. B2. Design the osteotomy cutting guide (green) to indicate several osteotomy lines, according to the osteotomy plan. B3. Transfer the positions of the mandibular reconstuction prosthesis screw holes to the osteotomy cutting guide. C1. Perform osteotomy according to the markings of the osteotomy cutting guide. C2. Install the customized mandibular reconstruction prosthesis; check the joint and occlusion. C3. Affix the autogenous graft bone block to the prosthesis with screws. C4. Complete the second phase dental implantation according to the preoperative design

inferior alveolar neurovascular bundle, shallowly excising the cortical bone along its edges
4. Distal osteotomy line: for safe resection of the lesion (Fig. 9.10, A2)
The above osteotomy lines will be used for designing the osteotomy positioning cutting guides.
   - Defect modeling: A model of the defect to be left after the osteotomies is obtained through digitally simulating resection of the lesion at the osteotomy lines. Some adjustment may need to be made with reference to the healthy side of the face, for facial symmetry. This model will be used in design of the mandibular reconstruction prosthesis and osteotomy cutting guides (Fig. 9.10, A3).

9.1.5.1 Digital design of mandibular reconstruction prosthesis and osteotomy cutting guides

- Mandibular reconstruction prosthesis size design: Design the mandibular reconstruction prosthesis (Fig. 9.10, B1) based on the defect model (Fig. 9.10, A3). The requirements are the same as in Chap. 8, Sect. 8.1.5, Digital design of customized TMJ-mandibular joint prosthesis in the general process of digital design (2) in the design of the prosthesis and the cutting guides.
- Mandibular reconstruction prosthesis shape design: As described before in Chap. 8, design the mandibular reconstruction prosthesis by taking the contralateral teeth as the reference for designing the dental implants as well as determining the ideal position of autogenous grafted bone. The shape of the mandibular reconstruction prosthesis is required to achieve retention strength for all of the grafted bone blocks as well as weight reduction and aesthetics of the face and teeth. This part of the design reflects the functional necessity for joint-mandibular-occlusal reconstruction.
Finally, the screw holes in the mandibular reconstruction prosthesis are designed so that the screw holes in the condylar portion of the prosthesis should be as far away from the articular surface as possible, while requiring that the reconstruction prosthesis will maintain stability with the condyle, the autogenous graft bone, and the residual mandible. Also, they must avoid the positions of the reserved implant screws, so that the second-stage dental implantation can be carried out.
- Osteotomy positioning cutting guides design: Based on the osteotomy line design (Fig. 9.10, A2), design the osteotomy positioning cutting guides (Fig. 9.10, B2). If the condylar osteotomy line is lower than the mandibular notch, a cutting guide can be designed to locate the osteotomy lines of the condylar end, the mandibular end, and the inferior alveolar neurovascular bundle (see Sect. 8.1.5.2 Prosthesis and Osteotomy Cutting Guide Design). If the condylar osteotomy line is near the condyle, in order to prevent the cutting guide from being too long, it can be designed as two cutting guides, one to locate the condylar osteotomy line and the other to locate the mandible and preserve the inferior alveolar neurovascular bundle osteotomy line.
Matching osteotomy cutting guides to mandibular reconstruction prosthesis screw holes: Overlay the images in Figs. 9.10, B1 and B2 to determine the screw hole locations on the cutting guides based on the screw holes of the mandibular reconstruction prosthesis. The result of this is that not only is the osteotomy precise, but the installation is also precise, simple, and fast, without the need for an intermaxillary ligation (Fig. 9.10, B3).
Design of the autogenous graft osteotomy cutting guide: The autogenous graft osteotomy cutting guide is designed according to the size and dimensions of the autogenous graft bone designed in the defect model.

9.1.6 Surgical Procedure

- Condylar and mandibular osteotomies (Fig. 9.10, C1):
   1. Condylar osteotomy: A modified anterior auriculotemporal incision is used to expose the condyle, but the joint capsule is not opened, and the lateral pterygoid muscle is preserved. The condylar osteotomy guide is placed in position to resect the neck just above the posterior extent of the condylar lesion.
   2. Mandibular osteotomy: Mandibular osteotomy involves fixing the mandible and preserving the positioning cutting guide for the inferior alveolar neurovascular bundle osteotomy. Subsequently, the inferior alveolar neurovascular bundle and mandibular osteotomy are performed in sequence. When performing the inferior alveolar neurovascular bundle osteotomy, only a single cortical bone is first cut, the osteotomy positioning cutting guide is removed, the bone chisel is used to cut the osteotomy line, and the diseased tissue above and below the nerve tube is removed in sections. If the disease invades soft tissue, attention should be paid to the integrity of the edges.
- Mandibular reconstruction prosthesis installation:
   1. Following the cutting guide screw holes, the mandibular reconstruction prosthesis and condyle are fixed in place; if only one screw can be fixed in place at first, it needs to have enough length to maintain interoperative stability.

2. The same reasoning fixes the mandibular reconstruction prosthesis to the mandibular stump while checking and satisfying occlusal stability of the remaining teeth and good condylar position (Fig. 9.10, C2).

- Autogenous graft bone implantation: the autogenous graft bone has been harvested and trimmed with the guidance of the cutting guide, and the autogenous graft bone block is seated and secured according to the design and embedded with the inferior alveolar neurovascular bundle (Fig. 9.10, C3).
- Occlusal reconstruction: restored in a second phase with dental implantation (Fig. 9.10, C4).

9.2 Application of Customized Mandibular Reconstruction Prosthesis Reconstruction Where the TMJ Can Be Preserved

Minjie Chen and Jisi Zheng

This section, through one clinical case of a Class IVb defect in Yang's new classification (mandibular lesion with salvageable joint), provides a complete review of the entire process from mandibular reconstruction prosthesis design and clinical application to follow-up 5 years later. The prosthesis which was applied was the simpler one (Fig. 9.8), since the lesion, though large, did not extend as far posterior as the back edge of the jaw and did not involve the condyle.

9.2.1 Case R Design and Application of a Mandibular Reconstruction Prosthesis Preserving the Condyle and Mandibular Lower Posterior Margin

- Patient information: male, 34 years old.
- Complaint: recurrence of ameloblastoma of the left mandible more than 1 year after curettage.
- History: the patient presented 4 years ago with recurrent mouth opening limitation and left mandibular swelling. Two years ago, he underwent open decompression surgery and curettage for a left mandibular mass in an outside hospital, and the postoperative pathology showed ameloblastoma of the left mandible, which recurred 1 year after the surgery.
- Past history: physically fit, denies history of systemic disease. History of drug and food allergies denied.
- Clinical examination: facial asymmetry, enlargement of the left parotid occlusal region, scarring of the submandibular region, bilateral symmetry of sensation in the mandibular region, and no abnormalities. There was no tenderness in the joints bilaterally (Fig. 9.11), and the mouth opening was 35 mm. There was no fistula in the mouth, and the occlusal relationship was stable (Fig. 9.12).
- Imaging examination: panoramic radiographs showed cystic displacement of the left coronoid process proximal to the articulation and involving part of the mandibular ramus and mandibular body, with obvious swelling

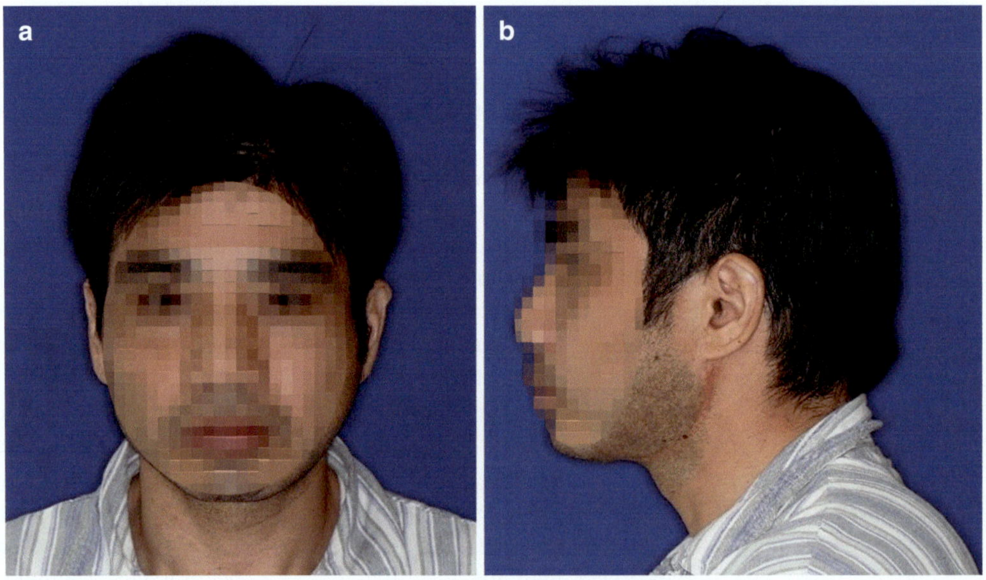

Fig. 9.11 Case R. Extraoral examination showing facial asymmetry, swelling in the left parotid and masseter region, and a scar on the left submandibular region from earlier surgery. (**a**) Frontal view. (**b**) Lateral view

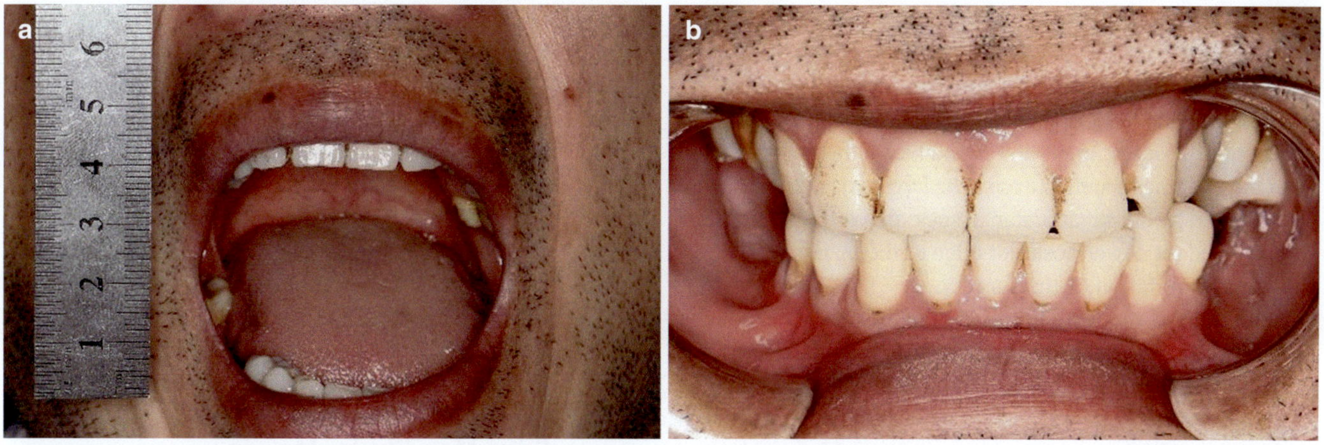

Fig. 9.12 Case R. Intraoral examination shows a 35 mm mouth opening and a stable occlusal relationship. (**a**) Open mouth. (**b**) Intraoral occlusal condition

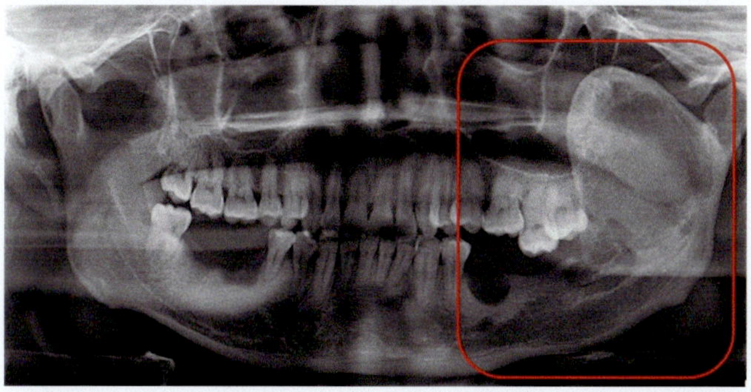

Fig. 9.13 Case R. Preoperative panoramic X-ray. The red box shows a cystic mass occupying the left mandible coronoid process and adjacent areas, but not the condyle

(Fig. 9.13). CT scan showed that the left mandibular body had bone defects, and the remnant mandibular ramus and mandibular body had swelling (the size of the lesion about 6 cm × 2.7 cm), with multiple cystic hypodense shadows and bone resorption, but no obvious abnormality of the surrounding soft tissues, and the posterior lower margin of the mandible was intact (Fig. 9.14).

- Diagnosis: recurrence of ameloblastoma of the left mandible.
- Postoperative pathology: microscopic description, bone tissue 6 cm × 4.5 cm × 4 cm, cystic wall-like tissue in the inner wall of the cavity, grayish-white and grayish-red with wall thickness 1 mm to 2 mm, and yellow tissue with grainy texture like dregs of soya bean pressing attached to the capsule in some areas. Pathology diagnosis: recurrent left mandible ameloblastoma with cystic degeneration.

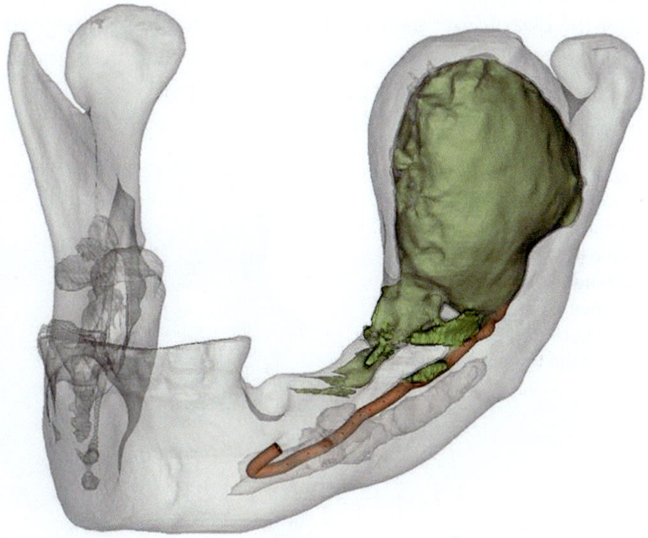

Fig. 9.14 Case R. Relationship of the mass (green) to mandible. The posterior lower edge of the mandible is intact, suggesting that it and the condyle may be preserved, and the inferior alveolar neurovascular bundle (orange) adjacent to the lower margin of the lesion may be retained since the lesion is a benign cystic lesion

9.2.2 Case R. Diagnostic Imaging

9.2.3 Case R. Treatment Plan

- Overall treatment plan: resection of the left mandibular lesion proximal to but not involving the joint, repair of the mandible with free iliac bone graft, and customized mandibular reconstruction prosthesis (condyle and mandibular posterior margin preservation type).

- Surgical resection design.

  Design of the resection scope: partial resection of the left coronoid process, mass and mandible; temporary removal of the zygomatic arch to excise the large mass beneath, with preservation of the articular tissues above the mandibular notch and the lower posterior edge of the mandible.
- Digital simulation of the surgery.

  Temporary osteotomy of the zygomatic arch: the anterior and posterior osteotomy lines of the zygomatic arch are identified, and the zygomatic arch is resected, preserving the joint capsule as well as the underlying attachments of the joint, which are pushed anteriorly and inferiorly (red arrows) to expose the coronal lesion (Fig. 9.15).

Resection of the lesion and modeling of the defect left after the osteotomy: the osteotomy lines should be designed to preserve the posterior lower mandibular margin as much as possible, as well as the condyle (Fig. 9.16).

- Autogenous graft bone design: Model the cranium as after resetting the zygomatic arch. Create an autogenous iliac bone graft design (bone cortex up for all pieces) with the goal of restoring the dentition, while planning to place the inferior alveolar neurovascular bundle mostly on the lateral side of the graft (Fig. 9.17).

9.2.4 Case R. Design and Processing of the Mandibular Reconstruction Prostheses and Osteotomy Positioning Cutting Guides with Preservation of the Condylar Process and Lower Edge Mandibular Margin

- Design of a mandibular reconstruction prosthesis with preservation of the condylar process and lower edge of mandibular margin.

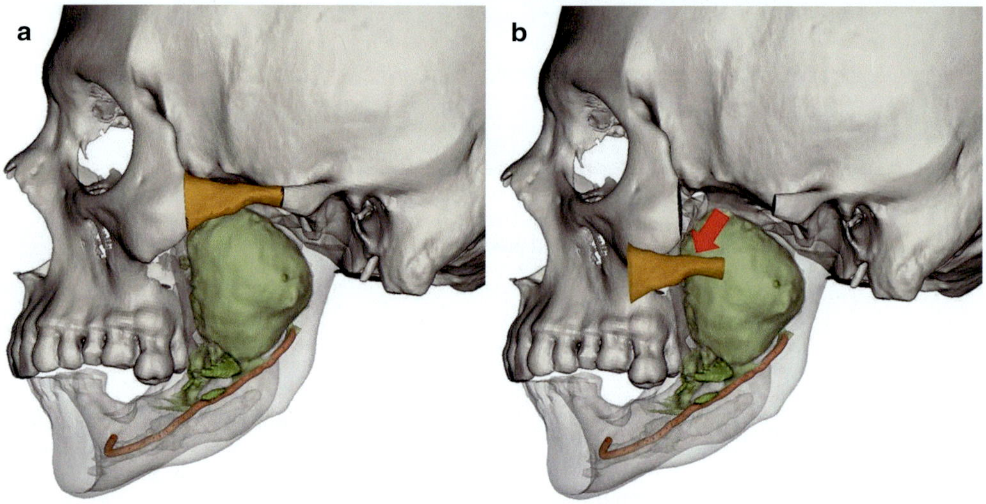

Fig. 9.15 Case R. Temporary zygomatic arch (yellow) osteotomy. (**a**) Zygomatic arch osteotomy lines. (**b**) Pushing the detached zygomatic arch forward and downward (red arrow) to expose the tumor (green)

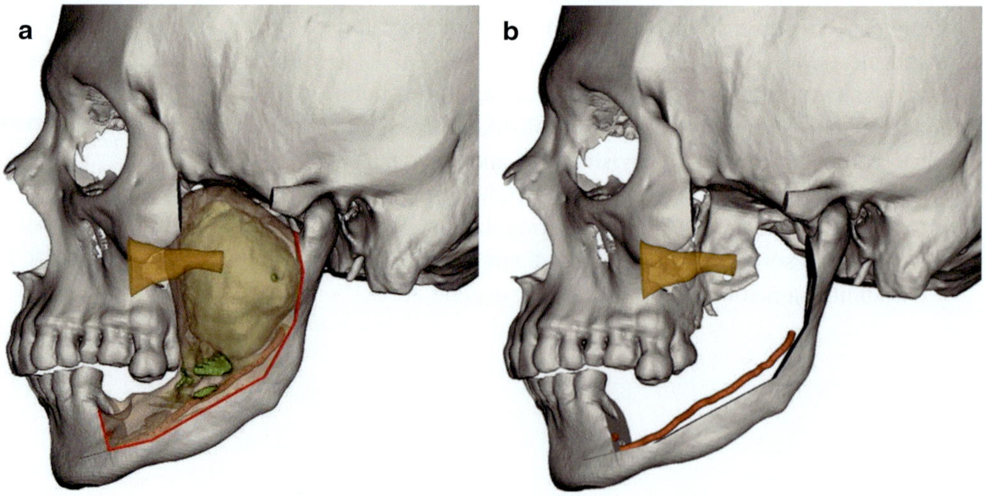

Fig. 9.16 Case R. Design of the osteotomy line preserving the back lower mandibular margin and the condyle. (**a**) Design of the osteotomy line (red line). (**b**) Model of the mandibular defect after osteotomy with the inferior alveolar neurovascular bundle (to be preserved) shown in orange

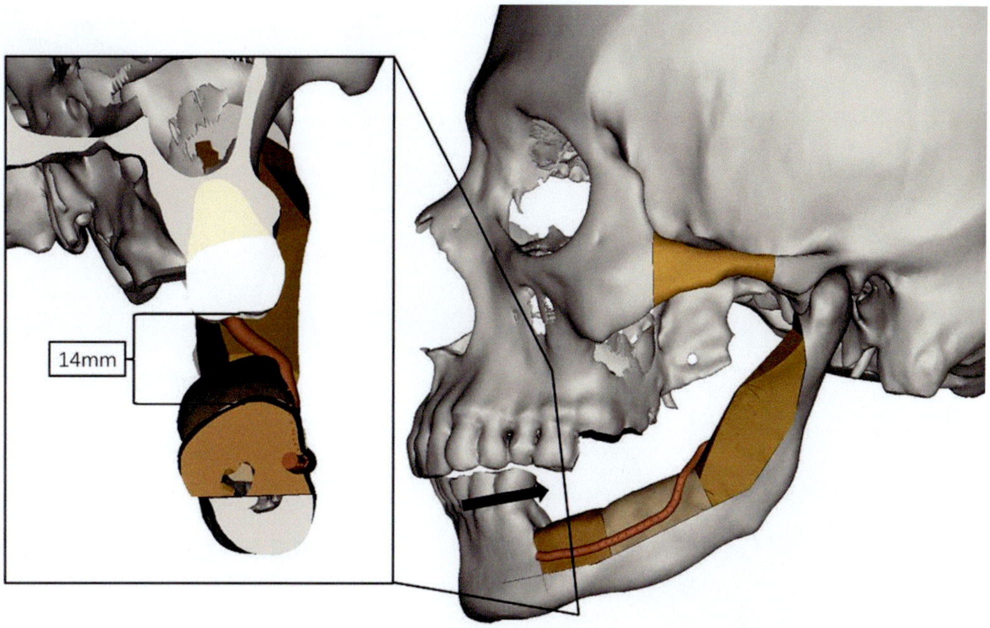

Fig. 9.17 Case R. Autogenous bone graft fixation design (in mm) (orange). The top of the grafted bone is 14 mm from the upper tooth root plane. The inferior alveolar neurovascular bundle is mostly set on the lateral side of the graft

Principles of mandibular reconstruction prosthesis design: based on the design of individualized TMJ and craniomandibular prostheses in Chap. 2, Sect. 2.4.2.

According to joint-craniomandibular stress analysis of the full normal cranial stress distribution, the mandibular stresses are mainly distributed along the external oblique line and the lower back border of the mandible. This suggests that the mandibular reconstruction prosthesis should be designed with the main bracket along the external oblique line and the posterior inferior border of the mandible and that the two brackets can be connected by an "X" bracket to spread the stresses more evenly (Fig. 9.18).

- Fabrication of the mandibular reconstruction prosthesis plate: The prosthesis is made of titanium alloy and fabricated using a metal 3D printer. After fabrication, the reconstruction plate is test fitted on a resin head model to check if the plate fits the bone surface and is stable (Fig. 9.19).
- Digital design of osteotomy positioning cutting guides

Design of the zygomatic arch osteotomy cutting guide: design the zygomatic arch cutting guide to follow the zygomatic arch osteotomy line (Fig. 9.20).

Mandibular osteotomy cutting guide: design the mandibular osteotomy cutting guide to follow the condylar osteotomy line, mandibular osteotomy line, and inferior alveolar neurovascular bundle lines for intraoperative positioning, precise osteotomy, and preservation of the neurovascular bundle (Fig. 9.20).

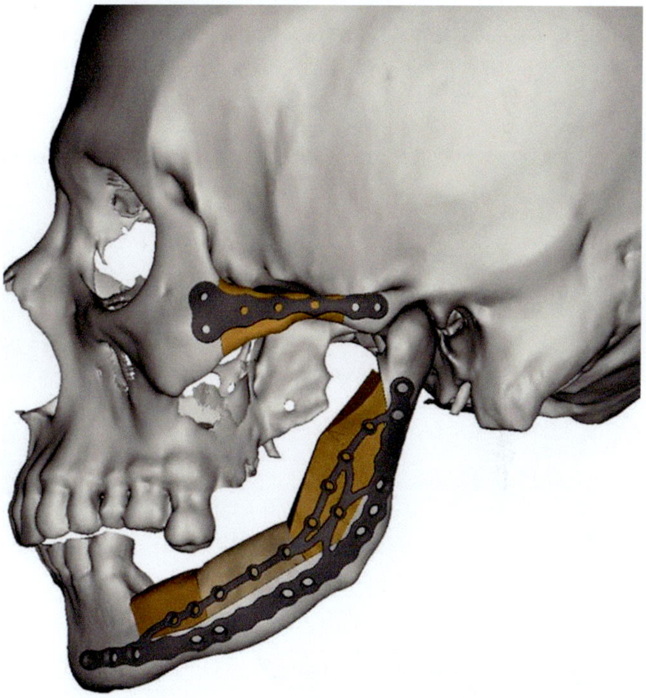

Fig. 9.18 Case R. Design of a mandibular reconstruction prosthesis (dark gray) serving for preservation of condyle and lower posterior mandibular edge, as well as fixation of autogenous bone graft. Plate to reattach the zygomatic arch is also shown

- Autogenous graft bone block osteotomy cutting guide design: after examining the shape of the ilium, determine the bone extraction area and design the osteotomy cutting guide (Fig. 9.21).

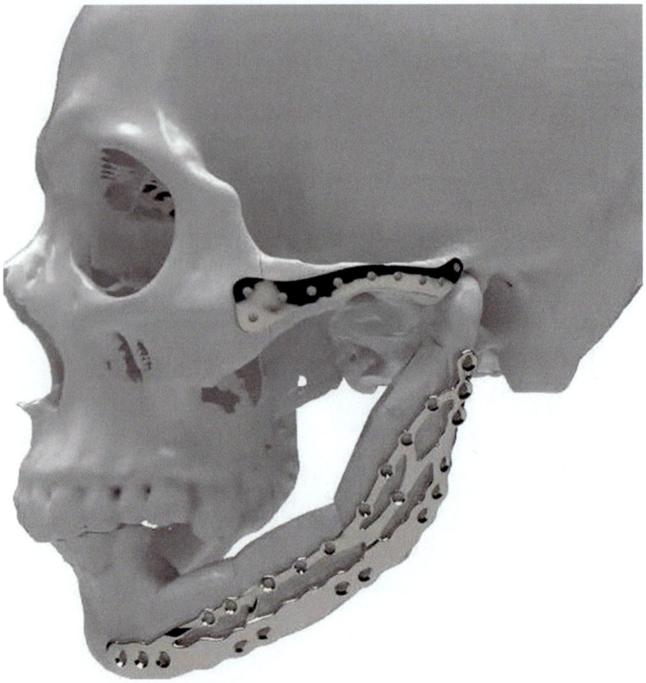

Fig. 9.19 Case R. Mandibular reconstruction prosthesis plate test fitting on a resin head model to check if the plate fits the bone surface and is stable

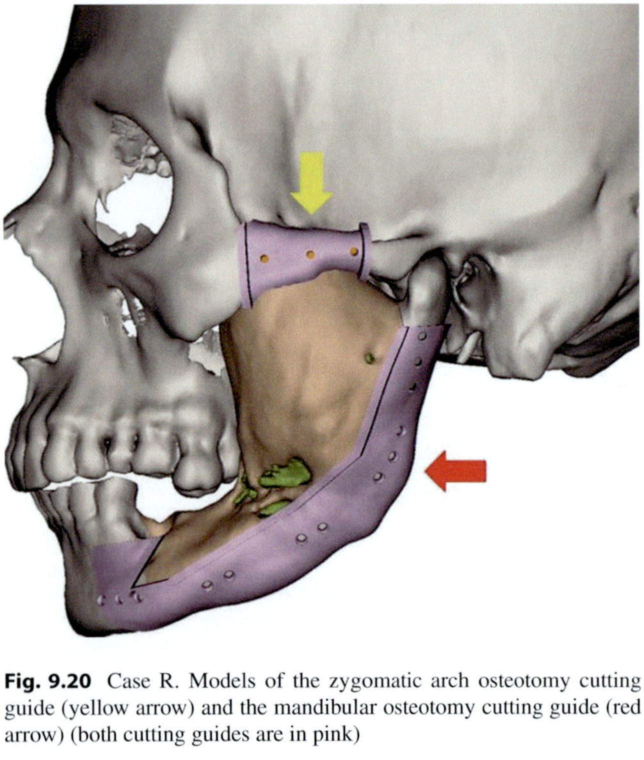

Fig. 9.20 Case R. Models of the zygomatic arch osteotomy cutting guide (yellow arrow) and the mandibular osteotomy cutting guide (red arrow) (both cutting guides are in pink)

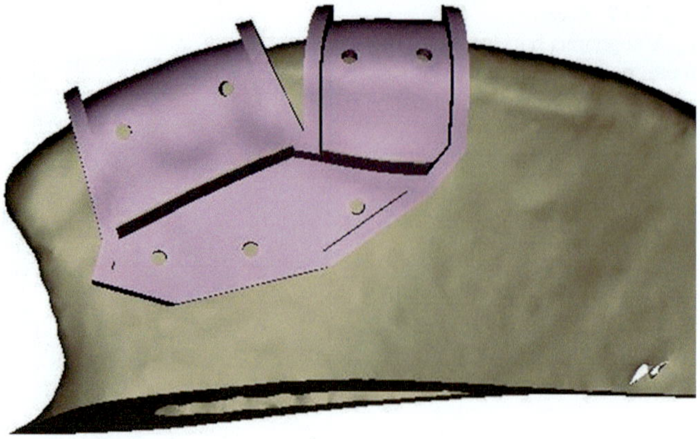

Fig. 9.21 Case R. Iliac osteotomy cutting guide (pink) design

9.2.5 Case R. Surgical Procedure

Preoperative laboratory tests: the same as described in "3.2.5 Case A. Surgical Procedure, Preoperative Laboratory Tests."

Preoperative preparation: prepare 400 mL of blood; other preparations, see "3.2.5 Case A. Surgical Procedure, Preoperative Preparation."

- Steps of the surgical procedure

Surgical approach: a modified anterior auriculotemporal incision connected with a submandibular incision was used to expose the joint, zygomatic arch, mandibular ramus, and mandibular body.

Zygomatic arch osteotomy: The zygomatic arch osteotomy cutting guide is installed and the zygomatic arch is temporarily severed, taking care not to detach the masseter attachments. The severed zygomatic arch is then retracted and the zygomatic arch, and the masseter muscle are put to one side, exposing the lesion while protecting the facial nerve (Fig. 9.22).

Resection of the lesion: using the mandibular osteotomy cutting guide to determine the lower border of the lesion, the inferior alveolar neurovascular bundle is isolated and preserved, and the lesion is completely removed, also preserving the lower posterior margin of the mandible (Figs. 9.23 and 9.24).

Autogenous iliac bone grafting: iliac osteotomy cutting guides are utilized to assist in bone harvesting (Fig. 9.25).

Installation of mandibular reconstruction prosthesis and fixation of iliac bone graft: installation of mandibular recon-

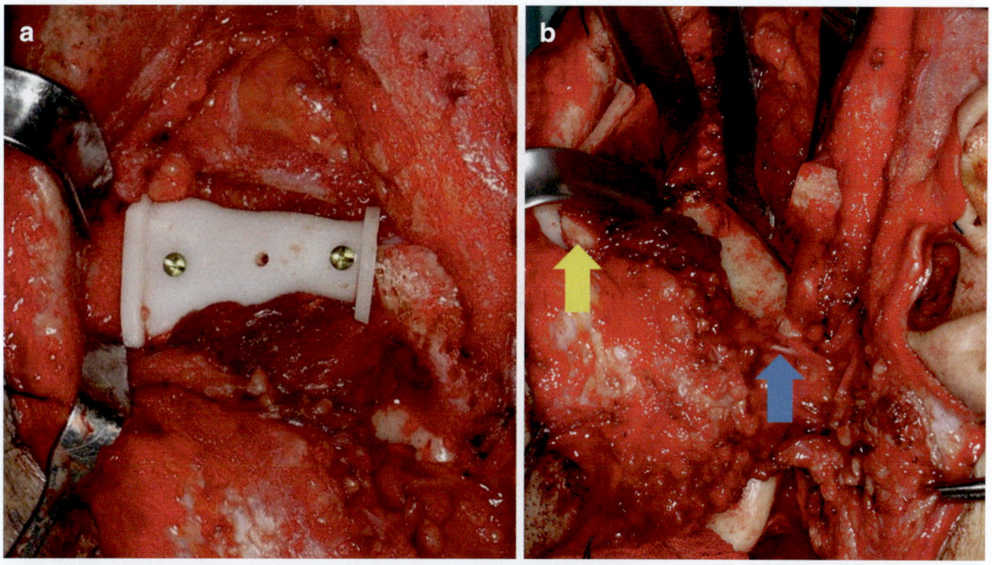

Fig. 9.22 Case R. Surgical approach and lesion exposure. Yellow arrow shows the severed zygomatic arch and the occlusal muscle, and blue arrow shows the facial nerve. (**a**) Temporary truncation of the zygomatic arch. (**b**) Exposure of the lesion

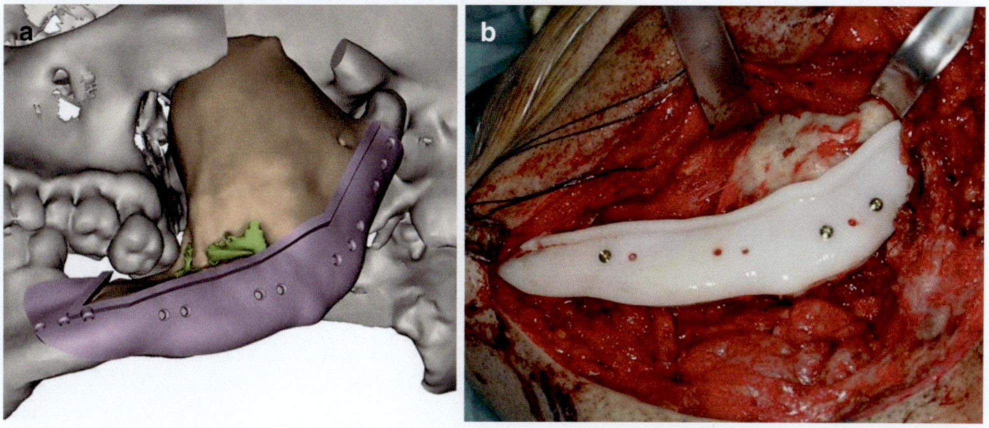

Fig. 9.23 Case R. Mandibular osteotomy cutting guide assists in the removal of the lesion with preservation of the inferior alveolar neurovascular bundle. (**a**) Design. (**b**) Actual

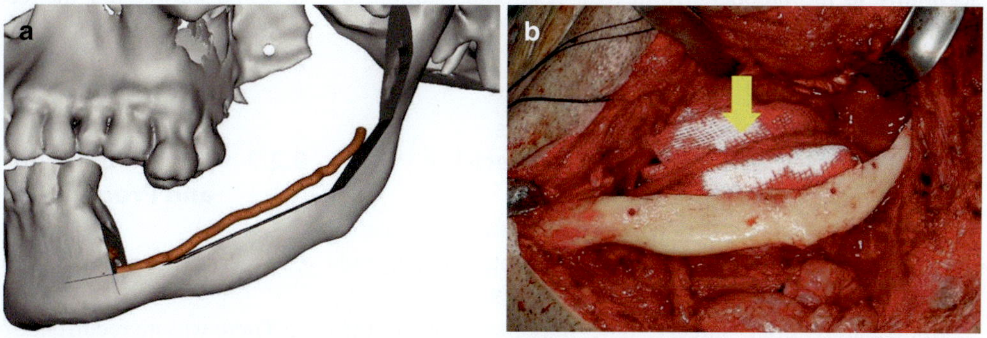

Fig. 9.24 Case R. Lesion resected while the inferior alveolar neurovascular bundle is preserved. (**a**) Design of the defect model (neurovascular bundle in orange). (**b**) Actual (yellow arrow points to the neurovascular bundle)

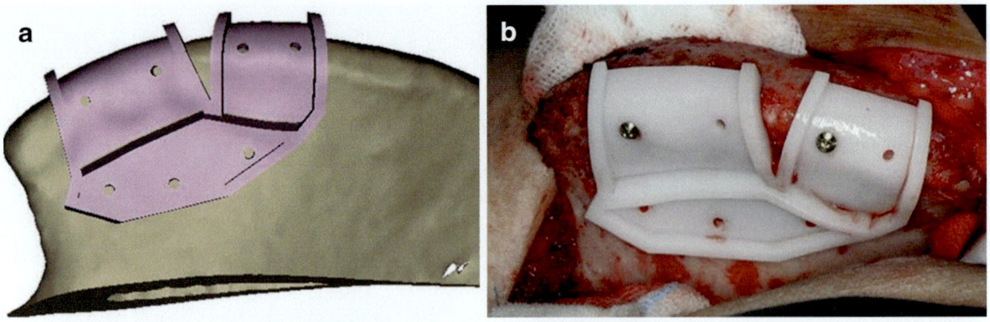

Fig. 9.25 Case R. Iliac osteotomy cutting guides for precise harvesting of the bone, in segments. (**a**) Design. (**b**) Actual

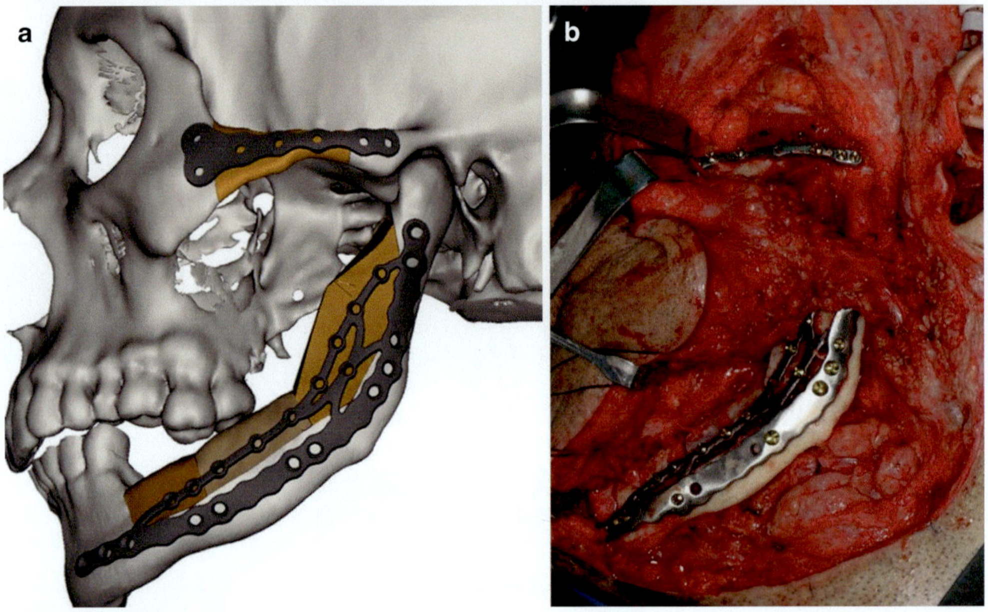

Fig. 9.26 Case R. Installation of the mandibular reconstruction prosthesis with autogenous graft bone fixation; also, zygomatic arch repositioning and fixation with titanium plate. (**a**) Design. (**b**) Actual

struction prosthesis and fixation of autogenous graft bone according to the preoperative design; reset and fixation of zygomatic arch also shown (Fig. 9.26).

9.2.6 Case R. Postoperative Analysis of Prosthesis Implantation Precision

Regular postoperative follow-up was performed for cosmetic (facial shape), functional (mouth opening, mouth shape), and reconstruction plate evaluation (safety, accuracy).

Immediately after surgery: The intraoperative cutting guide was accurately seated, and the mandibular reconstruction plate was installed smoothly (Fig. 9.27). A comparison between the preoperative design and the postoperative reconstruction showed that the reconstruction plate was accurately seated (Fig. 9.28); the reconstruction plate installation error was 1.14 mm (Fig. 9.29).

9.2.7 Case R. Long-Term Follow-Up and Prognosis

- 5-year postoperative follow-up

There was no recurrence of the tumor, good facial appearance without abnormalities, and no redness or other reactions in the surgical area. Normal eating.

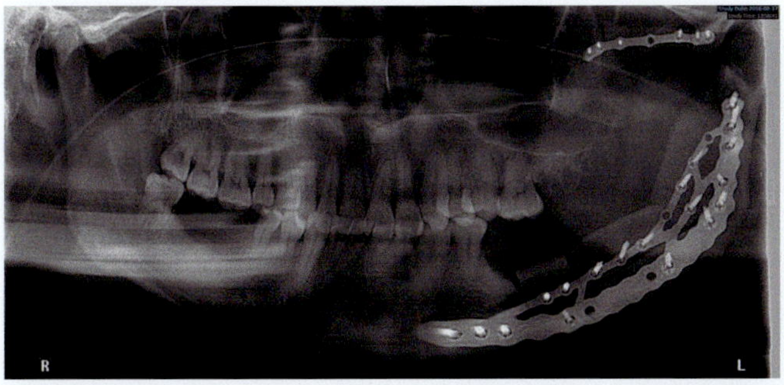

Fig. 9.27 Case R. Immediate postoperative panoramic X-ray shows that the prosthesis and the transplanted bone block are in place and stable, without displacement

The pain in the mandibular region disappeared, the VAS pain score dropped to 0, and the joint-mandibular-occlusal-facial pattern was harmonized with a stable occlusal relationship (Fig. 9.30).

The mouth opening improved to 38 mm, with 6 mm lateral motion on the affected side and 6 mm lateral motion on the healthy side, and the mouth opening pattern was even (Fig. 9.31).

Evaluation of the grafted bone and reconstruction plate: The panoramic view showed that the reconstruction plate had been removed, with good autogenous bone incorporation though with some localized autogenous bone resorption

Fig. 9.28 Case R. Postoperative CT reconstruction comparison showing accurate positioning of the mandibular reconstruction plate. (**a**) Preoperative design. (**b**) Immediate postoperative

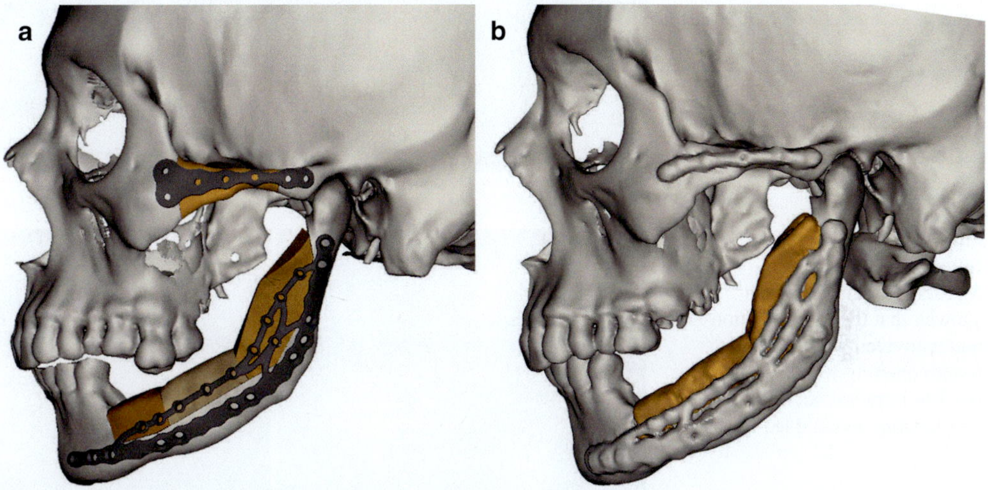

Fig. 9.29 Case R. Mandibular reconstruction prosthesis maximum error was 1.14 mm. (**a**) Lateral error. (**b**) Medial error

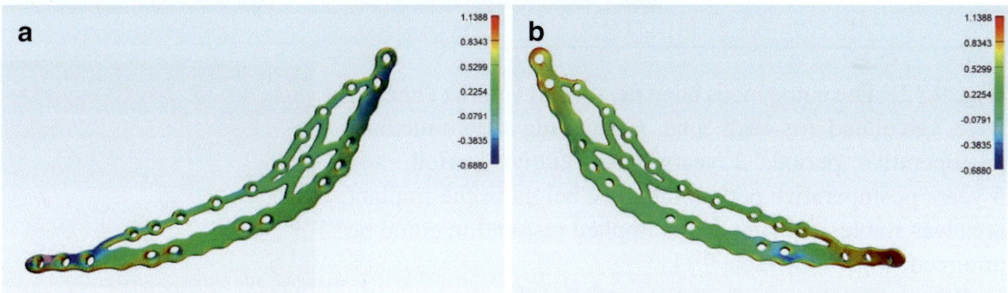

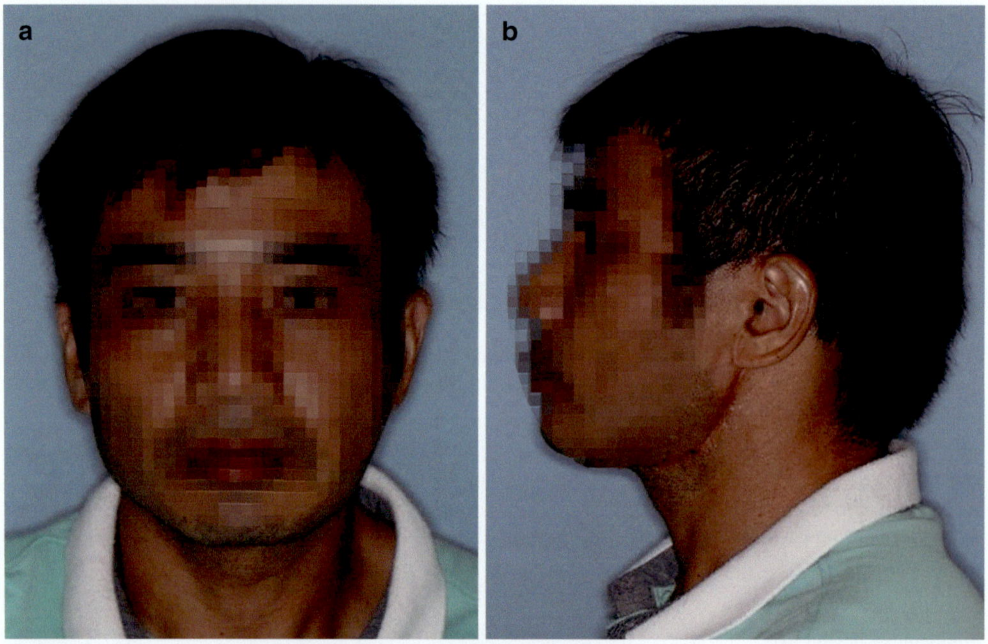

Fig. 9.30 Case R. The 5-year postoperative follow-up showed a good appearance with no abnormalities, and no reactions such as redness or swelling in the surgical area. (**a**) Front view. (**b**) Lateral view

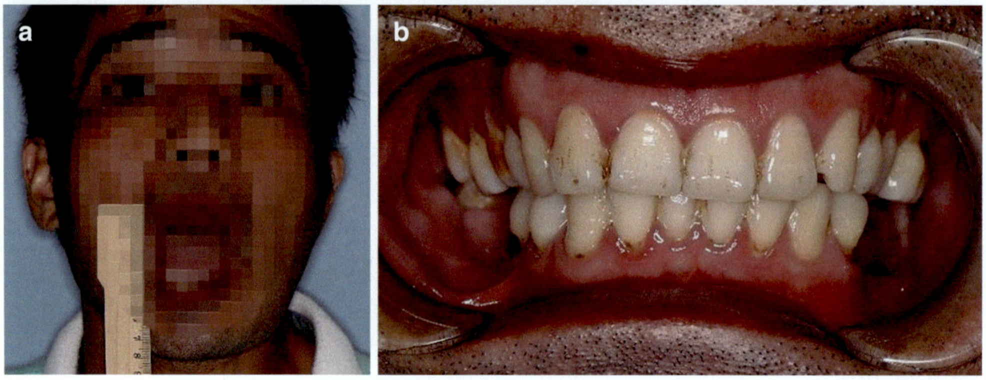

Fig. 9.31 Case R. A follow-up examination 5 years after the operation showed that the joint function had recovered well. (**a**) The mouth opening was 38 mm. (**b**) The intraoral occlusal relationship was stable

(Fig. 9.32). The autogenous bone height and volume changes were calculated for each time. Comparing the immediate postoperative period, 2 years postoperative period, and 5 years postoperative period, the bone height in the implant area was stable, and later dental implant restoration could be arranged (Fig. 9.33, Table 9.1).

Others: The degree of numbness of the lower lip basically returned to the preoperative level at 6 months postoperatively. The bone healed well after zygomatic arch replantation, indicating that zygomatic arch removal and replantation, preserving the masseter muscle attachment, does not induce bone resorption.

Volume in mm^3, surface area in mm^2, length in mm.

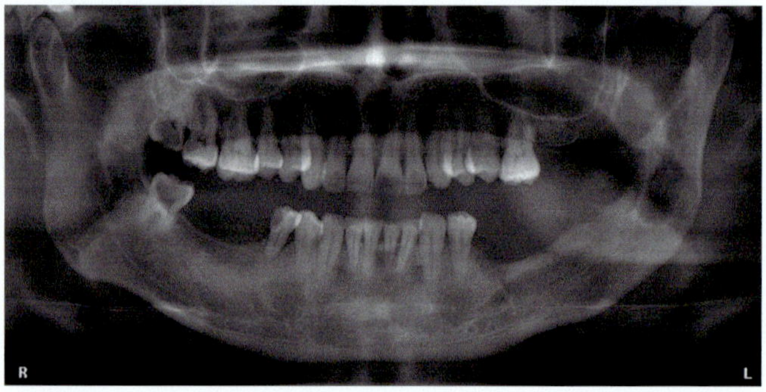

Fig. 9.32 Case R. Panoramic radiograph 5 years after surgery showed that the reconstruction plate had been removed, and the autogenous bone had been well integrated, though some autologous bone had been absorbed

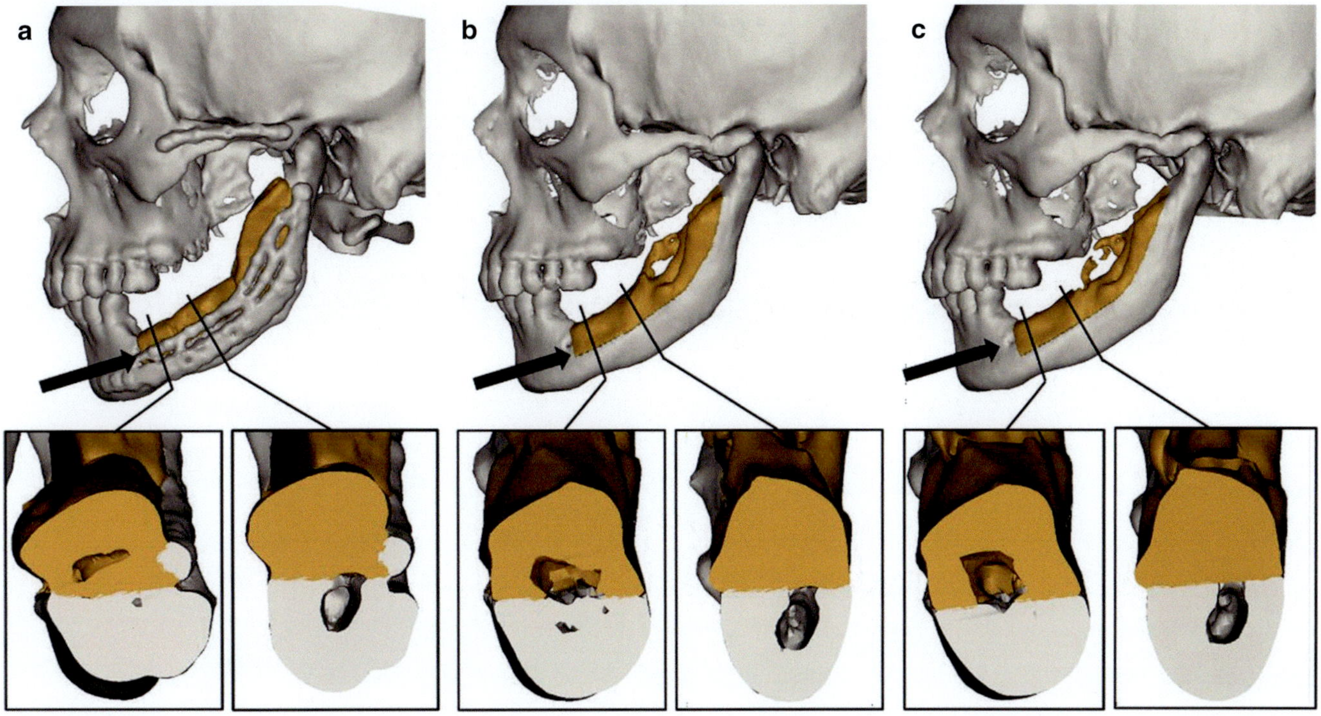

Fig. 9.33 Case R. Comparison of CT reconstruction of cross-sections of the mandible, showing good integration of original bone (white) and autogenous graft bone (orange). (**a**) Immediate postoperative period. (**b**) 2 years postoperatively. C. 5 years postoperatively

Table 9.1 Changes in bone mass volume, surface area, and height by follow-up time points

	Follow-up time		
Bone mass condition	Immediately after surgery	2 years after surgery	5 years after surgery
Bone mass volume	12,411.92	9955.11	9323.85
Surface area of a bone block	5945.04	4698.43	4545.18
Lower left 6 bone height in the implant area	12.03	11.81	11.76
Lower left 7 bone height in the implant area	12.11	12.02	11.97

9.2.8 Case R. Advantages and Disadvantages

- Advantages

The reconstruction plate is stable and reliable, as evidenced by the absence of adverse reactions and complications after a maximum of 5 years of follow-up.

Applying the stress distribution analysis, the design concept was more advanced in realizing the preservation of the condyle and the posterior lower edge of the mandible, maintaining the structure of the joint-mandibular-facial shape, which allows the restoration and balance of function.

High digital precision and numerical control of the entire process, including osteotomy, bone extraction, reconstruction design and manufacture, and installation. This customized mandibular reconstruction prosthesis is more useful in cases of restoration of mandibular defects with the condyle preserved to ensure that the condylar position and angle remain unchanged.

The dental implant area was composed of autogenous bone with cortex upward, effectively reducing bone resorption.

- Disadvantages

Free bone grafting is not indicated for infected lesions.

This bone graft design cannot be used in excessively long mandibular lesions.

An elective dental implantation was urgently needed, but the patient in this case refused.

Treatment for Condylar Dislocation

10

Chi Yang, Minjie Chen, and Zixiang Han

Condylar dislocation refers to the displacement of the condyle from the glenoid fossa due to spontaneous movement or external trauma, with anterior dislocation being the most common. The primary surgical treatment methods include: articular eminence augmentation, articular eminence reduction, and high condylectomy. However, these procedures share a common drawback—disruption of the joint structure and internal environment.

To avoid intracapsular surgery while maximizing joint integrity preservation, ensuring long-term stability, and achieving minimally invasive and efficient surgical execution, customized prostheses have emerged as the optimal solution for individualized condylar dislocation cases due to their highly tailored fit.

Design principles for such prostheses include:

1. Physiological motion retention: the prosthesis should permit condylar movement within normal physiological limits while preventing dislocation from the fossa.
2. Stability and durability: resistance to fracture and displacement.
3. Extracapsular placement: no violation of the joint capsule or intracapsular structures.
4. Ease of installation and precision: simplified yet accurate positioning.
5. Simplified design and fabrication: streamlined structure and manufacturing process.

The authors have developed two types of customized condylar dislocation prostheses, which, after over 2 years of clinical application, have successfully achieved the intended objectives.

10.1 Overview of Condylar Dislocation and Its Treatment

Chi Yang and Minjie Chen

This section will first review the definition of condylar dislocation and classify the various kinds of dislocation that are commonly seen in practice. The classification is made according to the farthest positions of the condyle in the open mouth (anterior) and closed mouth (posterior) positions, as seen in MRI examination. This section will continue with a summary of the traditional surgical treatments, as well as their advantages and disadvantages. It will introduce innovative kinds of titanium plate protheses for condylar dislocation treatment that have been applied in our clinical practice and how they are digitally measured to fit and be customized for the patient. Following, two clinical cases will be presented in two subsequent sections, one of each kind.

10.1.1 Definition of Condylar Dislocation

Condylar movement beyond the joint fossa, beyond the normal limits of joint movement, is called condylar dislocation or temporomandibular joint (TMJ) dislocation. Its clinical symptoms are mostly manifested as abnormal jaw movement, the jaw extended forward, the front teeth not meeting in occlusion with the lower teeth and with an open space or anterior crossbite, and a shallow depression can be felt in front of the ear when it is pressed (palpation examination). Aside from pain or discomfort, long-term or repeated dislocation often causes serious speech and eating difficulties for the patient.

Chi Y. (✉) · Minjie C · Zixiang H.
Shanghai Ninth People's Hospital, Shanghai Jiao Tong University
School of Medicine, Shanghai, China

© People's Medical Publishing House, PR of China 2025
Chi Y. (ed.), *Atlas of Customized TMJ-Cranio-Jaw Prosthesis*, https://doi.org/10.1007/978-981-95-0611-8_10

10.1.2 Classification of Condylar Dislocation

Condylar dislocations can be categorized into unilateral and bilateral dislocations according to their location; acute, recurrent, and old dislocations according to their nature; and anterior, posterior, superior, and lateral dislocations according to the direction and location of the dislocation, with anterior dislocations being the most common, and the latter three mainly due to traumatic injuries. This chapter focuses on recurrent and old dislocations that require surgical intervention.

10.1.2.1 Classification of Recurrent Condylar Dislocations

Recurrent condylar dislocation, also known as habitual dislocation, refers to condylar dislocation that occurs repeatedly during normal mandibular movement. The author has proposed a classification based on whether the articular disc is displaced or not, as can be seen through MRI imaging (Fig. 10.1). These are Class I, normal disc-condylar relationship in the mouth closed position and condylar dislocation in the maximum open position, and Class II, anterior displacement of the articular disc in the closed position and condylar dislocation in the maximum open position.

10.1.2.2 Classification of Old Condylar Dislocations

Whether it is an acute condylar dislocation or a recurrent condylar dislocation, if the jaw has not been reset for a period of several weeks, it is called an "old" dislocation. When the condyle has been dislocated out of the fossa for a long time, the local tissues of the joint become torn and squeezed, so there are often different degrees of connective tissue or bone tissue proliferation around the joint, especially in the posterior part of the condyle, and there are different degrees of spasticity in the corresponding muscles of mastication. The longer the dislocation, the more severe these changes are, and the more difficult it is to reset the joint. The author proposes the following classification, depending on the degree of destruction of the joint structure (Fig. 10.2): Class I old dislocation, but short dislocation time, no changes in the bone structure of the joint, and basically no adhesion in the joint cavity; Class II old dislocation, longer dislocation time (3–6 months), changes in the bone structure of the joint, condylar hyperplasia (increased cell production) can be seen, and there are hyperplasia and adhesions in the joint cavity; and Class III old dislocation, involving longer dislocation time (6 months or more), significant changes in the bone structure of the joint, with obvious spasticity of the chewing muscles, a large number of hyperplasia and adhesions in the joint cavity, and even the formation of joint ankylosis.

10.1.3 Traditional Methods for Condylar Dislocation

Traditional surgical methods for recurrent and old condylar dislocations mainly include articular eminence augmenta-

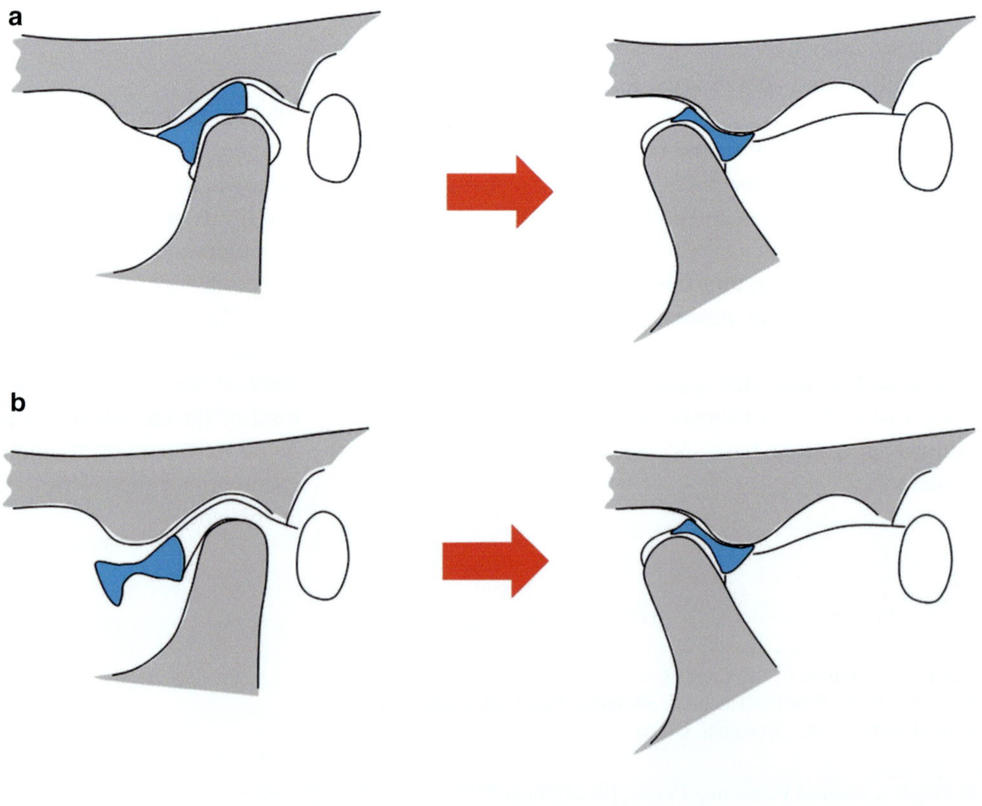

Fig. 10.1 Classification of recurrent condylar dislocations. Articular disc shown in blue. (**a**) Class I, normal disc-condylar relationship in the mouth closed position and anterior dislocation of the condyle in the mouth maximum open position. (**b**) Class II, anterior displacement of the disc in the closed position (left bottom figure) and condylar dislocation in the maximum open position

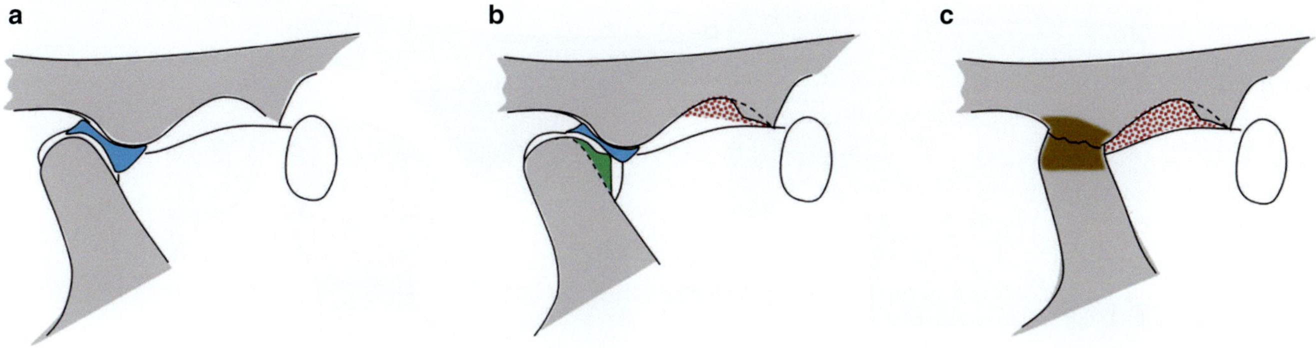

Fig. 10.2 Classification of old condylar dislocations. (**a**) Class I, articular disc (blue) has moved anteriorly past the articular eminence. (**b**) Class II shows deformed articular disc (blue), condylar hyperplastic bone (green), and adhesions in the articular cavity (red). (**c**) Class III, with brown showing the condyle with ankylosing and fusing bone, and red showing an ankylosing joint cavity with a great deal of hyperplasia and adhesions

tion, articular eminence flattening, high condylectomy, arthroplasty, articular disc repositioning, and articular ligament tightening. All these methods have some disadvantages.

10.1.3.1 Articular Eminence Augmentation

The forward motion of the condyle is checked by increasing the protrusion of the articular eminence. The most popular method is the Dautrey method (the zygomatic arch is cut obliquely and then reset lower), and some scholars have used the articular eminence bone split with inserted graft method, both of which come at the expense of the bone structure (Fig. 10.3). The author has proposed articular eminence augmentation with a small titanium plate, which preserves the articular structure, but with improvement through the use of a customized plate. In past practice, the small titanium plate was bent by the surgeon during the operation, but it was not possible to predict the natural trajectory of the condyle, and the material was relatively thin, so the plate could easily be fractured under repeated condylar impact (Fig. 10.4).

10.1.3.2 Articular Eminence Flattening

Articular eminence flattening was first utilized by Al-Kayat and Bramly in 1979 to remove obstructions in the route of condylar motion and allow it to move back and forth freely (Fig. 10.5). The biggest problem is that intracapsular resection of the joint disc will cause severe intracapsular adhesions and affect joint movement. Changes in the microenvironment of the articular cavity can also lead to degeneration.

10.1.3.3 High Condylar Resection

High condylectomy is mostly used in cases of old condylar dislocation with concomitant condylar hyperplasia. Condylar resection not only releases condylar entrapment in the mouth wide open position but also makes the condylar morphology more adapted to the articular fossa for stabilization after repositioning (Fig. 10.6). However, the loss of cartilage on the surface of the condyle after trimming makes it susceptible to secondary osteoarthropathy and ankylosis.

10.1.3.4 Joint Replacement with a Prosthesis

In patients with old dislocations secondary to severe osteoarthrosis or joint ankylosis, condylectomy and arthrodesis (replacement of the condylar extension with autologous bone or total joint prosthesis) are required to facilitate maintenance of mandibular ramus height and occlusion (Fig. 10.7).

10.1.3.5 Joint Disc Repositioning/Joint Ligament Tightening

For Class I recurrent dislocations with a normal closed disc-condylar relationship, tightening the ligament at the posterior side of the articular disc can be performed, so that the condyle does not move so far forward when the mouth is opened. For Class II recurrent dislocations, the disc is also displaced in the mouth-closed position, but the disc can be repositioned. These two methods of treatment are less invasive, but there is still a certain recurrence rate.

10.1.4 Innovative Repair Methods for Condylar Dislocation with Customized Prostheses

To resolve the many deficiencies and shortcomings of the traditional condylar dislocation surgical methods, the author's team has designed several prostheses to treat condylar dislocation, with application depending on the above classifications of recurrent and old condylar dislocations. The intention is to achieve a highly effective resolution for condylar dislocation, while maintaining the complete preser-

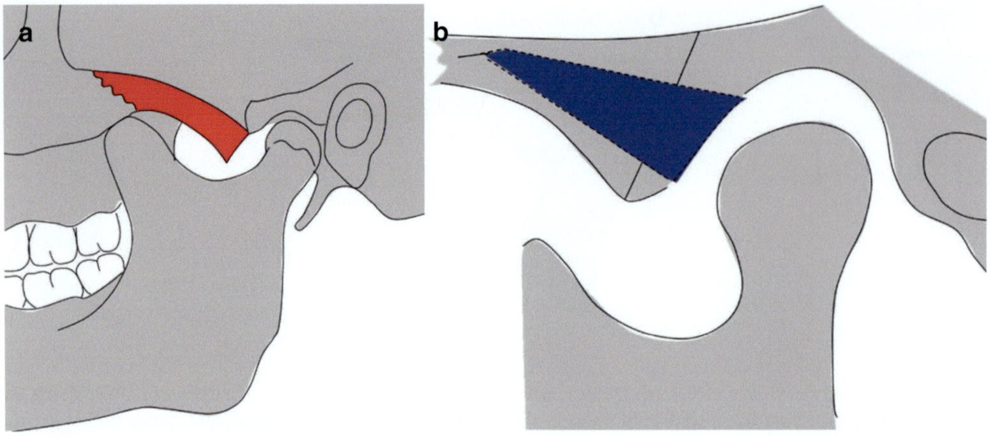

Fig. 10.3 Articular eminence augmentation. (**a**) Dautrey method (shifting the zygomatic arch downward), in which the zygomatic arch is cut obliquely, moved down, and reset (red) to increase the protrusion of the articular tubercle. (**b**) Split-articular implantation, in which the articular eminence is split from its posterior edge, obliquely, and a bone graft is placed at the site of the split (blue) to increase the protrusion of the articular eminence

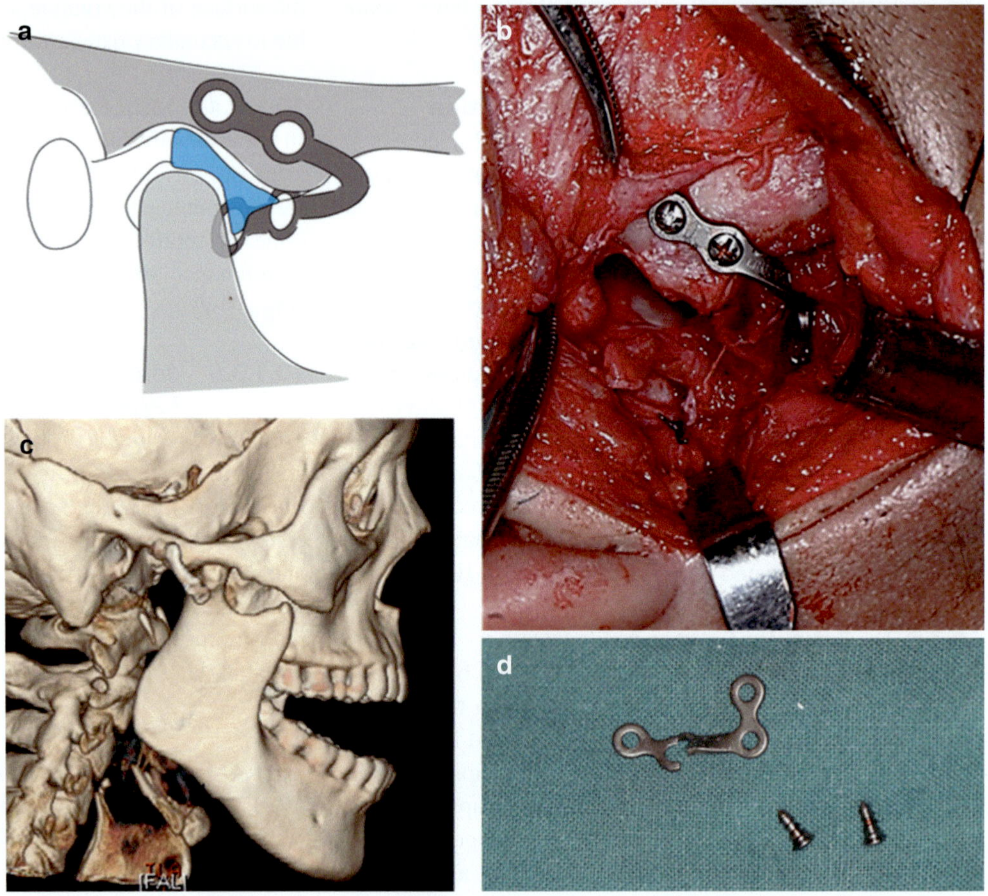

Fig. 10.4 Small titanium plate applied for articular eminence augmentation. (**a**) Schematic illustration of this method, in which a small titanium plate was implanted anterior to the articular eminence to increase its height and block the condyle. (**b**) Intraoperative implantation of the small titanium plate. (**c**) Postoperative review showing fracture of the small titanium plate and recurrence of the dislocation. (**d**) Fractured titanium plate that was removed through surgery

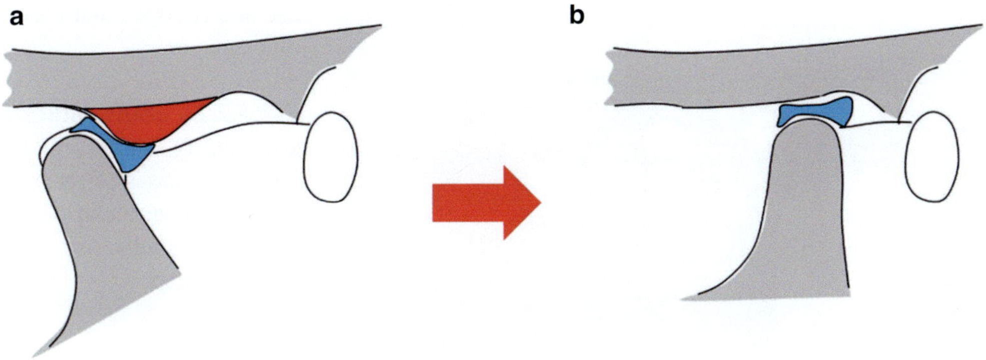

Fig. 10.5 Articular eminence flattening. This method removes the protrusion of the articular eminence (red) that blocks condylar motion, allowing the condyle to move back and forth freely. (**a**) Preoperative. (**b**) Postoperative

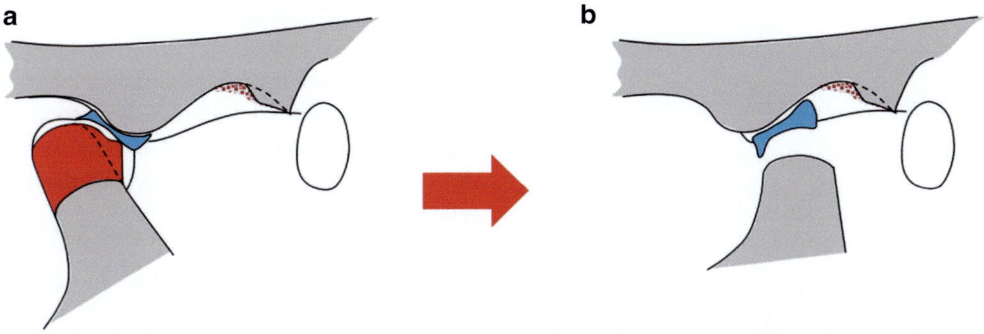

Fig. 10.6 High condylectomy. This approach resects and trims the condyle (red), which has become hyperplastic and deformed after an old dislocation. It entails the removal of the top 3–5 mm of the condylar head. This procedure releases the movement of the condyle and maintains postoperative stability. (**a**) Preoperative. (**b**) Postoperative

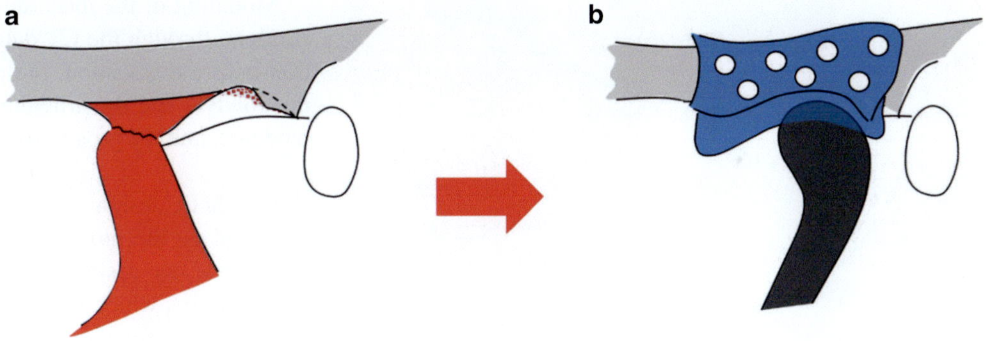

Fig. 10.7 Joint replacement with a prosthesis. This method removes the condyle and the ankylosed bone head (red) in a patient with old dislocation secondary to ankylosis and performs an arthroplasty, thereby maintaining the height of the mandibular ramus and occlusion. (**a**) Preoperative. (**b**) Postoperative

vation of the joint structure, the function of the joint, and the related musculo-neurological system.

10.1.4.1 Types of Prosthesis Designs for Condylar Dislocation

There are two types of condylar dislocation prostheses that have been designed so far, and there may be more in the future. They are distinguished by the fact that one type is designed to block excessive condylar movement, and it is named the "condylar dislocation blocker plate." The other type serves to increase the anterior area of the articular eminence at the level of the transverse crest, thus preventing the condyle from crossing the eminence, and it is named the "articular eminence extension prosthesis."

10.1.4.1.1 Condylar Dislocation Blocker Plate

The prosthesis blocks excessive condylar mobility by placing a transverse blocking plate anterior to and below the articular eminence (Fig. 10.8).

10.1.4.1.2 Articular Eminence Lengthening Prosthesis

This prosthesis serves to prevent the condyle from crossing the transverse ridge by providing a longitudinal extension within the zygomatic arch and temporal bone gap, which serves to increase the anterior area at the level of the transverse ridge of the articular eminence (Fig. 10.9). This also serves to provide a slightly longer range for condylar movement but puts a blocker at the end of the range.

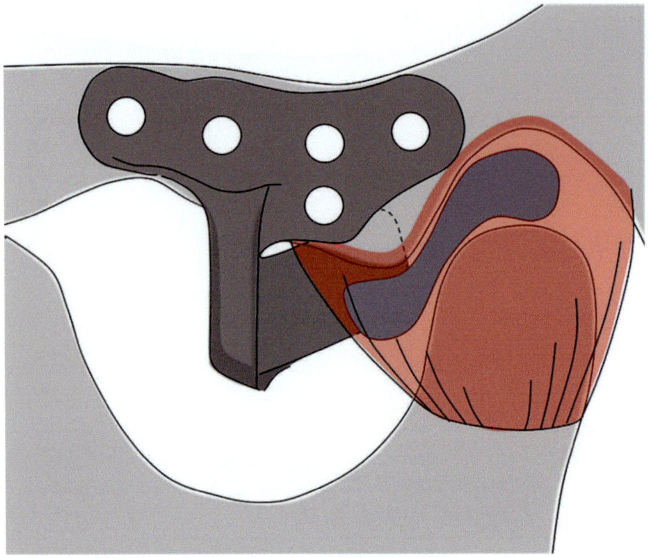

Fig. 10.8 Condylar dislocation blocker plate. Dark gray shows the condylar dislocation blocker plate, orange shows the joint capsule, and light gray marks the articular disc within the joint capsule

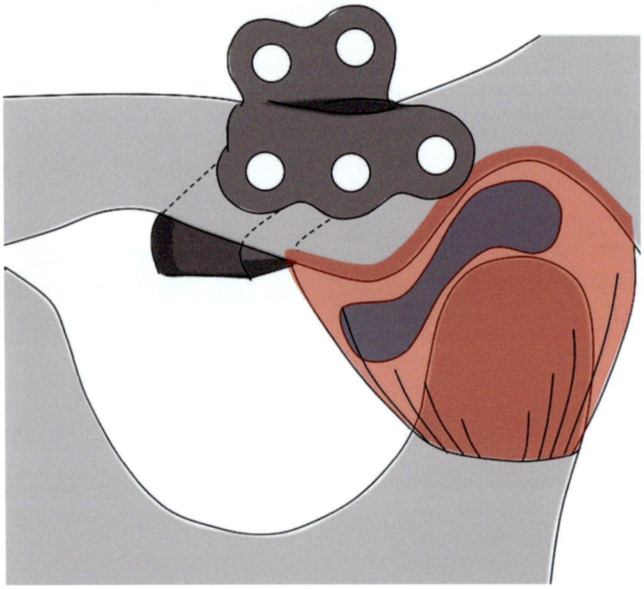

Fig. 10.9 Articular eminence lengthening prosthesis. Dark gray shows the articular eminence extension prosthesis, orange shows the joint capsule, and light gray marks the articular disc within the joint capsule

10.1.4.2 Indications and Contraindications for the Use of Prostheses for Condylar Dislocation

10.1.4.2.1 Indications

The prosthesis is recommended for recurrent and old condylar dislocations because it allows preservation of the articular disc and condyle, and these are expected to perform normal joint function.

10.1.4.2.2 Contraindications

Arthroplasty, i.e., surgical removal and replacement, is required in cases of recurrent and old condylar dislocations in which the articular disc and condyle are not preservable. For the remainder, see contraindications to total TMJ prostheses in Chap. 3.

10.1.5 General Process of Digitally Designing Customized Prostheses for Condylar Dislocation

In the case of the articular eminence lengthening prosthesis, for example, the total digital design process consists of three stages: simulation of the most anterior movement position of the condyle, prosthesis design, and design of the surgical procedure.

- Simulation of the most anterior movement position of the condyle

CT data acquisition: the patient was photographed in the closed mouth position and the maximal open mouth position before dislocation, and the CT data were received in DICOM format and inputted into the surgical design software.

Modeling of the most anterior movement position of the condyle: through the CT data of the maximal opening position before dislocation, the positional relationship between the condyle and the articular eminence in this position was modeled, and the prosthesis design was based on this model.

- Prosthetic design
  Based on the model of the most anterior motion of the condyle, we designed the articular eminence lengthening prosthesis, which logically consists of three parts according to their function:
  - Articular eminence lengthening part, to be installed in front of the articular tubercle, between the root of zygomatic arch and the temporal bone. The lower part is flush or slightly higher than the lowest point of the articular eminence, and the most anterior point is in line with the most anterior point of condylar movement. This component should not be wider than the gap between the root of the zygomatic arch and the temporal bone, to allow the insertion of the prosthesis into the gap.
  - Temporal bone fixation part, matching the contour of the temporal bone, designed with two to three screw

holes, each specified and labeled according to the designed depth of the screw holes in the bone.
 - Zygomatic arch fixation part, shaped in an inverted U shape following the contours of the upper edge of the zygomatic arch root, designed with two to three screw holes, each specified and labeled according to the designed depth of the screw holes in the bone.
- Design of the surgical procedure
  1. Surgical approach design: a modified preauricular anterior temporal incision is to be used to open the skin layer by layer, exposing the lateral aspect of the articular capsule, the zygomatic arch, the articular eminence, and part of the temporal bone.
  2. Installation of the prosthesis: the prosthesis is to be seated in the gap between the temporal bone and the root of the zygomatic arch, the fixation part is tightened against the temporal bone and the zygomatic arch, and the articular eminence lengthening component is tightened against the anterior oblique surface of the articular eminence and fixed with titanium screws.
  3. Validation of mouth opening: a mouthpiece block is placed in the mouth, and at maximum mouth opening the condyle is located below the articular eminence extension prosthesis without dislocation.

10.2 Customized Prosthesis to Treat Condylar Dislocation: The Blocker Plate

In the following sections, two clinical cases are presented to illustrate therapeutic considerations and prosthesis design points.

Case S shows the design and application of a "condylar dislocation blocker plate" (as shown in Fig. 10.8) manufactured from titanium alloy, designed to block excessive anterior movement of the condyle. The blocker plate was implanted anteriorly and lower at the front of the articular eminence using a modified anterior auriculotemporal incision.

In Case T, a modified prosthesis called the "articular eminence lengthening prosthesis" (as shown in Fig. 10.9) was implanted in the space between the zygomatic arch and the temporal bone. It was designed to increase the anterior area at the level of the transverse ridge of the articular tubercle, thus blocking excessive condylar movement.

10.2.1 Case S: Design and Application of a Condylar Dislocation Blocker Plate

- Patient information

  Patient: female, 32 years old.

  Complaint: repeated dislocation of the left jaw joint for more than 10years.

  History: the patient has suffered from recurrent dislocation of the left TMJ, which was treated 7 years ago with manipulation, bandage fixation and sclerotherapy, i.e., injection of a stiffening agent into the TMJ capsule. Six years ago, she underwent surgery that installed a small titanium plate to augment the articular eminence, and 1 year ago the dislocation recurred, and a CT scan showed a fracture in the small titanium plate.

  Past history: history of systemic disease was denied.

  Clinical examination: her face was basically symmetrical, no obvious pressure pain in the joint area bilaterally; mouth opening 40 mm, with left deviation of the mouth; permanent teeth in the mouth, stable occlusal relationship.

  Imaging: MRI of the joint (before implantation of the small titanium plate) showed excessive joint motion on the affected side; CT of the maxillofacial region showed that the small titanium plate was fractured and could not block the excessive gliding motion of the condyle, which led to recurrence of the dislocation (Figs. 10.10, 10.11 and 10.12).

  Diagnosis: left-sided recurrent condylar dislocation.

10.2.2 Case S: Treatment Plan

Overall treatment plan: left side TMJ, fractured titanium plate removal and installation of condylar dislocation blocker plate.

10.2.3 Case S: Design and Machining of the Condylar Dislocation Blocker Plate

- Condylar dislocation blocker plate design: find the most anterior safe position of the condyle

Modeling of the most anterior motion position of the condyle: Utilizing also the designer's experience, the patient's

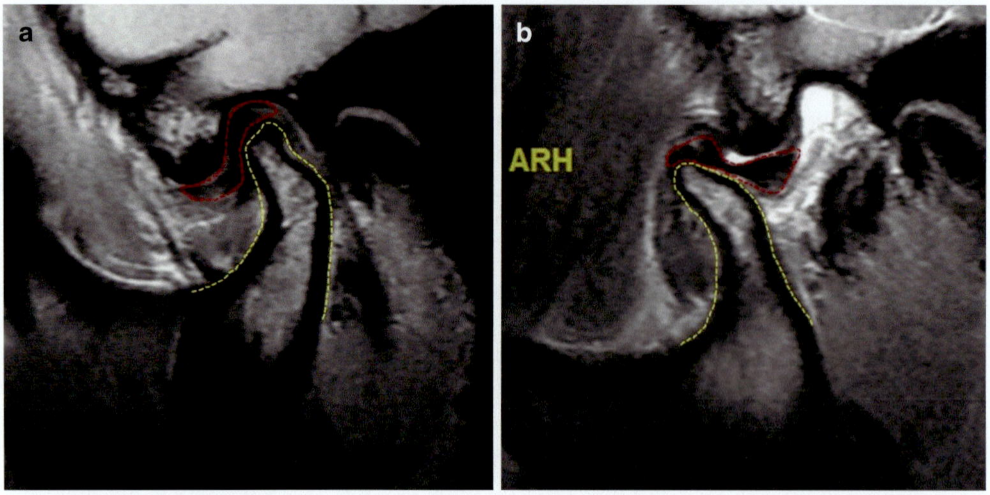

Fig. 10.10 Case S. MRI of the joint (before implantation of the small titanium plate). Hypermobility of the affected joint with a normal disc-condylar relationship (red dashed line shows the disc, yellow dashed line shows the condyle). (**a**) Closed position. (**b**) Open position

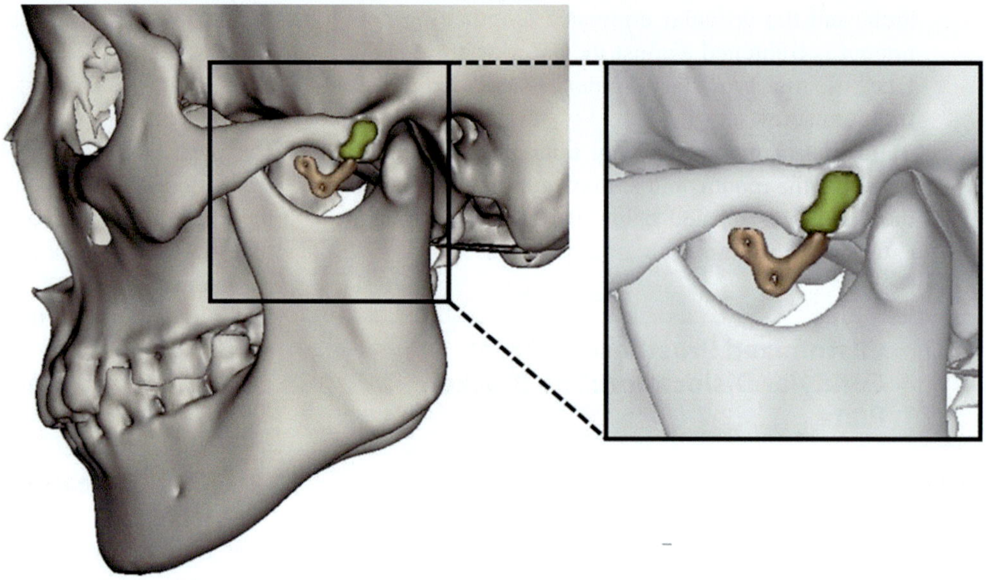

Fig. 10.11 Case S. Three-dimensional CT reconstruction showing fracture of the small titanium plate

maximum mouth opening safe from condylar dislocation (37 mm) was simulated in 3D design software. That is, the desired position of the condyle is the most anterior safe position of the condyle, and this position is used as the basis for modeling in the prosthesis the most anterior position of the condyle (Fig. 10.13).

- Blocker plate design
  The dark gray part is the main part of the blocker, which consists of two parts:
  1. The zygomatic arch retention component, which is convex on the front and concave on the back to fit the zygomatic arch contour.
  2. The blocker plate component, which is positioned immediately anterior to the articular eminence to limit excessive anterior and downward movement of the condyle (Figs. 10.14, 10.15, 10.16 and 10.17).
- Fabrication and test fitting of the blocker plate

Titanium alloy was chosen as the material and fabricated using a metal 3D printer. After fabrication, the blocker was test fitted on a resin head model to see if the blocker fit the bone surface and was stable (Fig. 10.18).

10.2.4 Case S: Surgical Procedure

- Preoperative laboratory tests: the same as described in Sect. 3.2.5.
- Preoperative preparation: see Chap. 3, Case A, preoperative preparation.
- Surgical sequence: the surgery was performed using a modified auriculotemporal anterior incision approach, fully exposing the articular eminence and part of the lat-

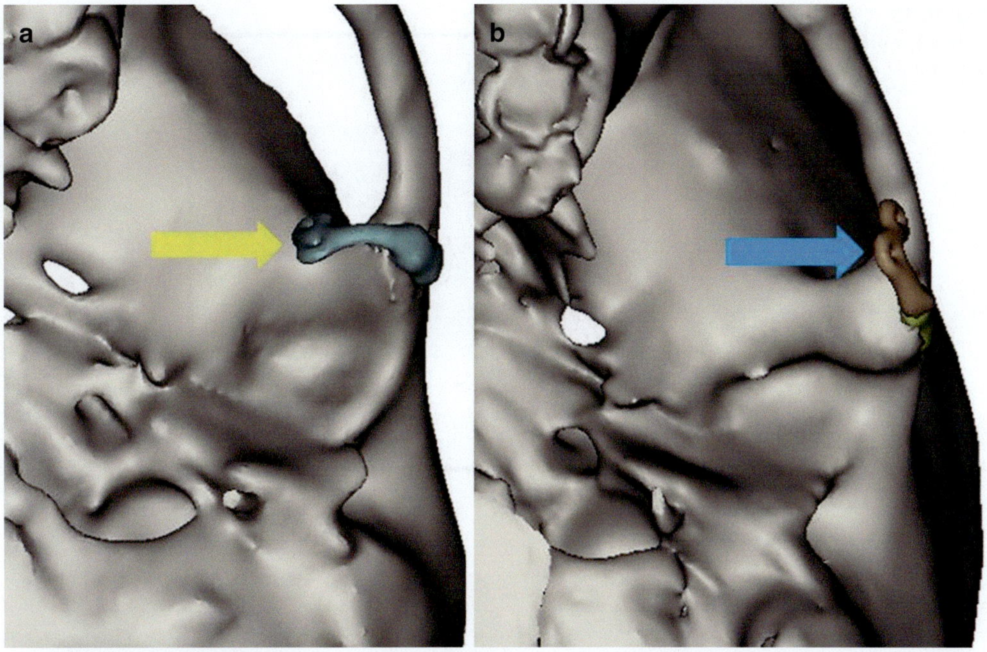

Fig. 10.12 Case S. Three-dimensional CT reconstruction of the skull base. (**a**) Routine implantation position of the small titanium plate (yellow arrow). (**b**) Six years after the operation, CT shows fracture and displacement of the small titanium plate (blue arrow)

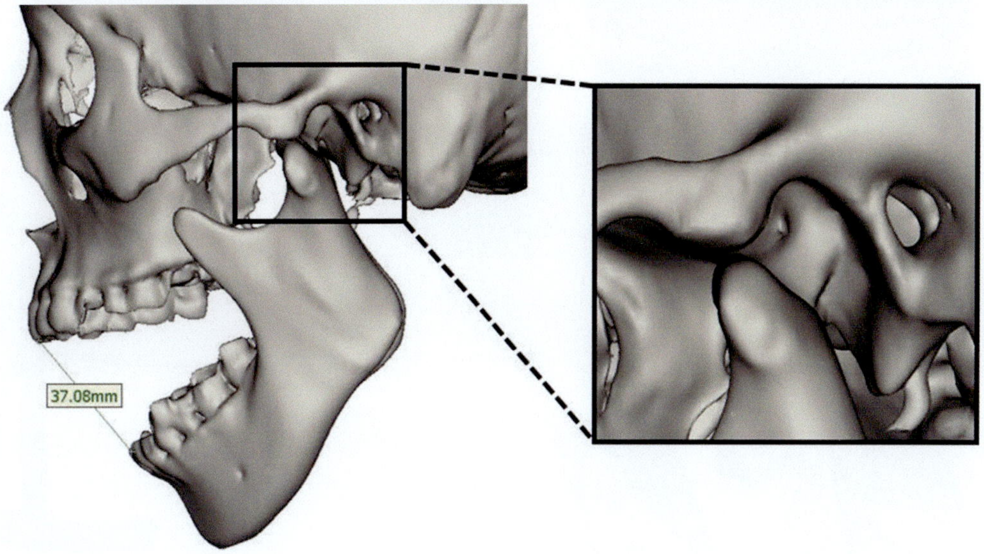

Fig. 10.13 Case S. Modeling of the most anterior movement position of the condyle that is safe from condylar dislocation

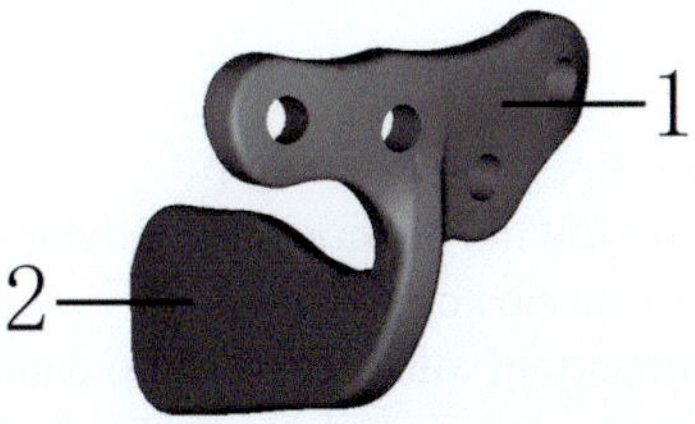

Fig. 10.14 Case S. Blocker plate design. (1) is the zygomatic arch fixation component and (2) is the blocker component

eral zygomatic arch without opening the joint capsule. The blocker plate was put in place and fixed with titanium screws following the preoperative design (Fig. 10.19).

- Postoperative advice and care: see postoperative advice and care in Case A in Chap. 3.

10.2.5 Case S: Follow-Up and Prognosis

Regular postoperative follow-up was performed for cosmetic (facial shape), functional (presence of subluxation recurrence, mouth opening, mouth opening pattern), and blocker plate evaluation (effect on condyle, bite, and lateral pterygoid muscles).

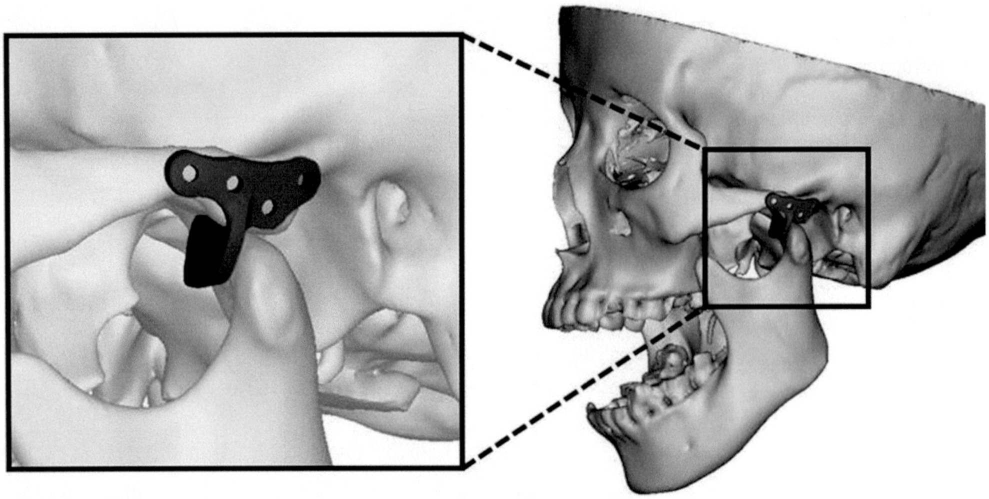

Fig. 10.15 Case S. Side view of blocker plate design location

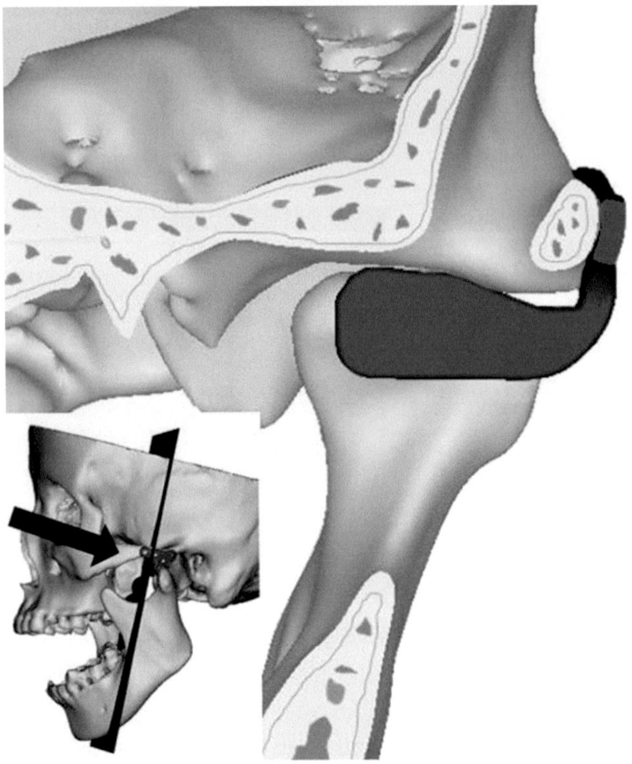

Fig. 10.16 Case S. Front and rear view of blocker plate design location

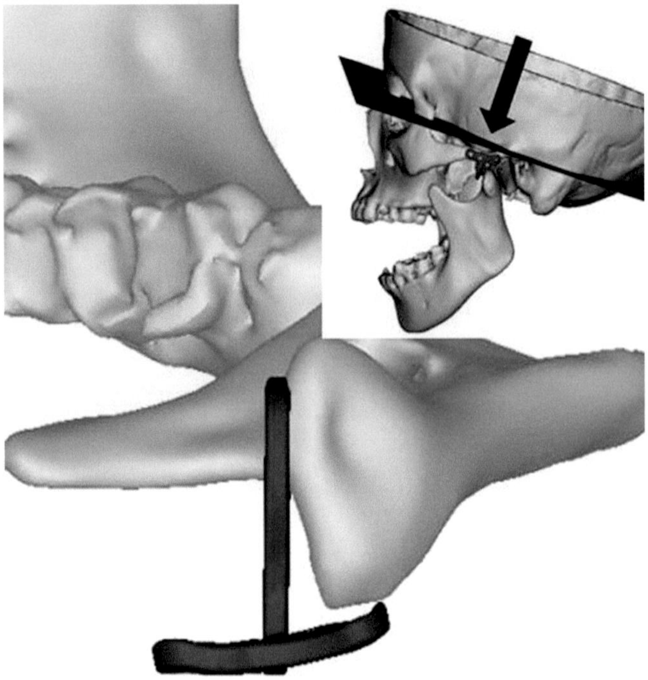

Fig. 10.17 Case S. Top view of the blocker plate design location

- Immediately postoperative follow-up
  The blocker plate was installed smoothly in the surgery, and a comparison of the preoperative design with the postoperative reconstruction showed that it was seated accurately (Fig. 10.20). Postoperative analysis of the positioning error showed a maximum error of 1.20 mm, a position that was slightly more anterior than the design position (Fig. 10.21).

- One-year postoperative follow-up
  - The patient did not experience condylar dislocation for at least 1 year postoperatively.
  - Good recovery of joint function, no pain or discomfort in the joint area, mouth opening distance 31 mm, mouth opening tilted 6 mm to the affected side, occlusion relationships stable.
  - Effect of the blocker plate on the bone quality of the affected condyle: comparison of preoperative and one-year postoperative CT examinations showed that the preoperative volume of the affected condyle was

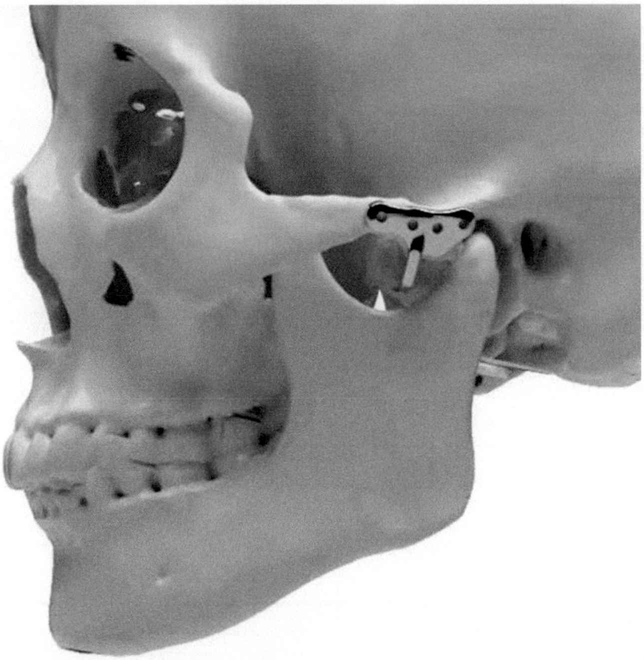

Fig. 10.18 Case S. Condylar dislocation blocker plate fabrication and test fitting

2737.71 mm^3, and at 1 year postoperatively, the volume of the affected condyle was 2720.51 mm, and there was no change in the affected condyle at 1 year postoperatively.

  - Effect of the blocker on the masseter muscle: comparison of preoperative and one-year postoperative CT examinations showed that the preoperative volume of the masseter muscle on the affected side was 24474.74 mm^3; and 1 year after surgery, the volume of the masseter muscle on the affected side was 19465.90 mm^3; and from this measurement, the masseter muscle on the affected side appeared to be atrophic at 1 year after surgery.
  - Effect of the blocker on the lateral pterygoid muscle: comparison of preoperative and one-year postoperative CT examinations showed that the preoperative volume of the lateral pterygoid muscle on the affected side was 8405.77 mm^3; and 1 year postoperatively, it was 8359.25 mm^3; and so there was no change in the affected side of the lateral pterygoid muscle in the one-year postoperative period.
- Three-year postoperative follow-up.
  - The patient did not experience condylar dislocation during at least 3 years after surgery.
  - The face was slightly asymmetrical from side to side, and the left area of the mastication muscles was reduced when compared with the preoperative period (Fig. 10.22).
  - The mouth opening improved to 33 mm, and the rest was the same as the one-year postoperative review (Fig. 10.23).
  - Effect of the blocker on the bone quality of the affected condyle: comparison of preoperative and 3-year postoperative CT examinations showed that the preoperative volume of the affected condyle was 2737.71 mm^3, and at 3 years postoperatively, the volume of the affected condyle was 2813.13 mm, so there was no change in the affected condyle after implantation (Fig. 10.24, Table 10.1).
  - Effect of the blocker plate on the masseter muscle: comparison of preoperative and 3-year postoperative CT examinations showed that the preoperative volume of the masseter muscle on the affected side was 24,474.74 mm^3; and 3 years after surgery, the volume of the masseter muscle on the affected side was 10,944.16 mm^3; and so the masseter muscle on the affected side showed significant atrophy at 3 years after surgery (Fig. 10.25, Table 10.2).
  - Effect of the blocker plate on the lateral pterygoid muscle: comparison of preoperative and 3-year postoperative CT examinations showed that the preoperative volume of the lateral pterygoid muscle on the affected side was 8405.77 mm^3; and 3 years postoperatively, it was 8195.30 mm3, and so there was no significant change in the affected masseter pterygoid muscle (Fig. 10.26, Table 10.3).

10.2.6 Case S: Advantages and Disadvantages

- Advantages
  - Efficacy: no recurrence of dislocation after three years of follow-up, proving its effectiveness.
  - Stability: imaging confirms that after three years the blocker is not broken and is in precise position.
- Disadvantages
  - Design:
    - The simulated design positioning of the blocker plate was not based on enough solid evidence, so the condyle was placed directly below the articular eminence in modeling in the CT reconstruction, which is not completely true to the real physiological situation.
    - The blocker plate came in contact with the condyle, and the positioning failed to consider the space reserved for the articular disc, so the outcome tended to excessively restrict condylar movement.
    - The blocker plate was placed too low, which theoretically might press on the lateral pterygoid muscle and affect its contraction and make it prone to atro-

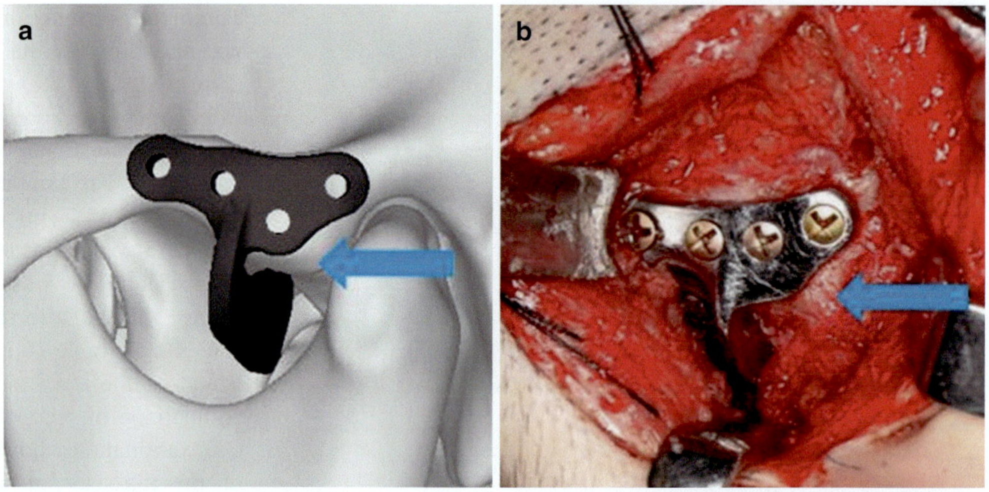

Fig. 10.19 Case S. Blocker plate implantation. Blue arrows show the left articular eminence. (**a**) Design. (**b**) Actual

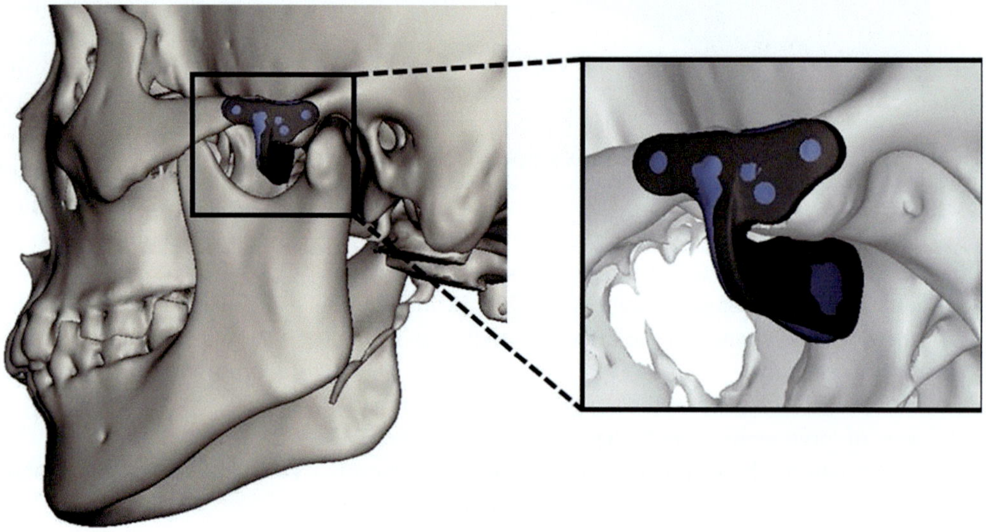

Fig. 10.20 Case S. CT reconstruction and comparison. Comparison of preoperative design position (dark gray) and postoperative position (blue) demonstrates accurate blocker plate implantation

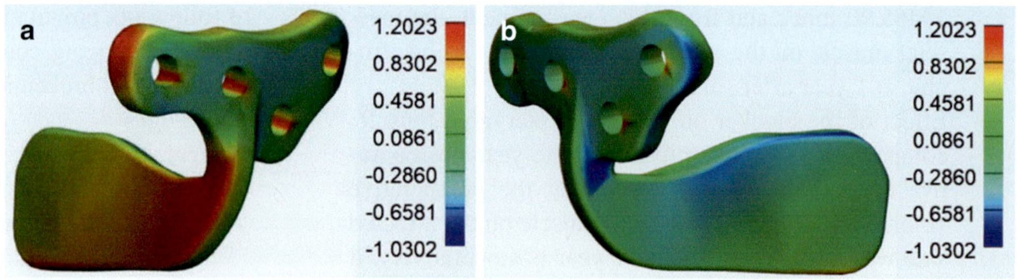

Fig. 10.21 Case S. Error analysis of positioning of the blocker plate. Maximum error 1.20 mm, slightly forward of design position. (**a**) Front lateral error. (**b**) Rear lateral error

phy. But in this case, there was no great change in the volume of the lateral pterygoid muscle, so the prosthesis had minimal effect on the lateral pterygoid muscle.

- The positioning of the blocker plate was not precise enough, and the fixation was prone to deviation.

– Postoperative adverse results:

- Condylar movement has been limited to some extent, presumably related to obstruction by the blocker plate.
- There has been some masseter muscle atrophy, presumably caused by the blocker plate compressing the masseter nerve, because the location of the blocker is on the nerve pathway, coupled with the fact that the positioning of the blocker was too low. This probably tended to create compression, and the effect could be clearly detected in neuromuscular electrical testing.

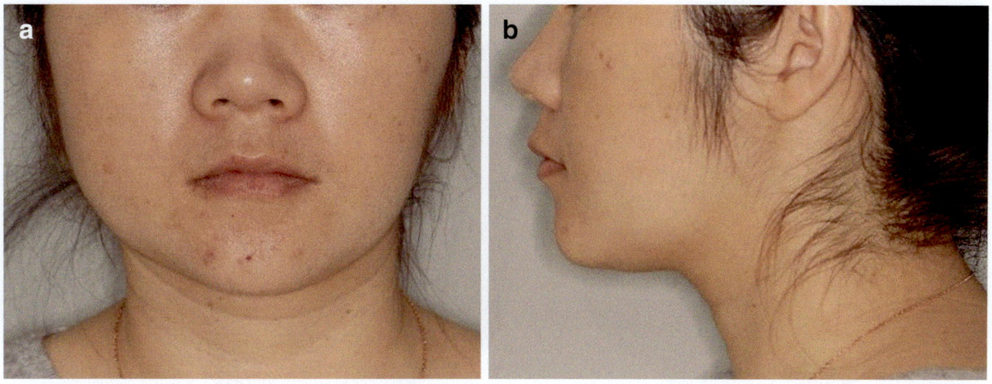

Fig. 10.22 Case S. Three-year postoperative review. Facial asymmetry, with the left cheek area depressed compared to the preoperative view. (**a**) Frontal view. (**b**) Lateral view

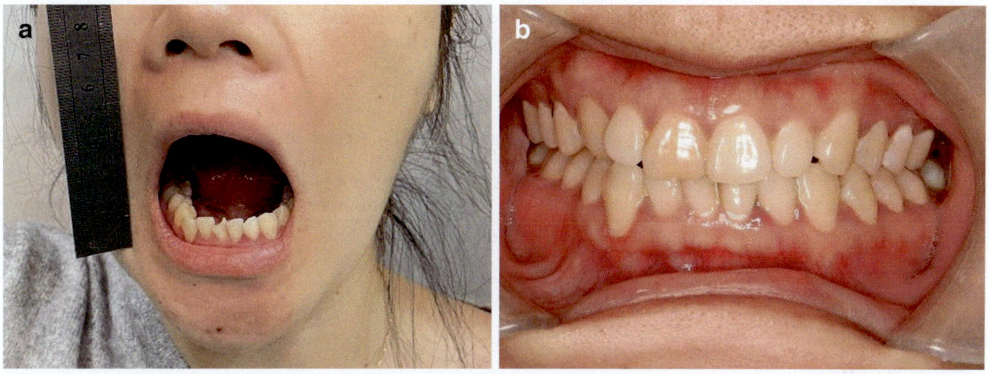

Fig. 10.23 Case S. Three-year postoperative review. (**a**) Mouth opening of 33 mm with left deviation. (**b**) Stable intraoral occlusal relationship

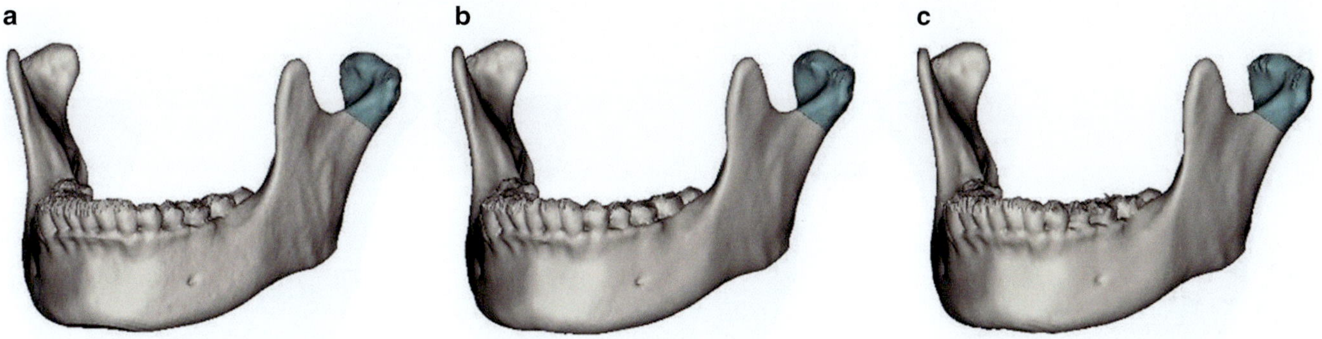

Fig. 10.24 Case S. No change in the quality of the affected condylar bone after surgery. (**a**) Preoperative. (**b**) One year postoperatively. (**c**) Three years postoperatively

Table 10.1 Case S. Comparison of the affected left condyle before and after surgery

	Follow-up time		
Left condylar situation	Preoperative	One year after surgery	Three years after surgery
Condylar internal and external diameter	22.08	21.77	21.63
Anteroposterior condylar diameter (anatomy)	8.68	8.99	9.08
Condylar volume	2737.71	2720.51	2813.13
Surface area of the condyle	1205.67	1200.60	1233.08

Length in mm, volume in mm^3, surface area in mm^2

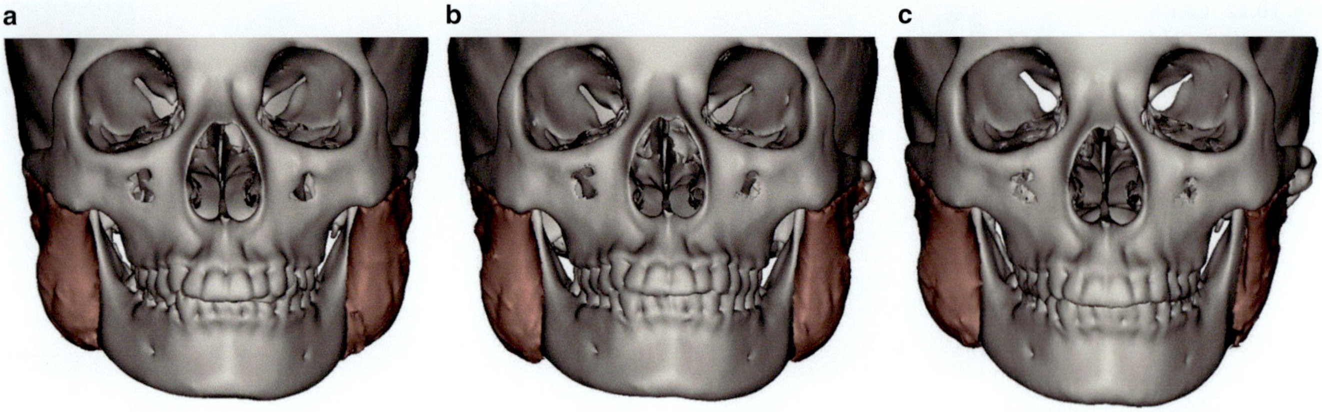

Fig. 10.25 Case S. Postoperative reduction in the volume of the affected masseter muscle. (**a**) Preoperative. (**b**) One year postoperative. (**c**) Three years postoperative

Table 10.2 Case S. Changes in the volume and surface area of the masseter muscles on the healthy and affected sides before and after surgery

	Follow-up time		
Condition of the mastication muscle	Preoperative	One year after surgery	Three years after surgery
Volume of the masseter muscle on the affected left side	24,474.74	19,465.90	10,944.16
Volume of the healthy right masseter muscle	24,906.41	24,716.10	24,664.99
Surface area of the masseter muscle on the affected left side	7192.40	6108.99	5115.22
Surface area of the healthy right masseter muscle	6725.87	6977.50	6676.10

Volume in mm^3, surface area in mm^2

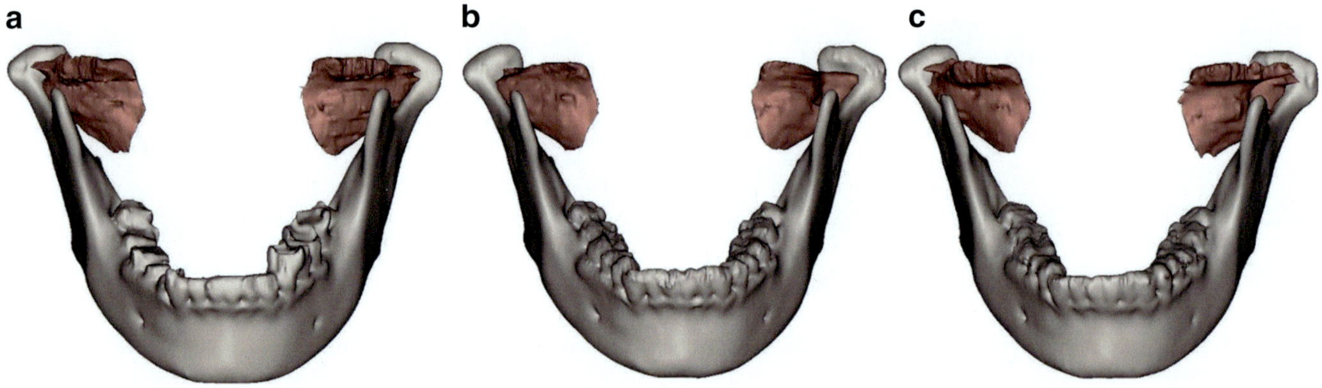

Fig. 10.26 Case S. No change in volume of the affected lateral pterygoid muscle after surgery. (**a**) Preoperative. (**b**) one year postoperatively. (**c**) Three years postoperatively

Table 10.3 Case S. Changes in volume and surface area of the pterygoid muscle on the healthy and affected sides before and after surgery

	Follow-up time		
Lateral pterygoid muscle condition	Preoperative	One year after surgery	Three years after surgery
Volume of the affected lateral pterygoid muscle	8405.77	8359.25	8195.30
Volume of healthy lateral pterygoid muscle	7712.29	7936.08	7892.67
Surface area of the affected lateral pterygoid muscle	3230.13	3301.94	3474.60
Surface area of the healthy lateral pterygoid muscle	3015.14	3107.50	3016.91

Volume in mm^3, surface area in mm^2

10.3 Customized Prosthesis for Treating Condylar Dislocation: Articular Eminence Lengthening Prosthesis

Minjie Chen and Zixiang Han

10.3.1 Case T: Design and Application of the Articular Eminence Lengthening Prosthesis

- Patient information.

  Patient: male, 17 years old.

  Complaint: repeated bilateral dislocation of condyles for more than 3 years.

  History: repeated dislocation of bilateral condylar joints over the past 3 years, which was treated with manipulation and bandage fixation, with inadequate effect.

  Past history: patient denied history of systemic diseases.

  Clinical examination: basic facial symmetry, no obvious pain on pressure for both joint areas, mild mandibular retraction; mouth opening of 41 mm, shape of mouth opening okay; permanent teeth in the mouth, occlusal relationship stable (Figs. 10.27 and 10.28).

  Imaging: MRI of the joint shows hypermobility of the TMJ, with an acceptable disc-condylar relationship (Fig. 10.29).

  Diagnosis: recurrent bilateral condylar dislocation.

10.3.2 Case T. Treatment Plan

Overall treatment plan: installation of bilateral articular eminence lengthening prostheses.

10.3.3 Case T. Design and Processing of the Articular Eminence Lengthening Prostheses

- Articular eminence lengthening prosthesis design

Determine the maximum mouth opening that is possible without causing dislocation of the condyle. First place an occlusal retention block in the patient's mouth to fix the mouth opening at a height of 35 mm; take CT and MRI in this position. Then construct a model of the relationship between the condyle and the articular eminence in this position, using the CT data of the maximal safe opening position without dislocation. Use this model as the basis for the prosthesis design (Figs. 10.30 and 10.31).

- Determination of the articular disc thickness and reservation of space for movement

The position of the disc and the measure of its thickness are obtained by matching CT and MRI images of the condyle in the most anterior position of motion (Fig. 10.32).

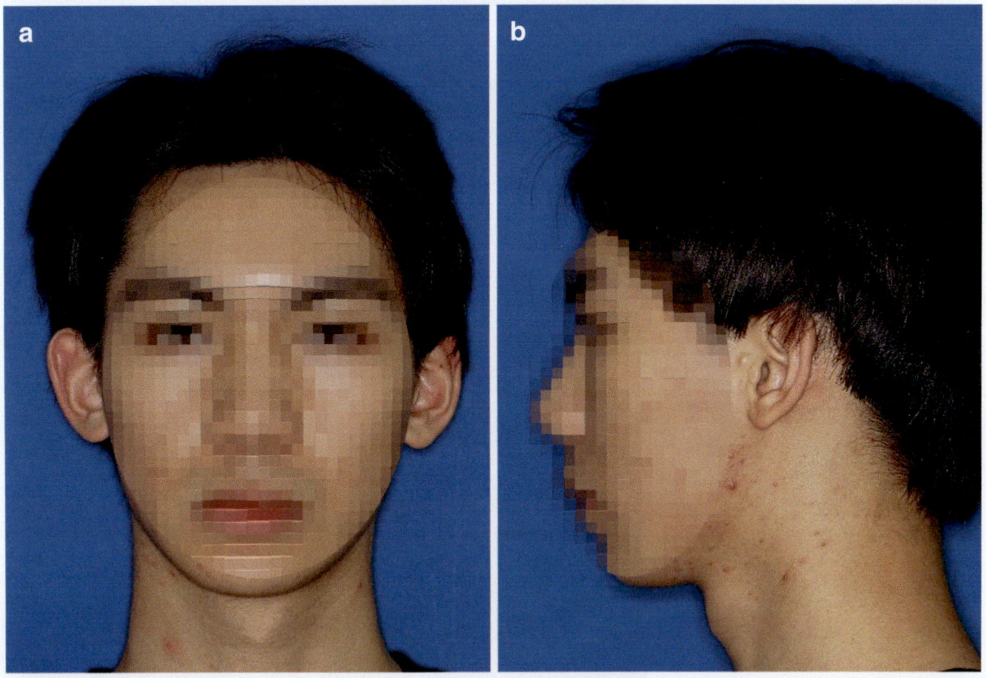

Fig. 10.27 Case T. Extraoral examination. (**a**) Frontal view. B. Lateral view

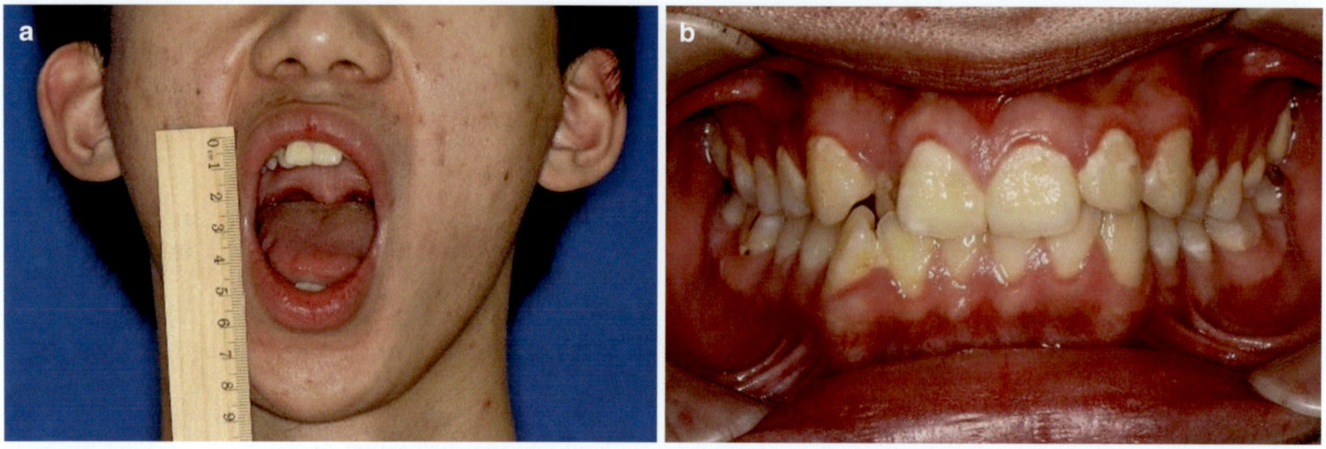

Fig. 10.28 Case T. Intraoral examination showing mouth opening of 41 mm and stable intraoral occlusal joints. (**a**) Mouth opening. (**b**) Occlusion

Fig. 10.29 Case T. MRI of the joint shows a possible disc-condylar relationship (red dashed line shows the articular disc, yellow dashed line shows the condyle). (**a**) Closed position. (**b**) Open position

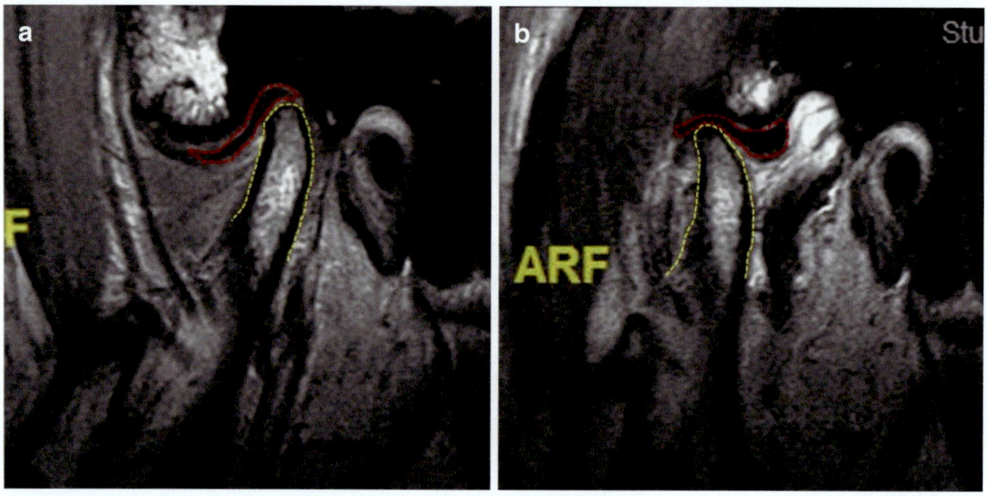

Fig. 10.30 Case T. Judgment of the most anterior motion of the condyle. The yellow arrow shows the occlusal retention block for fixation of the mouth opening at a height of 35 mm. (**a**) Frontal view. (**b**) Lateral view

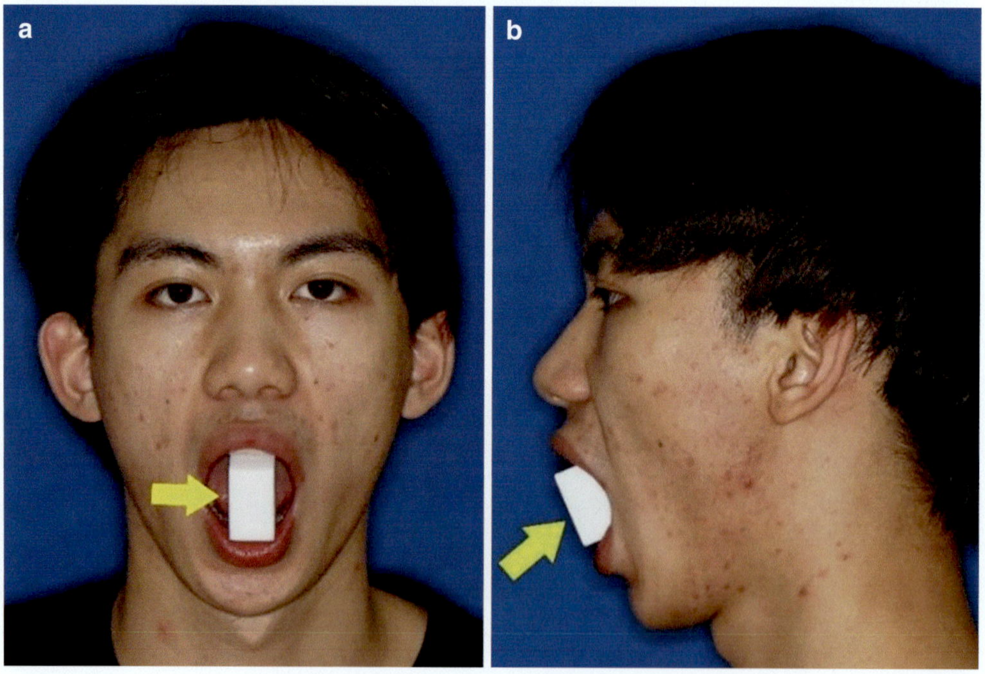

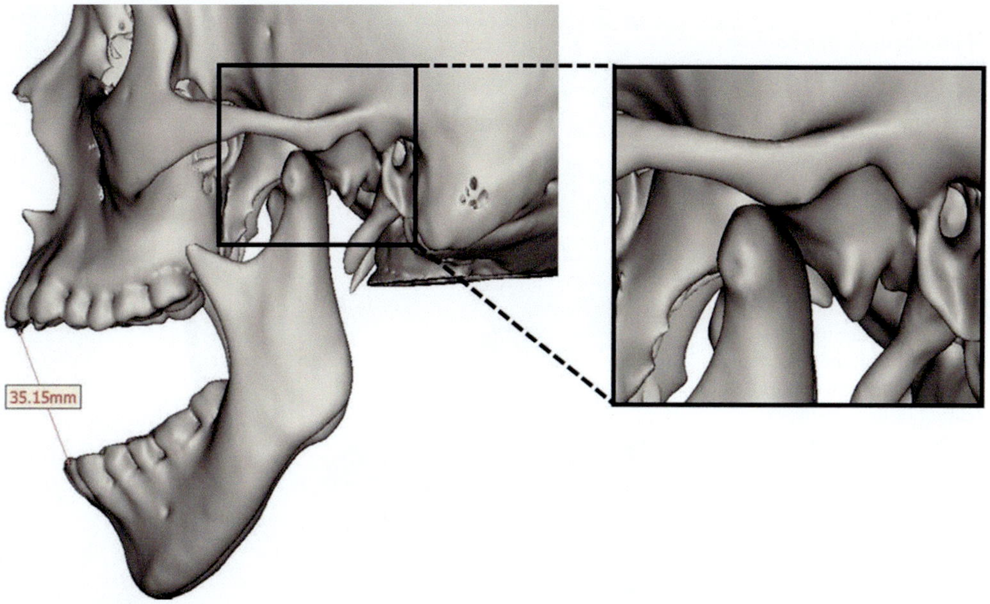

Fig. 10.31 Case T. Model of the most anterior movement position of the condyle that is safe and will not lead to dislocation

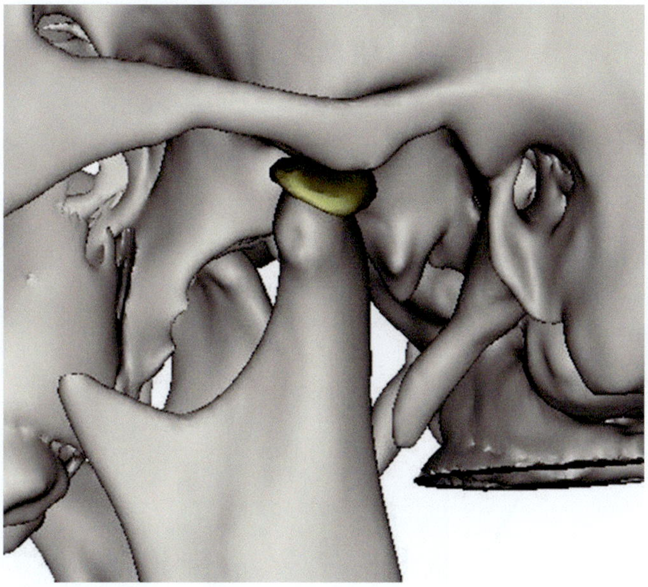

Fig. 10.32 Case T. Articular disc thickness measurement model, to measure the reservation of space for its movement

- Articular eminence lengthening prosthesis design
  The dark gray color is the main part of the prosthesis. The prosthesis consists of three parts:
  1. The temporal bone retention part, which fits the shape of the temporal bone and fixes the prosthesis to the temporal bone contour
  2. The zygomatic arch fixation part, which fits the shape of the zygomatic arch and fixes the prosthesis to the zygomatic arch
  3. The articular eminence extension, which spans the temporal bone scale and the zygomatic arch and ends anteriorly at the articular eminence, to prevent dislocation of the condyle due to excessive motion

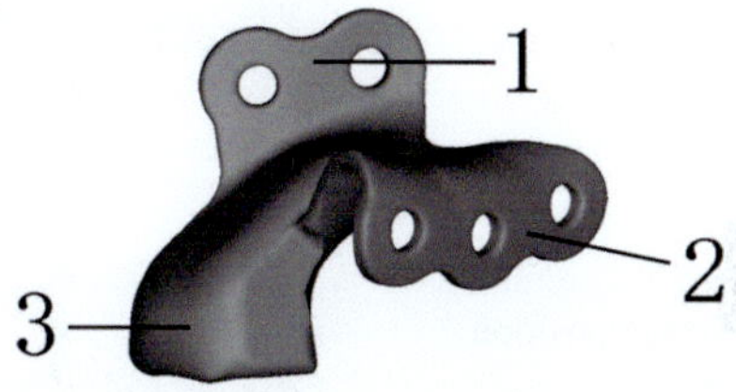

Fig. 10.33 Case T. Articular eminence lengthening prosthesis design. (1) is the temporal bone fixation component, (2) is the zygomatic arch fixation component, and (3) is the articular eminence extension component that blocks excessive condylar movement

  For the physical design, see Figs. 10.33, 10.34, 10.35, 10.36 and 10.37.
- Manufacturing and fitting of the prosthesis

The material used is titanium alloy, which is manufactured using a metal 3D printer. After fabrication, a trial fitting is performed on a resin head model to see if the prosthesis fits the bone contour well and is stable and whether there are gaps (Fig. 10.38).

10.3.4 Case T. Surgical Procedure

Preoperative laboratory tests: the same as described in Sect. 3.2.5.

Preoperative preparation: see Chap. 3, Case A, Preoperative Preparation.

Sequence of surgery: the surgery was performed using a modified anterior auriculotemporal incision to fully expose the anterior border of the articular tubercle, zygomatic arch,

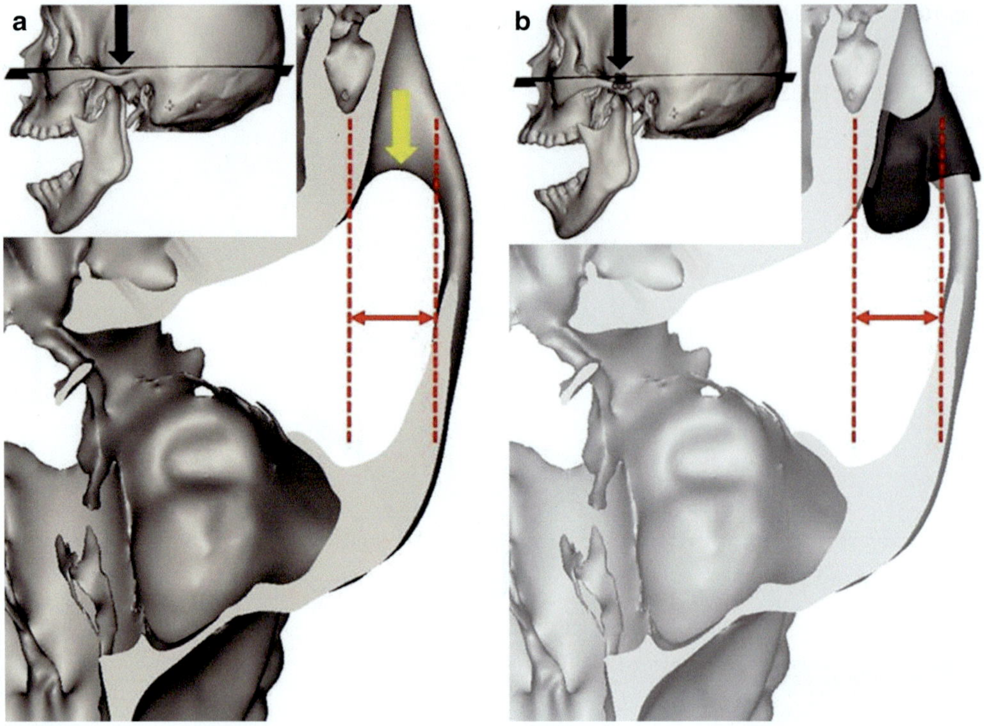

Fig. 10.34 Case T. Top view of prosthesis design position. The yellow arrow marks an overhead view of the gap between the temporal bone and the zygomatic arch; the external diameter of the articular eminence lengthening component must be smaller than the narrowest part of the gap (the area indicated by the red double arrows) in order to avoid creating a protuberance that would interfere with the seating of the prosthesis inside the gap. (**a**) Gap between the temporal bone and the zygomatic arch. (**b**) Prosthesis design position

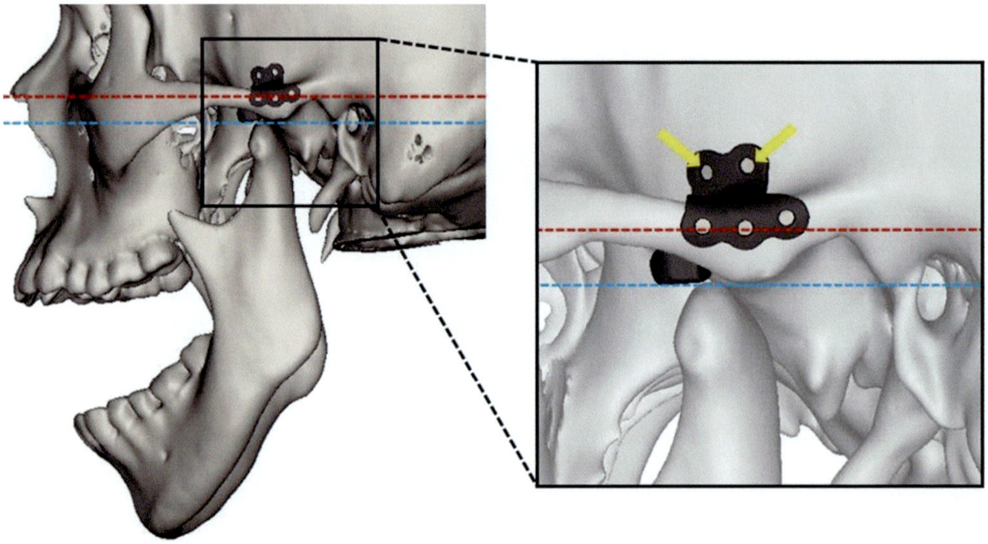

Fig. 10.35 Case T. Lateral view of the designed position of the prosthesis. Requirements: (1) the direction of the lower edge of the articular eminence extension (blue dotted line) is parallel to the orbital auricular plane (red dotted line), and the articular eminence extension is flush with or slightly above the lowest point of the articular tubercle; (2) the length of the temporal bone fixation screws (yellow arrows) should not extend past the medial bone cortex, in order to avoid adverse intracranial effects

and temporal bone scales without opening the joint capsule, and the prosthesis was seated and secured with titanium screws according to the preoperative design (Figs. 10.39 and 10.40).

Postoperative advice and care: see Case A in Chap. 3.

10.3.5 Case T. Follow-Up and Prognosis

Regular postoperative follow-ups were performed for cosmetic (facial shape), functional (presence or absence of dislocation recurrence, mouth opening, mouth shape), and prosthetic evaluation (for condylar function, occlusion, and effect on lateral pterygoid muscles).

- Immediately postoperatively

The prosthesis was fitted smoothly, and a comparison of the preoperative design with the postoperative reconstruction showed that the prosthesis was seated accurately (Fig. 10.41). The analysis of the postoperative prosthesis fitting error

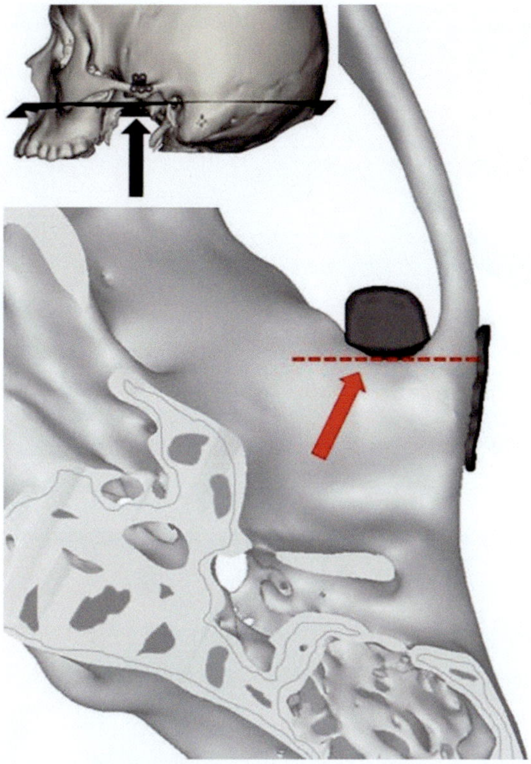

Fig. 10.36 Case T. Bottom view of the designed position of the prosthesis. The posterior edge of the articular eminence extension component must not impinge on the articular eminence (red arrow) and not protrude below it, to avoid creating an inverted concavity or disrupting the integrity of the joint capsule

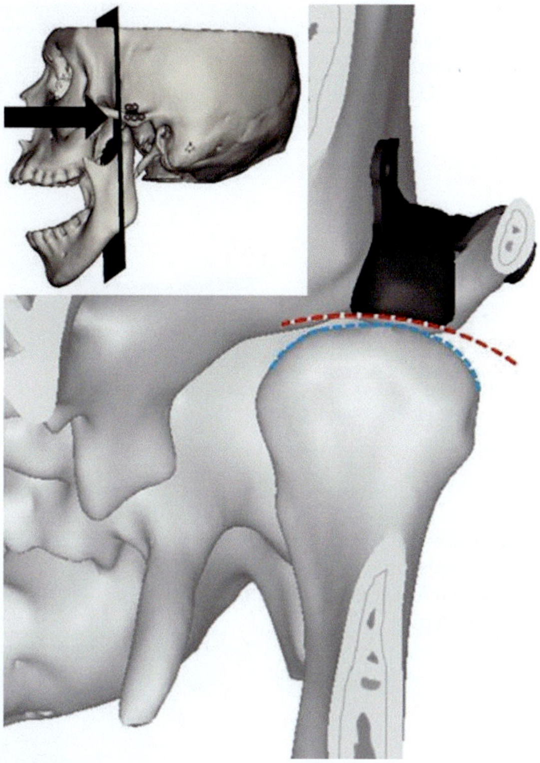

Fig. 10.37 Case T. Anteroposterior view of the designed position of the prosthesis. It is required that the bottom surface of the articular eminence lengthening component corresponds to the curvature of the superior edge of the condyle: the condylar apex is convex (blue dashed line), and the lengthening component has a bottom edge with a matching concave surface (red dashed line) to ensure that the articular eminence lengthening component does not cause localized compression on the condyle that could trigger bone destruction

showed a maximum error of 0.47 mm, with a position that was slightly higher than the design position (Fig. 10.42).

- Two-year postoperative follow-up.
  - No condylar dislocation occurred for the patient during at least 2 years after surgery.
  - The face was symmetrical from side to side with no change from preoperative appearance (Fig. 10.43).
  - The joint function recovered well, with no pain or discomfort in the joint area, a mouth opening of 33 mm, no deviation in the mouth opening pattern, and a stable occlusal relationship, with no change compared with the preoperative period (Fig. 10.44). CT examination two years after surgery showed that the patient's prosthesis could effectively prevent condylar dislocation (Fig. 10.45) in the maximum mouth opening position.
  - Effect of the prosthesis on condylar bone quality: comparison of preoperative and two-year postoperative CT examinations showed that the preoperative volume of the left condyle was 2217.60 mm^3, the right condyle was 1930.63 mm^3, and 2 years postoperatively the volume of the left condyle was 2271.06 mm^3, and the volume of the right condyle was 1965.80 mm^3, so it is

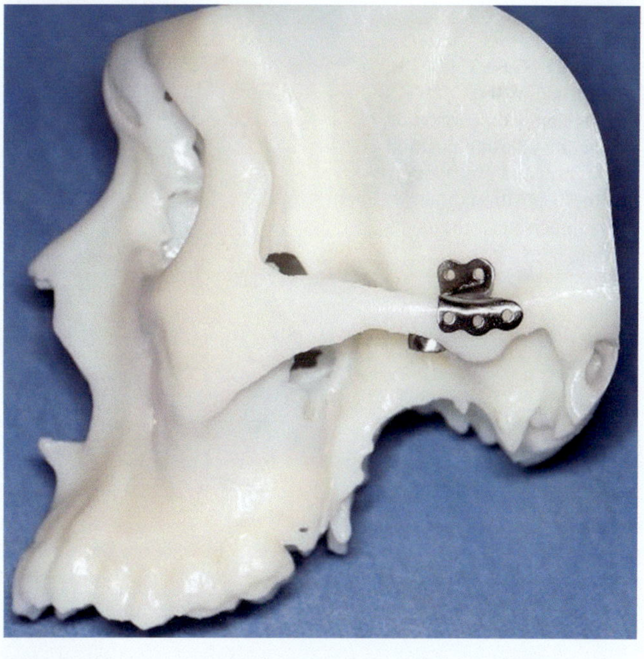

Fig. 10.38 Case T. Prosthesis fabrication and test fitting on a resin head model

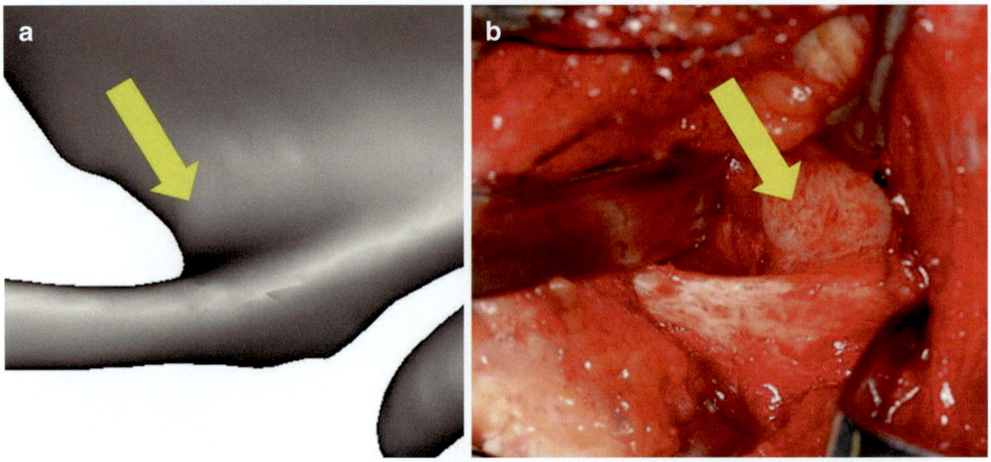

Fig. 10.39 Case T. Exposure of the implant area (yellow arrow) during prosthetic implantation. (**a**) Design. (**b**) Actual

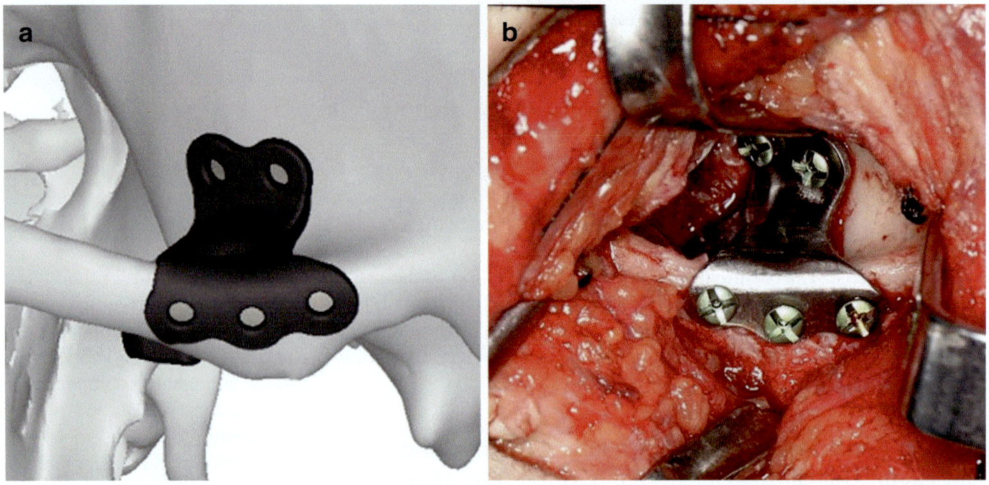

Fig. 10.40 Case T. Prosthesis implantation and fixation with titanium screws. (**a**) Design. (**b**) Actual

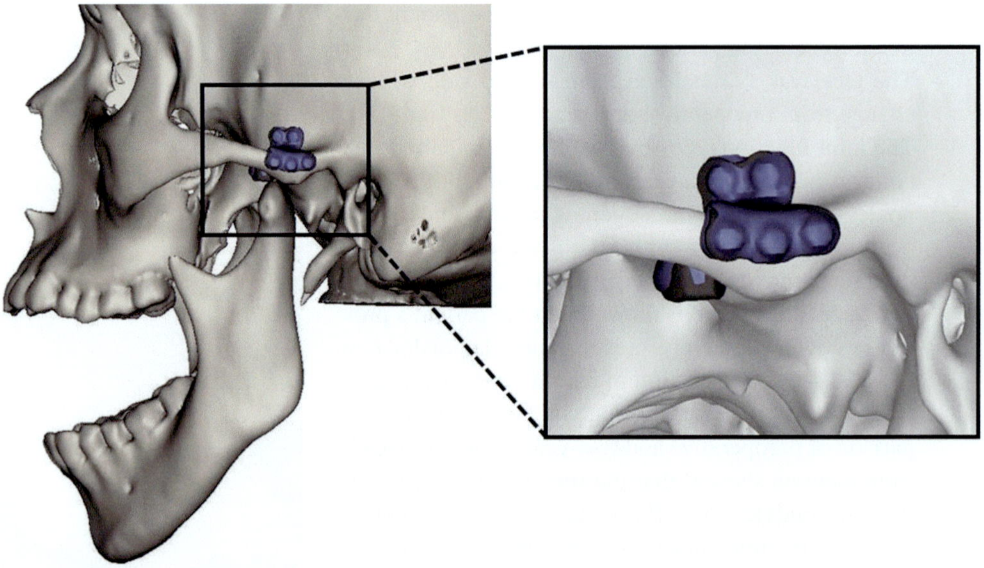

Fig. 10.41 Case T. CT reconstruction and comparison. Comparison of preoperative design position (dark gray) and postoperative prosthesis position (blue) shows precise prosthesis seating

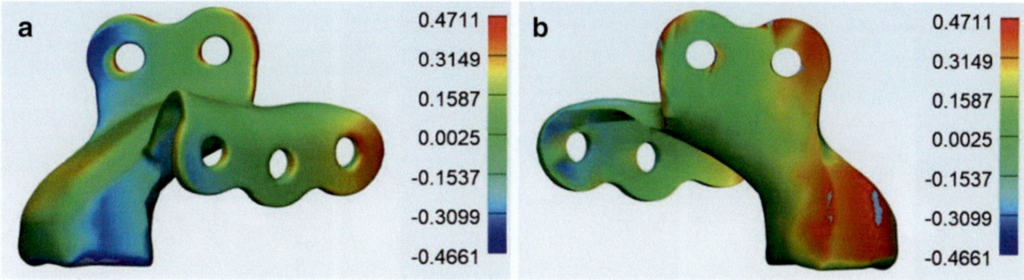

Fig. 10.42 Case T. Error analysis. Maximum error 0.47 mm, slightly higher than the design position. (**a**) Front lateral error. (**b**) Back medial error

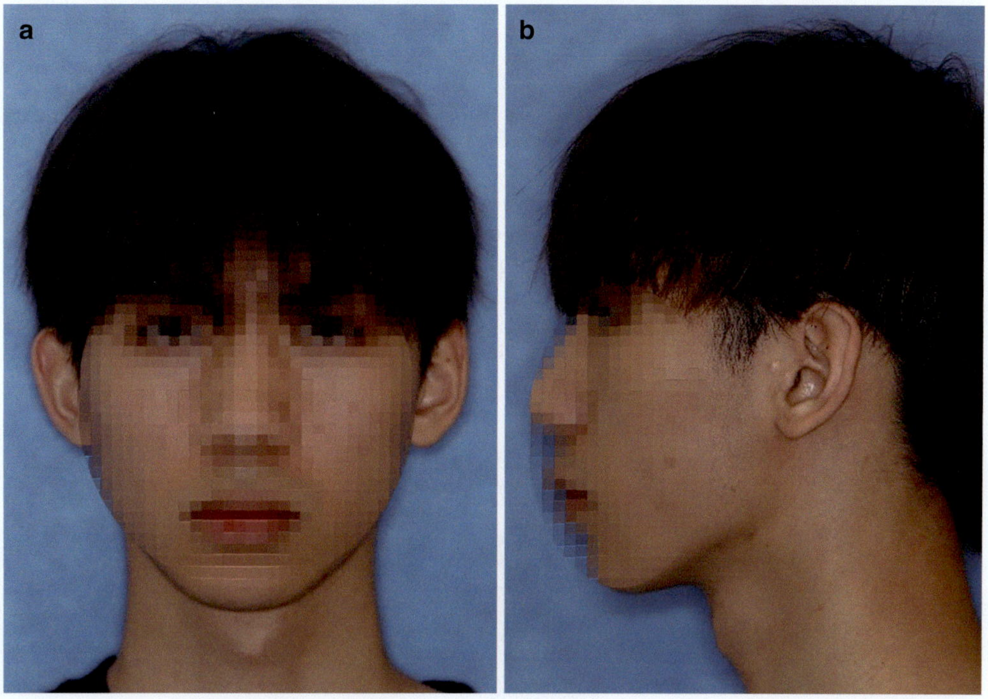

Fig. 10.43 Case T. Two years after surgery. The face is symmetrical from side to side, with no change from the preoperative period. (**a**) Front view. (**b**) Side view

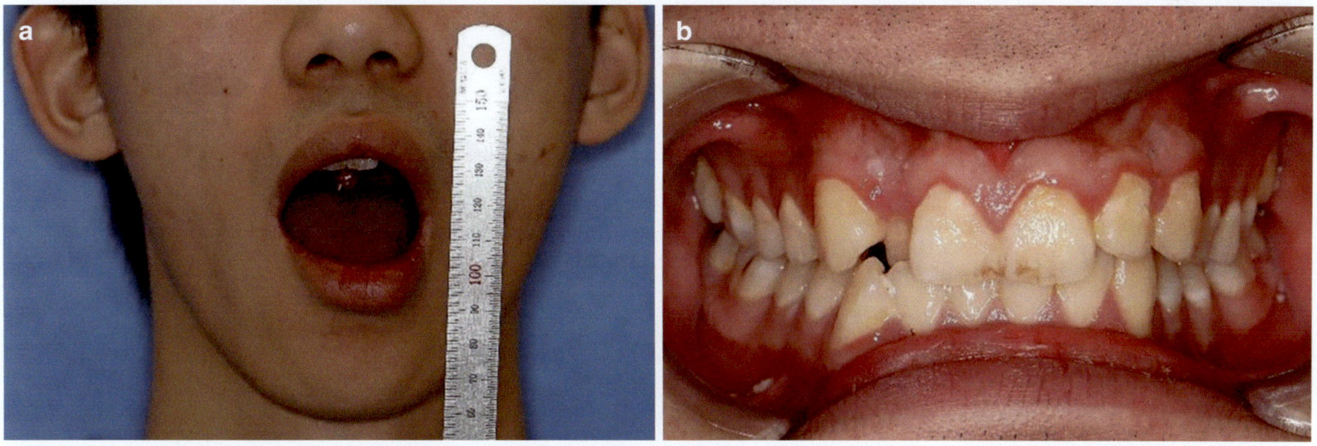

Fig. 10.44 Case T. Examination 2 years after surgery: (**a**) Mouth opening of 33 mm, no deviation in mouth opening shape. (**b**) Stable intraoral occlusal relationship, no change compared with preoperative period

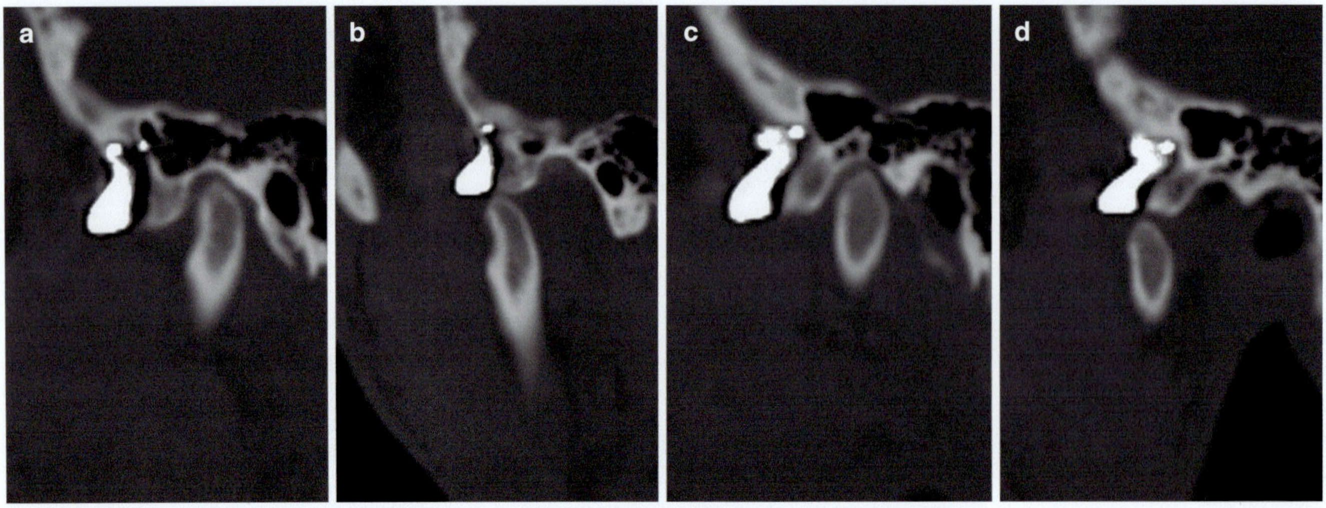

Fig. 10.45 Case T. 2-year postoperative CT review results. (**a**) Left occluded position. (**b**) Left open position. (**c**) Right occluded position. (**d**) Right open position

Fig. 10.46 Case T. Bilateral condylar bone quality is unchanged after surgery. (**a**) Preoperative. (**b**) Two years postoperatively

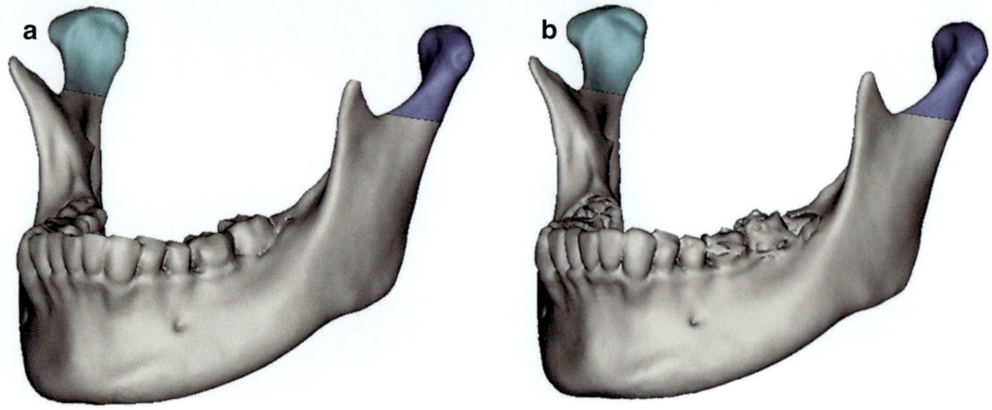

concluded that the implanted prostheses had no effect on the condyles (Fig. 10.46, Table 10.4).

- Effect of the prosthesis on the masseter muscle: comparison of preoperative and two-year postoperative CT examinations showed that the preoperative volume of the left masseter muscle was 22,715.09 mm^3 and the volume of the right masseter muscle was 22144.96 mm^3; and at 2 years after surgery, the volume of the left masseter muscle was 21,293.60 mm^3 and the volume of the right masseter muscle was 21,977.10 mm^3; and so the prosthesis had no effect on the masseter muscle; and there was no atrophy of the masseter muscle bilaterally (Fig. 10.47, Table 10.5).
- Effect of the prosthesis on the lateral pterygoid muscle: comparison of preoperative and two-year postoperative CT examinations showed that the preoperative

Table 10.4 Case T. Measurements of bilateral condyles before and after surgery

	Follow-up time	
Condylar measurements	Preoperative	Two years after surgery
Inside and outside diameter of the left condyle	18.37	18.22
Anteroposterior diameter of the left condyle	7.93	8.16
Left condylar volume	2217.60	2271.06
Surface area of the left condyle	1075.85	1103.58
Inside and outside diameter of the right condyle	19.81	20.08
Anteroposterior diameter of the right condyle	8.19	8.14
Right condylar volume	1930.63	1965.80
Surface area of the right condyle	998.91	1026.05

Length in mm, volume in mm^3, surface area in mm^2

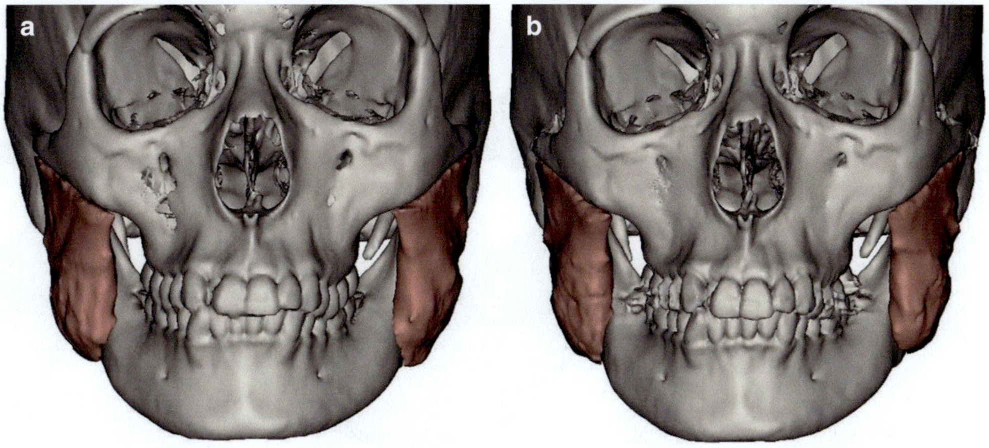

Fig. 10.47 Case T. No change in bilateral masseter muscles after surgery. (**a**) Preoperative. (**b**) Two years postoperatively

Table 10.5 Case T. Volume and surface area of bilateral masseter muscles before and after surgery

Condition of the mastication muscle	Follow-up time	
	Preoperative	Two years after surgery
Left mastication muscle volume	22,715.09	21,293.60
Volume of the right mastication muscle	22,144.96	21,977.10
Surface area of left mastication muscle	6926.58	7116.89
Surface area of the right mastication muscle	6730.36	6942.20

Volume in mm^3, surface area in mm^2

volume of the left lateral pterygoid muscle before surgery was 10,532.73 mm^3; and the volume of the right lateral pterygoid muscle was 9708.87 mm^3, while the volume of the left lateral pterygoid muscle was 10,540.60 mm^3; and the volume of the right lateral pterygoid muscle was 9118.94 mm^3. Apparently, the prostheses had no effect on the lateral pterygoid muscles, and there was no bilateral lateral pterygoid muscle atrophy (Fig. 10.48, Table 10.6).

10.3.6 Case T. Advantages and Disadvantages

- Advantages

With the goal of effective treatment of condylar dislocation, this prosthesis is implanted between the temporal bone scale and the zygomatic arch, which can effectively avoid damage to the integrity of the joint capsule and the joint-related areas, avoid adverse effects on condylar movement, and realize the complete preservation of the joint structure and function; at the same time, the design of this prosthesis can effectively avoid damage to the nerve of the masseter muscle, the lateral pterygoid muscle attachment, and other neuromuscular tissues, thus completely preserving the structure and function of the masticatory muscle.

- Disadvantages

In patients with a narrow gap between the temporal bone scales and the zygomatic arch, the internal and external diameters of the articular eminence lengthening component are reduced accordingly, which may affect the strength and durability of the articular eminence lengthening component.

In patients with dislocation, it is often difficult to determine the anterior movement distance of the dislocated condyle. For patients with a large anterior dislocation distance of the condyle, the anteroposterior diameter of the articular eminence lengthening component may be insufficient according to the conventional design of the prosthesis, which may result in the recurrence of the dislocation. Therefore, the anterior and posterior diameters of the articular eminence lengthening component should be lengthened accordingly in patients with a large anterior dislocated condyle.

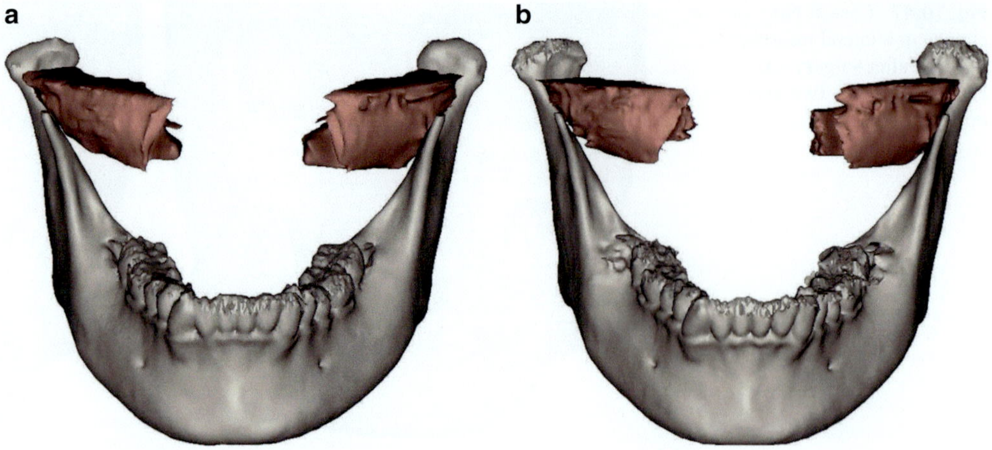

Fig. 10.48 Case T. No postoperative changes in the bilateral lateral pterygoid muscles. (**a**) Preoperative. (**b**) 2 years postoperatively

Table 10.6 Case T. Volume and surface area of bilateral lateral pterygoid muscles before and after surgery. Volume in mm^3, surface area in mm^2

	Follow-up time	
Lateral pterygoid muscle condition	Preoperative	Two years after surgery
Left lateral pterygoid muscle volume	10532.73	10540.60
Volume of right lateral pterygoid muscle	9708.87	9118.94
Surface area of left lateral pterygoid muscle	3732.06	4102.12
Surface area of the right lateral pterygoid muscle	3381.66	3618.21

11 Future Trends: For Prostheses in the Experimental Phase, Reflecting on Experience and Recognizing the Challenges

Chi Yang, Jisi Zheng, and Guo Bai

Clinical follow-up ranging from at least 2 years to a maximum of 8 years has yielded results that largely affirm the safety and efficacy of the various customized temporomandibular joint (TMJ) and craniomaxillofacial prostheses developed by our team. However, certain limitations remain evident, primarily manifested in the following aspects:

1. The core components of total joint prostheses and combined prostheses—namely, the articular fossa and condylar articular surfaces—are not fully personalized in design.
2. Functional mobility, including mouth opening, protrusion, and lateral movements, still falls short of normative values observed in healthy individuals.
3. Discrepancies persist between the prosthetic design and actual surgical outcomes, reflecting challenges in procedural precision.
4. Excessive thickness of the prosthetic fossa results in a lower-than-physiological axis of rotation, deviating from natural joint kinematics. The use of metal-to-nonmetal welding further exacerbates fossa thickness.
5. Large-scale joint-mandible composite prostheses have yet to achieve satisfactory clinical outcomes.
6. Broader clinical adoption and extended follow-up periods are necessary to substantiate the advantages of these prostheses and guide iterative improvements.

What defines the future trajectory of craniomaxillofacial joint prosthesis development? To address this, we must first establish the criteria for an ideal joint-craniomaxillofacial prosthesis. Our proposed standards are as follows:

1. Preservation or functional integration of physiological joint musculature, particularly the attachment of the lateral pterygoid muscle
2. High-level customization of core components, including size and kinematic pathways
3. Prosthetic articular surfaces that are smooth, wear-resistant, and semi-compliant (nonmetallic) to absorb excessive stress
4. Superior osseointegration at the bone-prosthesis interface for seamless structural unification
5. Compact and thin-profile designs that retain the biomechanical properties required to withstand extreme physiological loads
6. Biocompatible materials compliant with Class III implant standards

This "demand-driven" research paradigm will guide subsequent discussions on the design, material selection, and manufacturing techniques for personalized joint and craniomaxillofacial prostheses.

11.1 Future Directions in Personalized Prosthesis Design

Prosthetic design remains the primary challenge. To achieve true personalization of core functional components—particularly the articular surfaces—artificial intelligence (AI) must be leveraged. AI also serves as a powerful tool for optimizing extended prosthetic components and fixation screw hole design.

Currently, all internationally available joint prostheses are designed with osteotomy lines positioned below the condyle, often flush with the mandibular notch. This approach sacrifices the attachment of the lateral pterygoid muscle, a critical loss since this muscle provides the primary driving force for mandibular protrusion and lateral movements.

The future of prosthetic design must prioritize preservation of the lateral pterygoid muscle attachment to restore near-physiological joint kinematics.

Chi Y. (✉) · Jisi Z. · Guo B.
Shanghai Ninth People's Hospital, Shanghai Jiao Tong University School of Medicine, Shanghai, China

© People's Medical Publishing House, PR of China 2025
Chi Y. (ed.), *Atlas of Customized TMJ-Cranio-Jaw Prosthesis*, https://doi.org/10.1007/978-981-95-0611-8_11

11.1.1 AI-Driven Design of Personalized Prostheses

Exploring the ideal reconstruction strategy for bone and joint structural defects is an enduring topic in medical research. The craniomaxillofacial bone-joint complex, being one of the most sophisticated and delicate structures in the human body in terms of both anatomy and function, makes this endeavor particularly significant. As "no two leaves in the world are identical," the mission of this system is to provide each patient with a uniquely tailored reconstruction solution.

The concept of an AI-powered personalized prosthesis design system has long been envisioned. Its fundamental components include:

1. Establishment of a normative craniomaxillofacial bone-joint structure and motion database: through large-scale collection of imaging and kinematic data from healthy individuals, the AI system generates comprehensive libraries of joint structures, articular movements, and biomechanical parameters.
2. Customized joint design: by inputting the patient's craniomaxillofacial CT images, the system identifies the "most closely matched normative specimen" from the database, thereby determining the patient's ideal bone-joint architecture, kinematic patterns, and biomechanical characteristics, which informs the design of personalized core components and extension modules (Figs. 11.1 and 11.2).

11.1.2 Muscle-Function-Preserving Temporomandibular Joint and Craniomandibular Prostheses

A review of the literature and long-term follow-up data from our research team has confirmed that current commercially available joint prostheses often lead to postoperative complications such as restricted lateral and protrusive movements, as well as mandibular deviation during mouth opening. These issues primarily stem from: ① the complete resection of joint structures (including the articular disc, condyle, and condylar neck), which results in the loss of lateral pterygoid muscle attachment and consequent impairment of forward and contralateral movement and ② the coverage of the mandibular ramus angle by the prosthesis stem component, leading to insufficient masseter muscle attachment and partial loss of masticatory function.

The critical clinical challenge lies in profoundly optimizing the prosthetic design to preserve the attachments of both the lateral pterygoid and masseter muscles, thereby restoring normal mandibular movement and masticatory function. To address this, our team has leveraged the extensive preliminary research data, rich clinical experience, key surface modification technologies, and exceptional prosthetic design expertise from the Department of Oral Surgery at Shanghai Ninth People's Hospital, affiliated with Shanghai Jiao Tong University School of Medicine. We have developed a novel muscle-attachment-preserving temporomandibular joint prosthesis (Figs. 11.3 and 11.4). Its innovative design principles, modular components, surface architecture, and asso-

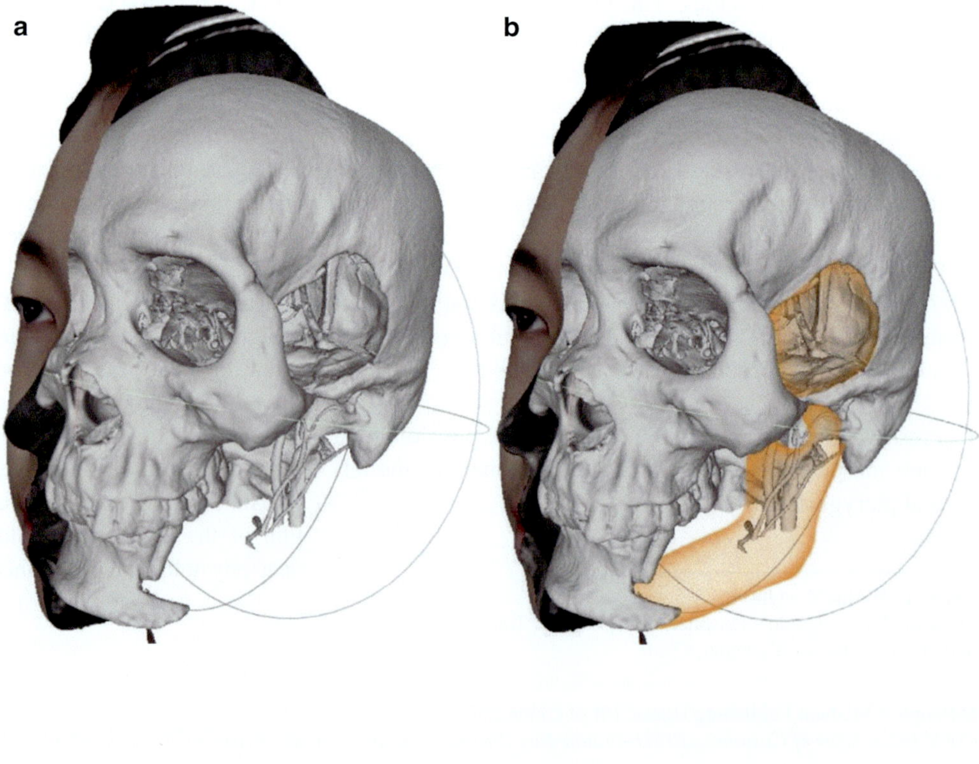

Fig. 11.1 Multimodal big database intelligent design matching of "the ideal normal person" to the individual and design of a customized prosthesis. (**a**) Multimodal data fitting. (**b**) Big data intelligent matching

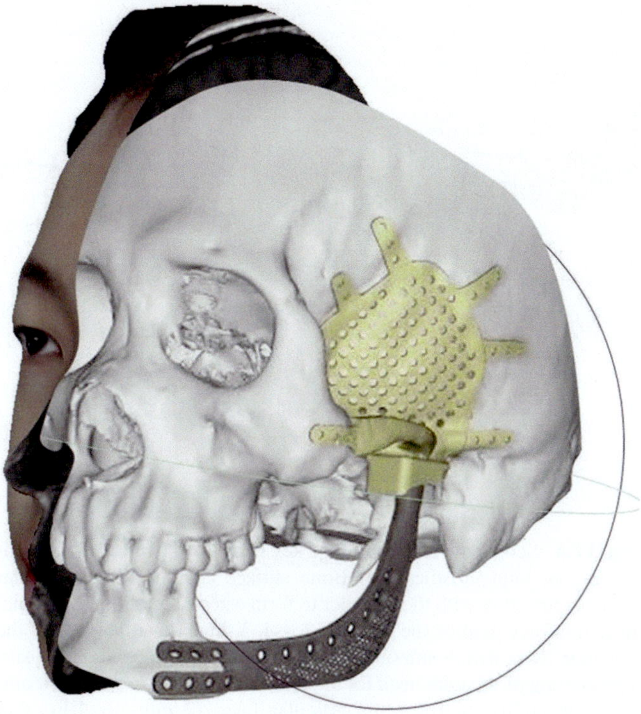

Fig. 11.2 Intelligent design of core components and extension components for the individualized prosthesis

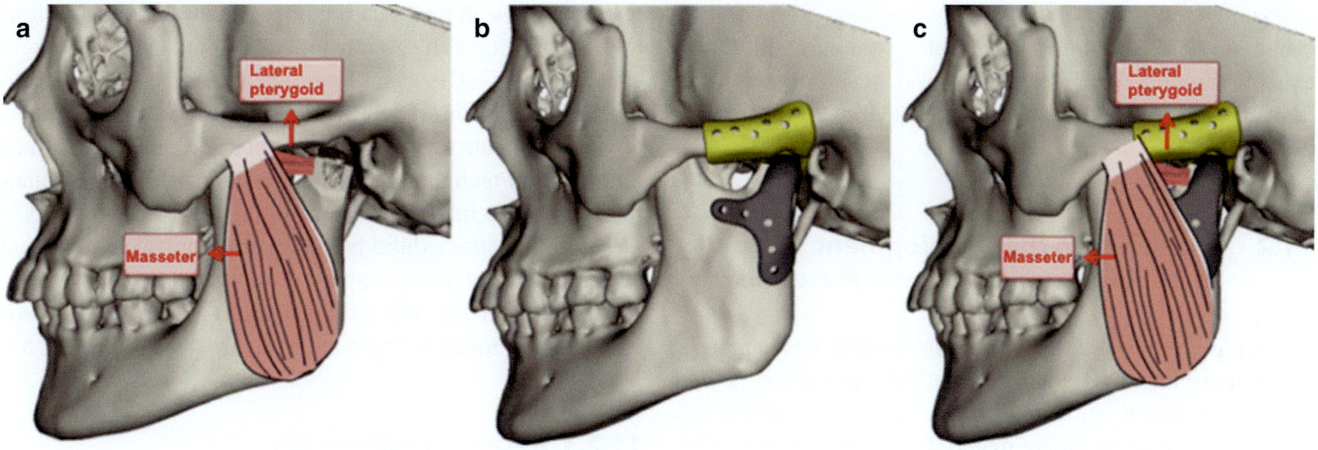

Fig. 11.3 TMJ prosthesis designed to preserve muscle function. (**a**) Excision of lesion with preservation of muscle insertions. (**b**) Design of modified prosthesis. (**c**) Restoration of original muscle insertions (right)

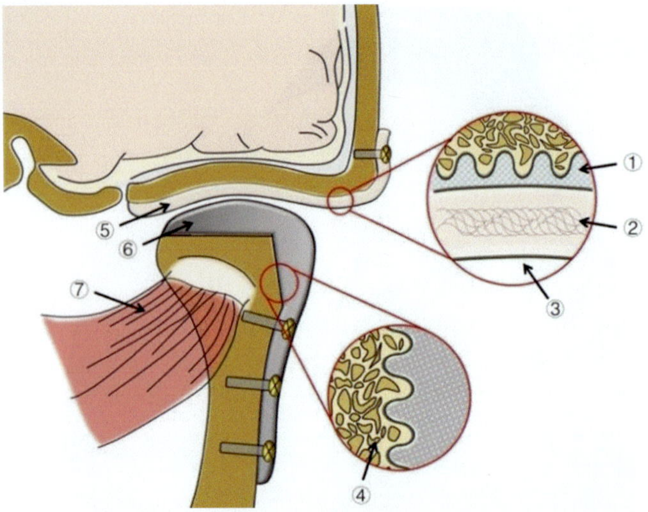

Fig. 11.4 Schematic diagram of the key features of a muscle-function-preserving joint prosthesis. 1. Bone surface coating of the articular fossa: connection with the polymer to form osteointegration. 2. Internal fiber reinforcement of the articular fossa. 3. Functional surface of the articular fossa with a smooth and wear-resistant surface. 4. Bone surface coating of the joint head for the joint-mandible prosthesis: osteointegration ability. 5. Ultra-thin articular fossa (2 mm). 6. Ultra-thin articular head (2 mm to 3 mm): high strength and wear resistance. 7. Retention of the lateral pterygoid muscle

ciated surgical techniques represent a paradigm shift from existing products and methodologies, positioning it as a next-generation prosthesis with high potential for rapid clinical translation.

11.2 Prospects in the Development of Personalized Prosthetic Materials

The bridge between design and manufacturing lies in materials, making material science one of the most dynamic and highly scrutinized fields in prosthetic innovation. While this is fundamentally a matter of materials and engineering, clinical end users can—and should—articulate performance-driven requirements and forward-looking concepts for high-performance biomaterials.

11.2.1 Wear-Resistant Ultra-Thin Materials

The development and application of highly wear-resistant, ultra-thin materials with superior mechanical properties hold significant promise for enhancing the performance of TMJ prostheses. For instance, such materials could enable the fabrication of ultra-thin artificial glenoid fossae or condylar heads, allowing the prosthetic joint's axis of motion to closely mimic natural physiological conditions. This advancement would also provide material support for the development of "muscle-preserving TMJ prostheses." Cobalt-based alloys and ceramic materials exhibit excellent wear resistance and mechanical properties, with established clinical success in total hip arthroplasty. Considering the biomechanical characteristics of the TMJ, if challenges such as the weak osteoinductive capacity of cobalt-based alloys and ceramics, as well as the brittleness of ceramics, can be addressed, novel wear-resistant, small-scale prosthetic joint surfaces made of pure cobalt-based alloys or ceramics may be developed. This would make surface replacement of the condyle and glenoid fossa feasible.

11.2.2 Lightweight Materials

Metallic materials have a high density, resulting in greater weight compared to natural bone structures of the same volume. Therefore, selecting lightweight materials to reduce prosthetic weight is essential. Polymeric materials, such as polyetheretherketone (PEEK), are increasingly being explored in joint prosthesis development. Extensive preclinical and clinical studies have demonstrated that PEEK exhibits properties similar to human bone. While PEEK has been clinically applied in non-load-bearing or low-stress bone regions, its use in load-bearing bones and joints remains limited. To overcome this, our team has employed high-strength carbon fibers (CFs) and carbon nanotubes (CNTs) to mechanically reinforce PEEK. Using 3D printing technology, we fabricate these composites and further apply surface modification techniques to enhance their osteogenic potential at the bone interface. The resulting CF-PEEK and CNT-PEEK composites exhibit both high mechanical strength and strong osseointegration capabilities, making them suitable for TMJ prostheses. We anticipate these materials will gradually replace metallic components in prostheses (Fig. 11.5).

11.2.3 Resorbable Materials

Resorbable materials have already been adopted in craniomaxillofacial surgery, including resorbable plates and screws, sutures, hemostatic agents, and bone substitutes. Currently, resorbable fixation systems are primarily fabricated from absorbable polymers such as polylactic acid (PLA) and are used for stabilizing non-load-bearing or low-stress bone segments. However, for load-bearing skeletal applications—such as orthognathic surgery, mandibular fractures, and condylar fractures—resorbable metallic materials have emerged as a key research focus, with magnesium (Mg) and zinc (Zn) being the most extensively studied.

Through strategies like alloying, surface coating, and microstructural modification, researchers aim to enhance the mechanical strength of these metals, precisely control their

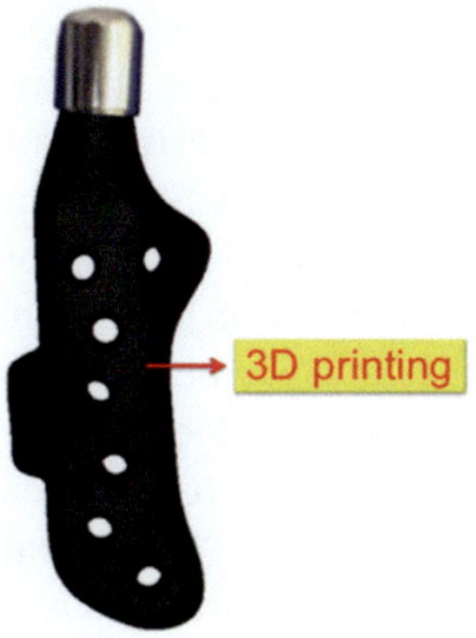

Fig. 11.5 The mandibular fixation component of titanium alloy was replaced by CF-PEEK or CNT-PEEK composite materials

degradation rates, and optimize their degradation byproducts. These advancements could enable their use in the rigid fixation of craniomaxillofacial bones and joints, as well as in the reconstruction of bone defects, ultimately achieving both stable mechanical support and progressive biodegradation.

11.3 The Future of Personalized Prosthesis Manufacturing Processes

Prosthesis design represents the conceptual framework, materials form the foundation, and manufacturing serves as the bridge that integrates the two to achieve personalized prostheses. Currently, our team employs 3D printing and five-axis machining as primary manufacturing techniques. However, to realize the novel designs proposed in Sect. 11.1 and the advanced materials discussed in Sect. 11.2, innovative manufacturing processes must be developed.

11.3.1 3D Printing Technology

3D printing has revolutionized manufacturing and breathed new life into the production of medical implants. Given the stringent requirements for dimensional accuracy, structural integrity, and biocompatibility in human implants, 3D printing not only meets these demands but also makes personalized treatment a tangible reality. Nevertheless, the clinical application of 3D-printed implants remains in its exploratory phase. The limited variety of clinically approved printing materials underscores the need for process optimization in the following areas:

1. Refinement of existing printing techniques: improvements in printer hardware and parameter settings to minimize defects such as porosity, voids, incomplete powder fusion, cracks, delamination, and inclusions.
2. Multi-material hybrid printing: co-printing of different metals, polymers, or metal-polymer combinations. Integration of resorbable and non-resorbable materials.
3. Biomimetic structure printing: printing of bone, cartilage, muscle, and ligament-like topological architectures. Fabrication of osteochondral composite structures, cortical-cancellous bone mimics, and bone-muscle/ligament interfaces.
4. Bioprinting: printing of bioactive scaffolds incorporating growth factors or stem cells. Development of tissue- or organ-like constructs.

Advances in these areas will significantly propel the field of medical implants forward.

11.3.2 Surface Coating Technologies

Surface coating involves depositing a functional layer onto a substrate to enhance its properties. Common techniques include electroplating, electroless plating, physical/chemical vapor deposition (PVD/CVD), thermal spraying, laser/electron beam cladding, and hot-dip coating. For prostheses, coating applications focus on three critical aspects:

1. Wear-resistant coatings for articulating surfaces: hard metals (e.g., cobalt-chromium) or ceramics are applied to friction-prone areas (e.g., glenoid fossa and condyle) to reduce wear, particularly for materials like titanium alloys with suboptimal tribological properties.
2. Osteoconductive coatings for bone interfaces: hydroxyapatite, tantalum, or titanium coatings on titanium or cobalt-chromium-molybdenum alloys promote osseointegration, ensuring long-term stability between the prosthesis and mandible.
3. Myogenic coatings for muscle interfaces: coatings incorporating hydroxyapatite or myoactive substances on muscle-contact surfaces (e.g., lateral pterygoid attachment sites) aim to restore functional muscle-prosthesis integration, addressing post-implant complications like mandibular deviation.

11.3.3 Connection of Dissimilar Materials

Hybrid material integration enables multifunctional prosthesis designs. For instance, this book highlights the metal/nonmetal bonding of ultrahigh-molecular-weight polyethylene (UHMWPE) and titanium alloys. Key joining methods—mechanical (e.g., riveting), chemical (e.g., covalent bonding), or thermal (e.g., welding)—are under exploration for:

1. Metal/nonmetal hybridization: UHMWPE-titanium composites fabricated via powder fusion under heat/pressure, enhancing interfacial bonding while minimizing prosthesis thickness.
2. Resorbable/non-resorbable hybridization: load-bearing frameworks (e.g., titanium, PEEK) combined with osteoinductive resorbable materials (e.g., PLA composites, Mg/Zn alloys) for integrated joint-bone reconstruction.

Example PEEK-hydroxyapatite-PLA composites via melt fusion, or titanium-magnesium/zinc hybrids via 3D printing/welding.

11.3.4 Tissue Engineering Technology

Tissue engineering represents a transformative approach for craniomaxillofacial bone and joint reconstruction. By seeding viable cells onto biocompatible scaffolds and culturing them ex vivo, engineered constructs can repair or replace damaged tissues/organs. Core elements include signaling factors (e.g., growth factors), functional cells, and scaffold matrices. Current advancements and future directions include:

1. Osteochondral condyle constructs: biphasic scaffolds loaded with chondrogenic/osteogenic factors and cells for condylar replacement.
2. Disc-condyle-muscle triphasic constructs: tri-layered scaffolds mimicking the articular disc, condyle, and lateral pterygoid muscle, potentially enabling whole-joint organoid transplantation.
3. Vascularized bone-nerve-muscle complexes: quadruple-functional scaffolds integrating jawbone, nerves, vasculature, and muscles for composite mandibular reconstruction.

While these goals present challenges, they are within the realm of achievable innovation.

11.4 The Bionic Joint-Mandible Integrated Prosthesis Concept

Among the various joint-craniomaxillofacial prostheses developed by our research team, the joint-mandible integrated prosthesis represents perhaps the most complex challenge. This is because such prostheses must account for not only joint functionality but also occlusal dynamics and the intricate attachment requirements of multiple masticatory muscles. Consequently, clinical trials of large-scale joint-mandible prostheses conducted by our team have yet to yield satisfactory outcomes.

Moreover, as the mandible is the only mobile bone in the craniomaxillofacial complex, its physiological importance cannot be overstated. A critical future direction lies in developing integrated prostheses whose structure and function more closely mimic natural joint-mandible systems—what we term "bionic joint-mandible reconstruction." Through the advancements in prosthesis design, materials science, and manufacturing processes outlined in the preceding three sections, our team aims to overcome two major challenges: "large-scale joint-mandible prostheses" and "physiomimetic joint-mandible reconstruction."

11.4.1 Large-Scale Joint-Mandible Integrated Prostheses

The reconstruction of Class IV and V joint-mandible defects (involving extensive bone and soft tissue loss) ranks among the most formidable challenges in craniomaxillofacial rehabilitation—a problem our team has not yet fully resolved. Over the past 5years, we performed large-scale joint-mandible reconstructions on three patients, all of whom experienced complications to varying degrees (Fig. 11.6). The shortcomings manifested as:

1. Prosthesis exposure or infection
2. Immediate postoperative stability issues
3. Muscle attachment challenges (compromising dynamic function and long-term stability)

To address these limitations, our new design framework prioritizes solutions for these three critical problems.

11.4.2 Muscle Attachment and Myodynamic Problems: The Physiology of Muscular Contraction

The successful reattachment of muscle tissue to the implant is a guarantee of long-term stability and a condition that allows the reconstructed articulating mandible to gain myodynamic power, thus ensuring the physiologic function of the joint and mandible (Fig. 11.7). This must be considered in the prosthesis and reconstruction design.

- Prosthesis design: the design of the grafting plate must minimize obstruction of the muscle tissue attachment area (Fig. 11.7, part (2)).
- Bone tissue at the muscle attachment: bone tissue is a fundamental condition for muscle attachment, so bone grafting at the muscle attachment area is necessary. To meet the needs of both dental implants and muscle attachment,

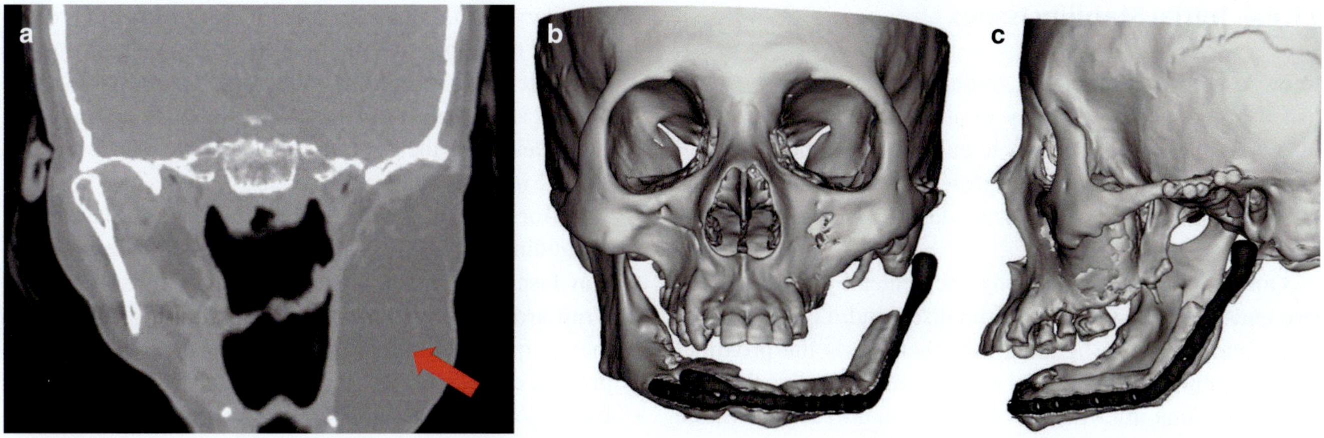

Fig. 11.6 Displacement of a large joint-mandible prosthesis after implantation of a Class IV joint-mandibular defect prosthesis. (**a**) Preoperative CT shows absence of muscle tissue on the affected left side, with only adipose tissue remaining (red arrow). (**b**) Front view, 6 months after implantation of a joint-mandibular prosthesis: the head of the condyle is outwardly and downwardly displaced. C. Lateral view: the head of the condyle can be seen to be posteriorly displaced as well

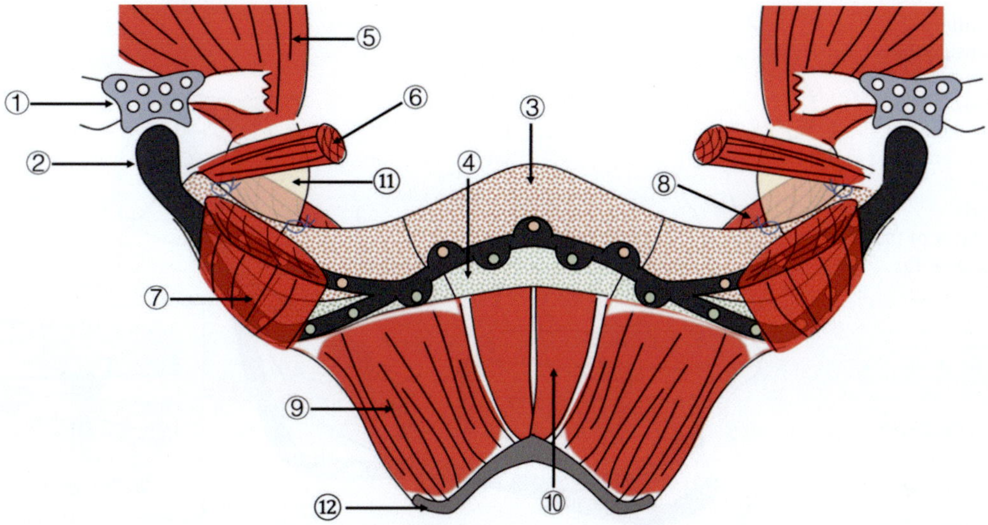

Fig. 11.7 Schematic diagram of a joint-mandibular Class V defect repair. The prosthesis is designed in the form of a bilateral reconstruction plate, and the bone grafts are shaped to the angle of the mandible and the chin for healing with the soft tissues and muscles to ensure the restoration of the mandibular muscle attachment. (1) Articular fossa prosthesis. (2) Biarticular joint-mandibular prosthesis. (3) Superior bone grafting, mostly fibula. (4) Lower bone grafting, ribs may be used. (5) Temporal muscle. (6) Lateral pterygoid muscle. (7) Masseter muscle. (8) Medial pterygoid muscle. (9) Mylohyoid muscle. (10) Geniohyoid muscle. (11) Tendon and temporal muscle suture and then suspended on the superior grafted bone. (12) Hyoid bone

a double-layer bone grafting design is usually utilized (Fig. 11.7, parts (3), (4)).

- Muscle dynamics: muscle tissues, especially the masticatory muscles, combined with the reconstructed joint-mandible, are the guarantee for long-term joint-mandible movement and functions such as mastication (Fig. 11.2, parts (5)–(11)).
- Future directions for research on muscle attachment problems: metal surface treatment to give the prosthesis the ability to bind with muscles or tendons, i.e., the bionic prosthesis, is the logical next step.

11.4.3 Non-exposure of Metallic Prostheses in Critical Areas

The chin and mandibular angle are the places on the mandible that protrude the most; these are also the most common areas where metal prostheses are exposed. For this reason, bone tissue must be present in these critical areas, and when musculoskeletal bonding is present here, it ensures that the metal prosthesis will not be exposed (Fig. 11.7 parts (3), (4)).

11.4.4 Initial Stability Issues

In the case of large defects, initial stability must be established intraoperatively, firstly to align the core components of the prosthesis and secondly to guide the postoperative processes of healing and bone regrowth. But stabilization is a tall order in the case of extensive defects; we have our concept of the task.

Our program of "stabilizing the center by grasping the two ends" means: One end is the distal end, i.e., occlusion, using intermaxillary ligation; the other end is the proximal end, i.e. joint(s), using fascial suspension. "Stabilize the center" means that after the two ends are stabilized, the whole mandible is naturally stabilized.

- Intermaxillary ligation protocol: With jaw clearance secured, an occlusal plate is designed and secured to the maxillary teeth, long screws are used to secure the reconstructed mandible, and the screws are secured to the occlusal plate as a means of obtaining distal stabilization (Fig. 11.8). The rigid screw ligature is removed at 2–4 weeks, and the ligation is switched to elastic traction for 1–2 months.
- Anterior and posterior articular ligament suspension: depending on the situation, anterior and posterior articular fascial suspension or anterosuperior and posterior wrap-around suspension may be used (Fig. 11.9) as a means of obtaining proximal-articular stabilization to prevent dislocation of the joint head.
- Bionic joint capsules and joint ligaments: technology imitating life is the future research direction.

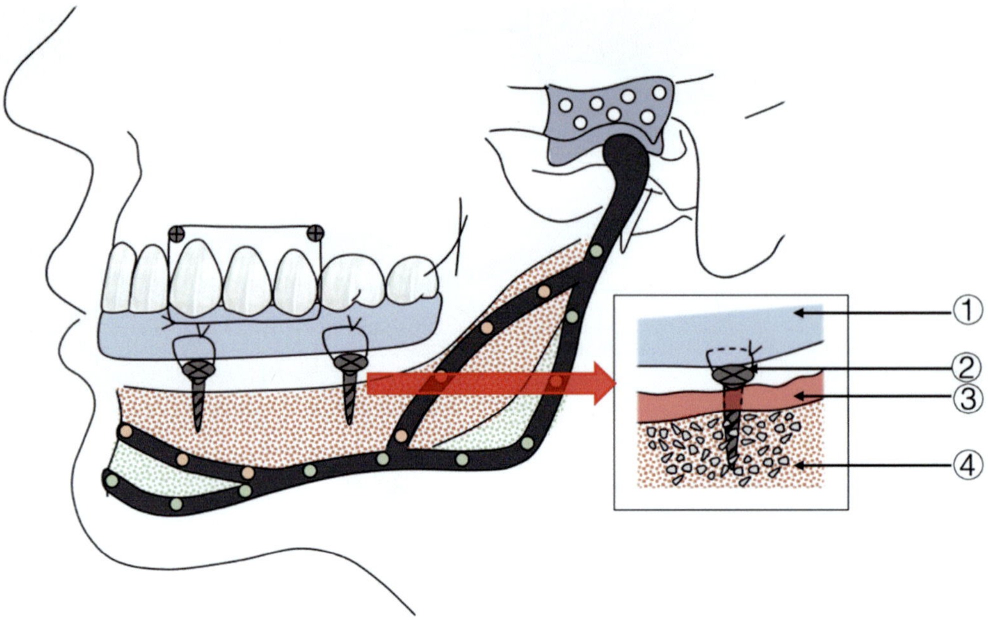

Fig. 11.8 Intermaxillary fixation is used to ensure the initial stability of the prosthesis. (1) Occlusal plate. (2) Long screws implanted in the upper layer of the graft. (3) The gum or mucous membrane is properly sutured. (4) Upper layer of the graft serves as an anchor for the occlusal plate

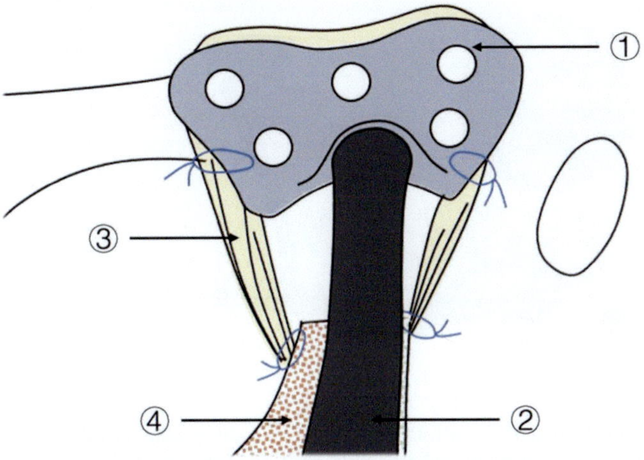

Fig. 11.9 Articular ligament suspension scheme to guarantee initial stability of the prosthesis. (1) Articular socket component of the prosthesis. (2) Mandibular extension component of the prosthesis. (3) Fascia or autologous ligaments. (4) Grafted bone

11.5 Visions of a Future with Regeneration of Multiple Tissues in Integration with Prostheses

Chi Yang, Jisi Zheng, and Guo Bai

11.5.1 Bionic Solutions for Load-Bearing of the Mandible, Especially for Large Prostheses

For large-scale defects of the joint-mandible, reconstruction of the joint-mandible-occlusion is the most challenging problem in the future. The future vision is to make the reconstruction with a bionic joint-mandible-occlusion complex. The main points for joint reconstruction are:

1. Force-bearing pillar: the force-bearing scaffold of the joint-mandible, restoring the joint structure and function, and providing the mechanical support of the mandible.
2. Dental implant scaffold: the alveolar bone repair scaffold, providing the alveolar bone repair and regeneration space; stimulating the regeneration of bone, blood vessels, and nerves; and obtaining the bionic and sufficient dental implant bone volume.
3. Muscle integration: the muscle attachment area is processed with a pro-osteo-integrative surface treatment, so as to re-attach the masseter muscle, the external pterygoid muscles, internal pterygoid muscles, mandibular hyoid muscle, etc.
4. Osteointegration: osteointegration-promoting surface treatment of the bone contact interface, so that the prosthesis or scaffold is connected with the autogenous bone to form a whole.
5. Preservation of original autogenous tissues: preservation of the original inferior alveolar nerve-vascular bundles and periosteum, to provide the microenvironment for bone regeneration and stimulation factors.

Through the above principles, a multifunctional composite joint-mandibular joint prosthesis with biological, mechanical, and kinetic properties close to the natural state is constructed, and ultimately the composite regeneration of multiple tissues such as bone, joints, muscles, nerves, and blood vessels is realized, saying goodbye to autogenous bone reconstruction, and going from outer form mimicry to functional mimicry (Fig. 11.10).

With this futuristic image of a bionic prosthesis, we complete our book on surgery for joint-mandible and cranial-mandibular defects. We hope that in the future we can offer our patients solutions that return them virtually to their pristine condition before the onset of disease. And that they may suffer much less in the process. We acknowledge and appreciate the contribution of these many patient cases to the advance of our ability to deal with these diseases. The solutions may require considerable advances in technology, but much of this technology is already within reach, and with the large scale of our hospital and long experience, we may be able to provide such a future. We hope our efforts are worthy of our scientific predecessor and visionary inventor Leonardo da Vinci.

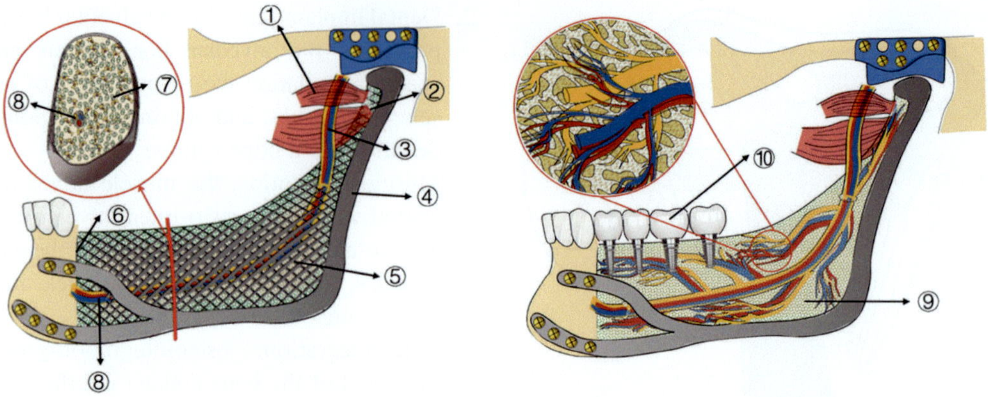

Fig. 11.10 Multifunctional bionic composite materials in the prosthesis of the future, a composite regenerative system that integrates multiple tissues such as bone, muscle, nerves, and blood vessels. (1) Upper head of the external pterygoid muscle. (2) Lower head of the external pterygoid muscle. (3) Inferior alveolar nerve and blood vessel bundle. (4) Bionic joint-metal part of the mandible joint prosthesis. (5) Bionic joint-biomaterial scaffold part of the mandible joint prosthesis. (6) Biological material and mandible joint. (7) Embedded biomaterial of the bionic joint-mandible prosthesis. (8) The inferior alveolar nerve and blood vessel bundle is completely preserved. (9) Good osseous remodeling after scaffold resorption. (10) Dental implants in the bone-simulating portion of the prosthesis

Bibliography

1. Aagaard E, Thygesen T. A prospective, single-centre study on patient outcomes following temporomandibular joint replacement using a custom-made Biomet TMJ prosthesis. Int J Oral Maxillofac Surg. 2014;43(10):1229–35.
2. Bai G, He D, Yang C, et al. Application of digital templates to guide total alloplastic joint replacement surgery with Biomet standard replacement system. J Oral Maxillofac Surg. 2014;72(12):2440–52.
3. Bai G, Yang C, He D, et al. Application of fossa bone graft to stabilize stock total joint prosthesis in temporomandibular joint surgery. J Craniomaxillofac Surg. 2015;43(8):1392–7.
4. Bai G, Yang C, Zheng ZW, et al. Mandible resection and reconstruction with preservation of 10 mm condyle and temporomandibular joint attachment. China J Oral Maxillofac Surg. 2016;14(2):144–8.
5. Baldridge OL, Henny FA. Condylectomy for the persistently painful temporomandibular joint. J Oral Surg. 1957;15(1):24–31.
6. Cai XY, Yang C, Chen MJ, et al. Arthroscopic management for synovial chondromatosis of the temporomandibular joint: a retrospective review of 33 cases. J Oral Maxillofac Surg. 2012;70(9):2106–13.
7. Cai YH, Lu C, He DM, et al. Analysis of the mandibular condylar fracture type leading to temporomandibular joint ankylosis in adults. China J Oral Maxillofac Surg. 2014;12(1):39–44.
8. Cardoso AB, Vasconcelos BC, Oliveira DM. Comparative study of eminectomy and use of bone miniplate in the articular eminence for the treatment of recurrent temporomandibular joint dislocation. Braz J Otorhinolaryngol. 2005;71(1):32–7.
9. Chen MJ, Yang C. Surgical treatment of chronic anterior dislocation of the temporomandibular joint. Shanghai J Stomatol. 2000;9(1):49–50.
10. Chen MJ, Yang C, Zhang SY, et al. Use of coblation in arthroscopic surgery of the temporomandibular joint. J Oral Maxillofac Surg. 2010;68(9):2085–91.
11. Chen MJ, Yang C, Qiu YT, et al. Local resection of the mass to treat the osteochondroma of the mandibular condyle: indications and different methods with 38-case series. Head Neck. 2014;36(2):273–9.
12. Chen M, Yang C, Qiu Y, et al. Superior half of the sternoclavicular joint pedicled with the sternocleidomastoid muscle for reconstruction of the temporomandibular joint: a preliminary study with a simplified technique and expanded indications. Int J Oral Maxillofac Surg. 2015;44(6):685–91.
13. Chen X, Wang Y, Mao Y, et al. Biomechanical evaluation of Chinese customized three-dimensionally printed total temporomandibular joint prostheses: a finite element analysis. J Craniomaxillofac Surg. 2018;46(9):1561–8.
14. Chen MJ, Yang C, Zheng JS, et al. Skull base erosion resulting from primary tumors of the temporomandibular joint and skull base region: our classification and reconstruction experience. J Oral Maxillofac Surg. 2018;76(6):1345–54.
15. Chen X, Mao Y, Zheng J, et al. Clinical and radiological outcomes of Chinese customized three-dimensionally printed total temporomandibular joint prostheses: a prospective case series study. J Plast Reconstr Aesthet Surg. 2021;74(7):1582–93.
16. Christensen RW. The temporomandibular joint prosthesis eleven years later. Oral Implantol. 1971;2(2):125–33.
17. Dautrey J. Surgery of the temporomandibular joint. Acta Stomatol Belg. 1975;72(4):577–81.
18. Dimitroulis G. The role of surgery in the management of disorders of the temporomandibular joint: a critical review of the literature. Part 2. Int J Oral Maxillofac Surg. 2005;34(3):231–7.
19. Dimitroulis G, Austin S, Sin Lee PV, et al. A new three-dimensional, print-on-demand temporomandibular prosthetic total joint replacement system: preliminary outcomes. J Craniomaxillofac Surg. 2018;46(8):1192–8.
20. Dong YJ, Hu SL, Zhong LS, et al. Preliminary report on the treatment of temporomandibular joint ankylosis by artificial temporomandibular joint semi-replacement. Stoma. 1983;1:30–1.
21. Driemel O, Braun S, Müller-Richter UD, et al. Historical development of alloplastic temporomandibular joint replacement after 1945 and state of the art. Int J Oral Maxillofac Surg. 2009;38(9):909–20.
22. Elledge R, Mercuri LG, Speculand B. Extended total temporomandibular joint replacements: a classification system. Br J Oral Maxillofac Surg. 2018;56(7):578–81.
23. Ferri J, Piot B, Ruhin B, et al. Advantages and limitations of the fibula free flap in mandibular reconstruction. J Oral Maxillofac Surg. 1997;55(5):440–8.
24. Gahhos F, Ariyan S. Facial fractures: hippocratic management. Head Neck Surg. 1984;6(6):1007–13.
25. Gu ZY, Wu QL, Cao ZQ, et al. Efficacy and mechanism of intra-articular irrigation and injection therapy for temporomandibular joint. Chin J Stomatol. 1996;31(2):78–80.
26. Hall HD. Intra-articular disc displacement part II: its significant role in temporomandibular joint pathology. J Oral Maxillofac Surg. 1995;53(9):1073–9.
27. He D, Yang C, Zhang S, et al. Modified temporomandibular joint disc repositioning with miniscrew anchor: part I--surgical technique. J Oral Maxillofac Surg. 2015;73(1):47.e41–9.
28. He D, Yang C, Zhu H, et al. Temporomandibular joint disc repositioning by suturing through open incision: a technical note. J Oral Maxillofac Surg. 2018;76(5):948–54.
29. Hong M. Discussion on the treatment of temporomandibular joint ankylosis by sigmoid osteotomy. Chin J Stomatol. 1986;21(5):289–91.
30. Hu QG, Qiu WL, Ha Q. Treatment of habitual dislocation of the temporomandibular joint with subsynovial injection of sclerosant through arthroscope. J Pract Stomatol. 1990;2:89–91.
31. Huo L, Han Z, Jiao Z, et al. Introduction of temporomandibular joint and skull base combined reconstruction by autogenous bone graft. Clin Oral Investig. 2023;27(6):2513–20.

© People's Medical Publishing House, PR of China 2025

Chi Y. (ed.), *Atlas of Customized TMJ-Cranio-Jaw Prosthesis*, https://doi.org/10.1007/978-981-95-0611-8

32. Ishii N, Shimizu Y, Ihara J, et al. Analysis of fibular single graft and fibular double-barrel graft for mandibular reconstruction. Plast Reconstr Surg Glob Open. 2016;4(8):e1018.
33. Jiao ZX, Zheng JS, Liu H, et al. The measurement data related to cranio -mandibular bones for research and development of total temporomandibular joint prosthesis. China J Oral Maxillofac Surg. 2015;13(2):151–4.
34. Johnson NR, Roberts MJ, Doi SA, et al. Total temporomandibular joint replacement prostheses: a systematic review and bias-adjusted meta-analysis. Int J Oral Maxillofac Surg. 2017;46(1):86–92.
35. Kumar BP, Venkatesh V, Kumar KA, et al. Mandibular reconstruction: overview. J Maxillofac Oral Surg. 2016;15(4):425–41.
36. Liu X, Zheng J, Cai X, et al. Techniques of Yang's arthroscopic discopexy for temporomandibular joint rotational anterior disc displacement. Int J Oral Maxillofac Surg. 2019;48(6):769–78.
37. Liu X, Abdelrehem A, Zheng J, et al. An arthroscopic technique for closure of perforations in temporomandibular joint retrodiscal tissues. Int J Oral Maxillofac Surg. 2022;51(5):669–76.
38. Long X, Li JR, Wang CD, et al. Arthroscopic examination and treatment of internal derangements of the temporomandibular joint. Chin J Stomatol. 1995;4:253.
39. Lu Y, Chen M, Yang C. Access to the infratemporal fossa: a modified transzygomatic approach with preservation of masseter attachment and a long-term follow-up period. J Stomatol Oral Maxillofac Surg. 2023;124(2):101336.
40. Lu C, Zhao J, Zhang X, et al. Comparison of disc position stability and condylar bone remodeling between two open disc repositioning surgeries: a retrospective single-Centre cohort study. Int J Surg. 2024;110(4):2187–95.
41. McCaffery C, Dodd M, Bekiroglu F, et al. Synovial chondromatosis of the temporomandibular joint with extension into the middle cranial fossa and internal carotid canal. Int J Oral Maxillofac Surg. 2017;46(7):867–70.
42. McCain JP, Sanders B, Koslin MG, et al. Temporomandibular joint arthroscopy: a 6-year multicenter retrospective study of 4831 joints. J Oral Maxillofac Surg. 1992;50(9):926–30.
43. Mercuri LG. Alloplastic temporomandibular joint reconstruction. Oral Surg Oral Med Oral Pathol Oral Radiol Endod. 1998;85(6):631–7.
44. Nicoli TK, Saat R, Kontio R, et al. Multidisciplinary approach to management of temporal bone giant cell tumor. J Neurol Surg Rep. 2016;77(3):e144–9.
45. Ohnishi M. Arthroscopic laser surgery and suturing for temporomandibular joint disorders: technique and clinical results. Arthroscopy. 1991;7(2):212–20.
46. Onoriobe U, Miloro M, Sukotjo C, et al. How many temporomandibular joint total joint alloplastic implants will be placed in the United States in 2030? J Oral Maxillofac Surg. 2016;74(8):1531–8.
47. Prasad SC, Piccirillo E, Nuseir A, et al. Giant cell tumors of the skull base: case series and current concepts. Audiol Neurootol. 2014;19(1):12–21.
48. Puelacher WC, Waldhart E. Miniplate eminoplasty: a new surgical treatment for TMJ-dislocation. J Craniomaxillofac Surg. 1993;21(4):176–8.
49. Qiu WL. Qiu Weiliu's Oral and maxillofacial surgery. Shanghai: Shanghai Scientific & Technical Publishing House; 2008.
50. Qiu WL, Pan JC, Pan KF, et al. Simultaneous surgical treatment of true ankylosis of the temporomandibular joint with severe respiratory obstruction. Chin J Stomatol. 1985;20(3):154–6.
51. Qiu YT, Yang C, Zhang XH. Primary granulocytic sarcoma of the mandibular condyle presenting with the characteristic green color. J Oral Maxillofac Surg. 2010;68(10):2575–9.
52. Qiu YT, Yang C, Chen MJ. Endoscopically assisted reconstruction of the mandibular condyle with a costochondral graft through a modified preauricular approach. Br J Oral Maxillofac Surg. 2010;48(6):443–7.
53. Quinn PD, Granquist EJ. Atlas of temporomandibular joint surgery. Wiley; 2015.
54. Rikhotso ER, Bobat MA. Total alloplastic joint reconstruction in a patient with temporomandibular joint ankylosis following condylar dislocation into the middle cranial fossa. J Oral Maxillofac Surg. 2016;74(12):2378.e1–5.
55. Ruiz Valero CA, Duran-Rodriguez G, Solano-Parra N, et al. Immediate total temporomandibular joint replacement with TMJ concepts prosthesis as an alternative for ameloblastoma cases. J Oral Maxillofac Surg. 2014;72(3):646.e1–e12.
56. Safaee M, Oh T, Sun MZ, et al. Pigmented villonodular synovitis of the temporomandibular joint with intracranial extension: a case series and systematic review. Head Neck. 2015;37(8):1213–24.
57. Sanders B, Buoncristiani R. Diagnostic and surgical arthroscopy of the temporomandibular joint: clinical experience with 137 procedures over a 2-year period. J Craniomandib Disord. 1987;1(3):202–13.
58. Shen P, Zhang SY, Yang C, et al. Stability study of total TMJ replacement on sheep. J Craniomaxillofac Surg. 2014;42(7):1265–70.
59. Shen Y, Ma C, Wang L, et al. Surgical management of giant cell tumors in temporomandibular joint region involving lateral skull base: a multidisciplinary approach. J Oral Maxillofac Surg. 2016;74(11):2295–311.
60. Shen P, Bai G, Xie Q, et al. Efficacy of arthroscopic discopexy on condylar growth in temporomandibular joint anterior disc displacement: a randomized clinical trial. Plast Reconstr Surg. 2023;154(3):544e–55e.
61. Song RY, Qian YC, Hu QM. Facial deformity and occlusal abnormality caused by hyperplasia of the mandibular condyle. Chin J Stomatol. 1957;5(3):194–201.
62. Song RY, Gao ML, Lai QS. Bilateral temporomandibular joint ankylosis and surgical treatment. Chin J Stomatol. 1964;10(4):266–8.
63. Wang X, Zhang ZK, Zhang XE. Orthognathic surgery. Jinan: Shandong Science and Technology Press; 1999.
64. Wang MJ, Chen TT, Si JW, et al. Application of virtual technology in the treatment of first and second branchial arch syndrome. China J Oral Maxillofac Surg. 2016;14(2):123–7.
65. Ward TG. Surgery of the mandibular joint. Ann R Coll Surg Engl. 1961;28(3):139–52.
66. Westermark A. Total reconstruction of the temporomandibular joint. Up to 8 years of follow-up of patients treated with Biomet(®) total joint prostheses. Int J Oral Maxillofac Surg. 2010;39(10):951–5.
67. Westermark A, Hedén P, Aagaard E, et al. The use of TMJ concepts prostheses to reconstruct patients with major temporomandibular joint and mandibular defects. Int J Oral Maxillofac Surg. 2011;40(5):487–96.
68. Westwood RM, Fox GL, Tilson HB. Eminectomy for the treatment of recurrent temporomandibular joint dislocation. J Oral Surg. 1975;33(10):774–9.
69. Wolford LM, Karras S, Mehra P. Concomitant temporomandibular joint and orthognathic surgery: a preliminary report. J Oral Maxillofac Surg. 2002;60(4):356–62.
70. Wolford LM, Mercuri LG, Schneiderman ED, et al. Twenty-year follow-up study on a patient-fitted temporomandibular joint prosthesis: the Techmedica/TMJ concepts device. J Oral Maxillofac Surg. 2015;73(5):952–60.
71. Wu XG, Hong M, Li YH. Review and prospect of the diagnosis and treatment of mandibular condylar fractures. Chin J Stomatol. 1991;26(5):312–4.
72. Xie Q, Yang C, He D, et al. Is mandibular asymmetry more frequent and severe with unilateral disc displacement? J Craniomaxillofac Surg. 2015;43(1):81–6.

73. Xie Q, Li P, Yang C, et al. Feasibility of simultaneous TMJ arthroscopy in ADDwoR patients undergoing orthognathic surgery for jaw deformity. J Craniomaxillofac Surg. 2024;52(3):347–54.
74. Xu YD, Xu BG, Cui YT, et al. Experimental and clinical study on the treatment of recurrent dislocation of the temporomandibular joint by extra-articular injection of sclerosant. Chin J Stomatol. 1992;27(3):148–50.
75. Yang C. Exploration of the relationship between anterior disc displacement of the temporomandibular joint and condylar bone resorption, as well as a combined diagnostic and therapeutic model. Chin J Stomatol. 2017;52(3):157–60.
76. Yang C, Qiu WL, Zhang WJ. A case report of osteoid osteoma in the temporomandibular joint. Chin J Stomatol. 1997;6:24.
77. Yang C, Qiu WL, Ha Q, et al. Long-term effectiveness of arthroscopic subsynovial sclerotherapy and suturing on recurrent dislocation of the temporomandibular joint. Chin J Stomatol. 1999;1:51–3.
78. Yang C, He DM, Chen MJ, et al. Treatment of intracapsular condyle fracture of the mandible. China J Oral Maxillofac Surg. 2010;8(2):112–8.
79. Yang C, Cai XY, Chen MJ, et al. New arthroscopic disc repositioning and suturing technique for treating an anteriorly displaced disc of the temporomandibular joint: part I--technique introduction. Int J Oral Maxillofac Surg. 2012;41(9):1058–63.
80. Ye ZX, Yang C, Chen MJ, et al. Digital resection and reconstruction of TMJ synovial chondrosarcoma involving the skull base: report of a case. Int J Clin Exp Med. 2015;8(7):11589–93.
81. Zeng RS, Ren CN, Shen Q. Preliminary experience in the surgical treatment of temporomandibular joint disturbance syndrome with endoscopy. Chin J Stomatol. 1995;6:367–9.
82. Zhang ZY. Oral and maxillofacial oncology. Jinan: Shandong Science and Technology Press; 2004.
83. Zhang ZY. Oral and maxillofacial surgery. 8th ed. Beijing: People's Medical Publishing House; 2020.
84. Zhang DS, Wang FP, Zhou SS. Report on the treatment of forty-seven cases of temporomandibular joint ankylosis. Chin J Stomatol. 1954;2(4):247–57.
85. Zhang GP, Sun YQ, Pan YH. Left mandibular condylar hyperplasia (with report of two cases). Chin J Stomatol. 1957;5(3):203–7.
86. Zhang ZK, Zhang XE, Ma XC, et al. Preliminary report on the application of disc repositioning/repair and discectomy with silicone disc implantation. Chin J Stomatol. 1987;22(2):78–81.
87. Zhang Y, He DM, Ma XC. Clinical characteristics and classification treatment of traumatic temporomandibular joint ankylosis. Chin J Stomatol. 2006;41(12):751–4.
88. Zhang S, Liu X, Yang X, et al. Temporomandibular joint disc repositioning using bone anchors: an immediate post surgical evaluation by magnetic resonance imaging. BMC Musculoskelet Disord. 2010;11:262.
89. Zhang D, Abdelrehem A, Luo Y, et al. Effect of arthroscopic discopexy on condylar growth in adolescents with temporomandibular joint disc displacement without reduction: a retrospective self-controlled case series study. J Craniomaxillofac Surg. 2024;52(2):157–64.
90. Zheng J, Chen X, Jiang W, et al. An innovative total temporomandibular joint prosthesis with customized design and 3D printing additive fabrication: a prospective clinical study. J Transl Med. 2019;17(1):4.
91. Zheng JS, Liu XH, Chen XZ, et al. Customized skull base-temporomandibular joint combined prosthesis with 3D-printing fabrication for craniomaxillofacial reconstruction: a preliminary study. Int J Oral Maxillofac Surg. 2019;48(11):1440–7.
92. Zheng JS, Liu XH, Ahmed A, et al. Endoscopically assisted fixation of the custom-made total temporomandibular joint prosthesis in TMJ Yang's system through a modified preauricular approach. Int J Oral Maxillofac Surg. 2020;49(2):224–9.
93. Zheng JS, Wei X, Jiao ZX, et al. Development and clinical application of custom-made temporomandibular joint-skull base combined prosthesis. Chin J Stomatol. 2021;56(7):627–32.
94. Zheng JS, Jiao ZX, Wei X, et al. Accuracy of digital templates for guidance of custom-made total temporomandibular joint replacement. Int J Oral Maxillofac Surg. 2022;51(10):1330–6.
95. Zheng J, Huo L, Jiao Z, et al. 3D-printed temporomandibular joint-mandible combined prosthesis: a prospective study. Oral Dis. 2024;30(3):1360–6.
96. Zhou SS, Ding HC, Chen RT, et al. Summary report on the treatment of sixty-four cases of temporomandibular joint ankylosis. Chin J Stomatol. 1959;7(6):350–3.
97. Zhu SS, Hu J. Combined treatment of temporomandibular joint ankylosis and secondary dentofacial deformities. Chin J Oral Maxillofac Surg. 2016;14(3):193–7.
98. Zou ZJ, Wu YT, Sun GX, et al. Observation on the X-ray modification and clinical efficacy of conservative treatment for condylar fractures. Chin J Stomatol. 1988;23(4):193–6.
99. Zou L, Zhao J, He D. Preliminary clinical study of Chinese standard alloplastic temporomandibular joint prosthesis. J Craniomaxillofac Surg. 2019;47(4):602–6.
100. Zou L, He D, Yang C, et al. Preliminary study of standard artificial temporomandibular joint replacement with preservation of muscle attachment. J Oral Maxillofac Surg. 2021;79(5):1009–18.

MIX
Papier aus verantwortungsvollen Quellen
Paper from responsible sources
FSC® C105338

If you have any concerns about our products,
you can contact us on
ProductSafety@springernature.com

In case Publisher is established outside the EU,
the EU authorized representative is:
Springer Nature Customer Service Center GmbH
Europaplatz 3, 69115 Heidelberg, Germany

Printed by Libri Plureos GmbH
in Hamburg, Germany